Signal Detection and Recognition by Human Observers

CONTEMPORARY READINGS

edited by JOHN A. SWETS

Chief Scientist
BBN Laboratories
Cambridge, Massachusetts

and

Lecturer on Clinical Epidemiology
Harvard Medical School
Boston, Massachusetts

PENINSULA PUBLISHING

LOS ALTOS, CALIFORNIA USA

Signal Detection and Recognition by Human Observers

1988 reprint edition published by
Peninsula Publishing
P.O. Box 867
Los Altos, California 94023
United States of America

Library of Congress Catalog Number 87-063305
ISBN 0-932146-21-X

Printed in the United States of America.

preface

Adding further qualifications to the title would have made it unwieldy, but I must acknowledge at the earliest opportunity that this collection of articles does not represent the entire field of signal detection and recognition by human observers. This book samples a single line of work on these topics.

The unifying theme of this collection is that all the articles derive directly from a theoretical development made in electrical engineering in the early 1950's. At that time some mathematicians and engineers saw the relevance of statistical decision theory to the general detection problem, and they combined decision theory with an elaboration of the concept of ideal observers, as used in radar theory, to frame the general theory of signal detectability.

The general theory of signal detectability specifies the mathematically ideal or optimal detection process; it was never intended to apply precisely to any realizable sensing device, and it was certainly constructed without regard for human sensory processes. It soon became apparent, however, that the general theory is a good approximation to a descriptive theory of human detection and recognition behavior. The general theory also serves as a guide for the study of human perceptual processes—it specifies the appropriate experimental methods, and it leads to substantive results by disclosing new problems and by providing new approaches to old problems.

The chapters in this book describe a variety of psychophysical applications of the general theory. They range from a straightforward treatment of idealized visual and auditory tasks, through implications for experimental design and measurement, through extensions of the theory and methods to deal with more complex sensory tasks, to the treatment of substantive problems in perception.

Until now, no reasonably complete treatment of the subject has been available in a single volume. The articles selected for this book, roughly half of those published, are scattered through diverse sources. It is exceptional when the journals in which they appear are housed in fewer than three libraries. One purpose of this collection, therefore, is to provide a convenient, thorough introduction to the subject. This collection should serve as such until a systematic textbook is prepared, and it will complement the text subsequently. The second purpose of this collection is to provide convenient reference for those already acquainted with the material.

The version of the general theory of signal detectability that inspired the psychophysical applications represented in this book was constructed by W. W. Peterson and T. G. Birdsall of the Electronic Defense Group, Electrical Engineering Department, University of Michigan. A majority of the senior authors represented in this collection have worked together in the Electronic Defense Group, in the psychophysical laboratory headed by W. P. Tanner, Jr., and the indebtedness and appreciation they feel to Peterson and Birdsall should be recorded here. The articles in this volume, with a few exceptions, were first collected as class notes for a special program I directed at M.I.T. in the summer of 1962. I had pursued related teaching and research interests at M.I.T. for six years before that, in the Department of Economics and Social Sciences and in the Research Laboratory of Electronics, and I am grateful for the free and supportive environment provided me there. Preparations for publishing this book were carried out during a leave of absence spent at Bolt Beranek and Newman Inc., where the assistance I needed was always quickly and generously supplied. I appreciate especially the contributions of Judith R. Harris, who compiled the index, and Cynthia Mullen, who prepared the manuscript. Geraldine C. Stone and Patricia A. Lemon of Harvard's Laboratory for Psychophysics read the proofs with me; I am indebted to Miss Stone for reviewing the entire manuscript at that stage and for doing much to clarify the exposition. I would also acknowledge, for myself and for my associates in this research activity, the decade of research support granted by the Operational Applications Laboratory of the United States Air Force, the Air Force Office of Scientific Research, the Office of Naval Research, the Army Signal Corps, and the National Science Foundation.

JOHN A. SWETS

Cambridge, Massachusetts
January 1964

preface to the reprint edition

In the original (1964) edition, this book was the first to bring together, in a structured and convenient form, a broad sample of the applications of modern signal-detection theory to human performance. It did so 10 years after the initial article on the subject, and included 33 of the 100 or so articles then available. It presented descriptions of the theory, implications for experimental method and data analysis, and applications to simple and complex sensory tasks in vision and audition.

This book showed extensively how decision factors are centrally involved in even the simplest detection task, and how sensory capacity can be assessed in a manner independent of those factors. It illustrated the value of the pure measure of sensory or discrimination capacity in several substantive problems in psychology, including the integration of sensory information, signal uncertainty, auditory frequency analysis, speech communication, vigilance, and recognition memory. Though the range of applications of signal detection theory is now seen to be still broader, the various problems treated in this book suffice to indicate the possibilities and to demonstrate a variety of concepts and methods that remain fundamental. A topical bibliography of applications of signal detection theory, updated to include more than 1000 references, has been added.

The original Preface hinted that a systematic textbook would also appear, and one did shortly (D. M. Green and J. A. Swets, *Signal Detection Theory and Psychophysics*, reprinted by Peninsula Publishing in 1988). But that Preface also suggested that the collection of primary articles should continue to be useful in its own right and as a supplement to the textbook. Support for that notion has come from the recent designation of this book as a "citation classic" (*Current Contents, Social & Behavioral Sciences*, October 21, 1985, *17*[42], 20).

In the first Preface, I thanked the persons and institutions that had been helpful to me and supportive of this line of work, and I notice that my indebtedness seems even greater now. Additionally, from my present perspective, I would like to dedicate the book to my mother and to the memory of my father.

J. A. S.

Cambridge, Massachusetts
January, 1988

contents

section one

GENERAL THEORY AND BASIC EXPERIMENTS

The articles in this section present aspects of the general theory of signal detectability relevant to human observers—with some redundancy, but also with substantial differences in emphasis. Together they contain detailed descriptions of the experiments that constitute the primary tests of the validity of the theory in its psychophysical application; attempts to explicate the coordination between theory, experiment, and behavioral process; and comparisons of alternative theoretical formulations.

In the article entitled "Decision Processes in Perception" [1], Swets, Tanner, and Birdsall present the theory and the results of the first experiments stimulated by it; these experiments employed visual signals. Green, in "Psychoacoustics and Detection Theory" [2], reviews the applications of the theory in audition, with emphasis on the shape of the psychometric function. Immediately following this article is a letter published by Green which contains some comments on, and a correction to, the article. Licklider, in "Theory of Signal Detection" [3], considers theory and experimental results from a metatheoretical point of view and carefully coordinates the physical and psychological referents of the theory. In the last article, "Is There a Sensory Threshold?" [4], Swets examines several alternative theories based on the threshold concept in relation to the results of certain critical experiments.

1

Decision Processes in Perception

John A. Swets, Wilson P. Tanner, Jr., and Theodore G. Birdsall

About five years ago, the theory of statistical decision was translated into a theory of signal detection.[1] Although the translation was motivated by problems in radar, the detection theory that resulted is a general theory for, like the decision theory, it specifies an ideal process. The generality of the theory suggested to us that it might also be relevant to the detection of signals by human observers. Beyond this, we were struck by several analogies between this description of ideal behavior and various aspects of the perceptual process. The detection theory seemed to provide a framework for a realistic description of the behavior of the human observer in a variety of perceptual tasks.

The particular feature of the theory that was of greatest interest to us was the promise that it held of solving an old problem in the field of psychophysics. This is the problem of controlling or specifying the criterion that the observer uses in making a perceptual judgment. The classic methods of psychophysics make effective provision for only a single free parameter, one that is associated with the sensitivity of the observer. They contain no analytical procedure for specifying independently the observer's criterion. These two aspects of performance are confounded, for example, in an experiment in which the dependent variable is the intensity of the stimulus that is required for a threshold response. The present theory provides a quantitative measure of the criterion. There is left, as a result, a relatively pure measure of sensitivity. The theory, therefore, promised to be of value to the student of personal and social

---

[1] For a formal treatment of statistical decision theory, see Wald (1950); for a brief and highly readable survey of the essentials, see Bross (1953). Parallel accounts of the detection theory may be found in Peterson, Birdsall, and Fox (1954) and in Van Meter and Middleton (1954).

processes in perception as well as to the student of sensory functions. A second feature of the theory that attracted us is that it is a normative theory. We believed that having a standard with which to compare the behavior of the human observer would aid in the description and in the interpretation of experimental results, and would be fruitful in suggesting new experiments.

This paper begins with a brief review of the theory of statistical decision and then presents a description of the elements of the theory of signal detection appropriate to human observers. Following this, the results of some experimental tests of the applicability of the theory to the detection of visual signals are described.

The theory and some illustrative results of one experimental test of it were briefly described in an earlier paper (Tanner and Swets, 1954). The present paper contains a more nearly adequate description of the theory, a more complete account of the first experiment, and the results of four other experiments. It brings together all of the data collected to date in vision experiments that bear directly on the value of the theory.[2]

THE THEORY

Statistical decision theory

Consider the following game of chance. Three dice are thrown. Two of the dice are ordinary dice. The third die is unusual in that on each of three of its sides it has three spots, whereas on its remaining three sides it has no spots at all. You, as the player of the game, do not observe the throws of the dice. You are simply informed, after each throw, of the total number of spots showing on the three dice. You are then asked to state whether the third die, the unusual one, showed a 3 or a 0. If you are correct—that is, if you assert a 3 showed when it did in fact, or if you assert a 0 showed when it did in fact—you win a dollar. If you are incorrect—that is, if you make either of the two possible types of errors—you lose a dollar.

How do you play the game? Certainly you will want a few minutes to make some computations before you begin. You will want to know the probability of occurrence of each of the possible totals 2 through 12 in the event that the third die shows a 0, and you will want to know the probability of occurrence of each of the possible totals 5 through 15 in the event that the third die shows a 3. Let us ignore the exact values of these probabilities, and grant that the two probability distributions in question will look much like those sketched in Fig. 1.

---

[2] Reports of several applications of the theory in audition experiments are available in the literature; for a list of references, see Tanner and Birdsall (1958).

Realizing that you will play the game many times, you will want to establish a policy which defines the circumstances under which you will make each of the two decisions. We can think of this as a *criterion* or a cutoff point along the axis representing the total number of spots showing on the three dice. That is, you will want to choose a number on this axis such that whenever it is equaled or exceeded you will state that a 3 showed on the third die, and such that whenever the total number of spots showing is less than this number, you will state that a 0 showed on the third die. For the game as described, with the a priori probabilities of a 3 and a 0 equal, and with equal values and costs associated with the four possible decision outcomes, it is intuitively clear that the optimal cutoff point is that point where the two curves cross. You will maximize your winnings if you choose this point as the cutoff point and adhere to it.

Now, what if the game is changed? What, for example, if the third die has three spots on five of its sides, and a 0 on only one? Certainly you will now be more willing to state, following each throw, that the third die showed a 3. You will not, however, simply state more often that a 3 occurred without regard to the total showing on the three dice. Rather, you will lower your cutoff point: you will accept a smaller total than before as representing a throw in which the third die showed a 3. Conversely, if the third die has three spots on only one of its sides and 0's on five sides, you will do well to raise your cutoff point—to require a higher total than before for stating that a 3 occurred.

Similarly, your behavior will change if the values and costs associated with the various decision outcomes are changed. If it costs you 5 dollars

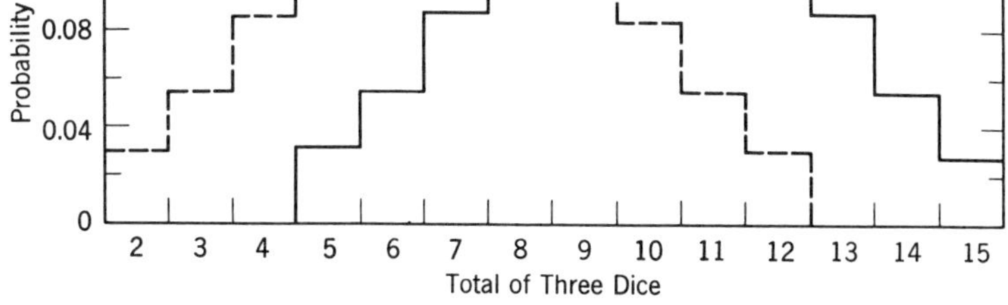

FIG. 1. The probability distributions for the dice game.

every time you state that a 3 showed when in fact it did not, and if you win 5 dollars every time you state that a 0 showed when in fact it did (the other value and the other cost in the game remaining at 1 dollar), you will raise your cutoff to a point somewhere above the point where the two distributions cross. Or if, instead, the premium is placed on being correct when a 3 occurred, rather than when a 0 occurred as in the immediately preceding example, you will assume a cutoff somewhere below the point where the two distributions cross.

Again, your behavior will change if the amount of overlap of the two distributions is changed. You will assume a different cutoff from the one you assumed in the game as first described if the three sides of the third die showing spots now show four spots rather than three.

This game is simply an example of the type of situation for which the theory of statistical decision was developed. It is intended only to recall the frame of reference of this theory. Statistical decision theory—or the special case of it which is relevant here, the theory of testing statistical hypotheses—specifies the optimal behavior in a situation where one must choose between two alternative statistical hypotheses on the basis of an observed event. In particular, it specifies the optimal cutoff, along the continuum on which the observed events are arranged, as a function of (*a*) the a priori probabilities of the two hypotheses, (*b*) the values and costs associated with the various decision outcomes, and (*c*) the amount of overlap of the distributions that constitute the hypotheses.

According to the mathematical theory of signal detectability, the problem of detecting signals that are weak relative to the background of interference is like the one faced by the player of our dice game. In short, the detection problem is a problem in statistical decision; it requires testing statistical hypotheses. In the theory of signal detectability, this analogy is developed in terms of an idealized observer. It is our thesis that this conception of the detection process may apply to the human observer as well. The next several pages present an analysis of the detection process that will make the bases for this reasoning apparent.[3]

[3] It is to be expected that a theory recognized as having a potential application in psychophysics, although developed in another context, will be similar in many respects to previous conceptions in psychophysics. Although we shall not, in general, discuss explicitly these similarities, the strong relationship between many of the ideas presented in the following and Thurstone's earlier work on the scaling of judgments should be noted (see Thurstone, 1927*a*, 1927*b*). The present theory also has much in common with the recent work of Smith and Wilson (1953) and of Munson and Karlin (1956). Of course, for a new theory to arouse interest, it must also differ in some significant aspects from previous theories—these differences will become apparent as we proceed.

Fundamental detection problem

In the fundamental detection problem, an observation is made of events occurring in a fixed interval of time, and a decision is made, based on this observation, whether the interval contained only the background interference or a signal as well. The interference, which is random, we shall refer to as *noise* and denote as N; the other alternative we shall term *signal plus noise, SN*. .In the fundamental problem, only these two alternatives exist—noise is always present, whereas the signal may or may not be present during a specified observation interval. Actually, the observer, who has advance knowledge of the ensemble of signals to be presented, says either "yes, a signal was present" or "no, no signal was present" following each observation. In the experiments to be reported, the signal consisted of a small spot of light flashed briefly in a known location on a uniformly illuminated background. It is important to note that the signal is always observed in a background of noise; some noise, as in the present case, may be introduced by the experimenter or by the external situation, but some is inherent in the sensory processes.

Representation of sensory information

In what follows we shall use the term *observation* to refer to the sensory datum on which the decision is based. We assume that this observation may be represented as varying continuously along a single dimension. Although there is no need to be concrete, it may be helpful to think of the observation as some measure of neutral activity, perhaps as the number of impulses arriving at a given point in the cortex within a given time. We assume further that any observation may arise, with specific probabilities, either from noise alone or from signal plus noise. We may

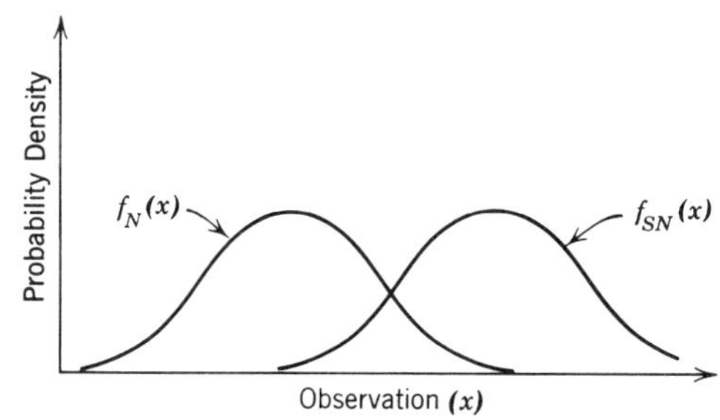

FIG. 2. The probability density functions of noise and signal plus noise.

portray these assumptions graphically, for a signal of a given amplitude, as in Fig. 2. The observation is labeled x and plotted on the abscissa. The left-hand distribution, labeled $f_N(x)$, represents the probability density that x will result given the occurrence of noise alone. The right-hand distribution, $f_{SN}(x)$, is the probability density function of x given the occurrence of signal plus noise. (Probability density functions are used, rather than probability functions, since x is assumed to be continuous.) Since the observations will tend to be of greater magnitude when a signal is presented, the mean of the SN distribution will be greater than the mean of the N distribution. In general, the greater the amplitude of the signal, the greater will be the separation of these means.

Observation as a value of likelihood ratio

It will be well to question at this point our assumption that the observation may be represented along a single axis. Can we, without serious violation, regard the observation as unidimensional, in spite of the fact that the response of the visual system probably has many dimensions? The answer to this question will involve some concepts that are basic to the theory.

One reasonable answer is that, when the signal and interference are alike in character, only the magnitude of the total response of the receiving system is available as an indicator of signal existence. Consequently, no matter how complex the sensory information is in fact, the observations may be represented in theory as having a single dimension. Although this answer is quite acceptable when concerned only with the visual case, we prefer to advance a different answer, one that is applicable also to audition experiments, where, for example, the signal may be a segment of a sinusoid presented in a background of white noise.

So let us assume that the response of the sensory system does have several dimensions, and proceed to represent it as a point in an m-dimensional space. Call this point y. For every such point in this space there is some probability density that it resulted from noise alone, $f_N(y)$, and, similarly, some probability density that it was due to signal plus noise, $f_{SN}(y)$. Therefore, there exists a likelihood ratio for each point in the space, $\lambda(y) = f_{SN}(y)/f_N(y)$, expressing the likelihood that the point y arose from SN relative to the likelihood that it arose from N. Since any point in the space, i.e., any sensory datum, may be thus represented as a real, nonzero number, these points may be considered to lie along a single axis. We may then, if we choose, identify the observation x with $\lambda(y)$; the decision axis becomes likelihood ratio.[4]

Having established that we may identify the observation x with $\lambda(y)$, let us note that we may equally well identify x with any monotonic transformation of $\lambda(y)$. It can be shown that we lose nothing by distorting the linear continuum as long as order is maintained. As a matter of fact we may gain if, in particular, we identify x with some transformation of $\lambda(y)$ that results in Gaussian density functions on x. We have assumed the existence of such a transformation in the representation of the density functions, $f_{SN}(x)$ and $f_N(x)$, in Fig. 2. We shall see shortly that the assumption of normality simplifies the problem greatly. We shall also see that this assumption is subject to experimental test. A further assumption incorporated into the picture of Fig. 2, one made quite tentatively, is that the two density functions are of equal variance. This is equivalent to the assumption that the SN function is a simple translation of the N function, or that adding a signal to the noise merely adds a constant to the N function. The results of a test of this assumption are also described later.

To summarize the last few paragraphs, we have assumed that an observation may be characterized by a value of likelihood ratio, $\lambda(y)$, i.e., the likelihood that the response of the sensory system y arose from SN relative to the likelihood that it arose from N. This permits us to view the observations as lying along a single axis. We then assumed the existence of a particular transformation of $\lambda(y)$ such that on the resulting variable, x, the density functions are normal. We regard the observer as basing his decisions on the variable x.

Definition of the criterion

If the representation depicted in Fig. 2 is realistic, then the problem posed for an observer attempting to detect signals in noise is indeed similar to the one faced by the player of our dice game. On the basis of an observation, one that varies only in magnitude, he must decide between two alternative hypotheses. He must decide from which hypothesis the observation resulted; he must state that the observation is a member of

---

[4] Thus the assumption of a unidimensional decision axis is independent of the character of the signal and noise. Rather, it depends on the fact that just two decision alternatives are considered. More generally, it can be shown that the number of dimensions required to represent the observation is $M - 1$, where M is the number of decision alternatives considered by the observer.

the one distribution or the other. As did the player of the dice game, the observer must establish a policy that defines the circumstances under which the observation will be regarded as resulting from each of the two possible events. He establishes a criterion, a cutoff x_c on the continuum of observations, to which he can relate any given observation x_i. If he finds for the *i*th observation, x_i, that $x_i > x_c$, he says "yes"; if $x_i < x_c$, he says "no." Since the observer is assumed to be capable of locating a criterion at any point along the continuum of observations, it is of interest to examine the various factors that, according to the theory, will influence his choice of a particular criterion. To do so requires some additional notation.

In the language of statistical decision theory the observer chooses a subset of all of the observations, namely the Critical Region A, such that an observation in this subset leads him to accept the Hypothesis SN, to say that a signal was present. All other observations are in the complementary subset B; these lead to rejection of the Hypothesis SN, or, equivalently, since the two hypotheses are mutually exclusive and exhaustive, to the acceptance of the Hypothesis N. The Critical Region A, with reference to Fig. 2, consists of the values of x to the right of some criterion value x_c.

As in the case of the dice game, a decision will have one of four outcomes: the observer may say "yes" or "no" and may in either case be *correct* or *incorrect*. The decision outcome, in other words, may be a *hit* ($SN \cdot A$, the joint occurrence of the Hypothesis SN and an observation in the Region A), a *miss* ($SN \cdot B$), a *correct rejection* ($N \cdot B$), or a *false alarm* ($N \cdot A$). If the a priori probability of signal occurrence and the parameters of the distributions of Fig. 2 are fixed, the choice of a criterion value x_c completely determines the probability of each of these outcomes.

Clearly, the four probabilities are interdependent. For example, an increase in the probability of a hit, $p(SN \cdot A)$, can be achieved only by accepting an increase in the probability of a false alarm, $p(N \cdot A)$, and decreases in the other probabilities, $p(SN \cdot B)$ and $p(N \cdot B)$. Thus, a given criterion yields a particular balance among the probabilities of the four possible outcomes; conversely, the balance desired by an observer in any instance will determine the optimal location of his criterion. Now the observer may desire the balance that maximizes the expected value of a decision in a situation where the four possible outcomes of a decision have individual values, as did the player of the dice game. In this case, the location of the best criterion is determined by the same parameters that determined it in the dice game. The observer, however, may desire a balance that maximizes some other quantity—i.e., a balance that is optimum according to some other definition of optimum—in which case a different criterion will be appropriate. He may, for example, want to maximize $p(SN \cdot A)$ while satisfying a restriction on $p(N \cdot A)$, as we typically do when as experimenters we assume an .05 or .01 level of confidence. Alternatively, he may want to maximize the number of correct decisions. Again, he may prefer a criterion that will maximize the reduction in uncertainty in the Shannon (1948) sense.

In statistical decision theory, and in the theory of signal detectability, the optimal criterion under each of these definitions of optimum is specified in terms of the likelihood ratio. That is to say, it can be shown that, if we define the observation in terms of the likelihood ratio, $\lambda(x) = f_{SN}(x)/f_N(x)$, then the optimal criterion can always be specified by some value β of $\lambda(x)$. In other words, the Critical Region A that corresponds to the criterion contains all observations with likelihood ratio greater than or equal to β, and none of those with likelihood ratio less than β.

We shall illustrate this manner of specifying the optimal criterion for just one of the definitions of optimum proposed above, namely, the maximization of the total expected value of a decision in a situation where the four possible outcomes of a decision have individual values associated with them. This is the definition of optimum that we assumed in the dice game. For this purpose we shall need the concept of *conditional probability* as opposed to the *probability of joint occurrence* introduced earlier. It should be stated that conditional probabilities will have a place in our discussion beyond their use in this illustration; the ones we shall introduce are, as a matter of fact, the fundamental quantities in evaluating the observer's performance.

There are two conditional probabilities of principal interest. These are the conditional probabilities of the observer saying "yes": $p_{SN}(A)$, the probability of a Yes decision *conditional upon*, or *given*, the occurrence of a signal, and $p_N(A)$, the probability of a Yes decision given the occurrence of noise alone. These two are sufficient, for the other two are simply their complements: $p_{SN}(B) = 1 - p_{SN}(A)$ and $p_N(B) = 1 - p_N(A)$. The conditional and joint probabilities are related as follows:

$$p_{SN}(A) = \frac{p(SN \cdot A)}{p(SN)}$$
$$p_N(A) = \frac{p(N \cdot A)}{p(N)} \tag{1}$$

where $p(SN)$ is the a priori probability of signal occurrence and $p(N) = 1 - p(SN)$ is the a priori probability of occurrence of noise alone.

Equation (1) makes apparent the convenience of using conditional rather than joint probabilities—conditional probabilities are independent of the a priori probability of occurrence of the signal and of noise alone. With reference to Fig. 2, we may define $p_{SN}(A)$, or the conditional probability of a hit, as the integral of $f_{SN}(x)$ over the Critical Region A, and $p_N(A)$, the conditional probability of a false alarm, as the integral of $f_N(x)$ over A. That is, $p_N(A)$ and $p_{SN}(A)$, respectively, represent the areas under the two curves of Fig. 2 to the right of some criterion value of x.

To pursue our illustration of how an optimal criterion may be specified by a critical value of likelihood ratio β, let us note that the expected value of a decision (denoted EV) is defined in statistical decision theory as the sum, over the potential outcomes of a decision, of the products of probability of outcome and desirability of outcome. Thus, using the notation V for *positive* individual values and K for costs or *negative* individual values, we have the following equation:

$$EV = V_{SN\cdot A}\,p(SN\cdot A) + V_{N\cdot B}\,p(N\cdot B) - K_{SN\cdot B}\,p(SN\cdot B) - K_{N\cdot A}\,p(N\cdot A) \tag{2}$$

Now if a priori and conditional probabilities are substituted for the joint probabilities in Eq. (2) following Eq. (1), for example, $p(SN)p_{SN}(A)$ for $p(SN\cdot A)$, then collecting terms yields the result that maximizing EV is equivalent to maximizing:

$$p_{SN}(A) - \beta p_N(A) \tag{3}$$

where

$$\beta = \frac{p(N)}{p(SN)}\cdot\frac{(V_{N\cdot B} + K_{N\cdot A})}{(V_{SN\cdot A} + K_{SN\cdot B})} \tag{4}$$

It can be shown that this value of β is equal to the value of likelihood ratio, $\lambda(x)$, that corresponds to the optimal criterion. From Eq. (3) it may be seen that the value β simply weights the hits and false alarms, and from Eq. (4) we see that β is determined by the a priori probabilities of occurrence of signal and of noise alone and by the values associated with the individual decision outcomes. It should be noted that Eq. (3) applies to all definitions of optimum. Equation (4) shows the determinants of β in only the special case of the expected-value definition of optimum.

Return for a moment to Fig. 2, keeping in mind the result that β is a critical value of $\lambda(x) = f_{SN}(x)/f_N(x)$. It should be clear that the optimal cutoff x_c along the x axis is at the point on this axis where the ratio of the ordinate value of $f_{SN}(x)$ to the ordinate value of $f_N(x)$ is a certain number, namely β. In the symmetrical case, where the two a priori probabilities are equal and the four individual values are equal, $\beta = 1$ and the optimal value of x_c is the point where $f_{SN}(x) = f_N(x)$, where the two curves cross. If the four values are equal but $p(SN) = 5/6$ and $p(N) = 1/6$, another case described in connection with the dice game, then $\beta = 1/5$ and the optimal value of x_c is shifted a certain distance to the left. This shift may be seen intuitively to be in the proper direction—a higher value of $p(SN)$ should lead to a greater willingness to accept the Hypothesis SN, i.e., to a more lenient cutoff. To consider one more example from the dice game, if $p(SN) = p(N) = 0.5$, if $V_{N \cdot B}$ and $K_{N \cdot A}$ are set at 5 dollars and $V_{SN \cdot A}$ and $K_{SN \cdot B}$ are equal to 1 dollar, then $\beta = 5$ and the optimal value of x_c shifts a certain distance to the right. Again intuitively, if it is more important to be correct when the Hypothesis N is true, a high, or strict, criterion should be adopted.

In any case, β specifies the optimal weighting of hits relative to false alarms; x_c should always be located at the point on the x axis corresponding to β. As we pointed out in discussing the dice game, just where this value of x_c will be with reference to the x axis depends not only upon the a priori probabilities and the values but also upon the overlap of the two density functions, in short, upon the signal strength. We shall define a measure of signal strength within the next few pages. For now, it is important to note that for any detection goal to which the observer may subscribe, and for any set of parameters that may characterize a detection situation (such as a priori probabilities and values associated with decision outcomes), the optimal criterion may be specified in terms of a single number, β, a critical value of likelihood ratio.[5]

Receiver operating characteristic

Whatever criterion the observer actually uses, even if it is not one of the optimal criteria, can also be described by a single number, by some value of likelihood ratio. Let us proceed to a consideration of how the observer's performance may be evaluated with respect to the location of his criterion, and at the same time we shall see how his performance may be evaluated with respect to his sensory capabilities.

---

[5] We have reached a point in the discussion where we can justify the statement made earlier that the decision axis may be equally well regarded as likelihood ratio or as any monotonic transformation of likelihood ratio. Any distortion of the linear continuum of likelihood ratio, that maintains order, is equivalent to likelihood ratio in terms of determining a criterion. The decisions made are the same whether the criterion is set at likelihood ratio equal to β or at the value that corresponds to β of some new variable. To illustrate, if a criterion leads to a Yes response whenever $\lambda(y) > 2$, if $x = [\lambda(y)]^2$ the decisions will be the same if the observer says "yes" whenever $x > 4$.

As we have noted, the fundamental quantities in the evaluation of performance are $p_N(A)$ and $p_{SN}(A)$, these quantities representing, respectively, the areas under the two curves of Fig. 2 to the right of some criterion value of x. If we set up a graph of $p_{SN}(A)$ versus $p_N(A)$ and trace on it the curve resulting as we move the decision criterion along the decision axis of Fig. 2, we sketch one of the arcs shown in Fig. 3. Ignore, for a moment, all but one of these arcs. If the decision criterion is set way at the left in Fig. 2, we obtain a point in the upper right-hand corner of Fig. 3: both $p_{SN}(A)$ and $p_N(A)$ are unity. If the criterion is set at the right end of the decision axis in Fig. 2, the point at the other extreme of Fig. 3, $p_{SN}(A) = p_N(A) = 0$, results. Between these extremes lie the criterion values of more practical interest. It should be noted that the exact form of the curve shown in Fig. 3 is not the only form which might result, but it is the form which will result if the observer chooses a criterion in terms of likelihood ratio, and the probability density functions are normal and of equal variance.

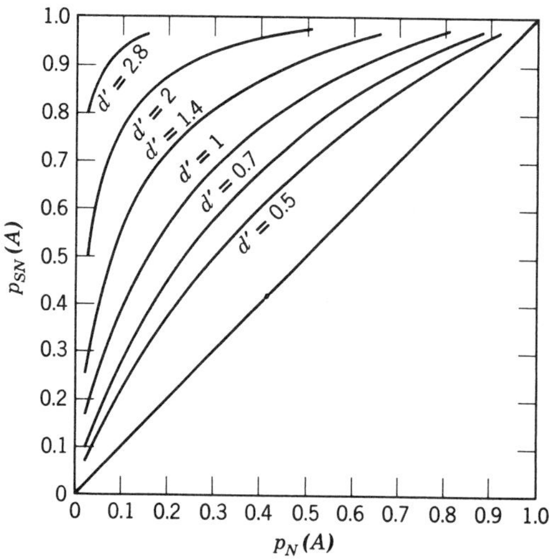

FIG. 3. The receiver-operating-characteristic curves. These curves show $p_{SN}(A)$ versus $p_N(A)$ with d' as the parameter. They are based on the assumptions that the probability density functions, $f_N(x)$ and $f_{SN}(x)$, are normal and of equal variance.

This curve is a form of the *operating characteristic* as it is known in statistics; in the context of the detection problem it is usually referred to as the *receiver-operating-characteristic*, or ROC, curve. The optimal "operating level" may be seen from Eq. (3) to be at the point of the ROC curve where its slope is β. That is, the expression $p_{SN}(A) - \beta p_N(A)$ defines a utility line of slope β, and the point of tangency of this line to the ROC curve is the optimal operating level. Thus the theory specifies the appropriate hit probability and false alarm probability for any definition of optimum and any set of parameters characterizing the detection situation.

It is now apparent how the observer's choice of a criterion in a given experiment may be indexed. The proportions obtained in an experiment are used as estimates of the probabilities, $p_N(A)$ and $p_{SN}(A)$; thus, the observer's behavior yields a point on an ROC curve. The slope of the curve at this point corresponds to the value of likelihood ratio at which he has located his criterion. Thus we work backward from the ROC curve to infer the criterion that is employed by the observer.

There is, of course, a family of ROC curves, as shown in Fig. 3, a given curve corresponding to a given separation between the means of the density functions $f_N(x)$ and $f_{SN}(x)$. The parameter of these curves has been called d', where d' is defined as the difference between the means of the two density functions expressed in terms of their standard deviation, that is:

$$d' = \frac{M_{f_{SN}(x)} - M_{f_N(x)}}{\sigma_{f_N(x)}} \tag{5}$$

Since the separation between the means of the two density functions is a function of signal amplitude, d' is an index of the detectability of a given signal for a given observer.

Recalling our assumptions that the density functions $f_N(x)$ and $f_{SN}(x)$ are normal and of equal variance, we may see from Eq. (5) that the quantity denoted d' is simply the familiar normal deviate, or x/σ measure. From the pair of values $p_N(A)$ and $p_{SN}(A)$ that are obtained experimentally, one may proceed to a published table of areas under the normal curve to determine a value of d'. A simpler computational procedure is achieved by plotting the points $[p_N(A), p_{SN}(A)]$ on graph paper having a probability scale and a normal deviate scale on both axes. We shall illustrate this procedure later.

We see now that the fourfold table of the responses that are made to a particular stimulus may be treated as having two independent parameters—the experiment yields measures of two independent aspects of the observer's performance. The variable d' is a measure of the observer's sensory capabilities, or of the effective signal strength. This may be thought of as the object of interest in classical psychophysics. The criterion β that is employed by the observer, which determines the $p_N(A)$ and $p_{SN}(A)$ for some fixed d', reflects the effect of variables which have been variously called the set, attitude, or motives of the observer. It is the ability to distinguish between these two aspects of detection performance that comprises one of the main advantages of the theory proposed here. We have noted that these two aspects of behavior are confounded in an experiment in which the dependent variable is the intensity of the signal that is required for a threshold response.

Relationship of d′ to signal energy

We have seen that the optimal value of the criterion, β, can be computed. In certain instances, an optimal value of d', i.e., the sensitivity of the mathematically ideal device, can also be computed. If, for example, the exact wave form and starting time of the signal are determinable, as in the case of an auditory signal, then the optimal value of d' is equal to $\sqrt{2E/N_o}$, where E is the signal energy and N_o is the noise power in a one-cycle band (Peterson, Birdsall, and Fox, 1954). A specification of the optimal value of d' for visual signals has been developed very recently.[6] Although we shall not elaborate the point in this paper, it is worth noting that an empirical index of detectability may be compared with ideal detectability, just as observed and optimal indices of decision criteria may be compared. The ratio of the squares of the two detectability indices has been taken as a measure of the observer's sensory efficiency. This measure has demonstrated its usefulness in the study of several problems in audition (Tanner and Birdsall, 1958).

Use of ideal descriptions as models

It might be worthwhile to describe at this point some of the reasons for the emphasis placed here on optimal measures, and, indeed, the reasons for the general enterprise of considering a theory of ideal behavior as a model for studies of real behavior.[7] In view of the deviations from any ideal which are bound to characterize real organisms, it might appear at first glance that any deductions based on ideal premises could have no more than academic interest. We do not think this is the case. In any study, it is desirable to specify rigorously the factors pertinent to the

---

[6] W. P. Tanner, Jr., and R. C. Jones, personal communication, November 1959.

[7] The discussion immediately following is, in part, a paraphrase of one in Horton (1957).

study. Ideal conditions generally involve few variables and permit these to be described in simple terms. Having identified the performance to be expected under ideal conditions, it is possible to extend the model to include the additional variables associated with real organisms. The ideal performance, in other words, constitutes a convenient base from which to explore the complex operation of a real organism.

In certain cases, as in the problem at hand, values characteristic of ideal conditions may actually approximate very closely those characteristics of the organism under study. The problem then becomes one of changing the ideal model in some particular so that it is slightly less than ideal. This is usually accomplished by depriving the ideal device of some particular function. This method of attack has been found to generate useful hypotheses for further studies. Thus, whereas it is not expected that the human observer and the ideal detection device will behave identically, the emphasis in early studies is on similarities. If the differences are small, one may rule out entire classes of alternative models, and regard the model in question as a useful tool in further studies. Proceeding on this assumption, one may then in later studies emphasize the differences, the form and extent of the differences suggesting how the ideal model may be modified in the direction of reality.

Alternative conceptions of the detection process

The earliest studies that were undertaken to test the applicability of the decision model to human observers were quite naturally oriented toward determining its value relative to existing psychophysical theory. As a result, some of the data presented below are meaningful only with respect to differences in the predictions based upon different theories. We shall, therefore, briefly consider alternative theories of the detection process.

Although it is difficult to specify with precision the alternative theories of detection, it is clear that they generally involve the concept of the *threshold* in an important way. The development of the threshold concept is fairly obscure. It is differently conceived by different people, and few popular usages of the concept benefit from explicit statement. One respect, however, in which the meaning of the threshold concept is entirely clear is its assertion of a limit on sensitivity. As we have just seen, the decision model does not include such a boundary. The decision model specifies no lower bound on the location of the criterion along the continuous axis of sensory inputs. Further, it implies that any displacement of the mean of $f_{SN}(x)$ from the mean of $f_N(x)$, no matter how small, will result in a greater value of $p_{SN}(A)$ than $p_N(A)$, irrespective of the location of the criterion.

To permit experimental comparison of decision theory and threshold theory, we shall consider a special version of threshold theory (Blackwell, 1953). Although it is a special version, we believe it retains the essence of the threshold concept. In this version, the threshold is described in the same terms that are used in the description of decision theory. It is regarded as a cutoff on the continuum of observations (see Fig. 2) with a fixed location, with values of x above the cutoff always evoking a positive response, and with discrimination impossible among values of x below the cutoff. This description of a threshold in terms of a fixed cutoff and a stimulus effect that varies randomly, it will be noted, is entirely equivalent to the more common description in terms of a randomly varying cutoff and a fixed stimulus effect. There are several reasons for assuming that the hypothetical threshold cutoff is located quite high relative to the density function $f_N(x)$, say at approximately $+3\sigma$ from the mean of $f_N(x)$. We shall compare our data with the predictions of such a "high threshold" theory, and shall indicate their relationship to predictions from a theory assuming a lower threshold. We shall, in particular, ask how low a threshold cutoff would have to be to be consistent with the reported data. It may be noted that if a high threshold exists, the observer will be incapable of ordering values of x likely to result from noise alone, and hence will be incapable of varying his criterion over a significant range.

If a threshold exists that is rarely exceeded by noise alone, this fact will be immediately apparent from the ROC curves (see Fig. 3) that are obtained experimentally. It can be shown that the ROC curves in this case are straight lines from points on the left-hand vertical axis—$p_{SN}(A)$—to the upper right-hand corner of the plot. These straight line curves represent the implication of a high threshold theory that an increase in $p_N(A)$ must be effected by responding "yes" to a random selection of observations that fail to reach the threshold, rather than by a judicious selection of observations, i.e., a lower criterion level. If we follow the usual procedure of regarding the stimulus threshold as the signal intensity yielding a value of $p_{SN}(A) = 0.5$ for $p_N(A) = 0.0$, then an appreciation of the relationship between d' and $p_N(A)$ at threshold may be gained by visualizing a straight line in Fig. 3 from this point to the upper right-hand corner. If we note which of the ROC curves drawn in Fig. 3 are intersected by the visualized line, we see that the threshold decreases with increasing $p_N(A)$. For example, a response procedure resulting in a $p_N(A) = 0.02$ requires a signal of $d' = 2.0$ to reach the threshold, whereas a response procedure yielding a $p_N(A) = 0.98$ requires a signal of $d' < 0.5$ to reach the threshold. A graph showing what threshold would be calculated as a function of $p_N(A)$ is plotted in Fig. 4. The calculated threshold is a strictly monotonic function of $p_N(A)$ ranging from infinity to zero.

The fundamental difference between the threshold theory we are considering and decision theory lies in their treatment of false alarm responses. According to the threshold theory, these responses represent guesses determined by nonsensory factors: i.e., $p_N(A)$ is independent of the cutoff which is assumed to have a fixed location. Decision theory assumes, on the other hand, that $p_N(A)$ varies with the temporary position of a cutoff under the observer's control; that false alarm responses arise for valid sensory reasons, and that therefore a simple correction will not eliminate their effect on $p_{SN}(A)$. A similar implication of Fig. 4 that should be noted is that reliable estimates of $p_{SN}(A)$ or of the stimulus threshold are not guaranteed by simply training the observer to maintain a low, constant value of $p_N(A)$. Since extreme probabilities cannot be estimated with reliability, the criterion may vary from session to session with the variation having no direct reflection in the data. Certainly, false alarm rates of 0.01, 0.001, and 0.0001 are not discriminable in an experimentally feasible number of observations; the differences in the calculated values of the threshold associated with these different values of $p_N(A)$ may be seen from Fig. 4 to be sizeable. The experiments reported in the following were designed, in large measure, to clarify the relationship that exists between $p_N(A)$ and $p_{SN}(A)$, to show whether or not the observer is capable of controlling the location of his criterion for a Yes response.

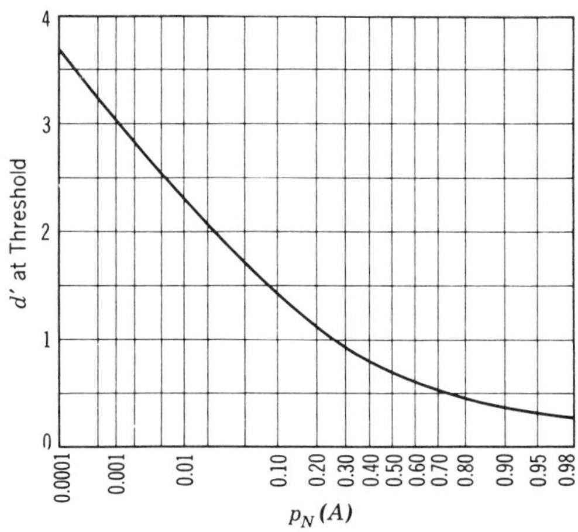

FIG. 4. The relationship between d' and $p_N(A)$ at threshold.

SOME EXPERIMENTS

Five experiments are reported here. They are the first experiments that were undertaken to test the applicability of decision theory to psychophysical tasks, and it must be emphasized that they were intended to explore only the general relationships specified in the theory. We shall refer also to more recent experiments conducted within the framework of decision theory. The later experiments, although not focused as directly on testing the validity of the theory, support the principal thesis of this paper.

The experiments reported here are devoted to answering the two principal questions suggested by a consideration of decision theory. The first of these may be stated in this way: is sensory information (or the decision axis) continuous, i.e., is the observer capable of discriminating among observations likely to result from noise alone? The alternative we consider is that there exists a threshold cut, on the decision axis, that is unlikely to be exceeded by observations resulting from noise, and below which discrimination among observations is impossible. The second question has two parts: is the observer capable of using different criteria, and, if so, does he change his criterion appropriately when the variables that we expect will determine his criterion (probabilities, values, and costs) are changed?

Three of the five experiments to be described pose for the observer what we have called the fundamental detection problem, the problem that occupied our attention throughout the theoretical discussion. Of these, two test the observer's ability to use the criterion that maximizes the expected value of a decision. The a priori probability of a signal occurrence and the individual values associated with the four possible decision outcomes are varied systematically, in order to determine the range over which the observer can vary his criterion and the form of the resultant ROC curve. A third experiment tests the observer's ability to maximize the proportion of hits while satisfying a restriction on the proportion of false alarms. This experiment is largely concerned with the degree of precision with which the observer can locate a criterion.

The remaining two experiments differ in that the tasks they present to the observer do not require him to establish a criterion, that is, they do not require a Yes or No response. They test certain implications of decision theory that we have not yet treated explicitly, but they will be seen to follow very directly from the theory and to contribute significantly to an evaluation of it. In one of these the observer is asked to report after each observation interval his subjective probability that the signal existed during the interval. This response is a familiar one; it is essentially a rating or a judgment of confidence. The report of "a posteriori probability of signal existence," as it is termed in detection theory, may be regarded as reflecting the likelihood ratio of the observation. This case is of interest since an estimate of likelihood ratio preserves more of the information contained in the observation than does a report merely that the likelihood ratio fell above or below a critical value. We shall see that it is also possible to construct the ROC curve from this type of response.

The other experiment not requiring a criterion employs what has been termed the temporal forced-choice method of response. On each trial a signal is presented in exactly one of n temporal intervals, and the observer states in which interval he believes the signal occurred. The optimal procedure for the observer to follow in this case, if he is to maximize the probability of a correct response, is to make an observation x in each interval and to choose the interval having the greatest value of x associated with it. Since decision theory specifies how the proportion of correct responses obtained with the forced-choice method is related to the detectability index d', the internal consistency of the theory may be evaluated. That is to say, if the observer follows the optimal procedure, then the estimate of the detectability of a signal of a given strength that is based on forced-choice data will be comparable to that based on yes-no data. The forced-choice method may also be used to make a strong test of a fundamental assumption of decision theory, namely, that sensory information is continuous, or that sensory information does not exhibit a threshold cutoff. For an experiment requiring the observer to rank the n intervals according to their likelihood of containing the signal, the continuity and threshold assumptions lead to very different predictions concerning the probability that an interval which is ranked other than first will be the correct interval.

All of the experiments reported in the following employed a circular signal with a diameter of 30 minutes of visual angle and a duration of 1/100 of a second. The signal was presented on a large uniformly illuminated background having a luminance of 10 foot-lamberts. Details of the apparatus have been presented elsewhere (Blackwell, Pritchard, and Ohmart, 1954).

Maximizing the expected value of a decision—an experimental analysis

A direct test of the decision model is achieved in an experiment in which the a priori probability of signal occurrence or the values of the decision outcomes, or both, are varied from one group of observations to another—in short, in which β (Eqs. 3 and 4) assumes different values. The observer, in order to maximize his expected value, or his payoff, must vary his willingness to make a Yes response, in accordance with the change in β. Variations in this respect will be indicated by the proportion of false alarms, $p_N(A)$. The point of interest is how $p_{SN}(A)$, the proportion of hits, varies with changes in $p_N(A)$, i.e., in the form of the observer's ROC curve. If the experimental values of $p_N(A)$ reflect the location of the observer's criterion, if the observer responds on the basis of the likelihood ratio of the observation, and if the density functions (Fig. 2) are normal and of equal variance, the ROC curve of Fig. 3 will result. If, on the other hand, the location of the criterion is fixed in such a position that it is rarely exceeded by noise alone, then the resulting ROC curve will be a straight line, as we have indicated. We shall examine some empirical ROC curves with this distinction in mind.

This experiment can be made to yield another and, in one sense, a stronger test of these two hypotheses, by employing several values of signal strength within a single group of observations, i.e., while a given set of probabilities and values are in effect. For in this case stimulus thresholds can be calculated, and correlational techniques can be used to determine whether the calculated threshold is dependent upon $p_N(A)$ as predicted by decision theory, or independent of $p_N(A)$ as predicted by what we have termed the high threshold theory. We will grant that presenting more than one value of signal strength, within a single group of observations to which fixed probabilities and values apply, is not, conceptually, the simplest experiment that could have been performed to test our hypotheses. Nevertheless, a little reflection will show that this experimental procedure is entirely legitimate from any of our present points of view. We simply associate several values of $p_{SN}(A)$ with a given value of $p_N(A)$, and thereby obtain at once a point on each of several ROC curves and an estimate of the stimulus threshold that is associated with that value of $p_N(A)$.

FIRST EXPECTED-VALUE EXPERIMENT. The first of the two expected-value experiments that were performed employed four values of signal strength.

Three observers, after considerable practice, served in sixteen 2-hour sessions. In each session, signals at four levels of intensity (0.44, 0.69, 0.92, and 1.20 foot-lamberts) were presented along with a "blank" or "no-signal" presentation. The order of presentation was random within a restriction placed upon the total number of occurrences of each signal intensity and the blank in a given session. Each of the signal intensities occurred equally often within a session. The proportion of trials on which a signal (of any intensity) was presented, $p(SN)$, was either 0.80 or 0.40 in the various sessions. In all, there were 300 presentations in each session—six blocks of 50 presentations, separated by rest periods. Thus each estimate of $p_N(A)$ is based on either 60 or 180 observations, and each estimate of $p_{SN}(A)$ is based on 30 or 60 observations, depending upon $p(SN)$.

In the first four sessions, no values were associated with the various decision outcomes. For the first and fourth sessions the observers were informed that $p(SN) = 0.80$ and, for the second and third sessions, that $p(SN) = 0.40$. The average value of $p_N(A)$ obtained in the sessions with $p(SN) = 0.80$ was 0.43, and, in the sessions with $p(SN) = 0.40$, it was 0.15—indicating that the observer's willingness to make a Yes response is significantly affected by changes in $p(SN)$ alone. In the remaining 12 sessions, these two values of $p(SN)$ were used in conjunction with a variety of values placed on the decision outcomes. In the fifth session, for example, the observers were told that $p(SN) = 0.80$ and were, in addition, given the following payoff matrix:

	No	Yes
Signal	-1 $K_{SN \cdot B}$	$+1$ $V_{SN \cdot A}$
No Signal	$+2$ $V_{N \cdot B}$	-2 $K_{N \cdot A}$

A variety of simple matrices was used. These included, reading from left to right across the top and then the bottom row: $(-1, +1, +3, -3)$ and $(-1, +1, +4, -4)$ with $p(SN) = 0.80$, and $(-1, +1, +2, -2)$, $(-1, +1, +1, -1)$, $(-2, +2, +1, -1)$, and $(-3, +3, +1, -1)$ with $p(SN) = 0.40$. By reference to Eq. (4), it may be seen that these matrices and values of $p(SN)$ define values of β ranging from 0.25 to 3.00. The observers were actually paid in accordance with these payoff matrices, in addition to their regular wage. The values were equated with fractions of cents, these fractions being adjusted so that the expected earnings per session remained relatively constant, at approximately one dollar.

The obtained values of $p_N(A)$ varied in accordance with changes in the values of the decision outcomes as well as with changes in the a priori probability of signal occurrence. Just how closely the obtained values of $p_N(A)$ approached those specified as optimal by the theory, we shall discuss shortly. For now, we may note that the range of values of $p_N(A)$

obtained from the three observers is shown in Fig. 5. The parts of this figure also show four values of $p_{SN}(A)$ corresponding to each value of $p_N(A)$; the four values of $p_{SN}(A)$, one for each signal strength, are indicated by different symbols. We have, then, in the parts of Fig. 5, four ROC curves.

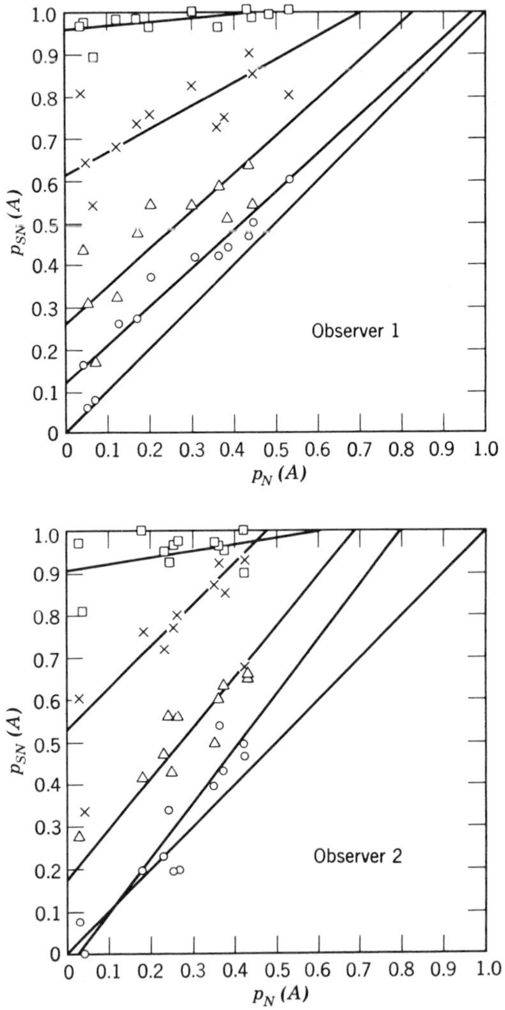

FIG. 5. Empirical receiver-operating-characteristic curves obtained from three observers in the first expected-value experiment.

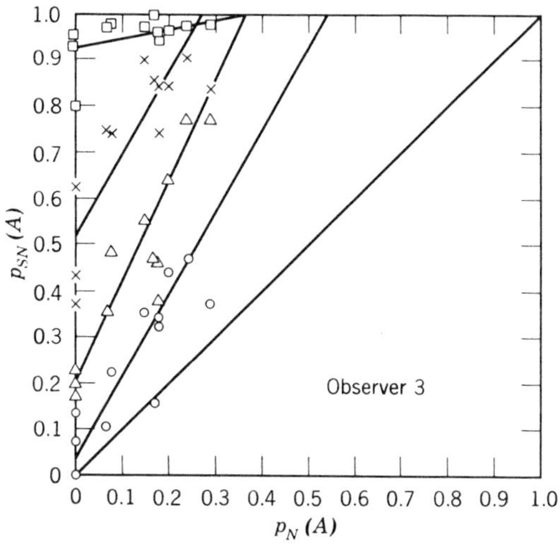

Although entire ROC curves are not precisely defined by the data of the first experiment, these data will contribute to our purpose of distinguishing between the predictions of decision theory and the predictions of a high threshold theory. It is clear, for example, that the straight lines fitted to the data do not intersect the upper right-hand corner of the graph, as required by the concept of a high threshold.

We have mentioned that another analysis of the data is of interest in distinguishing the two theories we are considering. As we have indicated earlier in this paper, and developed in more detail elsewhere (Tanner and Swets, 1954), the concept of a high threshold leads to the prediction that the stimulus threshold is independent of $p_N(A)$, whereas decision theory predicts a negative correlation between the stimulus threshold and $p_N(A)$. Within the framework of the high threshold model that we have described, the stimulus threshold is defined as the stimulus intensity that yields a $p_{SN}(A) = 0.50$ for $p_N(A) = 0.0$. This stimulus intensity may be determined by interpolation from psychometric functions—$p_{SN}(A)$ vs. signal intensity—that are normalized so that $p_N(A) = 0.0$. The normalization is effected by the equation:

$$p_{SN}(A)_{\text{corrected}} = \frac{p_{SN}(A) - p_N(A)}{1 - p_N(A)} \tag{6}$$

commonly known as the "correction for chance success." The intent of the correction is to remove what has been regarded as the spurious element of $p_{SN}(A)$ that is contributed by an observer's tendency to make a

Yes response in the absence of any sensory indication of a signal, i.e., to make a Yes response following an observation that fails to reach the threshold level. It can be shown that the validity of this correction procedure is implied by the assumption of what we have termed a high threshold. The decision model, as we have indicated, differs in that it regards sensory information as thoroughly probabilistic, without a fixed cutoff—it asserts that the presence and absence of some sensory indication of a signal are not separable categories. According to the decision model, the observer does not achieve more Yes responses by responding positively to a random selection of observations that fall short of the fixed criterion level, but by lowering his criterion. In this case, the chance correction is inappropriate; the stimulus threshold will not remain invariant with changes in $p_N(A)$.

The relationship of the stimulus threshold to $p_N(A)$ in this first experiment is illustrated by Figs. 6 and 7. The portion of data comprising each of the curves in these figures was selected to be relatively homogeneous with respect to $p_N(A)$. The curves are average curves for the three observers. Figure 6 shows $p_N(A)$ and $p_{SN}(A)$ as a function of the signal intensity, ΔI. The intercepts of the three curves may be seen to indicate values of $p_N(A)$ of 0.35, 0.25, and 0.04, respectively. Figure 7 shows the *corrected* value of $p_{SN}(A)$ plotted against signal intensity. It may be seen in Fig. 7 that the stimulus threshold—the value of ΔI corresponding to a

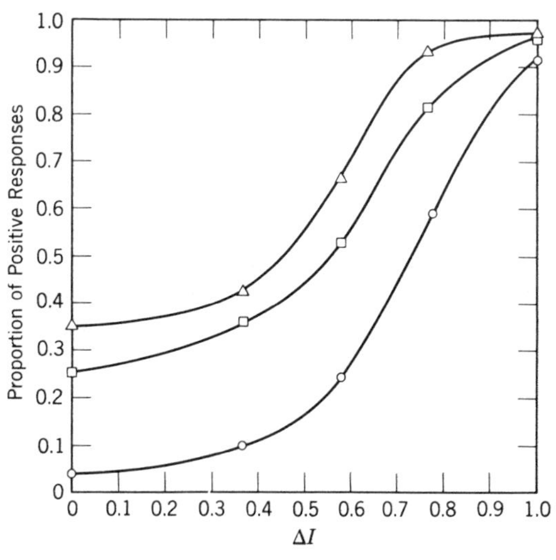

FIG. 6. The relationship between the stimulus threshold and $p_N(A)$ with the proportion of positive responses to four positive values of signal intensity, $p_{SN}(A)$, and to the blank or zero-intensity presentation, $p_N(A)$, at three values of $p_N(A)$.

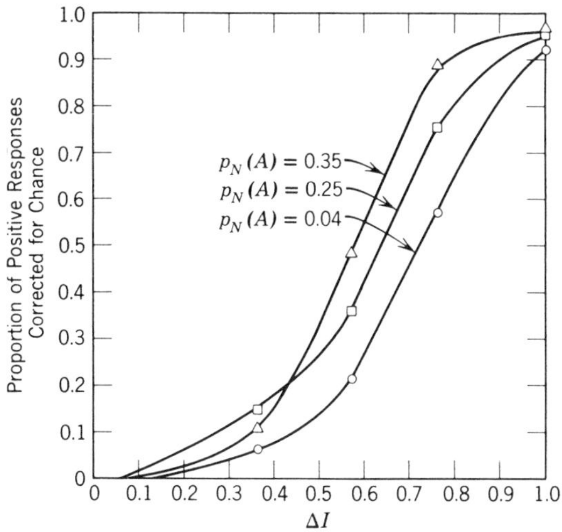

FIG. 7. The relationship between the stimulus threshold and $p_N(A)$ with the three curves corrected for chance success, by Eq. (6).

corrected $p_{SN}(A)$ of 0.50—is dependent upon $p_N(A)$ in the direction predicted by decision theory.[8]

Figures 6 and 7 portray the relationship in question in a form to which many of us are accustomed; they are presented here only for illustrative purposes. We can, of course, achieve a stronger test by computing the coefficients of correlation between $p_N(A)$ and the calculated threshold. We have made this computation, and have in the process avoided the averaging of data obtained from different observers and different experimental sessions. The product-moment coefficients for the three observers are $-.37$ ($p = 0.245$), $-.60$ ($p = 0.039$), and $-.81$ ($p = 0.001$), respectively. For the three observers combined, $p = 0.0008$. The implication of these correlations is the same as that of the straight lines fitted to the data of Fig. 5, namely, that a dependence exists between the conditional probability that an observation arising from SN will exceed the criterion and the conditional probability that an observation arising from N will exceed the criterion. Stated otherwise, the correlations indicate that the observer's decision function is likelihood ratio or some monotonic function of it, and that he is capable of adopting different criteria.

---

[8] ΔI is plotted in Figs. 6 and 7 in terms of the transmission values of the filters that were placed selectively in the signal beam to yield different signal intensities. These values (0.365, 0.575, 0.765, 1.000) are converted to the signal values in terms of foot-lamberts that we have presented above, by multiplying them by 1.20, the value of the signal in foot-lamberts without selective filtering.

SECOND EXPECTED-VALUE EXPERIMENT. A second expected-value experiment was conducted to obtain a more precise definition of the ROC curve than that provided by the experiment just described. In the second experiment greater definition was achieved by increasing the number of observations on which the estimates of $p_{SN}(A)$ and $p_N(A)$ were based, and by increasing the range of values of $p_N(A)$.

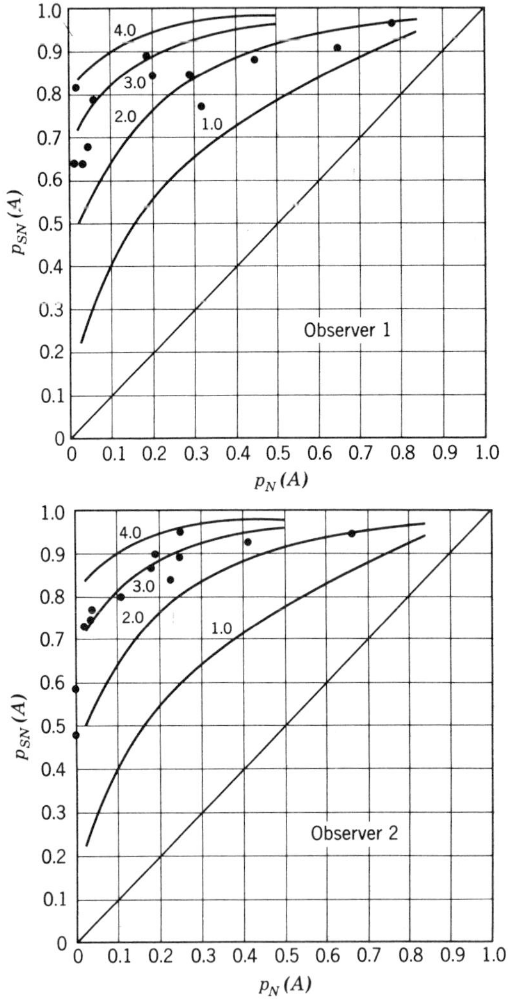

FIG. 8. Empirical receiver-operating-characteristic curves for four observers in the second expected-value experiment.

In this experiment only one signal intensity (0.78 foot-lamberts) was employed. Each of 13 experimental sessions included 200 presentations of the signal and 200 presentations of noise alone. Thus, $p(SN)$ remained constant at 0.50 throughout this experiment. Changes in the optimal criterion β, and thus in the obtained values of $p_N(A)$, were effected entirely by changes in the values associated with the decision outcomes. These values were manipulated to yield β's (Eq. 4) varying from 0.16 to 8.00. A different set of observers served in this experiment.

The results are portrayed in Fig. 8. It may be seen that the experi-

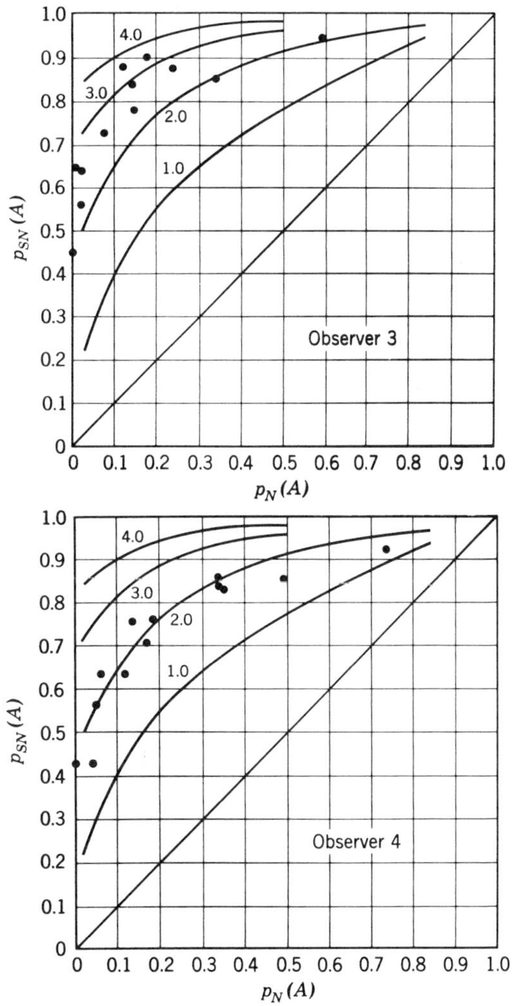

mentally determined points are fitted quite well by the type of ROC curve that is predicted by decision theory. It is equally apparent, excepting Observer 1, that the points do not lie along a straight line intersecting the point $p_N(A) = p_{SN}(A) = 1.00$, as predicted by the high threshold model.

One other feature of these figures is worthy of note. It will be recalled that in our presentation of decision theory we tentatively assumed that the density functions of noise and of signal plus noise, $f_N(x)$ and $f_{SN}(x)$, are of equal variance. Although we did not, in order to preserve the continuity of the discussion, we might have acknowledged at that point that the assumption of equal variance is not necessarily the best one. In particular, one might rather expect the variance of $f_{SN}(x)$ to be proportional to its mean. At any rate, the assumption made about variances represents a degree of freedom of the theory that we have not emphasized previously. We have, however, used this degree of freedom in the construction of the theoretical ROC curves of Fig. 8. Notice that these curves are not symmetrical about the negative diagonal, as are the curves of Fig. 3 which are predicated on equal variance. The curves of Fig. 8 are based on the assumption that the ratio of the increment of the mean of $f_{SN}(x)$ to the increment of its standard deviation is equal to 4, $\Delta M/\Delta\sigma = 4$. A close look at these figures suggests that ROC curves calculated from a still greater ratio would provide a still better fit. Since other data presented in the following bear directly on this question of a dependence between variance and signal strength, we shall postpone further discussion of it. We shall also consider later whether the exact form of the empirical ROC curves supports the assumption of normality of the density functions $f_N(x)$ and $f_{SN}(x)$. For now, the main point is that decision theory predicts the curvilinear form of the ROC curves that are yielded by the observers.

Forced-choice experiments

We have indicated previously that an extension of the decision model may be made to predict performance in a forced-choice test. On each trial of a typical forced-choice test, the signal is presented in one of n temporal intervals, and the observer selects the interval he believes to have contained the signal. It will be intuitively clear that, to behave optimally, in the sense of maximizing the probability of a correct response, the observer must make an observation x in each interval, and choose the interval having the greatest value of x associated with it. Equivalently, he may rank the intervals according to their values of likelihood ratio and choose that interval yielding the greatest value of likelihood ratio.

If the observer behaves optimally, then the probability that a correct answer will result, $p(c)$ for a given value of d', is expressed by

$$p(c) = \int_{-\infty}^{+\infty} [f(x)]^{n-1} g(x)dx \tag{7}$$

where $\mathrm{f}(x)$ is the area of the noise function to the left of x, $g(x)$ is the ordinate of the signal-plus-noise function, and n is the number of intervals used in the test. This is simply the probability that one drawing from the distribution due to signal plus noise is greater than the greatest of n-1 drawings from the distribution due to noise alone.

It is intuitively clear that if the signal produces a large shift in the noise function, i.e., if d' is large, then the probability that the greatest value of x will be obtained in the interval that contains the signal is also large, and conversely—indeed (for a fixed number of intervals) $p(c)$ is a monotonic function of d'. Equation (7) can be seen to be a function of d' by noting that, under the assumption of equal variance, the signal-plus-noise function is simply the noise function shifted by d', that is, $\mathrm{g}(x) = \mathrm{f}(x - d')$. Thus d' may be defined in a forced-choice experiment by determining a value of $p(c)$ for some signal intensity and then using Eq. (7) to determine d'. A plot of $p(c)$ versus d', for the case of four intervals, and under the assumption of equal variance, is shown in Fig. 9.

ESTIMATES OF SIGNAL DETECTABILITY OBTAINED FROM DIFFERENT PROCEDURES. According to detection theory, the estimates of d' for a

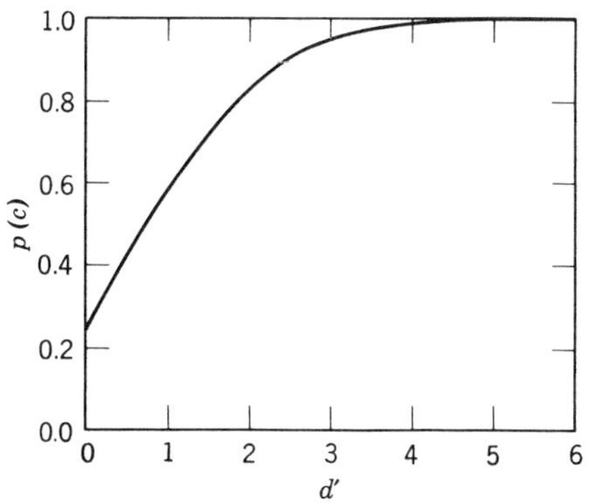

FIG. 9. The probability of a correct choice in a four-alternative forced-choice experiment as a function of d'.

signal and background of given intensities should be the same irrespective of the psychophysical procedure used to collect the data. Thus we may check the internal consistency of the theory by comparing estimates of d' based on yes-no and on forced-choice data. The results of such a comparison have been reported in another paper (Tanner and Swets, 1954). It was shown there that estimates of d' based on the data of the first expected-value experiment that we have presented above, and on forced-choice tests conducted in conjunction with it, are highly consistent with each other. Comparable estimates of d' have also been obtained in auditory experiments—from yes-no and forced-choice procedures, and from forced-choice procedures with from two to eight alternatives (Swets, 1959). Hence, decision theory provides a unification of the data obtained with different procedures; it enables one to predict the performance in one situation from data collected in another.

It is a commonplace that calculated values of the stimulus threshold are not independent of the psychophysical procedure that is employed (Osgood, 1953). Of particular relevance to our present concern is the finding that thresholds obtained with the forced-choice procedure are lower than those obtained with the yes-no procedure (Blackwell, 1953). This finding is accounted for, in terms of decision theory, by the fact that the calculated threshold varies monotonically with the false alarm rate (see Fig. 4)—with high thresholds corresponding to low false alarm rates such as were obtained in these experiments. The dependence of the stimulus threshold upon the false alarm rate, however the threshold is calculated, precludes the existence of a simple relationship between thresholds obtained with the yes-no procedure and those obtained with other response procedures. It is also the case that the normalization of the psychometric function provided by the correction for chance, or, equivalently, the normalization achieved by defining the threshold as the stimulus intensity yielding a proportion of correct responses halfway between chance performance and perfect performance, does not serve to relate forced-choice thresholds obtained with different numbers of alternatives.

THEORETICAL AND EXPERIMENTAL ANALYSIS OF SECOND CHOICES. As we have indicated, a variation of the forced-choice procedure—in which the observer indicates his second choice as well as his first—provides a powerful test of a basic difference between the decision model and the high threshold model. If the observer is capable of discriminating among values of the observations x that fail to reach what we have termed the threshold, i.e., a criterion fixed at approximately $+3\sigma$ from the mean of the noise function, then the proportion of second choices that are correct will be considerably higher than if he is not.[9]

According to the high threshold model, only very infrequently will more than one of the n observations of a forced-choice trial exceed the threshold. Since the observations which do not exceed the threshold are assumed by the model to be indiscriminable, the second choice will be made among the $n - 1$ alternatives on a chance basis. Thus, for a four-alternative experiment as described in the following, the high threshold model predicts that, when the first choice is incorrect, the probability that the second choice will be correct is 0.33. This predicted value, it may be noted, is independent of the signal strength.

Decision theory, on the other hand, implies that the observer is capable of ordering the four alternatives according to their likelihood of containing the signal. If this is the case, the proportion of correct second choices will be greater than 0.33. Should one of the samples of the noise function be the greatest of the four, leading to an incorrect first choice, the probability that the observation from the signal-plus-noise distribution will be the second greatest is larger than the probabilities that either of the observations of the noise distribution will be the second greatest. Again, it is intuitively clear that this probability is a function of d', or of signal strength—i.e., the probability that the observation of the signal-plus-noise value will be greater than two of the observations of noise increases with increases in d'. Specifically, the probability of a correct second choice in a four-alternative, forced-choice test, for a given value of d', is given by the expression:

$$\frac{3\int_{-\infty}^{+\infty} [f(x)]^2[1 - f(x)]g(x)\,dx}{1 - \int_{-\infty}^{+\infty} [f(x)]^3 g(x)\,dx} \tag{8}$$

where the symbols have the same meaning as in Eq. (7). This relationship is plotted in Fig. 10 under the assumptions that the density func-

[9] This experiment was suggested to us by R. Z. Norman. The general rationale of this experiment, and the results of its application to the perception of words exposed for short durations, have been presented by Bricker and Chapanis (1953) and by Howes (1954).

tions of noise and signal plus noise are Gaussian and of equal variance. (The function predicted by decision theory for the proportion of correct first choices in a three-alternative situation is included in Fig. 10 to show that this function is not the same as the predicted function of the probability of a correct second choice, given an incorrect first choice, for the four-alternative situation).

To distinguish between the two predictions, data were collected from four observers; two of them had served previously in the second expected-value experiment, whereas the other two had received only routine force-choice training. Each of the observers served in three experimental sessions. Each session included 150 trials in which both a first and second choice were required.

The resulting 12 proportions of correct second choices are plotted against d' in Fig. 10. The values of d' were determined by using the proportions of correct first choices as estimates of the probability of a correct choice, $p(c)$, and reading the corresponding values of d' from the middle curve of Fig. 10, which is the same curve shown in Fig. 9. Although just one value of signal intensity was used (0.78 foot-lamberts

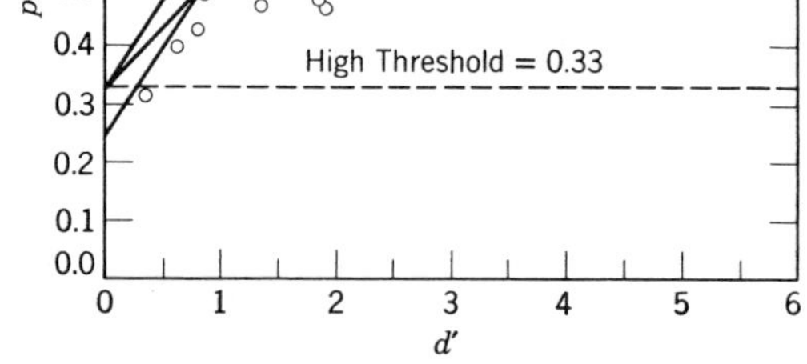

FIG. 10. The results of the second-choice experiment. The proportions of correct second choices are plotted against d'. The curve labeled "2nd Choice" represents the prediction of decision theory, assuming the density functions to be normal and of equal variance. The prediction of the high-threshold theory is shown by the dashed line.

as in the second expected-value experiment), the values of d' differed sufficiently from one observer to another to provide an indication of the agreement of the data with the two predicted functions. Additional variation in the estimates of d' resulted from the fact that, for two observers, a constant distance from the signal was not maintained in all three of the experimental sessions.

A systematic deviation of the data from a proportion of 0.33 clearly exists. Considering the data of the four observers combined, the proportion of correct second choices is 0.46. Further, a correlation between the proportion of correct second choices and d' is evident.

Two control conditions aid in interpreting these data. The first of these allowed for the possibility that requiring the observer to make a second choice might depress his first-choice performance. During the experiment, blocks of 50 trials in which only a first choice was required were alternated with blocks of 50 trials in which both a first and a second choice were required. Pooling the data from the four observers, the proportions of correct first choices for the two conditions are 0.650 and 0.651, a difference that is obviously not significant. A preliminary experiment in which data were obtained from a single observer for five values of signal intensity also serves as a control. In that experiment, 150 observations were made at each value of signal intensity. The relative frequencies of correct second choices for the lowest four values of signal intensity were, in increasing order of signal intensity: 26/117 (0.22), 33/95 (0.35), 30/75 (0.40), and 20/30 (0.67). For the highest value of signal intensity, none of five second choices was correct. In this experiment, then, the proportion of correct second choices is seen to be correlated with a physical measure of signal intensity as well as with the theoretical measure d'—this eliminates the possibility that the correlation found with a constant value of signal intensity, involving d' as one of the variables (Fig. 10), is an artifact of theoretical manipulation.

It may be seen from Fig. 10 that the second-choice data also deviate systematically from the predicted function derived from decision theory. This discrepancy, as will be seen, results from the inadequacy of the assumption—of equal variance of the noise and signal-plus-noise density functions—upon which the predicted functions in Fig. 10 are based. It has been pointed out that the data obtained in the second expected-value experiment (see Fig. 8 and accompanying text) indicate that a better assumption would be that the ratio of the increment in the mean of the signal-plus-noise function to the increment in its standard deviation is

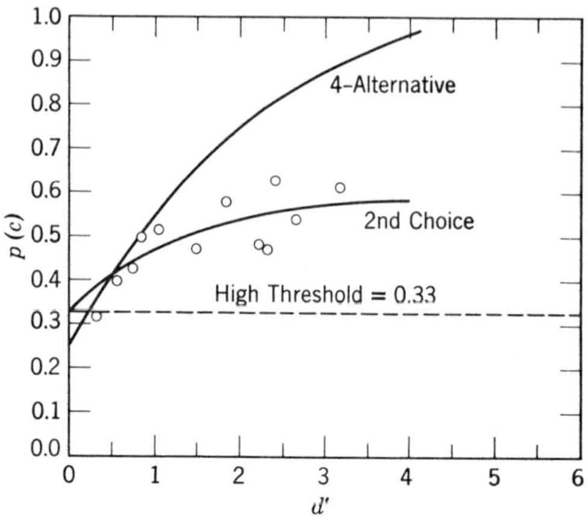

FIG. 11. The results of the second-choice experiment calculated under another assumption. The predictions from decision theory for first and second choices are plotted under the assumption that $\Delta M/\Delta\sigma = 4$.

equal to 4. Figure 11 shows the second-choice data and the predicted four-alternative and second-choice curves derived from the theory under this assumption that $\Delta M/\Delta\sigma = 4$. In view of the variance associated with each of the points (each first-choice d' was estimated on the basis of 300 observations and each second-choice proportion on less than 100 observations), the agreement of the data and the predicted function shown in Fig. 11 is quite good.

The conclusion to be drawn from these results of the second-choice experiment, though perhaps more obvious here, is the same as that drawn from the yes-no, or expected-value, experiments: the sensory information, or the decision axis, is continuous over a greater range than allowed for by the high threshold model. If a threshold cutoff, below which there is no discrimination among observations, exists at all, it is located in such a position that it is exceeded by much of the noise distribution.

Note on the variance assumption

Before considering the two remaining experiments, we should pause briefly to take up the problem of the relative sizes of the variances of the noise and signal-plus-noise distributions. We have seen, as indicated in the theoretical discussion, that an assumption concerning these variances may be tested by experiment. We have found that two sets of data, from yes-no and forced-choice experiments, support the assumption that the variance of the signal-plus-noise distribution increases with its mean. In particular, the assumption that $\Delta M/\Delta\sigma = 4$ is seen to fit those data reasonably well, and noticeably better than the assumption of equal variance. We should like to point out three aspects of this topic in the following paragraphs: first, that the assumption of $\Delta M/\Delta\sigma = 4$ is probably not generally applicable; second, that we have good reason to suspect in advance of experimentation, in the visual case, that the variance of the signal-plus-noise distribution is greater than that of the noise distribution; and, third, that the very assumption of unequal variances requires that we qualify a statement made earlier in this paper.

It will be apparent that if the variance of these sampling distributions is a function of sample size, then their variances will differ as a function of the duration and the area of the signal. The assumption of $\Delta M/\Delta\sigma = 4$ will probably not fit the results of experiments with different physical parameters. Further, as we have indicated, we have not explored the extent of agreement between other specific assumptions and our present data. It appears likely that more precise data will be required to determine the relative adequacy of different assumptions about the increase in variance with signal strength.

Peterson, Birdsall, and Fox (1954), after developing the general theory of signal detectability, spelled out the specific forms it takes in a variety of different detection problems. By way of illustration, we may mention the problems in which *the signal is known exactly*, *the signal is known exactly except for phase*, and *the signal is a sample of white Gaussian noise.* A principal difference among these problems lies in the shape of the expected ROC curve. For our present purposes, we may regard these problems as differing in the degree of variance contributed by the signal itself. For the first case mentioned, the signal contributes no variance—the signal-plus-noise distribution is simply a translation of the noise distribution, the two have equal variances. In the other two cases, the signal itself has a variability which increases with its strength.

Clearly, if we are to select one of the specific models incorporated within the theory of signal detectability to apply to a visual detection problem, we would not select the one that assumes that the signal is known exactly, for the visual signal does not contain phase information. Thus, the second model is more likely to be applicable than the first. Actually, the third model, which assumes that the signal is a sample of noise, is the best representation of a visual signal. The fundamental point here is that either of the last two models leads to predicted results quite similar to those that are predicted under the assumption that $\Delta M/\Delta\sigma = 4$. Further discussion of this point would lead us too far off the path; we would like simply to note here that a specific form of the theory of signal detectability, which on a priori grounds is most likely to be applicable to vision experiments, predicts results very similar to those obtained. It is interesting to note in this connection that the results of auditory experiments using pure tones as signals are in close agreement with the signal-known-exactly model, with the assumption of equal variance.

The discerning reader will have noted that the assumption of a variance of the signal-plus-noise distribution that increases with its mean is inconsistent with a statement made in the theoretical discussion. In particular, the assumption of a greater variance of $f_{SN}(x)$ than of $f_N(x)$ conflicts with the statement that the decision axis x may be regarded as a likelihood-ratio axis. It was stated (see the discussion following Fig. 2) that a multidimensional response of the sensory system, i.e., one that might be represented by a point y in a multi-dimensional space, could be mapped into a line by considering the likelihood that y arose from SN relative to the likelihood that y arose from N, or $\lambda(y) = f_{SN}(y)/f_N(y)$. We then stated that we could identify the observation variable x with some monotonic transformation of $\lambda(y)$. If, now, the variance of $f_{SN}(x)$ is greater than the variance of $f_N(x)$, then as x decreases from a high value, $\lambda(x)$ will decrease—but, at some point below the mean of the function $f_N(x)$, $\lambda(x)$ will begin to increase again, and will, as a matter of fact, become greater than unity. Thus, if we choose to maintain the assumption of a greater variance of $f_{SN}(x)$, then the variable x cannot be regarded, throughout its range, as a likelihood ratio. Given that we do want to maintain the assumption of increasing variance of $f_{SN}(x)$, for the time being at least, we may take any of several possible steps to correct the difficulty. We can, for example, assume that there exists a low threshold, near the mean of $f_N(x)$, such that values of x less than this threshold are not ordered by the observer, and hence the fact that x cannot be considered as a likelihood ratio below this point is of no consequence. Another alternative is to assume outright that the variable x is unidimensional, without recourse to the likelihood-ratio argument to make the assumption reasonable. Which particular solution we shall adopt will depend upon further experimentation.

Analysis of the rating scale

We have concluded from the experiments described that the observer's decision axis is continuous over a large range, i.e., that he can order observations likely to result from noise alone. We might expect then, in the language of decision theory, that he will be able to report the a posteriori probability of signal existence, i.e., that he will be able to state, following an observation interval, the probability that a signal existed during the interval. In more familiar terms, we are expecting that the observer will be capable of reporting a subjective probability, or of employing a rating scale. Experimental verification of this hypothesis is required, of course, for a reasonable doubt remains whether the observer will be able to maintain the multiple criteria essential to the use of a rating scale. If, for example, six categories of a posteriori probability are used, or a six-point rating scale, the observer must establish five criteria instead of just one as in the yes-no procedure—this may be considerably more difficult.

The ability to make a probability or rating response is of interest, in part, because such a response is highly efficient—in principle, a probability response retains all of the information contained in the observation. In contrast, breaking up the observation continuum into Yes and No sections is a process that loses information. From a procedure forcing a binary response, one learns from the observer only that the observation fell above or below a critical value, and not how far above or below. In some practical detection problems, the finer-grain information gained from a probability response can be utilized to advantage: the observer may record a posteriori probability so that Yes and No decisions concerning the action to be taken can be made at a later time, or by someone else who may be more responsible or who may possess more information about the values and costs of the decision outcomes.

More to the point in terms of our present interests, an experimental test of the ability to make a rating response contributes to the evaluation of decision theory, and also to distinguishing between the adequacy of decision theory and the high threshold theory. Since the data obtained with a rating procedure may be used to construct ROC curves, this experiment attacks the same problem as those already described, i.e., whether the observer can discriminate among observations likely to result from noise alone. It is also the case, as pointed out by Egan, Schulman, and Greenberg (1959), that the rating procedure generates ROC curves of a given reliability with a considerable economy of time, compared to the yes-no procedure. Therefore it is of interest, with respect to future applications of decision theory, to determine whether the observer can perform as well, as indexed by d', with the rating procedure as with the yes-no procedure.

The observer's task in this experiment was to place each observation in one of six categories of a posteriori probability. Four categories of equal size (0.2) were used in the range between 0.2 and 1.0; the other two categories were 0.0–0.04 and 0.05–0.19. The boundaries of the categories were chosen in conference with the observers; they believed that they would be able to operate reasonably within this particular scheme. Actually, the specific sizes of the categories used are not important for most purposes; we can as well think of a six-point rating scale and assume only the property of order.

The four observers in this experiment were those who served in the second expected-value experiment. Further, the same signal intensity (0.78 foot-lamberts) and the same a priori probabilities—$p(SN) = p(N) = 0.50$—that were employed in that experiment were employed in this one. The observers made a total of 1,200 observations in three experimental sessions.

RESULTS. The raw data for each observer consist of the number of observations of signal plus noise and the number of observations of noise alone that were placed in each of the six categories of a posteriori probability. Before proceeding with more complex analyses, we shall first make a rough determination of the validity of the observers' use of the categories, i.e., of whether we are, in fact, dealing with a scale. This may be achieved by computing the proportion of the total number of observations placed in each category that were actually observations of a signal. If the categories were used properly, this proportion will increase with increases in the probabilities that define the categories.

The results of this analysis are shown in Fig. 12. Five curves are plotted there, one for each of the four observers and one showing the

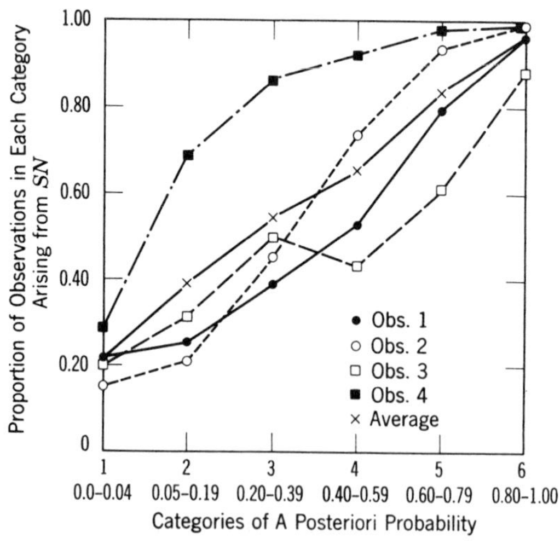

FIG. 12. The results of the rating experiment.

average result. We may note, as an aside, that Observer 4 is considerably more cautious than the others. A look at the raw data reveals that he used the lowest category twice to four times as often as the other observers; as a matter of fact, he placed 60 per cent of his observations in that category. We may look for this difference to reappear in other analyses of the data of this experiment. The major point here, however, is that three of the four individual curves are monotonic increasing, whereas the fourth shows only one reversal. This result indicates the feasibility of using a scaling procedure—it indicates that requiring an observer to maintain five criteria simultaneously in a detection problem is not unreasonable. The result is consistent with an ability to order completely the observations, those arising from noise alone as well as those arising from signal plus noise.

ROC CURVES OBTAINED FROM THE RATING DATA. ROC curves can be generated from data obtained with the rating procedure since these data can be compressed to those of the binary-decision procedure with any of several criterion levels. That is to say, we can calculate the pair of values, $p_N(A)$ and $p_{SN}(A)$, ignoring all but one of the (five) criteria, or category boundaries, employed by the observer. We successively calculate five pairs of these values, each time singling out a different criterion, and thus trace out an ROC curve. In particular, we first compute the conditional probabilities that observations arising from noise alone and from signal plus noise will be placed in the top category; then these probabilities are computed with respect to the top two categories, and so forth. We assume, in these calculations, that observations placed in a particular category would fall above the criteria that define a lower category.

The ROC curves so obtained are shown in the upper left-hand portions of each part of Fig. 13. (Ignore, for now, the other curves in Fig. 13.) We may note that the data are well described by the type of ROC curve predicted from decision theory. As is the case with the empirical ROC data from yes-no experiments, they cannot be fitted well by a straight line intersecting the point $p_{SN}(A) = p_N(A) = 1.0$, the prediction made from the high threshold theory. This result indicates that the observers can discriminate among observations likely to result from noise alone, and are capable of maintaining the multiple criteria required for the rating response.

COMPARISON OF ROC CURVES OBTAINED FROM RATINGS AND BINARY DECISIONS. It is intuitively clear that an estimate of d' of given reliability can be achieved with fewer observations by the rating procedure than by the yes-no procedure. This proposition is supported by a com-

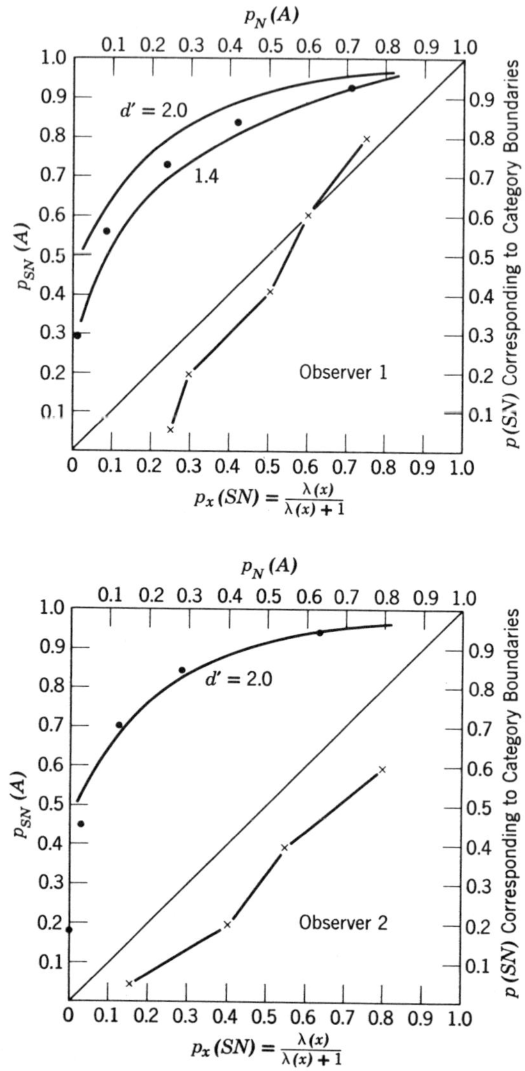

FIG. 13. Empirical receiver-operating-characteristic curves for four observers in the rating experiment. Two alternative presentations.

parison of the yes-no data shown in Fig. 8 with the rating data shown in Fig. 13—the rating data, which show considerably less variation, are based on 1200 observations whereas the yes-no data are based on approximately 5000 observations.

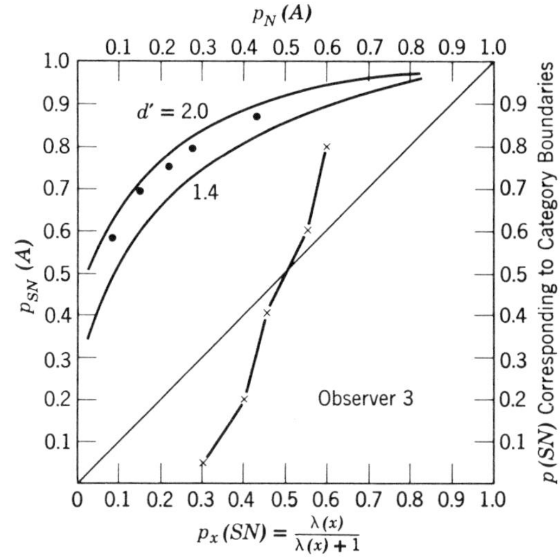

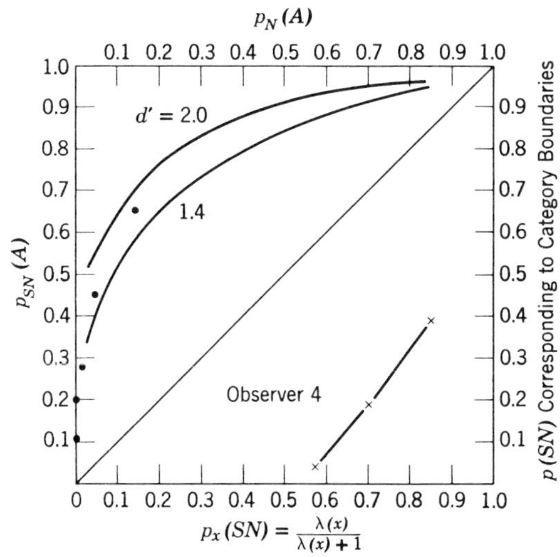

The economy provided by the rating procedure makes it desirable to determine whether the two procedures are equivalent means of generating the ROC curve. Unfortunately, to answer this question immediately, there are some clear differences between the ROC curves we have obtained with the two procedures. These differences are best illustrated by plotting the data on normal coordinates, i.e., on probability scales transformed so that the normal deviates are linearly spaced.

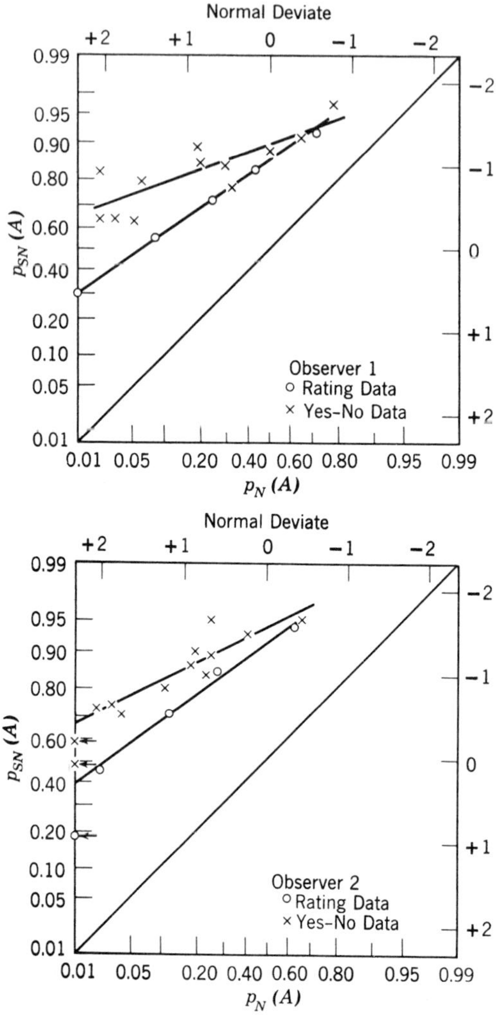

FIG. 14. Comparison of the receiver-operating-characteristic curves obtained from ratings and binary decisions.

These scales are convenient since on them the ROC curve specified by decision theory becomes a straight line. Further, the slope of this line represents the relative variances of the density functions, $f_N(x)$ and $f_{SN}(x)$, that underlie the ROC curve. In particular, it can be shown that the reciprocal of the slope (with respect to the normal deviate scales) is equal to the ratio $\sigma SN/\sigma N$.

The empirical ROC curves obtained with the rating and yes-no procedures are shown on normal coordinates in Fig. 14. It is immediately

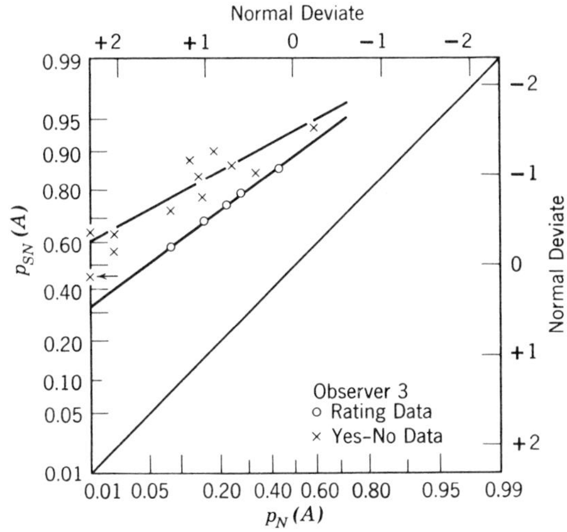

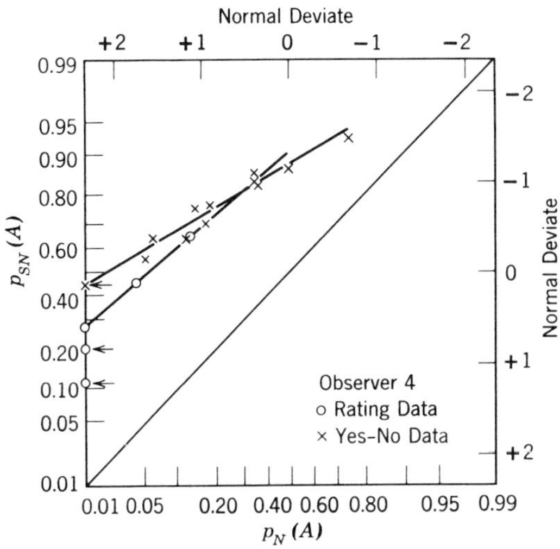

evident from this figure that a lower detectability resulted from the rating procedure for all four observers. We may see from the alternative presentations of these data in Figs. 8 and 13 that the values of d' range from 2.0 to 3.0 for the yes-no data and from 1.5 to 2.0 for the rating data.[10] It is further apparent in Fig. 14 that, consistent with the difference in d', the rating curve has a greater slope than the yes-no

[10] Values of d' can, of course, be computed from the normal deviate scales of the plots in Fig. 14. A problem arises, however, if the slope of the line fitted to the data is not unity. A solution to this problem is proposed by Clarke, Birdsall, and Tanner (1959).

curve. This difference is small—the greater variance of $f_{SN}(x)$ under the yes-no procedure did not show clearly in the plots on linear probability axes—but it is regular. We may also note again, as this way of plotting the data makes very clear, that the rating data show considerably less scatter than the yes-no data.

The values and costs associated with the decision outcomes in this situation make us hesitant, on the basis of the data we obtained, to reject the hypothesis that the rating and yes-no procedures are equivalent means of generating ROC curves. It is possible, of course, that some undetected difference existed between the experimental conditions in the two experiments; one was conducted after the other was completed. Such a difference might easily account for the relatively small discrepancies observed. Again, it has recently been shown in an auditory experiment that the two procedures result in essentially the same ROC curve, both with respect to d' and to slope (Egan, Schulman, and Greenberg, 1959). Still, we cannot discount the present results on the basis of the auditory experiment, for we have noted several differences between visual and auditory data that are likely to be real—one perhaps relevant to this issue is that the ROC curves obtained with pure tones have slopes that are uniformly near one. We should perhaps be content, at this point, with the admittedly weak conclusion that no data exist to support the hypothesis that the two procedures are equivalent in the case of visual stimuli.[11]

TEST OF THE NORMALITY OF THE DENSITY FUNCTIONS. At this juncture, it is convenient to turn briefly, but explicitly, to a topic first considered in the theoretical discussion. It was stated there that we would assume the density functions on the observer's decision axis to be Gaussian in form, but that the assumption was subject to experimental test. A test of this assumption is provided by plotting the empirical ROC curves on normal coordinates. Having now introduced plots of the data in this form in Fig. 14, we may use them for this purpose. If the observer's density functions are normal, then the empirical points of an ROC curve plotted on normal coordinates will be fitted best by a straight line. Clearly, a straight line provides an adequate description of the data in these figures. Thus the assumption of normality, an important one the sake of simplicity of analysis, is supported by the data.

---

[11] As this article goes to press we can report that in a repetition of this experiment with visual stimuli (unpublished) no reliable or regular differences were found between ROC curves obtained from ratings and binary decisions.

Approach to optimal behavior

In the presentation of experimental results thus far, we have concentrated on the continuity of the observer's decision axis, and on his ability to adopt various criteria along this axis. A remaining question is how closely the criteria he adopts correspond to those specified by decision theory as the optimal criteria. To answer this question we shall consider some further analyses of experimental results already described, and the results of an additional experiment.

It should be recalled that decision theory specifies as the optimal decision function either likelihood ratio, $\lambda(x)$, or some monotonic function of likelihood ratio, call it $\lambda(x)'$. That is to say, any transformation of the decision axis is acceptable as long as order is maintained. If the decision function is $\lambda(x)$, then the optimal criterion is the value of $\lambda(x)$ equal to β (Eq. 3). If the decision function is $\lambda(x)'$, then the optimal criterion is the value of this function that corresponds to β, call it β'. The monotonic relationship means that $\lambda(x)' > \beta' \leftrightarrow \lambda(x) > \beta$. Thus, to establish the applicability of decision theory, it is sufficient to demonstrate that the observer's criteria are monotonically related to β. If sampling error is taken into account, it is sufficient to demonstrate a significant correlation between the observer's criteria and β. It is of interest, however, to determine just how closely the observer's criteria do approach the optimal criteria as specified by β. In examining this question we shall make use of the fact that, in order to index the observer's criterion, it is not strictly necessary to compute a value of likelihood ratio from the proportions of hits and false alarms; it is more convenient, and for purposes of interpretation, more direct, to take simply the proportion of false alarms as the index.

CRITERIA EMPLOYED IN THE EXPECTED-VALUE EXPERIMENTS. In the first expected-value experiment, the observers were told only the a priori probabilities of signal and noise and the values of the various decision outcomes that were in effect during each experimental session. They were not told that any combination of these factors can be expressed by a single number (β) which, in conjunction with a value of d', specifies the optimal criterion or the optimal false-alarm rate. The rank-order correlations between β and the obtained proportions of false alarms that were computed from the data of this first study were .70, .46, and .71 for the three observers respectively. A correlation of .68 is significant at the .01 level of confidence. This result indicates that the observer did not merely vary his criterion from one session to another, but that his criterion varied appropriately with changes in β.

In the second expected-value experiment, the observers were told the optimal proportion of false alarms for each session as well as the a priori probabilities and decision values. This information was available to the experimenter since values of d' had previously been determined by the forced-choice procedure during a training period. Thus, in the second study, we were asking how closely the observer would approach the optimal false-alarm rate given knowledge of it. The rank-order correlations between the false-alarm rates announced as optimal and the false alarm rates yielded by the four observers were .94, .97, .86, and .98. Again, a coefficient of .68 is significant at the .01 level of confidence. Data obtained later in an auditory experiment showed coefficients of this magnitude—as a matter of fact, the rank-order coefficient based on five pairs of measures for each of two observers in the auditory experiment was 1.0—when the observers were *not* informed of the optimal false-alarm rate (Tanner, Swets, and Green, 1956).

SATISFYING A RESTRICTION ON THE PROPORTION OF FALSE ALARMS. A more direct attack on the question of the observer's ability to reproduce a given false-alarm rate is provided by an experimental procedure not previously described in detail, one involving a different definition of optimal behavior. Under this definition of optimal behavior, no values and costs are assigned the various decision outcomes; instead, a restriction is placed on the proportion of false alarms permitted. The optimal behavior is to maximize the proportion of hits while satisfying the restriction on false alarms. This, it will be recognized, is the procedure most popular among experimenters for testing statistical hypotheses.

An experiment using this procedure was conducted with a different set of four observers. The a priori probability of signal occurrence was 0.72 throughout the experiment. There were, then, 14 presentations of noise alone in a block of 50 presentations. There were four different experimental conditions, each extending over 18 blocks of 50 presentations. In each of these conditions, the observers were instructed to adopt a criterion that would result in Yes responses to approximately n or $n + 1$ of the 14 presentations of noise alone in a block of 50 presentations. For the four conditions of the experiment, n was equal to 0, 3, 6, and 9, respectively. Thus the acceptable range for the proportion of false alarms was .0–.07, .21–.28, .43–.50, or .64–.71. The primary data consist of four values of false-alarm rate for each observer; each value is based on 252 presentations of noise alone.

The data are shown in Fig. 15. The false-alarm rates obtained are plotted against the restricted ranges of false-alarm rate. The four observers are represented by different symbols; the vertical bars designate the acceptable range. It may be seen that the largest deviation from the

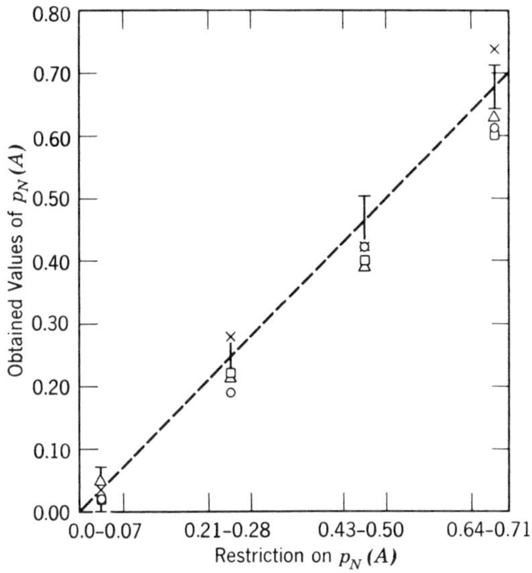

FIG. 15. The reproduction of a given false-alarm rate.

range stipulated is .04. This result suggests that the observer is able to adjust his criterion with considerable precision.

Two other pieces of information are needed, however, to interpret the data shown in Fig. 15. For, of course, if the observer were given information about the correctness of his response after each response, these data could be obtained even if the observer were unable to vary his criterion. The observer could then approximate any false-alarm rate by saying "yes" until the desired number of false alarms was achieved, and then by saying "no" on the remaining presentations. That procedure would entail a severe depression of d'. Actually, the observers were given information about correctness only after each block of 50 presentations, and the values of d' were not depressed. Thus the false-alarm rates that were obtained may legitimately be regarded as reflecting the observer's criteria.

CRITERIA EMPLOYED IN THE RATING SCALE EXPERIMENT. We may also investigate how closely the multiple criteria adopted by the observers in the rating scale experiment approach the optimal criteria. Stated otherwise, we may examine the relationship that existed between the subjective and objective probabilities of signal occurrence in that experiment. It may be noted in advance that an alternative presentation of the results, in Fig. 12, gives an indication of the extent of agreement we may expect.

As stated earlier, the a posteriori probability of signal existence is a monotonic function of likelihood ratio. In particular, the optimal relationship between the two is

$$p_x(SN) = \frac{\lambda(x)p(SN)}{\lambda(x)p(SN) + p(N)} \tag{9}$$

where $p_x(SN)$ denotes the probability that the signal existed given the observation x (i.e., the a posteriori probability), $\lambda(x)$ is the likelihood ratio, and $p(SN)$ and $p(N)$ are the a priori probabilities (Peterson, Birdsall, and Fox, 1954). For our experiment, with $p(SN) = p(N) = 0.50$, this equation reduces to:

$$p_x(SN) = \frac{\lambda(x)}{\lambda(x) + 1} \tag{10}$$

As described, a point on the ROC curve can be obtained for each of the boundaries of the six categories employed by the observer, i.e., for the five criteria he employed. Since, as we have also pointed out, the criterion value of $\lambda(x)$ corresponds to the slope of the ROC curve at the point in question, this criterion value of $\lambda(x)$ can be determined. Thus $p_x(SN) = \lambda(x)/[\lambda(x) + 1]$ can be computed for each of the criteria employed by the observer. Assuming now that the observer's decision function is likelihood ratio, then if he is behaving according to the optimal relationship between $p_x(SN)$ and $\lambda(x)$, the values of $\lambda(x)/[\lambda(x) + 1]$ computed from his data will correspond directly to probability values that were announced as defining the categories. In short, we know the values of $p_x(SN)$ that were announced as marking off the categories; by pursuing a route through the empirical ROC curve and $\lambda(x)$ we can calculate the values of $p_x(SN)$ that bound the categories the observer actually used—therefore we can assess how well the two sets of criterion values of $p_x(SN)$, the objective and subjective probabilities, agree.

The lower right-hand portions of Fig. 13 show the probability values that were announced as defining the categories, plotted against the probability values that characterize the criteria actually employed by the observers, i.e., against $p_x(SN) = \lambda(x)/[\lambda(x) + 1]$ as determined from the data. (Some points are missing since $\lambda(x)$ is indeterminate at very low values of $p_N(A)$. It is apparent from these plots that Observers 1, 2, and 3 are operating with a decision function similar to likelihood ratio and approximately according to the optimal relationship between $p_x(SN)$ and $\lambda(x)$. The pattern exhibited by Observers 1 and 3, that of overestimating small deviations from a probability of 0.50, will be familiar to those acquainted with the literature on subjective probability.

Observer 4, as we noted earlier, is quite different from the others. His tendency, also evidenced but to a far lesser extent by Observer 2, is to consistently underestimate the a posteriori probability, i.e., to set all of his criteria too high.

To summarize our discussion of how nearly the criteria adopted by the observers in these several experiments correspond to the optimal criteria, we may say that the observer, for want of a better term, behaves in an "optimal fashion." He is responsive to changes in both the a priori probability of signal occurrence and the values of the decision outcomes; the criteria he adopts are highly correlated with the optimal criteria. Subjective transformations of the real probability scale and of the "real" value scale do, of course, exist, and differ somewhat from one observer to another. Undoubtedly, values also play a role in those experiments in which no values are explicitly assigned by the experimenter. Nevertheless, we have seen that the observer can adopt successively as many as 10 different criteria, on the basis of different combinations of probabilities and values presented to him, that are almost perfectly ordered. He can maintain simultaneously at five least criteria that are a reasonable facsimile of the optimal criteria. If he is told the optimal false alarm rate, he can, provided it is not very large or very small, approximate it with a small error.

SUMMARY, CONCLUSIONS, AND REVIEW OF IMPLICATIONS

We imagine the process of signal detection to be a choice between two Gaussian variables. One, having a mean equal to zero, is associated with noise alone; the other, having a mean equal to d', is associated with signal plus noise. In the most common detection problem the observer decides, on the basis of an observation that is a sample of one of these populations, which of the two alternatives existed during the observation interval. The particular decision that is made depends upon whether or not the observation exceeds a criterion value; the criterion, in turn, depends upon the observer's detection goal and upon the information he has about relevant parameters of the detection situation. The accuracy of the decision that is made is a function of the variable d' which is monotonically related to the signal strength.

This description of the detection process is an almost direct translation of the theory of statistical decision. The main thrust of this conception, and the experiments that support it, is that more than sensory information is involved in detection. Conveniently, a large share of the nonsensory factors are integrated into a single variable, the criterion. There remains a measure of sensitivity (d') that is purer than any previously available, a measure largely unaffected by other than physical variables. This separation of the factors that influence the observer's attitudes from those that influence his sensitivity is the major contribution of the psychophysical application of statistical decision theory.[12]

We have indicated several times in the preceding that another conception of the detection process, one involving what we termed a "high threshold," is inconsistent with the data reported. It should be noted, however, that these data, to the extent analyzed in this paper, do not preclude the existence of a lower threshold. The analyses presented do not indicate explicitly how far down into the noise the observations are being ordered, i.e., how low a threshold must be relative to the noise distribution in order to be compatible with the data. As it happens, further analyses of the yes-no and forced-choice results show them to be consistent with a threshold slightly above the mean of the noise distribution. If, for example, we examine the empirical ROC curves of Figs. 8 and 13, we see that at values of $p_N(A)$ greater than 0.16, the curves are adequately fit by a straight line through the upper right-hand corner. Thus these data are consistent with a threshold cutoff that is located one sigma above the mean of the noise distribution.

Of course, a determination of the level at which a threshold may possibly exist is neither critical nor useful. A threshold well within the noise distribution is not a workable concept. Such a concept, since it is inconsistent with the correction for chance, complicates rather than facilitates the mathematical treatment of the data. Moreover, a threshold that is low is, for practical purposes, not measurable. The forced-choice experiment is a case in point; the observer conveys less information than he is capable of conveying if only a first choice is required. That the second choice contains a significant amount of information has

[12] It is interesting to note that the present account is not the first to model psychophysical theory after developments in the theory of statistical decision—as a matter of fact, Fechner was influenced by Bernoulli's suggestion that expectations might be expressed in terms of satisfaction units. As Boring (1950, p. 285) relates the story, Bernoulli's interest in games of chance led him to formulate the concept of "mental fortune"; he believed changes in mental fortune to vary with the ratio of the change in physical fortune to the total fortune. This mathematical relationship between mental and physical terms was the sort of relationship that Fechner sought to establish with his psychophysics. It should also be observed that Fechner anticipated the decision model under discussion in a much more direct way. His concept of "negative sensations," largely dismissed by subsequent workers in the field, denies the existence of a cut in the continuum of observations such that the magnitudes of observations below the cut are indiscriminable.

been demonstrated; in auditory experiments the fourth choice conveys information (Tanner, Swets, and Green, 1956). Thus it is difficult to determine when enough information has been extracted to yield a valid estimate of a *low* threshold. In addition, the existence of such a threshold is of little consequence for the application of the decision model—for example, yes-no data resulting from a suprathreshold criterion depend upon the criterion but are completely independent of the threshold value.

One of the major reasons for our concern with the threshold concept is that this concept supports several common psychophysical procedures that are invalidated by the results we have described. The correction for chance success has already been mentioned as a technique that stems from a high threshold theory, and one that is inconsistent with the data. This correction is frequently applied to data collected with the method of constant stimuli. It is used implicitly whenever the threshold is defined as the stimulus intensity that yields a probability of correct response halfway between chance and perfect performance. The method of adjustment and the standard method of serial exploration are also inappropriate, given the mechanism of detection described. When the method of serial exploration is used with the signal always present, or with insufficient "catch trials" to estimate the probability of a false alarm, the raw data will not permit separating the variation in the observer's criterion from variation in his sensitivity. Changes in an observer's criterion from one session to another can be estimated only if it is assumed that his sensitivity has not changed, and conversely. The same applies to data collected with the method of adjustment.

To be sure, unrecognized variations in the criterion are not important in many psychophysical measurements for they may be expected to contribute relatively little variation to the computed value of the threshold. Fairly large changes in the criterion will affect the threshold value by less than 3 db in the case of vision, and by no more than 6 db in the case of audition. This degree of reliability is acceptable in clinical audiometry, for example, in which the method of limits is usually employed. Neither would it distort appreciably curves of the course of dark adaptation. In many experiments, however—in experiments concerned with substantive as well as with theoretical problems—a reliability of less than 1 db is required, and in these cases a knowledge of the criterion used by the observer is essential.

To illustrate the problems in which the threshold concept and its associated procedures may have led to improper conclusions, we may single out one of current interest, that of "subliminal perception." In most of the studies of this phenomenon, the evidence for it consists of the finding that subjects who first report seeing no stimulus can then identify the stimulus with greater-than-chance accuracy when forced to make a choice.[13] We have mentioned as a typical result in psychophysical work that the forced-choice procedure yields lower threshold values than does the yes-no procedure. We have also suggested that this result may be accounted for by the fact that with the yes-no procedure the calculated value of the threshold varies directly with the observer's criterion, and that a strict criterion is usually employed by the observers under this procedure. That a strict criterion is usually used with the yes-no procedure is not surprising in view of the fact that observers are often instructed to avoid making false alarm responses. It is also likely that the stigma associated with "hallucinating" promotes the use of a strict criterion in the absence of an explicit caution against false alarms. Thus it may be expected that on many occasions when an observer does not choose to report the existence of the stimulus, he nevertheless possesses some information about it. It may be, therefore, that subliminal perception exists only when a high criterion is incorrectly identified as a limen.[14]

Having presented a theory of detection behavior and some detection experiments, and having just discussed the relationship of this work to "psychophysics," it remains to articulate with the title and the introductory paragraph of this paper, to consider the relationship of the work to the study of "perception."

In principle, the general scheme we have outlined may apply to perception as well as to detection. It seems reasonable to suppose that perception is also a choice among Gaussian variables. Consistent with the existence of many alternatives in the case of perception, we may imagine many critical regions to exist in the observation space. This space will have more dimensions than are involved in detection—as we have previously indicated, one less dimension than the number of alternatives considered. We may presume, in perception as in detection, that the boundaries of the critical regions are defined in terms of likelihood ratio, and are determined by the a priori probabilities of the alternatives and the relative values of the decision outcomes.

---

[13] This procedure was used explicitly in the earlier studies of subliminal perception; several of these studies are reviewed by Miller (1942). With minor variations, this procedure also underlies many of the more recent studies—see, for example, Bricker and Chapanis (1953).

[14] This analysis of the problem of subliminal perception has been elaborated by Goldiamond (1958).

It may also be contended that what we have been referring to as a detection process is itself a perceptual process. Certainly, if *perceptual processes* are to be distinguished from *sensory processes* on the grounds that the former must be accounted for in terms of events presumed to occur at higher centers whereas the latter can be accounted for in terms of events occurring within the receptor systems, then the processes with which we have been concerned qualify as perceptual processes. Since, in detecting signals, the observer's detection goal and the information he possesses about probabilities and values play a major role, we must assume either that signal detection is a perceptual process, or that the foregoing distinction between sensory and perceptual processes is of little value.

Thus the thesis of the present paper is, in one of its aspects, another stage in the history of the notion that the process of perceiving is not merely one of passively reflecting events in the environment, but one to which the perceiver himself makes a substantial contribution. Various writers have suggested that our perceptions are based upon unconscious inferences, that sensory events are interpreted in terms of unconscious assumptions about their probable significance, that our responses to stimuli reflect the influence of our needs and expectancies, that we utilize cues in selectively placing sensory events in categories of identity, and so forth. The present view differs from these in regarding the observer as relating his sense data to information he has previously acquired, and to his goals, in a manner specified by statistical decision theory. The approach from decision theory has the advantage that it specifies the perceiver's contribution to perception at other than the conversational level; it provides quantitative relationships between the nonsensory factors and both the independent and dependent variables.

We submit then that the present paper, although confined to detection experiments, is aptly named. We may view detection and perception as made of the same cloth. Of course, signal detection is a relatively simple perceptual process, but it is exactly its simplicity that makes the detection setting most appropriate to a preliminary examination of the value of statistical decision theory for the study of perception. Because detection experiments permit precise control over the variables specified by the theory as pertinent to the perceptual process, they provide the rigor desirable in the initial tests of a theory. Once these tests are passed, the theory may be extended and applied to more complex problems. Recent studies within the framework of decision theory include the recognition of one of two signals (Tanner, 1956), combined detection and recognition (Swets and Birdsall, 1956), problems in which a single decision is based on a series of observations (Swets, Shipley, McKey, and Green, 1959), problems in which the observer decides sequentially whether to make another observation before making a final decision (Swets and Green, 1961), and the recognition of speech (Decker and Pollack, 1958; Egan, 1957; Egan and Clarke, 1956; Egan, Clarke, and Carterette, 1956; Pollack and Decker, 1958).

ACKNOWLEDGMENTS

This paper is based upon Technical Report No. 40, issued by the Electronic Defense Group of the University of Michigan in 1955. The research was conducted in the Vision Research Laboratory of the University of Michigan with support from the United States Army Signal Corps and the Naval Bureau of Ships. Our thanks are due to H. R. Blackwell and W. M. Kincaid for their assistance in the research, and to D. H. Howes for suggestions concerning the presentation of this material. This paper was prepared in the Research Laboratory of Electronics, Massachusetts Institute of Technology, with support from the Signal Corps, Air Force (Operational Applications Laboratory and Office of Scientific Research), and Office of Naval Research. This article appeared as Tech. Rept. No. ESD-TR-61-20, and in Psychol. Rev., *1961,* **68,** *301-340.*

References

- Blackwell, H. R. Psychophysical thresholds: experimental studies of methods of measurement. *Bull. Eng. Res. Inst. U. Mich.*, 1953, No. 36.
- Blackwell, H. R., Pritchard, B. S., and Ohmart, T. G. Automatic apparatus for stimulus presentation and recording in visual threshold experiments. *J. opt. Soc. Am.*, 1954, **44,** 322–326.
- Boring, E. G. *A history of experimental psychology.* (2nd. ed.) New York: Appleton-Century-Crofts, 1950.
- Bricker, P. D., and Chapanis, A. Do incorrectly perceived tachistoscopic stimuli convey some information? *Psychol. Rev.*, 1953, **60,** 181–188.
- Bross, I. D. J. *Design for decision.* New York: Macmillan, 1953.
- Clarke, F. R., Birdsall, T. G., and Tanner, W. P., Jr. Two types of ROC curves and definitions of parameters. *J. acoust. Soc. Am.*, 1959, **31,** 629–630.
- Decker, L. R., and Pollack, I. Confidence ratings and message reception for filtered speech. *J. acoust. Soc. Am.*, 1958, **30,** 432–434.
- Egan, J. P. Monitoring task in speech communication. *J. acoust. Soc. Am.*, 1957, **29,** 482–489.
- Egan, J. P., and Clarke, F. R. Source and receiver behavior in the use of a criterion *J. acoust. Soc. Am.*, 1956, **28,** 1267–1269. [30]
- Egan, J. P., Clarke, F. R., and Carterette, E. C. On the transmission and confirmation of messages in noise. *J. acoust. Soc. Am.*, 1956, **28,** 536–550.
- Egan, J. P., Schulman, A. I., and Greenberg, G. Z. Operating characteristics determined by binary decisions and by ratings. *J. acoust. Soc. Am.*, 1959, **31,** 768–773. [7]

- Goldiamond, I. Indicators of perception: I. Subliminal perception, subception, unconscious perception: An analysis in terms of psychophysical indicator methodology. *Psychol. Bull.*, 1958, **55,** 373–411.
- Horton, J. W. *Fundamentals of sonar.* Annapolis: United States Naval Institute, 1957.
- Howes, D. H. A statistical theory of the phenomenon of subception. *Psychol. Rev.*, 1954, **61,** 98–110.
- Miller, J. G. *Unconsciousness.* New York: Wiley, 1942.
- Munson, W. A., and Karlin, J. E. The measurement of the human channel transmission characteristics. *J. acoust. Soc. Am.*, 1956, **26,** 542–553.
- Osgood, C. E. *Method and theory in experimental psychology.* New York: Oxford University Press, 1953.
- Peterson, W. W., Birdsall, T. G., and Fox, W. C. The theory of signal detectability. *Trans. IRE Professional Group on Information Theory,* 1954, PGIT-4, 171–212.
- Pollack, I., and Decker, L. R. Confidence ratings, message reception, and the receiver operating characteristic. *J. acoust. Soc. Am.*, 1958, **30,** 286–292. [31]
- Shannon, C. E. The mathematical theory of communication. *Bell Sys. Tech. J.*, 1948, **27,** 379–423.
- Smith, M., and Wilson, E. A. A model of the auditory threshold and its application to the problem of the multiple observer. *Psychol. Monogr.*, 1953, **67,** No. 9, Whole No. 359.
- Swets, J. A. Indices of signal detectability obtained with various psychophysical procedures. *J. acoust. Soc. Am.*, 1959, **31,** 511–513. [6]
- Swets, J. A., and Birdsall, T. G. The human use of information: III. Decision-making in signal detection and recognition situations involving multiple alternatives. *Trans. IRE Professional Group on Information Theory,* 1956, IT-2, 138–165.
- Swets, J. A., and Green, D. M. Sequential observations by human observers of signals in noise. In C. Cherry (Ed.), *Information theory.* London: Butterworth, 1961. [10]
- Swets, J. A., Shipley, E. F., McKey, M. J., and Green, D. M. Multiple observations of signals in noise. *J. acoust. Soc. Am.*, 1959, **31,** 514–521. [9]
- Tanner, W. P., Jr. A theory of recognition. *J. acoust. Soc. Am.*, 1956, **28,** 882–888. [19]
- Tanner, W. P., Jr., and Birdsall, T. G. Definitions, of d' and η as psychophysical measures. *J. acoust. Soc. Am.*, 1958, **30,** 922–928. [5]
- Tanner, W. P., Jr., and Swets, J. A. A decision-making theory of visual detection. *Psychol. Rev.*, 1954, **61,** 401–409.
- Tanner, W. J., Jr., Swets, J. A., and Green, D. M. Some general properties of the hearing mechanism. University of Michigan: Electronic Defense Group, 1956, Technical Report No. 30.
- Thurstone, L. L. A law of comparative judgment. *Psychol. Rev.*, 1927*a*, **34,** 273–286.
- Thurstone, L. L. Psychophysical analysis. *Am. J. Psychol.*, 1927*b*, **38,** 368–389.
- Van Meter, D., and Middleton, D. Modern statistical approaches to reception in communication theory. *Trans. IRE Professional Group on Information Theory,* 1954, **PGIT-4,** 119–145.
- Wald, A. *Statistical decision functions.* New York: Wiley, 1950.

2

Psychoacoustics and Detection Theory

David M. Green

There are two very striking characteristics of the field of psychoacoustics. One is the breadth and variety of research skills and techniques used to study hearing. The techniques range from hydrodynamic studies of the cochlea to analysis of the perception of vowel forms. This multidisciplinary approach is a fortunate one since it reduces the chances that any really significant aspect of the sensory system is being overlooked. However, it creates a diversity which makes integration of these areas most difficult.

A second characteristic of the field is the lack of any integrative structure from which to view the rapidly expanding experimental literature. If some basic theoretical structure existed, these new data might easily be integrated with the old. Psychoacoustics, however, does not have any complete comprehensive theory. A reflection of this deficit is the lack of consensus on methodology. Often, even where a general consensus seems to exist in some area of the field, a new paper may force a complete reexamination of the entire measurement procedure. A recent example of the latter may be found in the exchanges of Garner (1958) and Stevens (1959) on the quantitative scale of loudness. Such a situation compounds the problem of integration.

This paper, therefore, makes no attempt at broad coverage. The author hopes that by concentrating on one rather limited topic some positive contribution can be made. This topic is the detection of signals in noise. In recent years a general theoretical structure (detection theory) has been used to analyze such experiments. Unfortunately, there appears to be some confusion both about the theory itself and the manner of its application. The main objective of this paper will be to clarify these two questions. Part of the confusion about the theory arises from the fact that detection theory is a combination of two distinct theoretical structures: decision theory and the theory of ideal observers. Before we begin a detailed discussion of these two aspects of detection theory, we will briefly outline them and relate them to psychoacoustic problems.

Decision theory provides an analysis of the process which generates the dichotomy between stimuli the subject reports he does and does not hear. The theory recognizes that a priori probabilities, values and costs of correct and incorrect decisions, as well as the physical parameters of the signal, play a decisive role in establishing this dichotomy. We will find that this dichotomy is determined by an adjustable criterion. The theory shows how a quantitative estimate of the criterion can be obtained from the data.

There are many psychoacousticians whose only interest in this criterion is as a constant parameter from which to obtain substantive relations between two physical parameters, for example, the absolute threshold energy as a function of frequency, or the just-detectable change in power as a function of power (ΔI vs. I). To them this aspect of detection theory will be of methodological interest only. Yet clearly, if factors such as a priori probability, values, and costs do play a role in determining the threshold, their control in substantive experiments is imperative.

The second part of detection theory is more directly related to substantive matters—it is the theory of ideal observers. Briefly, the theory provides a collection of ideal mathematical models which relates the detectability of the signal to definite physical characteristics of the stimulus. There is a collection of such models because one may make different restrictions on the nature of the detection device. These theoretical observers are rarely used as actual models of the hearing mechanism. Most often, they are used for the sake of comparing human performance with that of the ideal observer in order to specify the nature and amount of discrepancy. This comparison, in turn, suggests either a new and hopefully more accurate representation of the hearing mechanism, or new experiments to clarify further the exact nature of the discrepancy. This will be illustrated in a later section of this selection.

DECISION THEORY

We shall demonstrate, under quite general assumptions, how a transformation of the subject's responses can be utilized to determine both the subject's criterion and the detectability of the signal. This analysis requires an understanding of several basic concepts which are rather complex. We might skip over these fundamentals and start, as some previous expositions have, with some assumptions about Gaussian distributions and parameters of these distributions. Such a procedure would be unfortunate because it robs the analysis of its generality and implies that strong assumptions are needed to justify its applicability. Such is not the case.

Typically, psychoacousticians try to analyze the subject's responses by making some assumptions about the way in which the sound is processed by the hearing mechanism. One assumes, for example, that the cochlea either makes a frequency analysis of the waveform or that it does not, etc. We wish to postpone temporarily such substantive issues. Let us, for the present, merely assume that each sound may be represented by a series of numbers. These numbers might be the values of a series of attributes, or various states of the nervous system. Whatever the representation, let us call this abstraction an *observation*.

The problem we wish to consider is this: Given an observation, what response alternative should be chosen? What is a good choice and how can we analyze these choices? We shall attempt to answer these questions by considering a single example. The example is obviously specific; the generality rests in the concepts. The single motive in presenting this example is to enable us to discuss these concepts—*likelihood ratio*, *decision rule*, and *criterion*—with some precision and yet avoid formalism.[1] After this theoretical discussion, we shall investigate the applicability of these concepts to a psychoacoustic experiment.

An example of decision theory

Let us assume we have ten observations, each observation (X_i) represented by three numbers [$X_i = (x_1,x_2,x_3)$], and that we have two hypotheses (H_1, H_2) about the observations. Given an observation, we wish

---

[1] These concepts come from the topic of statistical decision theory and the theory of inference. Most of the key theorems were first presented by Wald (1950), who extended the basic principle which originated with Neyman and Pearson (1933).

to decide whether the observation is an instance of H_1 or H_2.[2] We shall assume we have complete information about the probability of each observation given each hypothesis.

By limiting the example to ten observations we can work with probabilities directly. The reader should note that the three numbers (x_1,x_2,x_3) could have been extended to three hundred. Everything that follows is independent of the dimensionality of the observation. The variables (x) of the observation could be quantitative (integers or real numbers) or qualitative (red, blue, or green). They are simply descriptions of the observation.

LIKELIHOOD RATIO. In Table I, we have listed the observations and the three numbers corresponding to each observation. The next two columns provide the data on the probabilities of each observation on each hypothesis. The final column is simply the ratio of the fifth column to the sixth and represents the likelihood ratio. The likelihood ratio, then, is the probability that a particular observation resulted from H_1 divided by the probability that it resulted from H_2. The likelihood ratio gives what some call the "odds." If we have X_6 we should be willing to wager nine cents to one that H_1 is correct. Note that the likelihood ratio is a *number*, not a probability, and that this number is a function of three variables (x_1,x_2,x_3). Thus we have taken an observation which is specified by three values (x_1,x_2,x_3), and related it to a single variable $l(x_1,x_2,x_3)$.

The reason we have performed this transformation is simply stated: We can make optimum decisions if we use the likelihood ratio. We have not stated what we mean by optimum, but let us take up this point a little later. First, let us show how we might use the likelihood ratio in making decisions.

DECISION RULE. If someone asked us to make a decision about a particular observation, whether it is an instance of H_1 or H_2, we would probably guess it was H_1 if the probability of that observation was greater on H_1 than on H_2. Such a statement is called a decision rule. In terms of likelihood ratio this decision can be expressed as follows: Choose H_1 if $l(X) \geqslant 1$. In effect, we have specified our decision rule by choosing one number; in this case, the number "one." This number is called a criterion, or, more precisely, a likelihood-ratio criterion.

[2] For a concrete interpretation of the example, the reader might think of the observation as a sealed package, the three numbers as the length, width, and depth of the package, and the hypothesis as whether the package contains a toy car or animal. The problem, then, is this: Given the measurements of a package, guess whether it contains a car or an animal. Alternatively, one might think of the observation as a sound which can be specified by three numbers or attributes. The problem is: Decide from the three numbers whether the sound is a consonant or a vowel.

Suppose that, independent of any specific observation, H_2 was ten times as likely as H_1. Clearly, we would not maintain our previous criterion; even without knowing the characteristics of the observation, the odds are ten to one in favor of H_2. It turns out in this case that we should choose H_1 only if $l(X) \geqslant 10$. That is, we should choose H_1 only if, in our example, the specific observation is $X = (4,3,3)$.

Similarly, if one places asymmetrical values and costs on the various correct and incorrect decisions, we should change our criterion or likelihood ratio accordingly.

MONOTONIC FUNCTIONS OF LIKELIHOOD RATIO. While we can state our decision procedure in terms of likelihood ratio, there are other exactly equivalent ways of stating the decision rules. In the example, it so happens that the product x_1 times x_2 minus x_3 is also an optimum decision quantity. This is true because this quantity is monotonic with the likelihood ratio. The criterion number is not the same as that we would use on a likelihood-ratio scale, but there is always some number on this

TABLE I. DESCRIPTION OF THE OBSERVATIONS (X_i) AND THE PROBABILITY OF OBTAINING THAT OBSERVATION GIVEN EITHER HYPOTHESIS (H_1 or H_2)

Observation	x_1	x_2	x_3	$P_{H_1}(x_1,x_2,x_3)$	$P_{H_2}(x_1,x_2,x_3)$	$l(x_1,x_2,x_3) = \dfrac{P_{H_1}(x_1,x_2,x_3)}{P_{H_2}(x_1,x_2,x_3)}$
X_1	4	3	3	0.14	0.01	14.00
X_2	3	3	5	0.01	0.01	1.00
X_3	2	2	4	0.03	0.30	0.10
X_4	3	3	3	0.30	0.10	3.00
X_5	2	3	3	0.02	0.04	0.50
X_6	5	2	2	0.09	0.01	9.00
X_7	2	5	5	0.10	0.08	1.25
X_8	3	4	5	0.20	0.05	4.00
X_9	3	2	5	0.06	0.30	0.20
X_{10}	4	2	5	0.05	0.10	0.50
			Total	1.00	1.00	

monotonic scale which corresponds to the criterion number on likelihood ratio. For example, suppose we select the alternative H_1 if $l(x_1,x_2,x_3) \geqslant 1.25$; then we would make identical decisions using the decision rule, select H_1 if $(x_1 \cdot x_2 - x_3) \geqslant 5.00$.

In many cases, such as the application of this theory to psychoacoustics, the decision axis is unobservable, and hence we are only interested in equivalent decision procedures. To say the observer uses an optimum decision procedure means only that he is using a monotonic transformation of likelihood ratio.

OPTIMUM NATURE OF LIKELIHOOD RATIO. We turn now to the very important question of the optimum nature of likelihood ratio. Clearly a decision procedure based on likelihood ratio is only optimum if it best attains some specific objective. Let us list some of these objectives to indicate their generality: (1) maximize the expected value of decisions (Peterson, Birdsall, and Fox, 1954), (2) minimize risk (Anderson, 1958), (3) estimate a posteriori probability (Woodward, 1955), (4) maximize the percentage of correct decisions (Anderson, 1958), and (5) set the error rate on some decision alternative at some constant and maximize the number of correct decisions for the other alternative (Neyman and Pearson, 1933). The impressive fact is that a decision criterion based on likelihood ratio is optimum under all the above objectives. Naturally this criterion may be different for different objectives. The references listed with the objectives contain a more detailed explanation of each objective and prove how a decision rule based on likelihood ratio, or some monotonic transformation of that quantity, may be used to make the best decisions.[3]

TABLE II. PROBABILITY UNDER EACH HYPOTHESIS THAT $l(X)$ WILL HAVE A CERTAIN VALUE

$l(X)$	$P_{H_1}[l(X)]$	Cumulative	$P_{H_2}[l(X)]$	Cumulative
14.00	0.14	0.14	0.01	0.01
9.00	0.09	0.23	0.01	0.02
4.00	0.20	0.43	0.05	0.07
3.00	0.30	0.73	0.10	0.17
1.25	0.10	0.83	0.08	0.25
1.00	0.01	0.84	0.01	0.26
0.50	0.07	0.91	0.14	0.40
0.20	0.06	0.97	0.30	0.70
0.10	0.03	1.00	0.30	1.00

DISTRIBUTION OF LIKELIHOOD RATIO. We have seen how each observation, independent of the number of attributes included in the observa-

[3] To estimate a posteriori probability no criterion is involved. In this case the best estimate of a posteriori probability is a simple monotonic transformation of likelihood ratio.

tion, can be reduced to a single quantity—likelihood ratio. Likelihood ratio is simply a function of several variables and for any single observation is simply a number. We may then properly consider a probability defined on the variable likelihood ratio. Let us consider, in particular, the probability that we shall obtain a particular value of likelihood ratio under H_1 and H_2 of the preceding example. Table II shows these probabilities and the corresponding cumulative distributions for both hypotheses of our example. The likelihood ratio is ranked from largest to smallest to facilitate the explanation of the ROC curve.[4]

ROC CURVES AND THEIR PROPERTIES. We shall use Table II to construct an ROC (receiver-operating-characteristic) curve. To do this, let us assume the decision rule is to accept H_1 if $l(x_1,x_2,x_3) \geqslant k$. If $k = 14$ we find that the probability of accepting H_1 when it is true $[P_{H_1}(H_1)]$ is 0.14 and the probability of accepting H_1 when it is false $[P_{H_2}(H_1)]$ is 0.01. By decreasing k, we change both probabilities. The upper curve shown in Fig. 1 shows how the probabilities change as a function of k, and is called an ROC curve. The two probabilities completely represent the stimulus-response matrix in a two-alternative detection task since the complements of $P_{H_1}(H_1)$ and $P_{H_2}(H_1)$ are the two remaining cells in the stimulus-response matrix.

What if some decision procedure were used which was less than optimum? Let us consider an extremely poor decision procedure. The lower curve of the figure was generated by using the decision rule accepting H_1 if $l(x_1,x_2,x_3) \leqslant k$ for all k. This is the exact opposite of the first decision rule and hence generates the ROC curve for the worst possible decision rule.

The area included between the upper and lower bounds on performance represents attainable performance using any decision procedure in this task. Obviously any single decision is either right or wrong, but any decision rule whatever, in the long run, will produce some probability of "hit" and some probability of "miss" which lie within the bounds illustrated.[5] Other decision procedures do not necessarily involve likelihood ratio. One procedure would be to flip a coin and select the first alternative if the coin landed heads; if the coin were unbiased, this

---

[4] Note that since two observations yield a likelihood ratio of 0.50, we have added the probabilities under both hypotheses to obtain the probability of that likelihood ratio.

[5] It should also be noted that the lines connecting the points in the ROC curve do in fact represent attainable performance. For example, a point located midway between the points (7, 43) and (17, 73) is attainable by using a mixed-decision procedure, where H_1 is accepted if $l(X) > 3$, each alternative is selected half the time by some random procedure if $l(X) = 3$, and H_2 is selected if $l(X) < 3$.

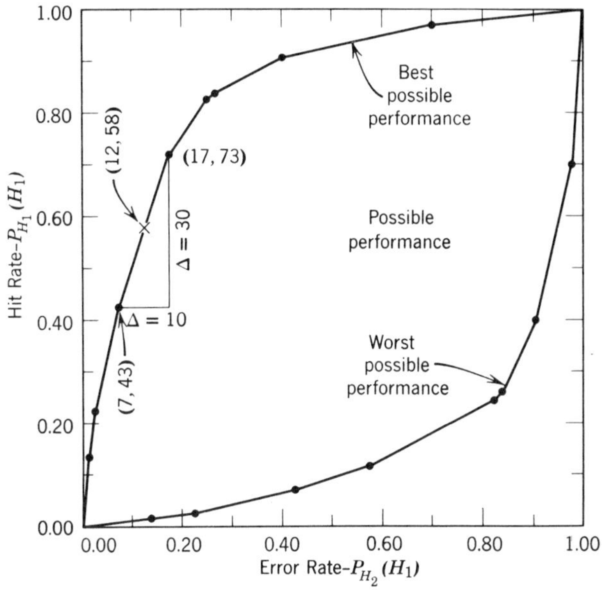

FIG. 1. The receiver-operating-characteristic (ROC) curve of the example. The axes are $P_{H_1}(H_1)$, which is the probability of responding H_1 if the observation was from H_1, and $P_{H_2}(H_1)$, which is the probability of responding H_1 if the observation was from H_2. The points were plotted from Table II.

decision rule would achieve an error and hit rate of 0.5. Should the coin be biased, this decision procedure would produce performance located somewhere along the center diagonal of Fig. 1.

Another point to be noted involves the slope of the ROC curve based on the optimum decision axis. Notice that the slope between any two consecutive points is equal to the likelihood ratio of the higher point. Thus the slope must clearly diminish because each successive point represents a lower value for likelihood ratio. Any ROC curve which does not show a monotonically decreasing slope implies an incorrect decision rule. This means that the decision maker is accepting the first hypothesis when the likelihood exceeds a certain value and yet accepting the other hypothesis when likelihood ratio is some greater value. Any such inversion in slope for any ROC curve implies that better performance might be achieved by interchanging some of the points on the decision axis.

ROC CURVE AND PER CENT CORRECT USING FORCED CHOICE. The ROC curve is useful in a situation where the subject's response is limited to selecting one or the other alternative. There are other ways in which the detection task may be structured; one involves the class of forced-choice procedures. For simplicity, we will consider a two-alternative forced-choice task. The extension to larger numbers of alternatives should be clear from the following discussion. A two-alternative forced-choice procedure is one in which two stimuli are presented, one from each class, and the subject is asked, in effect, what was the order of the stimuli, H_1H_2 or H_2H_1?

We shall calculate the probability of a correct decision based on the following rule: Select the alternative H_1H_2 if the likelihood ratio on the first observation is greater than on the second. In effect, this rule says to pick the larger likelihood ratio and say H_1 for that observation. The reason for considering only this particular decision rule is that this assumption is often made in the analysis of forced-choice tests.[6]

Assuming the subject picks the larger of two likelihood ratios and says the likelihood ratio was produced by H_1, we shall be correct if the larger likelihood was in fact produced by H_1 and the smaller was in fact produced by H_2. The probability of this occurrence is $P_{H_1}[l_1(X)] \cdot P_{H_2}[l_2(X)]$ where $l_1(X) > l_2(X)$. In fact, if the larger likelihood ratio is equal to k, the probability of a correct choice is simply[7]

$$P_{H_1}[l(X) = k] \cdot \sum_i P_{H_2}[l_i(X) < k]$$

To obtain the final result we need only summate over all the values of k, since any of these values might be the largest, except the lowest value of likelihood ratio itself.

Table III gives these calculations and the final answer (0.8042). Though the method of calculating this probability is straightforward, often, especially in psychoacoustic experiments, one does not have numerical distribution on a likelihood-ratio scale. Two approaches could be used in these situations. The first, and the safest, since it makes no additional assumptions, would be to compute the probability from an experimentally determined ROC curve. If you look at Table III closely, you will see that the quantities used in the calculation are simply $\Delta P_{H_1}(H_1)$ times $[1 - P_{H_2}(H_1)]$ for each successive point on the ROC curve (Fig. 1).

---

[6] Were we to give a complete analysis of this situation we would first list all possible stimulus pairs (S_iS_j). Next we would consider the probabilities on the hypothesis that the pairs represented instances of H_1H_2 or H_2H_1, compute a likelihood ratio, and, in fact, derive an ROC curve based on these computations.

[7] If more than two, say M, alternatives are used in the forced-choice test, the equation becomes

$$P(\text{correct}) = \sum_k P_{H_1}(l_i = k)[\sum_i P_{H_2}(l_i < k)]^{M-1}$$

Obviously, the accuracy of such a procedure is heavily determined by the accuracy of the experimental estimate of the ROC curve. The merit of the technique is that no assumptions beyond that of the decision rule are necessary to predict forced-choice behavior from the ROC data.

A second procedure, one which has often been used, is to make some assumptions about the distributions which generated the ROC curve

TABLE III. CALCULATION OF THE PROBABILITY OF A CORRECT RESPONSE IN A FORCED-CHOICE TEST

k	$P_{H_1}[l_1(X) = k]$	$P_{H_2}[l_2(X) < k]$	Product
14	0.14	0.99	0.1386
9	0.09	0.98	0.0882
4	0.20	0.93	0.1860
3	0.30	0.83	0.2490
1.25	0.10	0.75	0.0750
1.00	0.01	0.74	0.0074
0.50	0.07	0.60	0.0420
0.20	0.06	0.30	0.0180
0.10	0.03	0.00	0.0000
		Sum	0.8042

and then use these assumptions in predicting behavior in the forced-choice experiment. The most popular set of assumptions is that the distribution of observations on the likelihood-ratio axis, or some monotonic function of that axis, is normal or Gaussian under both hypotheses. The distributions are assumed to differ only in their means and, sometimes, in their standard deviations. Let us assume, for simplicity, that standard deviations are equal under both hypotheses; then the ROC curve can be characterized by one parameter, the difference in the means divided by the standard deviation ($\Delta M/\sigma$). This parameter is usually denoted by $d' = \Delta M/\sigma$. The calculations of the probability of a correct detection in a two-alternative forced-choice situation if these assumptions are made is quite simple. The probability that one likelihood is larger than another is the probability that the difference is greater than zero. Since, by assumption, some transformation of $l(X)$ is normal, the difference distribution is normal with a mean of ΔM and a variance equal to the sum of the original variances. Hence the probability of a correct decision is

$$P(\text{correct, 2-alternative}) = \Phi[\Delta M/(\sigma_1^2 + \sigma_2^2)^{\frac{1}{2}}] = \Phi[d'/(2)^{\frac{1}{2}}]$$

The probability of being correct for any number of alternatives is given by Elliott (1959).

We have now reviewed all the essential aspects of how detection theory uses decision theory in analyzing the process of detection. Let us now turn to some experimental results and see to what extent these notions are supported. Following this review of the experimental studies, we shall conclude this section with a discussion of the implications of these studies for psychoacoustic procedures in general.

Experimental Results

ROC CURVE. One of the earlier studies (Tanner, Swets, and Green, 1956) simply sought to determine experimentally the shape of the ROC curve in a simple psychoacoustic task. The signal was a 1/10 segment of a 1000-cps sinusoid. White noise, the masking stimulus, was present continuously throughout the experimental session. A light occurred to mark the observation interval. During this interval either the signal was added to the noise (SN) or only the noise was presented (N): these were the two hypotheses of the detection task. The subject gave one of two possible responses; he pressed one button if he believed the signal was present ("yes") or pressed a second button if he believed no signal was present ("no"). The physical parameters of the situation, including noise and signal levels, were held constant. The independent variable was the probability (a priori) of a signal being present. Five levels of a priori probability were selected (0.1, 0.3, 0.5, 0.7, 0.9) and the one used for a given session of 300 observations was announced to the subject. After the subject responded, he was given immediate information as to whether or not the signal had in fact been presented. The subject was awarded some fraction of a cent for each correct answer and fined an equal amount for each incorrect answer. He was instructed to make as much money as possible.

The results for one of the subjects are presented in Fig. 2. The general trend of the data supports the decision-theory analysis. The curve drawn is generated by assuming the distributions on likelihood ratio are normal under both hypotheses. The normalized difference between the means is 0.92.

THRESHOLD MODEL AND THE ROC CURVE. Before considering whether or not the subjects adopted the proper criterion so as actually to maximize their payoff, let us consider one alternative explanation of the data. This is the so-called threshold model. The essentials of this model are that the signal, when added to the noise, augments some process within the organism, such that if the increment reaches a critical level called the threshold, the signal is heard and can be correctly detected. So far, we note no great difference with the decision-theory analysis except in

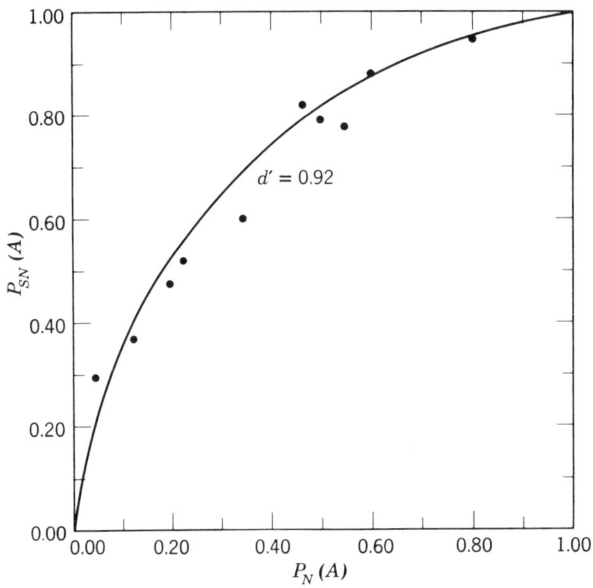

FIG. 2. A sample of the ROC curve from an auditory detection experiment (Tanner, Swets, and Green, 1956). $P_N(A)$ is the probability of responding "yes" when noise alone was presented. $P_{SN}(A)$ is the probability of saying "yes" when signal-plus-noise was presented. These probabilities were estimated from the stimulus-response matrix. See text for details of the experiment.

semantics. If one calls the decision-theory criterion a threshold and the hypothetical process likelihood ratio, the correspondence is complete. The differences between the models appear when one considers "subthreshold" events and the procedures used to deal with these events The threshold model assumes that should the signal increment fail to reach the threshold, the subject can only make a pure guess as to whether or not the signal is present. This is surely true since anything below the threshold is just that. If ordering is preserved below the threshold, the word has no meaning. The difference in terminology between criterion and threshold is important, for to say the subject adopts a criterion is to simply say an arbitrary cut point on a continuum is used as the decision rule.

Given that the subject guesses about events which are "subthreshold," he may, if blanks are ever employed, report the signal present when it is not (false-positive response). Two techniques, both consistent with the threshold assumption, might be employed if this occurs. One procedure widely used is to instruct the subject to be more careful; this can be interpreted as an attempt to instruct the subject to respond negatively to all "subthreshold" events. The implication of this procedure will be discussed in a later section. Another procedure, equally valid from the assumptions of this model, would be to employ a correction for guessing. This correction procedure assumes the guessing mechanism and the sensory mechanisms are independent. The excellent experiments of Smith and Wilson (1953) were the first, I believe, to show the inadequacy of this second procedure. This fact led them to reconsider the entire notion of the threshold and they presented, as an alternative model, one very similar to that suggested by decision-theory analysis. (See especially Sec. IV of Smith and Wilson, 1953). Munson and Karlin (1954), using an information-theory analysis, investigated the detection process under "absolute threshold conditions." In order to deal with false-positive responses, they proposed a "discriminant-level model." This model is also very similar to that suggested by decision-theory analysis.

The threshold model could still attempt to account for the data shown in Fig. 2. The argument would run as follows: Suppose the subject achieves some hit and false-alarm rate. If the situation is changed in some way, he can modify his behavior by simply giving more "yes" responses. Since this guessing rate is independent of the stimulus conditions (both noise and signal-plus-noise events are below the threshold) this will increase, by the same *relative* amounts, both the hit and false-alarm rates. In short, a linear function will result. In the extreme, the subject says "yes" all the time, hence this linear function must go through the point in the upper right-hand corner [$P_N(A) = 1.00$, $P_{SN}(A) = 1.00$]. Thus the threshold prediction for the data is a collection of lines having the upper right-hand corner as the common intercept, and a slope depending upon the detectability of the signal. No linear function which has this intercept as one value can fit more than a few of the data points for any value of the slope. The results of this first experiment, then, seriously conflict with this version of the threshold model and give some measure of support to the decision-theory analysis.

The conflict between some version of the threshold model and the decision analysis has been the subject of considerable experimental effort. There are other experimental results more damaging to the threshold position. These experiments attack the threshold concept directly because they suggest that ordering below the threshold value is indeed possible (Tanner, Swets, and Green, 1956). We shall drop this conflict and proceed to other questions.

ACTUAL CRITERION AND OPTIMUM CRITERION. Let us now return to the results displayed in Fig. 2 and discuss the question of the optimum criterion. It turns out that if one wishes to select an optimum criterion on likelihood ratio, it is equal to $\beta = P(N)/P(SN)$, where β is the criterion value on likelihood ratio and $P(N)$ and $P(SN)$ are the a priori probabilities of noise alone and signal-plus-noise, respectively. We can, of course, obtain a rough measure of the subject's criterion by measuring the slope of the ROC curve at the point nearest the experimental data point. This rough comparison is displayed in Fig. 3. Note that while there is a strong relation between the estimated and optimal criterion values, there is also a consistent departure from an exact correspondence. The general trend might be summarized by saying the subjects are conservative; they tend to adopt criteria which are not as different from $\beta = 1$ as they should be. This result is almost an inevitable consequence of the procedure. The way in which expected values change for various criterion levels is the crux of the problem. This topic is discussed in more detail in the Appendix.

Since these earlier investigations, other procedures have been utilized to vary the subject's criterion. One which seems more straightforward and is certainly successful is simply to instruct the subject verbally to adopt different criteria such as *lax* or *very strict*, or even to instruct the subject to maintain a certain value for $P_N(A)$ (Egan, Schulman, and Greenberg, 1959).

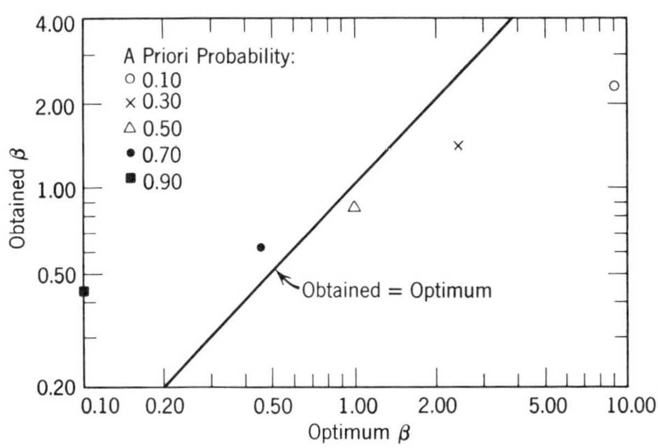

FIG. 3. Comparison of the optimum and obtained criterion levels. This criterion level, β, is the equivalent of the criterion level on likelihood ratio. The optimum criterion is obtained by assuming normal statistics for both hypotheses. It is equal to $[1 - P(SN)]/P(SN)$, where $P(SN)$ is the a priori probability of the signal.

MEASURE OF DETECTABILITY. Let us turn now from the question of the criterion and its adjustment to another aspect of detection-theory analysis, the measure of detectability, and more specifically, whether or not this measure remains relatively invariant over different experimental procedures. How one can compare different measurements obtained using different experimental procedures is an important question, not only for psychoacousticians, but for any scientific enterprise. Let us review the evidence on the extent to which detection-theory analysis has permitted such a comparison. If we make the usual assumption that the distribution of likelihood is normal with equal variance on both hypotheses, as in the situation outlined in the first experiment, then the measure of detectability is d'.

A paper by Swets (1959) has considered the applicability of this detectability index for yes-no and forced-choice procedures; he has also compared predicted and obtained results using two, three, four, six, and eight alternatives in the forced-choice procedure. In general, these predictions based on d' hold up remarkably well. The worst failure reported seems to be about 1 db; no consistent error trend is evident in the data.

Another method of generating ROC curves, first suggested by Swets, Tanner, and Birdsall (1955), has been employed. Egan, Schulman and Greenberg (1959) tested and compared this method with the standard yes-no procedure. In the single observation or yes-no procedure, the decision-theory analysis claims that the subject adopts a single criterion and this determines a "yes" or "no" response. The experimenter, then, is employing the subject as a threshold device. Alternatively, the experimenter could have the subject report a number after each observation such as likelihood ratio; from these numbers, the experimenter could construct an ROC curve by placing various criteria on the likelihood ratios reported.

The rating procedure is a compromise between these two extremes. The subject in the rating procedure is asked to place each observation in one of several categories; the top one being used for sureness of a signal's presence, the next for a lesser degree of sureness, and so forth. ROC curves are subsequently constructed. One can then compare the measure of signal detectability obtained from these two procedures, yes-no and rating. Egan, Schulman, and Greenberg (1959) found these two measures differed for their three subjects by 0.3, 0.4, and 0.1 db, differences probably well within the experimental error.

In summary, then, we have seen how decision analysis allows one to predict within a fairly wide range of psychoacoustic procedures. The forced-choice procedures using two to eight alternatives and a single-interval procedure using two to four categories of response can be summarized by a single measure of detectability, a measure which, for practical purposes, is invariant.

IMPLICATIONS FOR PSYCHOACOUSTIC METHODS. The more traditional methods of psychoacoustics utilize some parameter of the signal such as the threshold energy. This value is obtained by an analysis of the subject's responses. Many of these methods do not allow one to determine directly the subject's criterion and in most methods it is presumed to be constant.

Let us investigate how variation in the subject's criterion, if it occurs, will affect the estimate of the threshold energy. Variation of the subject's criterion affects the false-alarm rate $P_N(A)$. Figure 4 shows how the probability distribution for signal-plus-noise must be varied as the false-alarm rate $P_N(A)$ is changed to maintain a constant value of signal detection $P_{SN}(A)$. We have assumed Gaussian distribution and equal variance to construct the solid line of the figure. The insert displays the essentials of the calculations and shows how a change in $P_N(A)$ of from 0.10 to 0.01 necessitates a change in the mean of the signal distribution

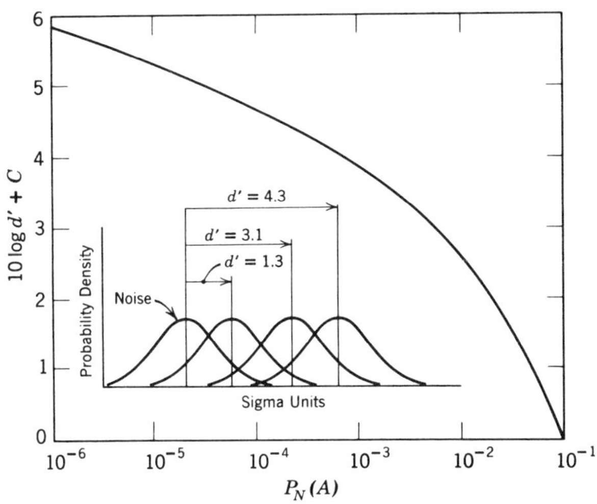

FIG. 4. Evaluation of how a change in criterion will influence the size of the "threshold" signal. $P_N(A)$ is the false-alarm rate: a "yes" response to no signal. The hit rate, $P_{SN}(A)$, was held constant at 0.5. The mean of the signal distribution was varied (see insert) to achieve this hit rate for various values of $P_N(A)$. The constant, C, was chosen so that $10 \log 1.3 + C = 0$.

from 1.3 to 3.1 in order to maintain $P_{SN}(A) = 0.50$. This value of $P_{SN}(A)$ is a reasonable one since it is often used as the estimate of "threshold." Very small values of false-alarm rate were used because most methods control this parameter to the extent of keeping it very low.

We cannot say *generally* how this change in the mean of the signal distribution is related to any signal parameter. However, for sinusoidal signals in noise, d' is roughly proportional to signal energy; thus the "estimated threshold" may vary over a 6-db range depending on the criterion of the subject. (In other experiments d' varies with signal voltage—hence the range might be 12 db. See Fig. 7 and the discussion.)

This change in the estimated threshold, of say 6 db, will occur only if the subject's criterion changes. One may be willing to assume that it is approximately constant over the course of the experiment.[8] Then this number, 6 db, could be interpreted as a tolerable difference in comparing two sets of different measurements. The theory, then, is consistent with the rather widespread view in psychoacoustics; namely, that results obtained using different methods should not be expected to show exact congruence. Whether these differences are large enough to warrant concern depends both on the particular nature of the problem and the precision desired.

DECISION ANALYSIS AND SPEECH RESEARCH. The use of ROC curves and the measure d' has not been limited to detection experiments. Since some confusion has been generated by the multiplicity of d' measures, this issue deserves some attention.

Figure 5 displays an ROC curve taken from a report by Egan (1957). The similarity between this figure and Fig. 2 is apparent, even though measures employed to construct this graph differ greatly. The procedure here is as follows: A word is presented in noise to a listener who writes down the word he thinks was presented. He then checks whether or not he believes the identification response was correct. The conditional probabilities of the receiver's saying he was correct on those words where he in fact was, and was not, correct define the ordinate and abscissa, respectively, of Fig. 5.

Egan's ROC curve, then, is constructed from a table of response-response contingencies rather than from stimulus-response contingencies,

---

[8] Obviously one can only assume it is constant because one cannot directly measure probabilities of the order 10^{-3}. If one is not willing to make this assumption, one must raise the false-alarm rate to a measurable value, $P_N(A) > 10^{-1}$, or use one of the other techniques discussed in the previous section. The signal energy necessary to obtain a certain d', say $d' = 1$, could then be used as the counterpart of the threshold energy.

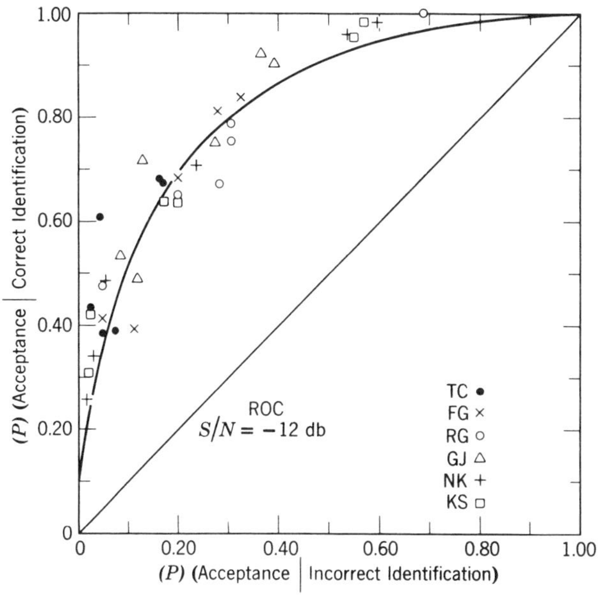

FIG. 5. Some data taken from Egan (1957). The signal-to-noise ratio refers to the peak signal power of the word compared with the noise power. The points represent different subjects. The subject listens to a word in noise, guesses what word it was, and then grades that response as being either correct (acceptance) or incorrect (rejection). The abscissa and ordinate refer to the probability of acceptance, given that the word was correctly or incorrectly identified.

as was the ROC curve presented earlier. This difference, from the standpoint of analysis, is by no means trivial. The method used by Egan is really a two-stage decision process. First, the observer has to select (from several possibilities) the most likely word; second, he must evaluate this decision with respect to all other possibilities. Such a process produces mathematical expressions virtually impossible to evaluate except under the most doubtful set of simplifying assumptions.

This difficulty does not, of course, prevent one from summarizing the data presented in Fig. 5 by a single parameter. The line drawn to the data points is that generated by moving a criterion along two normal deviates of the same variance which differ only in means. This measure was, unfortunately, initially labeled d' because of its analogy to the detection measure. It is unfortunate because the detection measure d' has often been specifically related to physical measurements of signal and noise. No such identification was ever intended in speech work, and therefore these measures obtained in speech research are presently denoted by various subscripts.[9]

The importance and usefulness of such measures is reviewed thoroughly in the monograph by Egan (1957) and in the work of Pollack (1959*b*), Pollack and Decker (1958), and Decker and Pollack (1959). Basically, these measures are all aimed at specifying the subject's criterion. For an interesting example of how this value of the criterion affects the substantive conclusion one might draw, the paper by Pollack (1959*c*) is recommended. A recent paper by Clarke (1960) has illustrated how confidence ratings may be utilized to supplement the usual articulation index.

THEORY OF IDEAL OBSERVERS

In the most general sense, an ideal observer is simply a function relating an observation to the likelihood of that observation. Thus we have already specified an ideal observer for our simple example, since Table I accomplishes this task. This is not an interesting example, however, because the observations were already specified in terms of the probabilities under each hypothesis. A more interesting example of an ideal observer arises where the observations are waveforms and where the characteristics of the waveform differ under each hypothesis. The task of the ideal observer is — given a waveform — to calculate likelihood ratio or some monotonic transformation of that quantity.

The ideal observer, strictly speaking, need not make any decisions. If likelihood ratio is computed, the problem of what decision rule to employ is determined by the specific objective in making the decisions. Various possible objectives have been discussed in the previous sections, where it was pointed out that these objectives could be attained by using a decision rule based on likelihood ratio. Although the calculation of likelihood ratio specifies the ideal observer for a given problem, such information is of little value unless we can evaluate this observer's performance. One general method of evaluating the ideal observer's performance is to determine ROC curves, but to obtain an ROC curve we must calculate two probabilities. Thus to completely evaluate the ideal

[9] As yet, no standard notation has evolved. The following list of references contains many of the proposals that have been advanced to clarify this confusion. At present, one must very carefully determine how the detectability measure is defined in each experiment. Even subscripted measures, d'_e in particular, are defined differently in different experiments. See Clarke, Birdsall, and Tanner (1959); Egan, Greenberg, and Schulman (1959*a*); and Pollack (1959*a*).

observer we actually have to specify not only how likelihood is calculated but the probability distribution of likelihood ratio on both hypotheses.

Having established the general background of this problem, let us consider a specific example: the ideal observer for conditions of a signal known exactly.

Ideal observer for the signal known exactly (SKE)

Two hypotheses actually define this special case in which, given a waveform, one must select one of the following hypotheses:

H_1—the waveform is a sample of white Gaussian noise $n(t)$ with specified bandwidth (W) and noise power density (N_0).

H_2—the waveform is $n(t)$ plus some specified signal waveform $s(t)$. Everything is known about $s(t)$ if it occurs: its starting time, duration, and phase. It need not be a segment of a sine wave as long as it is specified, i.e., known exactly.

From these two hypotheses we wish to calculate likelihood ratio, and, if possible, derive the probability distribution of likelihood ratio on both hypotheses. Obviously such calculations will be of little use unless the final results can be fairly simply summarized in terms of some simple physical measurement of signal and noise. Happily, such is the case.

We shall not present the derivation here since it is not in itself particularly instructive and can be obtained elsewhere (Peterson, Birdsall, and Fox, 1954). One assumption of the derivation will, however, be discussed, since an objection to this assumption has been recently raised — that an objection seriously questions the legitimacy of applying this result to any psychoacoustic experiment which has yet been conducted. Unfortunately, the alternative assumption suggested has a different but equally serious flaw.

Representation of the waveform

The assumption concerns the representation of the waveform. In order to compute likelihood ratio, one must find the probability of a certain waveform on each hypothesis. Since the waveform is simply a function of time, one must somehow associate a probability with this waveform, or somehow obtain a set of measures from the waveform and associate a probability with these measures.

But what exactly is the nature of the waveform? In order to compute these various probabilities we must make some very specific assumptions about the class of waveforms we will consider.

Peterson, Birdsall, and Fox (1954) assumed that the waveforms were Fourier series-band limited. If the waveform is of this class it can be represented by $n = 2WT$ measures, where W is the "bandwidth" of the noise and T is the duration of the waveform. A series representation in terms of sine and cosine might be used. There are, of course, many equivalent ways of writing this series to identify the n parameters, but these are all unique, and if the original waveform is indeed Fourier series-band limited, they will reproduce exactly the waveform in the interval $(0,T)$. Accepting this assumption, we find that a monotonic transformation of likelihood ratio (the logarithm) is normal under both hypotheses.

H_1: $\log l(x)$ is normal with mean $- E/N_0$, variance E/N_0

H_2: $\log l(x)$ is normal with mean $+ E/N_0$, variance E/N_0

$d' = \Delta M/\sigma = (2E/N_0)^{1/2}$ where E is the signal energy, $\int_0^T [s(t)]^2 dt$, and N_0 is the noise power density. Naturally, if this assumption about the waveform is not made, the preceding result is invalid. Mathews and David (1959) have considered a slightly different assumption. They assumed the waveforms are Fourier integral-band limited. The conclusion resulting from this assumption is that the signal is perfectly detectable in the noise independent of the ratio E/N_0, as long as it is not zero. In short, d' is infinite for any nonzero value of E/N_0. Which of these assumptions is the more reasonable or applicable to a psychoacoustic experiment?

Neither assumption can be completely justified. In almost all psychoacoustic experiments, the noise voltage is actually produced by a special tube. The voltage produced by this tube is amplified and filtered. Such noise is not Fourier series-band limited, for the noise is clearly not periodic.[10] Although a Fourier series might serve as an excellent approxi-

[10] It is somewhat unfair to imply that Peterson, Birdsall, and Fox assumed the noise was periodic. Their assumption, strictly speaking, was that each waveform could be represented by a finite set of numbers. The way they obtained these numbers is through a sampling plan, which we cannot discuss in detail. It was not a simple Fourier expansion in terms of *sine* and *cosine*. This is a difficult and complex topic; for a discussion of the details in this area see Peterson, Birdsall, and Fox (1954), Slepian (1958), and Davenport and Root (1958). Precise analysis of the situation where the noise is filtered, i.e., where the power spectrum of the noise is a polynomial, can be worked out in principle. The analysis is complex and exact answers can be obtained only in certain simple cases. One can show in general, however, that for practical situations the detectability of the signal is finite (Davenport and Root, 1958).

mation to these waveforms in the interval $(0,T)$, it would not be an *exact* representation of the waveform. Similarly, an assumption of a Fourier integral limitation of the bandwidth cannot be correct, because the waveform does not have a sharp cutoff in the Fourier integral sense. If it did, the waveform would be analytic. If it were analytic, the ideal observer could sample at one point in time, obtain all the derivatives at that point, and know the exact form of the wave for all time. Such a result leads to the conclusion that the ideal observer, by observing one sample of the waveform at any time can, immediately, in principle, make his decision about all the waveforms the experimenter has presented in the past and all those he may ever decide to produce. This approach is therefore of little practical use.

The issue, while obviously only an academic one, has indicated one very important aspect of the problem. The ideal observer is, like all ideal concepts, only as good as the assumptions that generate it. Clearly, any such idealization of a practical situation is based on certain simplifying assumptions. It is always extremely important to understand what these assumptions are and even more important to realize the implications of a change in these assumptions. In short, there are many ideal observers, each generated by certain key assumptions about the essential nature of the detection task.

For the discussion which follows, we shall use the Peterson, Birdsall, and Fox (1954) approach and assume that the waveforms can be completely represented by a finite number of measurements. A similar treatment is given by Van Meter and Middleton (1954). As more progress is made with the theory of ideal observers we should be able to state quite precisely how detection will vary if certain definite restrictions are imposed on the manner in which the observer operates. Peterson, Birdsall, and Fox have, in fact, considered several such cases and their results. Each case provides us with a framework from which we may evaluate and assess the performance of the subject. Such a comparison provides both qualitative and quantitative guides for further research (Tanner and Birdsall, 1958). There are several areas we might select to illustrate this approach. The one we have selected was chosen because it is a general topic and because it has been slighted somewhat in psychoacoustics.

Shape of the psychophysical function

The psychophysical function is generally defined as the curve relating the percentage of correct detections of the signal (the ordinate) to some physical measure of the signal (the abscissa). If some variant of the constant stimuli method is used, the curve rises monotonically from zero to 100 per cent as the signal level is increased.

Generally, hypotheses about the form of this function arise from assumptions about the process of discrimination. Often these assumptions are sufficient to allow one to deduce the form of the psychophysical function to within two or three parameters which are then determined experimentally. Obviously, it is extremely important for the model to specify the exact transformation of the physical stimulus which is used as the abscissa of the psychophysical function; without such specification, the theory is incomplete.

In psychoacoustics, there has been comparatively little concern with the form of this function. Most theories of the auditory process have been content with attempting to predict only one parameter of the psychophysical curve, usually the mean or threshold. As a result, it is nearly impossible to obtain from the literature information on the actual form of the psychophysical function.

The notable exception to the preceding statement is the neural-quantum hypothesis (Stevens, Morgan, and Volkmann, 1941). The authors of this theory say that it "enables us to predict the form and the slope of certain psychometric functions." It can be demonstrated from the model that the form of the function should be linear and this linear function is specified to within one parameter. The physical measure is never mentioned in the derivation of the theory, and we find only after the data is presented that sound pressure and frequency are the appropriate physical measures. The authors remark in their paper that "strictly speaking, data yielding rectilinear psychometric functions when plotted against sound pressure do not show absolute rectilinearity when expressed in terms of sound energy, but calculation shows that the departure from rectilinearity is negligible." It is certainly true that pressure, pressure squared, and indeed pressure cubed, are all nearly linear for small values of pressure—but that is not entirely the point.

It is the location of this function that plays a crucial role in the theory. If the subject employs a two-quantum criterion then, according to the theory, the psychophysical function must be zero up to one quantum unit, show a linear increase to 100 per cent at two quantum units, and maintain this level for more quantum units. Where the curve breaks from 0 per cent reports and where it reaches 100 per cent reports is precisely specified by the theory. In general, if the subject requires n quanta to produce a positive report, the increasing linear function must extend from n to $n + 1$ quantal units. Now clearly, what appears to be a two-quantum subject (0 per cent at one pressure unit, 100 per cent at two pressure units), when the data are plotted in pressure units, cannot be interpreted as a two-quantum subject in energy units. In fact, he cannot be interpreted as an any-number-of-quantum subject. This is true no matter how small the values of pressure.

This criticism of the rather post hoc treatment of the physical scale is by no means limited to the neural-quantum hypothesis. Many hypotheses about the shape of the psychophysical function, including some formulations of the Gaussian hypothesis, neglect this rather crucial factor.

Detection theory stands in marked contrast with these theories. Models based on the ideal observer concept predict the form of the psychophysical function exactly. The proper physical dimensions are completely specified and there are no free parameters.

Obviously, one would not be surprised to find human observers somewhat less than optimum, but hopefully, the shape of the psychophysical function might at least be parallel to that obtained from the model. Often, however, the obtained psychophysical function does not parallel that predicted by the model and this discrepancy deserves some discussion.

SIGNAL UNCERTAINTY AND IDEAL DETECTORS.[11] In Fig. 6, we have plotted the percentage of correct detections in a two-alternative forced-choice procedure versus $\mathcal{E}\text{-}\mathfrak{N}_0$ for a typical subject and a series of mathematical models. The problem in all cases is simply to detect a sinusoidal signal added to a background of white noise.

We say "typical subject" because the shape of this function is remarkably invariant over both subjects and a range of physical parameters. For signal durations of 10 to 1000 msec (Green, 1959) and signal frequencies from 250 to 4000 cps (Green, McKey, and Licklider, 1959), there appears to be no great change in the shape of the function when plotted against the scale shown in Fig. 6. Naturally, the exact location of the curve depends on the exact physical parameters of the signal, but except for this constant, which is a simple additive constant in logarithmic form the shape is remarkably stable. The striking aspect of this function is its slope. We notice the slope of the observed function is steeper than most of the theoretical functions depicted in Fig. 6.

[11] The analysis of detection data from the viewpoint of signal uncertainty is very similar to some ideas expressed by W. P. Tanner, Jr. Although several details of the analysis differ, the essentials are the same. The author is indebted to Dr. Tanner for many long and lively conversations on this topic.

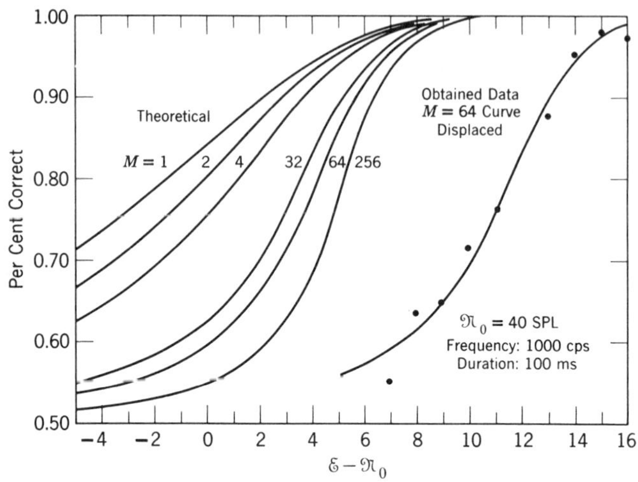

FIG. 6. The theoretical psychophysical functions for the ideal observer detecting one of M orthogonal signals. The parameter M is the number of possible orthogonal signals. The ideal detector need only detect the signal, not identify it. The abscissa is ten times the logarithm of signal energy to noise power density. The ordinate is the per cent correct detection in a two-alternative forced-choice test. The obtained data are compared with the theoretical function shifted about 10 db to the right.

The class of theoretical functions is generated by assuming the detector has various uncertainties about the exact nature of the signal.[12] Each function is generated by assuming the detector knows only that the signal will be one of M orthogonal signals. If the signal is known exactly ($M = 1$) there is no uncertainty. For sinusoidal signals, the nature of the uncertainty might be phase, time of occurrence of the signal, or signal frequency. The degree of uncertainty is reflected by the parameter M. As this uncertainty increases, the psychophysical function increases in slope. It therefore appears that there may exist a model with sufficient uncertainty about the signal to generate a function which is very similar to that displayed by the human observer.

[12] The details of this model may be found in Peterson, Birdsall, and Fox (1954), p. 207. This particular model was selected because it has been presented in the literature. There are other models which assume signal uncertainty but which differ in details about the decision rule. The psychophysical functions produced by these models are similar to those displayed in Fig. 6, although the value of the parameter (M) would be changed somewhat.

Accepting for the moment the assumption that the extreme slope of the human observer's psychophysical function is due to some degree of uncertainty about the signal, we might try to manipulate this slope by various experimental procedures.

PREVIEW TECHNIQUE. One general class of procedures would attempt to reduce the uncertainty by supplying the missing information through some form of cueing or preview technique. If, for example, the observer is uncertain about the frequency of the signal we might attempt to reduce this uncertainty by presenting the signal briefly at a high level just prior to the observation interval. Similarly, if the time of occurrence of the signal is uncertain we might increase the noise during the observation interval. If the noise was increased for all trials, whether or not the signal was presented, it would provide no information about the signal's presence but would convey direct information about the signal's starting time and duration. Both of these techniques have been utilized with only partial success. While it is impossible to assert that there was no change (the null hypothesis) the amount of change was very small, although in the proper direction.[13]

Another class of procedures which has been utilized to attempt to reduce the subject's uncertainty about the signal parameters involves changing the detection task so that some information is directly supplied. The procedures are like the preceding but actually include the information in the observation interval. For example, to remove frequency uncertainty, we might add a continuous sine wave to the noise. The continuous sine wave is adjusted to a level such that it is clearly evident in the noise. The signal is an increment added to this sine wave, and the task is to detect this increment. The procedure definitely changes the slope of the subject's psychophysical function—it becomes less steep and the signal is easier to detect.[14]

This procedure of making the signal an increment to a continuous sine wave provides good frequency information but does not remove temporal uncertainty. Another procedure which minimizes practically all uncertainty is in fact a modification of a standard procedure used to investigate the *j.n.d.* for intensity. A two-alternative forced-choice procedure is employed. Two gated sinusoids occur in noise, one at standard level, the other at this level plus an increment. The subject's task is to select the interval containing the increment. If the standard signal is adjusted to a power level about equal to the noise-power density, the psychophysical

---

[13] Unpublished work of the author. Also see Marill (1956) and Licklider and Flanagan, "On a methodological problem in audiometry" (unpublished).

[14] W. P. Tanner, Jr., J. Bigelow, and D. M. Green (unpublished). [See 16]

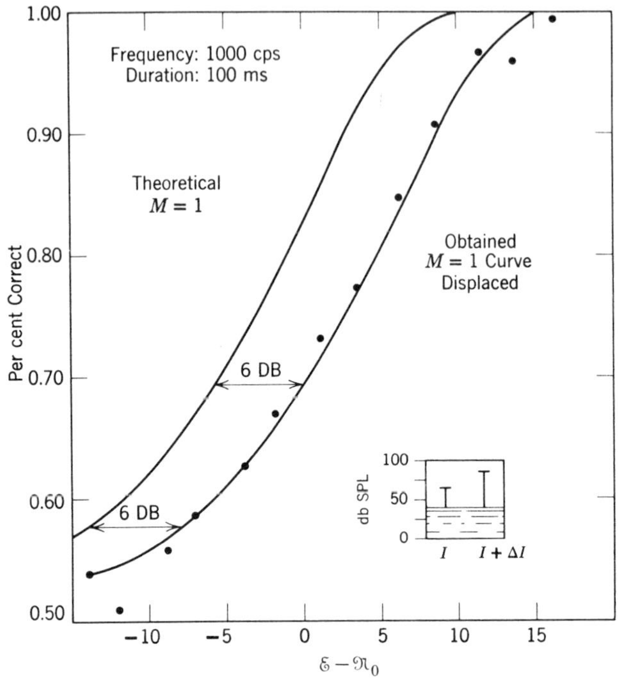

FIG. 7. Observed data in the ΔI versus I experiment and the signal-known-exactly observer ($M = 1$). The abscissa and ordinate are the same as in Fig. 6, but note the change in scale of the abscissa. The two curves differ by 6 db at each value of per cent correct. The apparent convergence of the two curves at low values of per cent correct is illusory. The insert shows the level of the noise; the lines show the level of I in power, and the maximum $I + \Delta I$ power.

function actually parallels that expected for the signal-known-exactly case (Tanner, 1958). It is from 3 to 6 db off optimum in absolute value, depending on the energy of the standard. (See Fig. 7. Note the change in scale between Figs. 6 and 7.)

Let us, at least tentatively, accept as the conclusion of these last results that the shape of the psychophysical function is in fact due primarily to various uncertainties about the signal parameter. If this is true, then we still have the problem of explaining the lack of success evidenced when the previous techniques were employed. Should not a preview of the signal, preceding an observation, serve to reduce frequency uncertainty? The answer might be that such procedures do reduce uncertainty, but not enough relative to the uncertainty still remaining. From Fig. 6 we note that, as we introduce signal uncertainty, the slope of the psychophysical function increases very rapidly for small changes in uncertainty; then, as the uncertainty increases, the slope approaches some asymptotic value. A change in uncertainty from $M = 256$ to 64 may hardly affect the psychophysical function. This fact also probably explains why the psychophysical functions do not appear to change very much for a variety of signal parameters, such as signal duration and signal frequency. Undoubtedly, as the signal duration increases, the uncertainty about the time of occurrence of the signal is reduced. Due to the large initial uncertainty, this change is too small to be detected in the data.

UNCERTAIN SIGNAL FREQUENCY. Still another manner of checking this general model is to vary the uncertainty of the signal and determine how this affects the subject's performance. One might, for example, select several different sinusoidal signals and select one at random as the signal used on a particular trial. The subject is simply asked to *detect* a signal, not identify it. Depending on the frequency separation and the number of signals used, one can directly manipulate signal uncertainty.

This in fact was a procedure used in an earlier study by Tanner, Swets, and Green (1956). A small decrement (1.0 to 1.5 db) in detectability was found if one compared a situation where a *single* fixed sinusoid was the signal and a situation where the signal was one of *two* sinusoids. Later results (Veniar, 1958a, 1958b; Creelman, 1959) show, however, that the decrement did not increase very much as more components were included in the set of possible signals. This result is consistent with the theoretical model we have been discussing. Figure 8 shows how, for a constant detectability, one must change the signal level as uncertainty (M) is increased. The decrement in signal detectability as a function of signal uncertainty changes very slowly after M reaches a value of 50 or so. The 1.5 db per octave decrement, suggested by some of the earlier models to account for the uncertain frequency data, (Green, 1958; Tanner, Swets, and Green, 1956; Creelman, 1959) is only a reasonable approximation for a rather limited range of M.[15]

While the preceding argument that the shape of the psychophysical function is largely due to signal uncertainty has some appeal, there still remain some problems with this interpretation. Another way to attack

[15] Egan, Greenberg, and Schulman (1959*b*) have investigated the way that temporal uncertainty affects signal detectability. In one condition they present a fixed-frequency sinusoidal signal of 0.25-sec duration somewhere in an 8-sec interval. They did not report the results in detail, but the decrement in detectability due to temporal uncertainty was small (1 or 2 db).

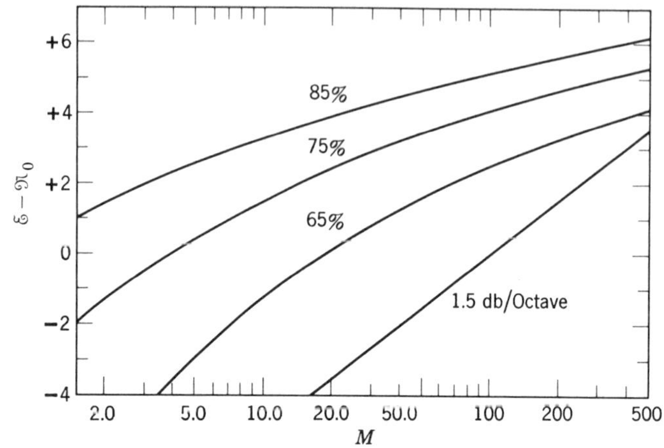

FIG. 8. The variation of signal-to-noise level for some constant per cent correct as a function of M. This curve is the same information presented in Fig. 6 with M as the variable and per cent correct as the parameter.

this problem of signal uncertainty is to use a signal where little information about the waveform is known, and compare the subject's performance with the theoretical optimum model in this situation. A specific case arises where the signal is a sample of noise, The most one can specify about the signal is the frequency region, starting time, duration, and power. The ideal detector for this signal can be specified—it simply measures signal energy in the signal band. But the psychophysical functions obtained with this type of signal are also slightly steeper than those predicted by the model (Green, 1960). Either partial time uncertainty still remains or signal uncertainty alone is not a sufficient explanation. The author feels that a better model would assume that the human observer utilizes some nonlinear detection rule. This assumption, coupled with the uncertainty explanation, could probably explain most of the results obtained thus far. The mathematical analysis of such devices is, however, complex.

INTERNAL NOISE. Before summarizing, one final point must be considered. Often it is a temptation to invoke the concept of internal or neural noise when discussing the discrepancy between an ideal model and the human observer. There are good reasons for avoiding this temptation. While it would take us too far afield to cover this point in detail, the following remarks will illustrate the point.

Only if the model is of a particularly simple form can one hope to evaluate the specific effects of the assumption of internal noise. The signal-known-exactly observer is of this type. Here one can show how a specific type of internal noise can simply be treated as adding noise at the input of the detection device. Thus one can evaluate the psychophysical function and it will be shifted to the right by some number of decibels (see Fig. 6) due to the internal noise. But, of course, such an assumption can immediately be rejected since no shift in the psychophysical function can account for the data displayed in the figure.

With more complicated models, it is usually difficult to say exactly what internal noise will do. While it will obviously lower discrimination, the specific effects of the assumption are often impossible to evaluate. Unless these specific effects can be evaluated, the assumption simply rephrases the original problem of the discrepancy.

I am not suggesting that the human observer is perfect in any sense, nor attempting to minimize the importance of the concept of internal noise. What I am emphasizing is that the concept must be used with great care. If the concept is to have any importance, we have to (1) state exactly what this noise is, i.e., characterize it mathematically, (2) specify in what way it interacts with the detection or discrimination process, and (3) evaluate specifically what effect it will have on performance. Unless these steps can be carried out, the ad hoc nature of the assumption vitiates its usefulness.

SUMMARY AND CONCLUSION

The main emphasis in this paper has been to explain detection theory and to illustrate how such a theory has been applied to certain areas of psychoacoustics. This method of analysis is simply one of many that are currently being used in an attempt to understand the process of hearing.

Two main aspects of this approach have been distinguished. The first, decision theory, emphasizes that the subject's criterion as well as the physical properties of the stimulus play a major role in determining the subject's responses. The theory both indicates the class of variables which determines the level of the criterion, and, more importantly, suggests an analytic technique for removing this source of variation. This technique leaves a relatively pure measure of the detectability of the signal. The invariance of this measure over several psychophysical procedures has already been demonstrated.

The second aspect, the theory of ideal observers, has also been discussed in some detail. The usefulness of such an analysis was illustrated by considering the form of the psychophysical function. No ideal observer provides a complete or comprehensive model even for the rather limited areas of psychoacoustics that we have discussed in this paper. The model provides a source of hypotheses and a standard against which experimental results can be evaluated. It is too early to attempt any complete evaluation of this approach. The mathematical models are relatively new and the application of these models to a sensory process began with Tanner and Swets only about five years ago (Tanner and Swets, 1954). There remain many problems to be solved, both of a mathematical and experimental nature. As more progress is made in both areas, the theory should become more specific and concrete, then perhaps it will be able to interact more directly with the research from several other areas in psychoacoustics.

APPENDIX

The inherent difficulty of comparing the optimum criterion value and that employed by the subject is the shape of the expected-value function. Let us investigate in detail a typical situation. We have assumed that the distribution on likelihood ratio is normal under both hypotheses, that the mean separation is one sigma unit, and that the values and costs of the various decision alternatives are all the same. From these assumptions we have constructed Fig. 9. This figure shows how the expected value

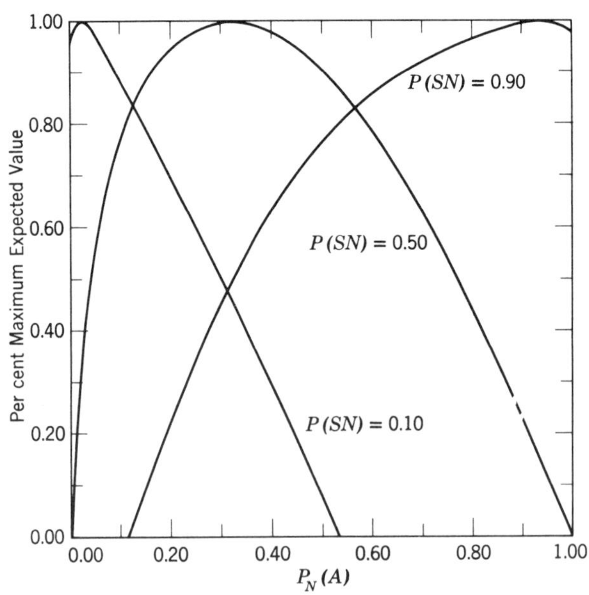

FIG. 9. The normalized expected value as a function of changes in criterion. This is a theoretical curve based on the data presented in Figs. 2 and 3. The appendix lists the assumptions used to construct the curve.

varies with changes in a priori probability of signal $P(SN)$ and false-alarm rate $P_N(A)$. We see immediately that for extreme values of a priori probability, e.g., $P(SN) = 0.10$, the difference between optimum expected-value behavior $[P_N(A) = 0.004]$ and a pure strategy $[P_N(A) = 0.000]$ is less than 3 per cent. In fact, the curves in the figure were somewhat exaggerated to allow one to see the location of the maximum. Since most subjects are instructed to avoid pure strategies in psychoacoustic experiments, this tends to force the subject to adopt more moderate values of $P_N(A)$ for extreme conditions.

On the other hand, if more moderate a priori probabilities are employed in the experiment [e.g., $P(SN) = 0.50$], we see that any value of $P_N(A)$ within a range from 0.15 to 0.50 will achieve at least 90 per cent of the maximum expected payoff. Thus any attempt to investigate, in more than a correlational sense, the correspondence between obtained and optimal criteria appears extremely difficult.

ACKNOWLEDGMENTS

This article was prepared in the Research Laboratory of Electronics of the Massachusetts Institute of Technology, with support from the Operational Applications Laboratory of the U. S. Air Force. This article appeared as Tech. Rept. No. AFCCDD TR-60-20, and in J. acoust. Soc. Am., *1960,* **32,** *1189–1203.*

References

- Anderson, T. W. *An introduction to multivariate statistical analysis.* New York: Wiley, 1958.
- Clarke, F. R. Confidence ratings, second-choice responses, and confusion matrices in intelligibility tests. *J. acoust. Soc. Am.,* 1960, **32,** 35–46. [33]
- Clarke, F. R., Birdsall, T. G., and Tanner, W. P., Jr. Two types of ROC curves and definitions of parameters. *J. acoust. Soc. Am.,* 1959, **31,** 629–630.
- Creelman, C. D. Detection of signals of uncertain frequency. University of Michigan: Electronic Defense Group, 1959, Technical Memorandum No. 71.
- Davenport, W. B., and Root, W. L. *Random signals in noise.* New York: McGraw-Hill, 1958.
- Decker, L. R., and Pollack, I. Multiple observers, message reception, and rating scales. *J. acoust. Soc. Am.,* 1959, **31,** 1327–1328.
- Egan, J. P. Message repetition, operating characteristics, and confusion matrices in speech communications. Indiana University: Hearing and Communication Laboratory, 1957, Technical Report No. AFCRC TR 57–50.
- Egan, J. P., and Clarke, F. R. Source and receiver behavior in the use of a criterion. *J. acoust. Soc. Am.,* 1956, **28,** 1267–1269. [30]
- Egan, J. P., Greenberg, G. Z., and Schulman, A. I. Operating characteristics, signal detectability, and the method of free response. Indiana University: Hearing and Communication Laboratory, 1959*a*, Technical Report No. AFCRC-TR-59-58. [See 15]

- Egan, J. P., Greenberg, G. Z., and Schulman, A. I. Detection of signals presented at random times. *J. acoust. Soc. Am.*, 1959*b*, **31,** 1579. (Abstract)
- Egan, J. P., Schulman, A. I., and Greenberg, G. Z. Operating characteristics determined by binary decisions and by ratings. *J. acoust. Soc. Am.*, 1959, **31,** 768–773. [7]
- Elliott, P. B. Tables of *d'*. University of Michigan: Electronic Defense Group, 1959, Technical Report No. 97. [34]
- Garner, W. R. Advantages of the discriminability criterion for a loudness scale. *J. acoust. Soc. Am.*, 1958, **30,** 1005–1012.
- Green, D. M. Detection of multiple component signals in noise. *J. acoust. Soc. Am.*, 1958, **30,** 904–911. [25]
- Green, D. M. Detection of a pulsed auditory signal in noise as a function of duration and frequency. *J. acoust. Soc. Am.*, 1959, **31,** 836. (Abstract)
- Green, D. M. Auditory detection of a noise signal. *J. acoust. Soc. Am.*, 1960, **32,** 121–131. [27]
- Green, D. M., McKey, M. J., and Licklider, J. C. R. Detection of a pulsed sinusoid in noise as a function of frequency. *J. acoust. Soc. Am.*, 1959, **31,** 1446–1452. [26]
- Marill, T. Psychophysics and signal detection theory. Massachusetts Institute of Technology: Research Laboratory of Electronics, 1956, Technical Report No. 319.
- Mathews, M. V., and David, E. E. On signal detection, signal perception, and ideal observers. *J. acoust. Soc. Am.*, 1959, **31,** 834. (Abstract)
- Munson, W. A., and Karlin, J. E. The measurement of human channel transmission characteristics. *J. acoust. Soc. Am.*, 1954, **26,** 542–553.
- Neyman, J., and Pearson, E. S. On the problem of the most efficient tests of statistical hypotheses. *Phil. Trans. Roy. Soc. London, Ser. A,* 1933, **231,** 289.
- Peterson, W. W., Birdsall, T. G., and Fox, W. C. The theory of signal detectability. *Trans. IRE Professional Group on Information Theory,* 1954, **PGIT-4,** 171–212.
- Pollack, I. On indices of signal and response discriminability. *J. acoust. Soc. Am.*, 1959*a*, **31,** 1031.
- Pollack, I. Message uncertainty and message reception. *J. acoust. Soc. Am.*, 1959*b*, **31,** 1500–1508.
- Pollack, I. Message repetition and message reception. *J. acoust. Soc. Am.*, 1959*c*, **31,** 1509–1515.
- Pollack, I., and Decker, L. R. Confidence ratings, message reception, and the receiver operating characteristic. *J. acoust. Soc. Am.*, 1958, **30,** 286–292. [31]
- Slepian, D. Some comments on the detection of Gaussian signals in Gaussian noise. *Trans. IRE Professional Group on Information Theory,* 1958, **PGIT-4, 65–68.**
- Smith, M., and Wilson, E. A. A model of the auditory threshold and its application to the problem of the multiple observer. *Psychol. Monogr.*, 1953, **67,** No. 9, Whole No. 359.
- Stevens, S. S. On the validity of the loudness scale. *J. acoust. Soc. Am.*, 1959, **31, 995–1003.**

- Stevens, S. S., Morgan, C. T., and Volkmann, J. Theory of the neural quantum in the discrimination of loudness and pitch. *Am. J. Psychol.*, 1941, **54,** 315–335.
- Swets, J. A. Indices of signal detectability obtained with various psychophysical procedures. *J. acoust. Soc. Am.*, 1959, **31,** 511–513. [6]
- Swets, J. A., Tanner, W. P., Jr., and Birdsall, T. G. The evidence for a decision-making theory of visual detection. University of Michigan: Electronic Defense Group, 1955, Technical Report No. 40. [See 1]
- Tanner, W. P., Jr. A re-evaluation of Weber's law as applied to pure tones. University of Michigan: Electronic Defense Group, 1958, Technical Report No. 47.
- Tanner, W. P., Jr., and Birdsall, T. G. Definitions of d' and η as psychophysical measures. *J. acoust. Soc. Am.*, 1958, **30,** 922–928. [5]
- Tanner, W. P., Jr., and Swets, J. A. A decision-making theory of visual detection. *Psychol. Rev.*, 1954, **61,** 401–409.
- Tanner, W. P., Jr., Swets, J. A., and Green, D. M. Some general properties of the hearing mechanism. University of Michigan: Electronic Defense Group, 1956, Technical Report No. 30.
- Van Meter, D., and Middleton, D. Modern statistical approaches to reception in communication theory. *Trans. IRE Professional Group on Information Theory,* 1954, **PGIT-4,** 119–145.
- Veniar, F. A. Signal detection as a function of frequency ensemble, I. *J. acoust. Soc. Am.*, 1958*a*, **30,** 1020–1024.
- Veniar, F. A. Signal detection as a function of frequency ensemble, II. *J. acoust. Soc. Am.*, 1958*b*, **30,** 1075–1078.
- Wald, A. *Statistical decision functions.* New York: Wiley, 1950.
- Woodward, P. M. *Probability and information theory with applications to radar.* New York: McGraw-Hill, 1955.

Some Comments and a Correction of "Psychoacoustics and Detection Theory"

David M. Green

Dr. S. S. Stevens has very kindly pointed out two items in my paper, "Psychoacoustics and Detection Theory" (Green, 1960 [2]), that require further comment in order to avoid misunderstanding.

I called the function relating the percentage of correct detection responses to the physical intensity of the stimulus the *psychophysical* function. It is true that this function is more often called the *psychometric* function, a term probably introduced by Urban (1908).

Originally Fechner added up successive just-noticeable-differences (jnd's) to determine the relation between the magnitude of sensation and the physical intensity of the stimulus. The resulting relation is commonly called the psychophysical function. Since Fechner's time many other techniques for determining this relation have been devised and the results are also called psychophysical functions (e.g., Stevens' power law, 1957). The newer methods do not involve determining jnd's and are not obtained by using any simple variant of the classical methods of psychophysics. We are therefore faced with the anomaly that psychometric functions are obtained by using psychophysical methods and psychophysical functions are now determined by other, different techniques.

Personally I find the designation used in vision—frequency-of-seeing curve—even more distasteful than the term psychometric function. Some change in terminology would be most welcome. I am open for suggestions.

The second item is more crucial and concerns my remarks about the neural-quantum theory. I asserted that data that appear to indicate a two-quantum observer when plotted against pressure units cannot be interpreted as any kind of quantum observer when plotted against energy units. There is, however, a very straightforward interpretation of the scales of pressure and energy that makes this assertion incorrect. Unfortunately, this interpretation had never occurred to me, and I thereby did injustice to the authors of the neural-quantum theory. Let me explain this interpretation and the scale of pressure and energy units that I had in mind when I made my remarks.

In the neural-quantum procedure we have a continuous sinusoidal stimulus (call it the standard). At specific times we increase briefly the amplitude of this sinusoid and the observer's task is to detect these increments. If we measure the pressure of the standard, call it p, and measure the pressure of the standard plus the increment, call it $p + \Delta p$, then by subtracting the former from the latter we obtain on a pressure scale values of Δp. We may call this quantity Δp the increment of pressure.

Similarly, if we measure the power of the standard, a quantity proportional to p^2, and the power of the standard plus the increment, a quantity proportional to $(p + \Delta p)^2$, we might subtract the former from the latter, and (since the constants of proportionality are the same) obtain the quantity $(p^2 + 2\Delta pp + \Delta p^2 - p^2) = (2\Delta pp + \Delta p^2)$. The latter quantity is also proportional to energy, since the increment is of constant duration, and we may call this quantity the increment of energy. The important result is that these two quantities, the increment in pressure and the increment in energy, are nearly linear for values of Δp much less than p. If some data are exactly consistent with the predictions of the neural quantum theory on one scale, they would very nearly be consistent on the other scale.

When I made my remarks, I had in mind data plotted on a scale of *signal* pressure or *signal* energy. By *signal* I mean the wave form added to the standard that the observers are asked to detect. In this terminology, the pressure of the signal is proportional to Δp and the energy of signal is proportional to that quantity squared, Δp^2. Only data plotted on a scale of signal pressure as I have now defined it are in agreement with the predictions of neural quantum theory.

Part of the reason for my oversight undoubtedly arose from the fact that this measure of signal energy Δp^2 is the quantity I used in presenting some of the data reported later in my paper. There is, however, no inherent reason for using my particular measure of the stimulus and I should have made my reference clear.

In some cases the two different scales of energy obtained from the pressure scale would be exactly the same. This would happen if the standard and signal were incoherent, that is, if the middle term in the square of $(\Delta p + p)$ were zero. An example of this would be an increment in white noise. In the case at hand, this is not true, and the quantity that I have called increment in energy and the quantity that I called signal energy are quite different.

The general point I was trying to make is that the neural-quantum theory does not specify in advance how the physical stimulus should be measured. It was my position that it is important for a theory of psychophysics to specify how the physical scale is related to the expected psychological results. This position is apparently not widely endorsed. I am particularly impressed with the number of theories that suggest that the psychometric function is Gaussian, log-Gaussian, Poisson, rectilinear, or logistic, but cannot specify in advance what particular transformation of the physical scale will yield these results. It is not hard to envision different circumstances in which all these assertions are true at least in the sense that deviations are within the range of experimental error. Somehow there never seems to be any resolution to these different findings.

One can, of course, simply ignore all this and go on measuring only one arbitrary parameter of the psychometric function such as the "threshold" value. While this position obviously has the merit of convenience, it would also appear important to demonstrate how all of these different results might come about from one single general theory. To accomplish the latter task one must have a theory which carefully specifies the physical part of the psychophysical theory.

The preparation of this letter was supported by the U. S. Army Signal Corps, the Air Force (Operational Applications Office and Office of Scientific Research), and the Office of Naval Research. It appeared as Technical Note No. ESD TN 61-56 and in *J. acoust. Soc. Am.*, **33,** 965, 1961.

References

• Stevens, S. S. On the psychophysical law. *Psychol. Rev.*, 1957, **64,** 153–181.

• Urban, F. M. *The application of statistical methods to the problems of psychophysics.* Philadelphia: Psychol. Clinic Press, 1908.

3

Theory of Signal Detection

J. C. R. Licklider

The specific theory of signal detection upon which we shall focus is the one presented by Tanner, Swets, and Green (1956). Let us call it TSG. It is a formulation in terms of statistical-decision theory, and it is presented as a preferred alternative to the conventional theory based upon fixed thresholds.

SUMMARY OF THE THEORY

TSG is formulated in such a way as to be applicable[1] to detection trials in each of which (1) a signal, of specifications known more or less completely by the listener, is either presented [s, with probability $P(s)$] or not presented [$\bar{s}$, with probability $P(\bar{s})$], and (2) a listener makes a response [S or $\bar{S}$] signifying whether or not, according to his judgment, the signal was presented.

The listener is assumed to know the a priori probabilities $P(s)$ and $P(\bar{s})$ governing signal presentation and to make his decision in relation to them and to a payoff matrix, or risk function, as well as to his sensory data. The payoff matrix M defines the values to the listener of the four possible pairings of stimulus and response events in Table I.

---

[1] TSG is applicable also to experiments in which the signal is located in one of several intervals of space or time and the subject's task is to specify which one. (Stevens calls these forced-location experiments instead of forced-choice experiments because the subject is forced to make a choice also in experiments using other procedures.) TSG can be extended to most clearly defined detection situations. We shall limit the discussion here for the sake of brevity.

TABLE I. THE PAYOFF MATRIX*

Response	Stimulus s	Stimulus $\bar{s}$
S	V_{sS}	$V_{\bar{s}S}$
$\bar{S}$	$V_{s\bar{S}}$	$V_{\bar{s}\bar{S}}$

* V_{sS} is the value of a correct positive report ("hit"); $V_{s\bar{S}}$ of an incorrect negative report ("miss"), $V_{\bar{s}S}$ of an incorrect positive report ("false alarm"), and $V_{\bar{s}\bar{S}}$ of a correct negative report. Usually V_{sS} and $V_{\bar{s}\bar{S}}$ are positive values, $V_{s\bar{S}}$ and $V_{\bar{s}S}$ negative values or positive costs.

When it is presented, the signal is superposed upon noise. Some of the noise may be introduced by the experimenter or the external situation. But part of it is inherent in the sensory process; it is added to the signal clues that are delivered from the receptors to the decision process. The auditory channel between the receptors and the decision process has, in TSG, a "narrow-band property." At any moment, only a single, narrow frequency band of the external signal and noise, and of the internal noise, is delivered to the decision process. Although TSG is not entirely explicit about how the center frequency and the width of the band are selected or controlled—the theory specifies a narrow-band scanning filter, the center frequency of which can remain fixed or sweep along the frequency scale—we may assume, in the case of a long-duration sinusoidal[2] signal, that the narrow band centers itself on the signal frequency and has the smallest width the auditory system can provide at that frequency.

The listener's decision is governed, according to TSG, by a decision process that uses in an optimal manner the a priori probabilities, the payoff matrix, and the sensory data. The decision process is extremely simple, but it is necessary to go through a rather complicated argument to show why such a simple process is admissible. In due course, we shall

[2] Sinusoidal is the generic term for waves of simple harmonic motion. Sinusoids are physically pure tones. Cosine waves ($|\Theta| \cos 2\pi ft$) and sine waves [$|\Theta| \sin 2\pi ft = |\Theta| \cos (2\pi ft - \pi/2)$] are sinusoids. So is any other wave of the same shape [$|\Theta| \cos (2\pi ft + \phi)$]. The maximum amplitude of the oscillation is $|\Theta|$. The cyclic frequency is f. The argument $(2\pi ft + \phi)$ is the phase angle, of which, ordinarily, $2\pi ft$ is the varying and ϕ is the fixed part. The maximum amplitude (usually shortened simply to amplitude), the frequency, and the fixed part of the phase angle (often referred to simply as "the phase") are the three real numbers that specify the three "dimensions" of a sinusoid.

represent the listener's sensory datum by a single number $\mathfrak{L}$ and his criterion by another single number $\mathfrak{L}_c$, and we shall have him say S, "signal presented," if $\mathfrak{L} \geq \mathfrak{L}_c$, and $\bar{S}$, "signal not presented," if $\mathfrak{L} < \mathfrak{L}_c$. It will be that simple. But we shall have to make a detour through signal space and the maximum likelihood criterion before we reach that point.

It may clarify matters to point out here, as Marill (1956) has suggested, that what Tanner, Swets, and Green, and their colleagues have done in TSG is to discover and call attention to the applicability of an existing mathematical structure to a body of empirical observations. The mathematical structure itself has inherently nothing to do with signals, with detection, or with psychophysics. It has to do with statistical hypothesis testing, with deciding between alternative hypotheses. At the simplest level, the problem with which it deals is the following: given a sample and two hypotheses, each of which determines a sampling distribution, make the best choice between the hypotheses. What is meant by "best"? The answer given by Neyman and Pearson is that, in any single instance, it has no definite meaning, but that one may follow a rule of behavior which, if followed consistently, will lead in the long run to maximization of certain expected values. If he adopts a definite payoff matrix, then he can find a rule that will maximize the expected payoff. The rule is: calculate the likelihood of the sample on each of the two hypotheses, take the ratio, and accept the first hypothesis if the ratio exceeds a given constant. We shall consider a little later the determination of the constant. Here let us note that the result is general and profound, that nothing is said about normality, homogeneity of variance, signals, or noise, and that the number of alternative hypotheses is exactly two.

The main obstacle standing in the way of connecting the mathematical structure of statistical hypothesis testing to the substantive observations of signal detection and psychophysics is that, in the latter, the "samples" of signals and noises are seen at first as continuous functions of time and not as discrete numbers or categorizable events. A way around that obstacle is provided by a theorem widely used in electrical engineering, the "sampling theorem" or the "2 WT theorem." In the following paragraphs, we shall first employ that theorem to give ourselves quantities to which statistical decision theory can readily be applied, and then we shall consider its application.

Signal space is a space of n dimensions in which a particular signal is represented by n coordinates. It is a standard mathematical-engineering concept, a part of the general theory of signal detection and of other theories, also. In order to have it make sense, it is necessary to see why any time function whose spectrum is limited to a definite interval Δf of frequency and whose duration is Δt can be specified by $2 \cdot \Delta f \cdot \Delta t$ coefficients.[3]

If the signal lasts Δt seconds, we can repeat it over and over, $1/\Delta t$ times per second (see Fig. 1). The waveform thus produced is periodic and its spectrum[4] is, therefore, made up entirely of harmonics (integral multiples) of $1/\Delta t$. Because of the restriction of the spectrum to the interval Δf, only those harmonics in the interval Δf have coefficients that need to be specified. There are, therefore, $\Delta f/(1/\Delta t) = \Delta f \cdot \Delta t$ such harmonics, with coefficients $\Theta_j = \alpha_j + i\beta_j$. The α's and the β's are independently specifiable numbers. Consequently, there are $n = 2 \cdot \Delta f \cdot \Delta t$ numbers to specify in order to determine the periodic wave uniquely. Determining it uniquely is, of course, equivalent to specifying the original Δt-sec segment uniquely.

The signal space for signals Δt long and Δf wide is then a space of $n = 2 \cdot \Delta f \cdot \Delta t$ dimensions, and any specified signal of the class is represented by a point in the space. The "signal" could of course be a segment of tone. Equally well, it could be a segment of noise. Or it could be a segment of tone added to a segment of noise.

If we specify only certain parameters of a distribution from which a sample signal is drawn—not the precise waveform or the spectrum of the particular sample—we do not say what point in the space corresponds to the sample. But we provide the information from which a person can pick out various points in the space and calculate from the specified parameters that it is this point with this probability (or probability density), that point with that probability, and so on. We thus specify a probability function throughout the space. For the important class of noises called Gaussian-process noises,[5] the distribution in the space is an n-dimensional, normal (Gaussian) density sphere, centered on the origin. (If $n = 2$, it is the familiar, normal, zero-correlation surface, illustrated

---

[3] Actually, the restrictions to Δf and Δt are incompatible, but it is rigorously true that a signal restricted to a frequency interval Δf cycles per second wide can be specified by $2 \cdot \Delta f$ numbers per second, and the "$2 \cdot \Delta f \cdot \Delta t$ rule" is usually approximately correct.

[4] The spectrum $\Theta(f)$ that corresponds to a waveform $\theta(t)$ is a complex function that specifies either the cosine and sine amplitudes or the resultant amplitude and phase of each of the sinusoids (see footnote 2) that add together to produce the waveform. The concept of paired waveforms and spectra is based on Fourier series and integrals, which are discussed in standard textbooks of mathematics.

[5] The random or "white" noise familiar in psychoacoustic laboratories is approximately a Gaussian-process noise. A Gaussian process is defined as a process that generates signals for which the joint probability density distribution of any m coefficients is an m-dimensional normal distribution.

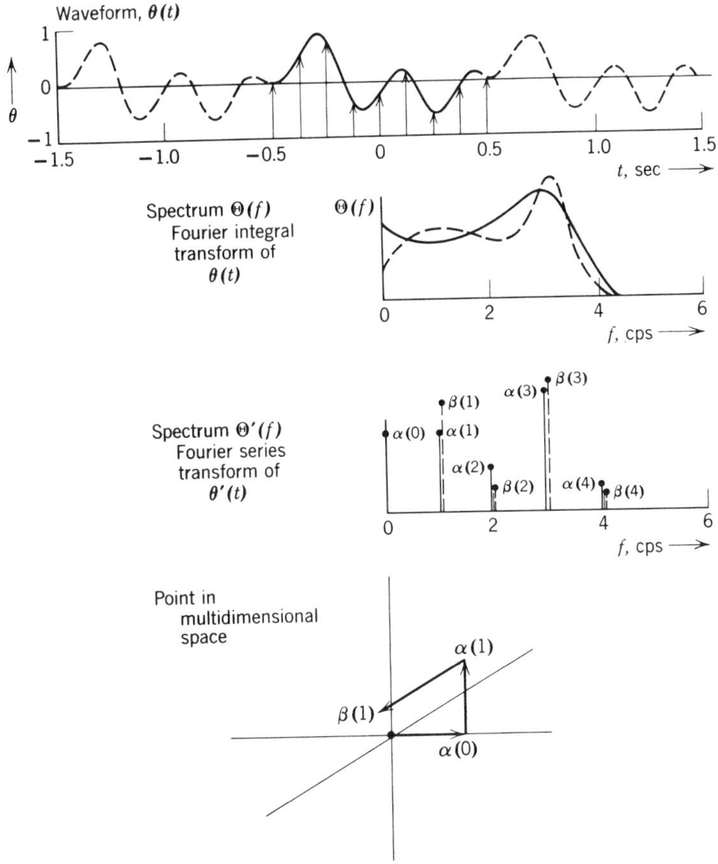

FIG. 1. Schematic illustration of the $2 \cdot \Delta f \cdot \Delta t$ theorem. We start with the waveform $\theta(t)$ shown as a solid curve at the top. It has nonzero values only within an interval 1 sec long. Its spectrum is $\Theta(f)$, a complex function of frequency, represented below the waveform. The solid line is the real part, the dashed line the imaginary part, of the spectrum. The spectrum is limited approximately to the band 0 to 4.5 cycles per second. In order to obtain a representation of $\theta(t)$ and $\Theta(f)$ in terms of a finite number of coefficients, we replicate the waveform over and over throughout all time, as suggested by the dashed extension of $\theta(t)$. The spectrum of the resulting periodic waveform $\theta'(t)$ is $\Theta'(f)$, a function with real (or cosine) coefficients only at zero cycles per second and integral multiples of the fundamental frequency and with imaginary (or sine) coefficients only at integral multiples. The coefficients at frequencies above 4 cycles per second are insignificant because of the band limitations of $\Theta(f)$. There are, therefore, $9 = 2 \cdot \Delta f \cdot \Delta t$ coefficients. The lowermost graph shows three of them represented by a point in three-dimensional space and suggests how the original signal, $\theta(t)$, can be represented as a point in *nine*-dimensional space. Shannon's (1949) sampling theorem shows that the $2 \cdot \Delta f \cdot \Delta t$ sample values of $\theta(t)$ indicated by the equally spaced arrows in the uppermost graph provide an equivalent representation of the wave. They may be used as the coordinates in an alternative n-dimensional space.

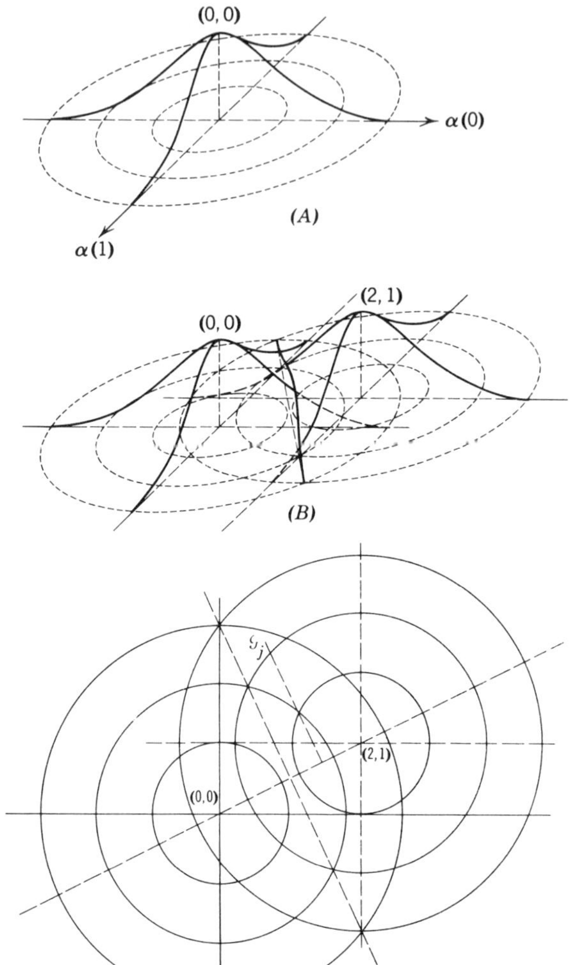

FIG. 2. Representation in signal space. For the sake of simplicity, only two of the dimensions of Fig. 1 are carried over into this figure. A shows the probability density function, in those two dimensions, of the noise alone. $\alpha(0)$ and $\alpha(1)$ are plotted in an oblique plane, and probability density is represented on the vertical scale. The figure is a normal zero-correlation surface centered on the origin (0,0). The dotted rings are one standard-deviation unit apart. B shows simultaneously the probability density function that obtains on the condition that noise alone was presented and the probability density function that obtains on the condition that signal plus noise was presented. The signal point is (2,1). The effect of the noise in the signal-plus-noise case is to spread the probability in the way specified by the right-hand normal surface.

in Fig. 2. If $n = 3$, it can be visualized as a sunlike sphere, centered upon a particular point in the space and having its greatest density at that point, but extending indefinitely outward from the center with density decreasing according to a negative-exponential function.) Adding a precisely known signal to the noise moves the n-dimensional sphere to a new center, the point (which we shall call $\mathfrak{S}$) corresponding to the precisely known signal.

Suppose that, on a particular trial of an experiment, a particular waveform is presented to the listener. In the model, the corresponding thing is a particular point $\mathcal{P}_j$ in the space. The experimenter knows whether he made the waveform by ($\bar{s}$) selecting a sample of noise alone or by (s) adding to a sample of noise a sample of tone. Let us suppose, for the time being, that the listener's sensory channels lose none of the information. Then the listener knows that he has made the observation $\mathcal{P}_j$, that the probabilities governing the experimenter's action were $P(s)$ for tone plus noise and $P(\bar{s})$ for noise alone, and that he is operating under the payoff matrix M. His task is to decide whether to report S or $\bar{S}$. The listener can do no more than figure out how likely it is that $\mathcal{P}_j$ came from s and how likely it is that $\mathcal{P}_j$ came from $\bar{s}$. He therefore examines the two probability density spheres mentioned earlier—the one centered at $\mathfrak{S}$ and the one centered at the origin—and reads off the two values of probability density that pertain to his point $\mathcal{P}_j$. The ratio of the two values, which is the likelihood ratio, is the measure that he compares with the criterion in making his decision.

The likelihood ratio $\mathfrak{l}$ is the ratio of the likelihood (or probability density) $p_s(\mathcal{P}_j)$ that $\mathcal{P}_j$ would stem from s to the likelihood $p_{\bar{s}}(\mathcal{P}_j)$ that $\mathcal{P}_j$ would stem from $\bar{s}$. It depends only upon the relative locations of $\mathcal{P}_j$, $\mathfrak{S}$, and the origin in signal space, and upon the size or spread of the

---

On the left-hand side of the separating curve, the ordinates of the noise function are greater than those of the signal-plus-noise function, and on the right-hand side of the separating curve the ordinates of the signal-plus-noise function are the greater. On any given trial, the observation yields a point in the space [on the plane of $\alpha(0)$, $\alpha(1)$, in this reduced representation], and the information it offers the ideal observer as a basis for his report is the ratio of the two ordinates. This ratio of the probability densities is the likelihood ratio. In C, the $\alpha(0)$, $\alpha(1)$ plane is the plane of the paper, and only the rings are shown to represent the probability density functions. The observation is represented by the point $\mathcal{P}_j$, which is about 2.3 standard-deviation units from the mean of the signal-plus-noise distribution and about 2.7 standard-deviation units from the origin or mean of the noise distribution. The ratio of the probability densities is 3.5, which is, in fact, the ratio of the probability densities anywhere along the projection from $\mathcal{P}_j$ to the line through (0,0) and (2,1). The problem is now to imagine all this in a space of n dimensions, instead of only two.

noise density sphere. For various points $\mathcal{P}$, there are various values of $\mathfrak{l}$, though some different values of $\mathcal{P}$ have the same $\mathfrak{l}$. The important thing is, it is only the value of $\mathfrak{l}$, and nothing else about $\mathcal{P}$ or $\mathfrak{S}$ or the noise sphere or the signal space, that, in making his judgment, the model listener uses as a measure of the stimulation. And $\mathfrak{l}$ is simply a number. The dimension on which it varies is called the decision axis. The only question is whether $\mathfrak{l}$ is greater than or less than the criterion number $\mathfrak{l}_c$.

How is $\mathfrak{l}_c$ determined? Clearly, if the a priori probabilities $P(s)$ and $P(\bar{s})$ are equal and if the payoff matrix is homogeneous $V_{sS} = V_{\bar{s}\bar{S}} = -V_{s\bar{S}} = -V_{\bar{s}S}$, then the decision should be S if $p_s(\mathcal{P}_j) > p_{\bar{s}}(\mathcal{P}_j)$ and $\bar{S}$ if $p_{\bar{s}}(\mathcal{P}_j) > p_s(\mathcal{P}_j)$. The critical value of $\mathfrak{l}$ is therefore $\mathfrak{l}_c = 1$. But if the a priori probabilities $P(s)$ and $P(\bar{s})$ are unequal, or if the payoff matrix is not homogeneous, then it is necessary to determine the value of $\mathfrak{l}_c$ that maximizes the *expected* payoff, the average of the values in the payoff matrix weighted by their probabilities of being applied. Peterson and Birdsall (1953) and Peterson, Birdsall, and Fox (1954) showed how a priori probabilities and the payoff function combine in the maximization. The cutoff point $\mathfrak{l}_c$ must be chosen to maximize $P_s(S) - \gamma P_{\bar{s}}(S)$ where $P_s(S)$ is the conditional probability that, if the signal actually was presented, the listener reports (correctly) that it was presented, $P_{\bar{s}}(S)$ is the conditional probability that, if the signal actually was not presented, the listener reports (incorrectly) that it was presented, and

$$\gamma = \frac{P(\bar{s})}{P(s)} \frac{V_{\bar{s}\bar{S}} - V_{\bar{s}S}}{V_{sS} - V_{s\bar{S}}}$$

The cutoff value that effects the maximization is $\mathfrak{l}_c = \gamma$.

TSG assumes that the distribution of the values of the logarithm $\mathfrak{L}$ of $\mathfrak{l}$ for the no-signal trials is normal with variance σ^2—and that the distribution of $\mathfrak{L}$ for the signal trials is also normal with variance σ^2, as illustrated in Fig. 3. (It is not essential that the distributions of the *logarithm* of $\mathfrak{l}$ be normal. It is essential only that the distributions of some monotonic function of $\mathfrak{l}$ be normal. We are making the assumption for the logarithm of $\mathfrak{l}$ for the sake of specificity.)

The distance between the means of the two density functions in Fig. 3 divided by the standard deviation σ is called d' in TSG. It is the fundamental measure of effective signal strength. To each value of d' corresponds (for an optimal decision process, which the listener is assumed to have) a single-valued function relating $P_s(S)$ and $P_{\bar{s}}(S)$. Under fixed

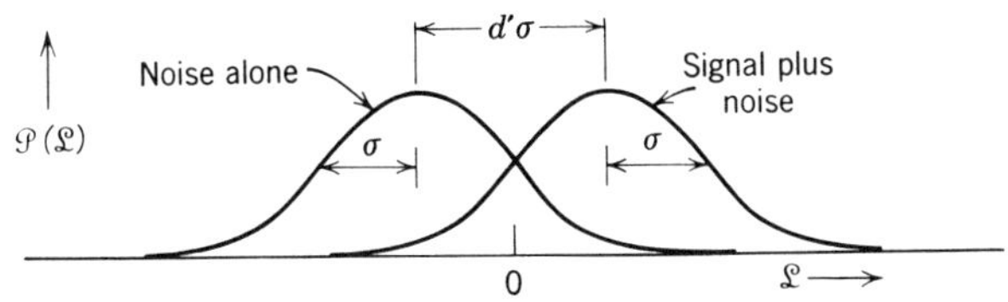

FIG. 3. Probability density functions of $\mathcal{L}$, the logarithm of the likelihood ratio, on the decision axis. The likelihood ratio is the ratio of the two probability density ordinates at $\mathcal{P}_j$, in Fig. 2. As $\mathcal{P}$ takes on various values from trial to trial, we have two probability density functions for the ratio, and therefore, two for its logarithm $\mathcal{L}$. One is for the trials on which noise alone is presented, the other for trials on which signal plus noise is presented. If the noise is Gaussian-process noise, the two probability density functions for $\mathcal{L}$ are normal, as indicated, and their means are separated by the interval $d'\sigma = d'N^{1/2}$. N is the power density of the noise, and d' turns out, in the case of the ideal observer who knows exactly the specifications of the signal and the statistical parameters of the noise, to be $(2E/N)^{1/2}$, where E is the signal energy. Thus $d'\sigma$ is proportional to the rms sound pressure of the signal, σ is proportional to the rms sound pressure of the noise, and d', a dimensionless parameter, is $\sqrt{2}$ times the rms signal-noise ratio.

experimental conditions, therefore, the value of d' can be estimated from the relative frequencies of hits and false alarms.

As we noted earlier, TSG assumes the degrading of the sensory message by internal or neural noise and the restriction of the frequency bandwidths of both signal and noise by a filterlike action of the sensory mechanism. It leaves open for experimental investigation the possibility that information is lost in other ways in the sensory process. This requires an important revision of our thus far too simplified summary of the theory. The revision is required because there are two signal spaces, one in which the acoustic stimulus is located and another in which is located the message that, via the listener's sensory channels, reaches his (assumedly ideal) decision process.[6]

The dimensionality of the stimulus signal space is determined by the experimenter or the external environment that presents the signals. The dimensionality of the listener's internal signal space, on the other hand, is determined by characteristics of the auditory sensory and perceptual system. Both the auditory Δf and the auditory Δt *may* be adjusted by the listener to match the stimulus Δf and the stimulus Δt. The values of the auditory Δf and Δt are not assumed; they are left open to experimental investigation.

[6] This distinction between the two signal spaces is not made explicitly in TSG. I am emphasizing it here because not seeing it at first caused me considerable difficulty.

The points in the auditory signal space corresponding to $\mathcal{S}$ and $\mathcal{P}_j$ in stimulus signal space we may call $\mathcal{S}'$ and $\mathcal{P}_j'$. $\mathcal{S}'$ is the hypothetical point that would arise if the signal were presented alone, without external noise, and if the neural noise were turned off without affecting the auditory bandwidth or examination interval. $\mathcal{P}_j'$ is the point that represents the message actually received at the perceptual display region on trial j. The theory TSG is then essentially a restatement of the story given earlier, but with prime marks inserted to indicate that the listener's decision process operates on likelihood ratios derived from auditory signal space.

The value of d' for an ideal detector is readily derived for the case of a signal known exactly and presented in a uniform spectrum Gaussian-process noise.[7] If E is the energy of the signal and N is the power density (power per unit bandwidth)[8] of the noise, $d' = (2E/N)^{1/2}$. With the aid of that formula, TSG permits ready comparison between the performance of a human detector and the performance, under the same stimulus conditions, of an ideal detector. One simply estimates d' for the human detector from the relative frequencies of hits and false alarms and calculates d' for the ideal detector from $d' = (2E/N)^{1/2}$. The ratio of the two values of d' is an index of the human listener's efficiency, which in TSG is called η.

This summary of TSG has indicated how d' may be inferred from data of experiments based on a particular paradigm, has shown how d', the a priori probabilities $P(s)$ and $P(\bar{s})$, and the payoff matrix M govern the behavior of an optimal detector, and has given an idea of the nature of the decision process assumed to be used by listeners. Supporters of the theory trust that, in interaction with experiment, those parts of the theory concerned with parameters of the auditory system will take fuller shape and become quantitative. Some progress has been made in that direction and in the direction of relating the fundamental ideas of statistical-decision theory to other experimental paradigms, particularly the multilocation forced-choice paradigm.

---

[7] It has been derived, also, for several other sets of conditions (Fox, 1953; Peterson and Birdsall, 1953; Peterson, Birdsall, and Fox, 1954).

[8] Power density is analogous to probability density. It is the limit, as the bandwidth approaches zero, of the ratio of power in the band to width of the band. The unit of power is an erg per second. The unit of bandwidth is a cycle per second or, since the cycle itself is dimensionless, simply "per second." The unit of power density is therefore an erg; the seconds cancel. This makes $2E/N$ dimensionless.

THE VARIABLES OF THE THEORY OF SIGNAL DETECTION

In the theory just outlined, most of the following variables were defined explicitly.

Systematic independent variables

$\mathfrak{s}$	A binary variable with the values s (signal presented) and $\bar{s}$ (signal not presented).
$P(s)$	The probability of s. $P(\bar{s}) = 1 - P(s)$.
$\mathfrak{S}$	A variable of n dimensions, a particular value[9] of which is selected by the experimenter as the signal (which he may or may not present on any given trial).
E	The energy of the signal.
f	Frequency.
Δf	The frequency bandwidth within which the signal lies (also, the bandwidth of the noise).
t	Time.
Δt	The duration of the signal (also, the duration of the noise).
n	$n = 2 \cdot \Delta f \cdot \Delta t$.
$\mathfrak{N}$	A variable of the n dimensions, a particular value $\mathfrak{N}_j$ of which is selected at random from a given distribution to constitute the noise on a particular trial j.
j	The trial index.
N	The power density of the noise. N is a function $N(f)$ of f.
$\mathcal{P}$	A variable of the n dimensions, a particular value $\mathcal{P}_j$ of which is the quantity actually presented on trial j. $\mathcal{P}_j = \mathfrak{S} + \mathfrak{N}_j$ if s; $\mathcal{P}_j = \mathfrak{N}_j$ if $\bar{s}$.
$p_s(\mathcal{P})$	The conditional probability density of $\mathcal{P}$ on the condition s; the likelihood that $\mathcal{P}$ will result if s.
$p_{\bar{s}}(\mathcal{P})$	The conditional probability density of $\mathcal{P}$ on the condition $\bar{s}$; the likelihood that $\mathcal{P}$ will result if $\bar{s}$.
M	A payoff matrix of values V.
$V_{\mathfrak{s}\mathfrak{r}}$	The value to the listener of making response $\mathfrak{r}$ if $\mathfrak{s}$ ($\mathfrak{s}$ is either s or $\bar{s}$).

---

[9] In a more advanced version of the theory, the signal may be drawn from a distribution of values of $\mathfrak{S}$.

Systematic intervening variables

$\mathfrak{S}'$	A variable of n' dimensions derived from $\mathfrak{S}$ by restricting the experimenter's signal to the $\Delta f'$ and $\Delta t'$ characteristic of the auditory system. To an approximation, $\Delta t' = \Delta t$ and $\Delta f'$ is the bandwidth of an "auditory filter." If we call the transfer operation of the filter $\mathcal{F}$, then $\mathfrak{S}' = \mathcal{F}\mathfrak{S}$.
$\mathfrak{N}''$	"Neural" noise, a variable of the n' dimensions.
$\mathcal{P}'$	A variable of the n' dimensions, $\mathcal{P}' = \mathcal{F}\mathcal{P} + \mathfrak{N}''$.
$\mathfrak{l}(\mathcal{P}')$	The likelihood ratio of $\mathcal{P}' : \mathfrak{l}(\mathcal{P}') = p_s(\mathcal{P}')/p_{\bar{s}}(\mathcal{P}')$.
$\mathfrak{L}(\mathcal{P}')$	The logarithm of the likelihood ratio of $\mathcal{P}' : \mathfrak{L}(\mathcal{P}') = \ln \mathfrak{l}(\mathcal{P}')$.
$p_s(\mathfrak{L})$	The conditional probability density of $\mathfrak{L}(\mathcal{P}')$ on the condition s; the likelihood that $\mathfrak{L}(\mathcal{P}')$ will be the value of $\mathfrak{L}$ on a given trial if the signal is presented on that trial.
$p_{\bar{s}}(\mathfrak{L})$	The conditional probability density of $\mathfrak{L}(\mathcal{P}')$ on the condition $\bar{s}$; the likelihood that $\mathfrak{L}(\mathcal{P}')$ will be the value of $\mathfrak{L}$ on a given trial if no signal is presented on that trial.
$\mathfrak{L}_c$	The cutoff or critical value of $\mathfrak{L}$ on the basis of which the listener makes his decision.

Systematic dependent variables

$\mathfrak{r}$	A binary variable with the values S (response signifying listener judges signal was presented) and $\bar{S}$ (response signifying listener judges signal was not presented): $\mathfrak{r} = S$ if $\mathfrak{L} \geq \mathfrak{L}_c$, $\mathfrak{r} = \bar{S}$ if $\mathfrak{L} < \mathfrak{L}_c$.
$P_s(S)$	The conditional probability of the response S on the condition s.
$P_{\bar{s}}(S)$	The conditional probability of the response S on the condition $\bar{s}$.

MODE OF DEFINITION. As we see from inspection of the list, the primary definitions of the independent variables give only their mathematical characteristics. The references to experimenter, the nervous system ("neural"), etc., I have introduced only as mnemonic aids. Calling j the "trial index," for example, is a shorthand way of stating that it is a variable that takes on successive integral values from 1 to some number that is characteristic of an experiment. In effect, the *systematic* or *structural* independent variables have only mathematical properties.

It may be helpful, at this point, to examine somewhat more closely the concept of spectrum that plays such a basic role in the specification of the stimulus. We have used it as little as possible thus far, but it was essential to the discussion of the dimensionality of signal space and of the filtering operation performed upon the signal.

Any monaural acoustic stimulus can be specified, we said, by its waveform [time function $\theta(t)$] or, entirely equivalently, by its spectrum [frequency function $\Theta(f)$]. Since it represents an acoustical wave, the time function $\theta(t)$ is assumed to be real and single-valued. The spectrum $\Theta(f)$, the Fourier transform of $\theta(t)$, is in general complex. Its real part $\alpha(f)$ and its imaginary part $i\beta(f)$ are both functions of frequency. The real and imaginary coefficients, combined in two different ways, give first the amplitudes and second the phases of the sinusoids into which any stimulus may be analyzed, and thus specify the stimulus in terms that make immediate sense in relation to frequency analysis, which is the central auditory problem.

The spectrum specifies the amplitudes and phases of the sinusoidal components in this way: $\alpha(f)$ is the maximum amplitude (or simply amplitude) of a cosine wave $\alpha(f) \cos 2\pi ft$ of frequency f. $\beta(f)$ is the maximum amplitude of a sine wave $\beta(f) \sin 2\pi ft$ of frequency f. The single sinusoidal component of frequency f is the sum of the cosine wave and the sine wave, $\alpha(f) \cos 2\pi ft + \beta(f) \sin 2\pi ft$. This sum is $|\Theta(f)| \cos [2\pi ft + \phi(f)]$. The maximum amplitude of the sum is $|\Theta(f)| = [\alpha^2(f) + \beta^2(f)]^{1/2}$ and the phase angle of the sum is $\phi(f) = \tan^{-1}[\beta(f)/\alpha(f)]$. The stimulus waveform $\theta(t)$ is thought of as the result of adding together (superposing) a number of these elementary components of the form $|\Theta(f)| \cos [2\pi ft + \phi(f)]$, one for each frequency f. In a (conceptual) pure tone, there is only one such component, specified by its amplitude $|\Theta|$, its frequency f, and its phase $2\pi ft + \phi$ at an arbitrary time. In a compound tone, there are several elementary components, each with its three parameters. In a sample of speech or of "random noise," there is an infinite number of components, and in principle it is necessary—if one is to specify the sample uniquely—to give the amplitude $|\Theta(f)|$ and the phase angle $\phi(f)$ as functions of frequency. However, the phase curve is often too complicated to handle. In a true random noise, all the phase angles are random, anyway, and only the amplitude curve is specified. Usually it is given in squared form, $N(f) = |\Theta(f)|^2 = [\alpha(f) + i\beta(f)]\,[\alpha(f) - i\beta(f)]$.

A bothersome problem arises when we try to handle with a simple, constant notation the spectra of sounds that differ in certain ways. We may think of a sound either as having a finite duration or as existing throughout infinite time. A sound of the latter kind can be truly periodic (the waveform consisting of identical segments coming one after another in endless succession), but it need not be. In a rigorous discussion, the three different classes of sounds—finite duration, aperiodic; infinite duration, aperiodic; infinite duration, periodic—must be handled with techniques particularly suitable for them. But the distinctions are not wholly essential for our discussion, and we shall, therefore, not go much further than to observe that all the sounds with which we actually deal can in principle be synthesized from very (i.e., infinitely) many sinusoids of very small but appropriately selected amplitudes and appropriately selected phase angles. Since the actual sound is of finite duration and has finite energy, each of the elementary sinusoids has only infinitesimal energy. If we conceive of an aperiodic sound of infinite duration, we have to attribute to each elementary sound infinitesimal energy per unit time, or infinitesimal power. Only if the conceptual sound is periodic can we think of the elementary sinusoids (harmonics) as having finite power.

The foregoing excursion into the spectral sphere leaves us with the notion that, if we choose to make them so, the sinusoidal components can be our stimulus elements. As we saw, any monaural acoustic stimulus can be represented by a set of these elements, or simply by their amplitudes and phases given as functions of their frequencies. The only trouble with this way of looking at things is that the elements are timeless—or, more precisely, they extend over all time—and we often want to speak of changing the acoustic stimulus. There are elegant ways out of the difficulty, and some of them are very important for auditory theory. In the interest of getting on with the story, however, we shall try to get along without the elegance. Let us take comfort from the thought that, although each sinusoidal component runs from $t = -\infty$ to $t = \infty$, by adding together an infinitude of them we can make, for example, a wave that begins at $t = 0$ and stops at $t = 1$.

To be general, one must specify two spectra (or two waveforms) in order to define a binaural stimulus. Often, however, the main difference between the waves at the two ears is a difference in time of arrival. If the leading wave $\theta_r(t)$ reaches the right ear and the following wave $\theta_l(t) = \theta_r(t - \tau)$ reaches the left ear τ seconds later, the corresponding spectra are $\Theta_r(f) = |\Theta_r(f)| \cos [2\pi ft + \phi_r(f)]$ and $\Theta_l(f) = |\Theta_r(f)| \cos [2\pi ft + \phi_r(f) - 2\pi f\tau]$. This transforms the time difference into a phase difference, a shift (proportional to frequency) of the phases $\phi_r(f)$.

With an infinitude of stimulus elements and no constraints on how many of them we add together to make a stimulus, we can see at once that we can easily swamp ourselves with stimulus patterns. The preoccupation with pure tones, referred to earlier, was in part an effort to avoid the swamping. The current popularity of "white" noise as a stimulus is in part an overreaction: if we are going to have complexity, let us go all the way and have all possible components (up to some cutoff frequency f_c) in equal strength and random phase.

The systematic intervening variables are defined as functions of the systematic independent variables or of other (preceding) intervening variables. The operator $\mathfrak{F}$ I have introduced to provide a bridge between stimulus signal space and intervening signal space. TSG does not stress that distinction, as I said. But TSG clearly assumes that a sweepable auditory bandpass filter intervenes between the stimulus and the signal space. The numerous primes (except for the one in d') are my intrusions, also.

The single systematic dependent variable is defined as a go-no-go function of the intervening variables $\mathfrak{L}$ and $\mathfrak{L}_c$. That completes the structure in purely mathematical, functional form.

The only structural linkages that are not completely specified are $\mathfrak{F}$ and $\mathfrak{N}''$. They are the main objects of experimental investigation. Everything else is determined when the experimenter substitutes specific values for the variables under his control. Note, however, that the determination is that of a rigid formula (except for the randomness of $\mathfrak{N}''$) operating upon a random input. Perhaps one should not stress the word "rigid": the properties of $\mathfrak{F}$ may turn out to vary with time or with systematic independent variables.

INITIAL EVIDENTIAL GROUNDS FOR ASSUMPTIONS

The main initial grounds for the assumptions were not evidential, but there was some evidence. Most of it was evidence *against* the rival formulation based on thresholds. It seems to me that most of this evidence can properly be directed against only a very limited concept of threshold which I think most of my contemporary colleagues have not held, but it is nevertheless true that the evidence had something to do with the adoption of the model based on statistical decision theory.

The main evidence against "the threshold" was that thresholds vary. It was suspected, but only later shown clearly, that a listener[10] could tell something more about the signals he reported absent ($\bar{S}$) than that he had decided to report them absent. He could, for example, say how confident he was that they were absent, and it turned out that he was more confident of the correctness of his $\bar{S}$ on $\bar{s}$-trials than on s-trials.

It has seemed to me, as I implied, that the evidence just mentioned is not critical against a modern version of the threshold concept. To set up

[10] I am using the word "listener" to maintain connection with auditory theory, but actually the theory was applied first (Tanner and Swets, 1954*a*,*b*,*c*) in vision.

an example of the latter, let us assume that we want to detect a segment of tone in fluctuating random noise. We do not know what absolute phase or level to expect, but we know the frequency and the duration that will characterize the signal if it comes. We construct a detector in which the input wave is passed through an amplifier with automatic gain control to stabilize its level against fluctuations of the noise and then into two narrow-band filters, identical except that one is centered on the frequency of the expected signal and the other is set off to one side. (We chose filters with bandwidths equal approximately to the reciprocal of the expected signal duration.) The output of each filter we pass to an envelope-detecting circuit, and we subtract the envelope of the second filter channel from that of the first. Finally, now, we apply the difference time-function to a threshold circuit. It is a nonlinear device that yields output 1 if its input time-function is greater than some value γ', output 0 if its input is less than γ'. Does γ' have to be constant? No, we can arrange to make γ' adjustable by turning a knob, so that we can encourage the device to report 1 if it is very important not to miss the signal, or discourage it from reporting 1 if false alarms are very costly. My engineering friends build devices similar to the one just described, and they refer to the nonlinear circuit as a threshold circuit and speak of adjusting its threshold. The evidence against "the threshold concept" does not react against the idea that a human listener may process his input signal in a way analogous to the detector with a threshold circuit. In fact, one might say that the operation in the TSG model that makes $\mathrm{r} = S$ if $\mathfrak{L} \geq \mathfrak{L}_c$ and $\mathrm{r} = \bar{S}$ if $\mathfrak{L} < \mathfrak{L}_c$ is precisely that of a threshold operator.

In recent discussions with Tanner, Swets, and Green, I have discovered that they distinguish between "sensory" and "response" thresholds and oppose only the former. The distinction seems valuable. The threshold mechanism described in the last paragraph is a "response" mechanism. As a result of the discussions, moreover, I have been forced to recognize that the too limited concept is not just a straw man. The evidence that the listener knows something—which he can later report—about the signal he judges "not presented" indicates that the nonlinear circuit is located at a point following a path of access to his memory. It thus reveals very clearly the flaw in "correction for chance guessing." The fact that that correction has been widely used convinces me that the rigid concept of threshold has in fact been widely held.

In order to talk about evidence for or against a theory, we must know to what empirical independent and dependent variables the systematic dependent and independent variables are related, and by what linkages or identifications. In the present instance, the correspondences are probably so obvious as to require no discussion—or so technical as to inhibit discussion. Let us, therefore, pass over most of the possible treatment of this area and dwell only upon two points that may be unclear.

The empirical signal that corresponds to $\mathfrak{S}$ is typically the result of transducing with an earphone the gated[11] output of a signal generator (usually an oscillator, a generator of sinusoidal signals of controlled frequency and amplitude). The oscillation may be turned on as it crosses the zero-voltage axis and then, at the end of an integral number of half-periods, off again as it again crosses zero. The bandwidth of such a signal is ideally infinite, but of course not practically infinite, since most of its energy is in the neighborhood of the nominal frequency, the frequency of the original, ungated oscillation. In fact, most of its energy lies in the frequency band within $1/\Delta t$ cycles per second of the nominal frequency.

That may raise a question concerning the dimensionality of the signal. We assumed that $\mathfrak{S}$ had n dimensions, where $n = 2 \cdot \Delta f \cdot \Delta t$, and we did not limit Δf or Δt. The fact is that, since the waveform of the signal is fixed by its mode of generation, it has no dimensions of free variability. It is completely specified, and it is in principle no harder to specify it in the space in which the noise is specified than it is in the space of fewer dimensions to which it appears to be confined by the fact that $2 \cdot \Delta f \cdot \Delta t = 4$ when $\Delta f = 2/\Delta t$.

The empirical signal that corresponds to $\mathfrak{N}$ is the filtered output, transduced into sound by an earphone, of a random noise generator. The source of the voltage fluctuations is the thermal motion of electrons in a resistor or the almost equally haphazard motion of ions in a gas tube. Those fluctuations are as nearly purely random as anything is likely to be in a real world. The bandwidth of the noise is ordinarily limited to some value such as 6000 cycles per second by an electrical filter before the noise is delivered to the earphone. That is mainly to facilitate determining the noise power density, however, because the earphone itself acts as a low-pass filter with a cutoff (typically) of 7000 cycles per second.

Usually no attempt is made to specify the empirical item corresponding to $\mathfrak{N}_j$, the particular noise wave on any given trial. The only things that require specification are the probability density functions corresponding to $p_s(\mathcal{P})$ and $p_{\bar{s}}(\mathcal{P})$. The usual procedure is (1) to measure the overall noise power in a band perhaps 1000 cycles per second wide, centered on the signal frequency, (2) to check the uniformity of the power density spectrum $N(f)$ with the aid of a narrow-band scanning filter,

[11] Switched on for a specified interval Δt, then off.

(3) to determine the power density by dividing the overall power by the 1000-cycle-per-second bandwidth, and (4) to check that the distribution of instantaneous noise voltages is approximately normal. The power density is then known rather accurately. The n-dimensional normality corresponding to $p_s(\mathcal{P})$ and $p_{\bar{s}}(\mathcal{P})$ is never checked, I think, but the experimenter is usually nonetheless confident because of faith in the linearity of his equipment and in the power of the central limit theorem.

On the side of the dependent variable, the empirical situation is an experimenter's delight. There is either a double-throw switch or two buttons. The empirical correlates of S and $\bar{S}$ flow from them into relay scoring circuits or into an IBM card puncher.

CONSTRUCTION OF FUNCTION FORMS

The functions that relate succeeding variables to preceding variables are of two kinds. First, there are the operator $\mathfrak{F}$ and the operation of superposing $\mathfrak{F}\,\mathcal{P}$ upon the neural noise $\mathfrak{N}''$. These "functions" are prescribed in rough outline by TSG, but their details are left for experimental study. In contrast are the operations performed upon the variables of the internal signal space. Those operations are wholly specified by the theory.

Actually, all TSG says about $\mathfrak{F}$ is that it involves, as one step, the passage of the external signal through a sweepable bandpass filter of width $\Delta f'$. Implicit, however, is the idea that $\mathfrak{F}$ involves other operations in addition to the filtering. One of them involves loss of some of the information about the phase pattern of $\mathcal{P}$ or, alternatively, of $\mathfrak{S}$.

The overall level and spectral distribution of the neural noise $\mathfrak{N}''$ are left open for experimental investigation, but a feature of the probability density function of $\mathfrak{N}''$ is prescribed indirectly by the assumption that the logarithms $\mathfrak{L}_{\bar{s}}(\mathcal{P})$ and $\mathfrak{L}_s(\mathcal{P})$—or at least some monotonic functions of the likelihood ratios of $\mathfrak{F}\mathfrak{N} + \mathfrak{N}''$ and $\mathfrak{F}(\mathfrak{S} + \mathfrak{N}) + \mathfrak{N}''$—are normally distributed with equal variances.

The forms of the other functions in TSG are specified in full by the assumption that the human decision process is optimal. The decision process derives from the observation point $\mathcal{P}$ and the probability density functions $p_s(\mathcal{P})$ and $p_{\bar{s}}(\mathcal{P})$ the value of $\mathfrak{L}$, and it derives from $P(s)$ and M the value of $\mathfrak{L}_c$, in each instance following without any error or deviation at all the functions we have examined for those operations. It then compares $\mathfrak{L}$ with $\mathfrak{L}_c$ and triggers off the response S or the response $\bar{S}$. Probably an appropriate reaction to these assumptions is that they are too stringent to be realistic for a model of human judgment. It hardly seems reasonable to suppose that while the sensory system loses information the decision process is ideal. Actually, however, Tanner, Swets, and Green are entirely willing to qualify the assumption of idealness as soon as the experimental work progresses far enough to permit discrimination between sensory losses of information and losses due to uncertainties in the decision process. They point out, however, that the latter cannot be far from ideal in some situations, for the over-all performance of the human detector is sometimes only a little less good than that of an optimal device.

MEASUREMENT OF INDEPENDENT AND DEPENDENT VARIABLES

The procedures specified by TSG for the measurement of the independent and dependent variables are wholly quantitative and consistent with the requirements of the functions of the theory in every point except the payoff matrix M. The quantitative specification of the stimulus and response variables presents no problems, as we have noted, other than purely technical ones that are handled effectively with the aid of modern electroacoustic instrumentation. It is not yet possible, however, to measure or control with full authority the value system of the listener. That fact has led to an emphasis, in experimental work related to TSG, of the method of forced choice among alternative positions or intervals.

In the multilocation forced-choice method, almost all the assumptions about the values in the payoff matrix are neutralized or canceled. The one very plausible assumption that is not thus eliminated is that the values $V_{\mathfrak{s}r}$ remain constant throughout the duration of a trial. In general, there are in a forced-choice trial m alternative stimulus intervals or positions. The listener's task is to report in which one of them the signal $\mathfrak{S}$ appeared. According to the theory, as developed to apply to this situation, the listener derives m values of $\mathfrak{L}$, corresponding to the m intervals, and reports the number of the interval for which $\mathfrak{L}$ is greatest. If m were large, this would place a burden upon his memory, but m is usually 2, and rarely greater than 4. TSG includes a procedure for calculating d' from the percentage of correct responses in m location forced-choice tests, and thereby permits comparison between forced-choice results and yes-no results.

Within the context of the multilocation forced-choice method, we may say that TSG has essentially no serious measurement difficulties. It is quantitatively specific to as high a degree as most theories in physical science.

FORMAL ORGANIZATION OF THE SYSTEM

In a sense, TSG is organized on a high level of axiomatization, for the published account presents eleven formal postulates. The question is, what kinds of deduction or derivation do the postulates support?

There are three answers to that question, depending upon the extent to which we read into the theory substantive properties of $\mathcal{F}$ and $\mathfrak{N}''$. Without definite assumptions about these two functions, the postulates specify the *form* into which stimulus information is converted for digestion by the decision process, but not the *quantity*. With only the definite statements made in the postulates (that $\mathcal{F}$ involves a sweepable band-pass filter characteristic, that $\mathfrak{N}'' > 0$), only very nonspecific, nonquantitative deductions can be made. With statements about $\mathcal{F}$ and $\mathfrak{N}''$ of the type that are beginning to emerge from the experimental work, it should eventually be possible to build a quantitative auditory theory.

The situation just outlined suggests this characterization of TSG: It is a formal, axiomatized recipe for studying the auditory process. It is the bare beginning of a substantive theory. The main exceptions to that generalization are points upon which the formal theory makes statements about substantive properties of hearing; for example, that the auditory system involves a sweepable filter (instead of a manifold of filters with fixed center frequencies), and that the decision process is ideal. These points the theory might better have left for empirical study, for they will be so studied, in any case.

Inasmuch as it is unusual to find postulates in auditory theories, we might ask what led to the formality of the treatment. Almost surely, it was the unusual circumstance of finding, ready-made, a structure that appeared to have relevance to sensory processes. The initial task of the theorists was to discover how the structure of statistical decision theory could be lined up with the procedure of sensory experiments. That led to deliberate manipulation of the several pieces of the puzzle. When a promising alignment was achieved, it was quite natural to make a series of statements relating the corresponding parts. That was done first for vision. The auditory theory followed the same pattern. The formality of the auditory theory thus appears to be related to the fact that statistical-decision theory had already evolved and achieved formality in another field. If it is true that axiomatization is more valuable as a way of compressing an established theory for storage than as a way of bringing theory into contact with experiment, then we may see TSG lose some of its formality for a time.

SCOPE OF THE SYSTEM

PRESENT AND INTENDED SCOPES. The theory we have been calling TSG is actually the auditory part of what the group at Michigan views as a general sensory theory. There has been no need to say how general, but certainly the possible scope includes all the senses and functions other than detection per se.

A natural extension of the theory that we have examined involves relaxation of the assumption that the same signal, $\mathcal{S}$, is the signal for each trial. The mathematics has been worked out (Peterson and Birdsall, 1953; Peterson, Birdsall, and Fox, 1954) for detection in situations in which the signal (exclusive of the noise) is selected at random from a set of orthogonal signals. This is close to the basic paradigm for communication. The function of identifying the received signal as a particular one of the transmitted signals is usually called recognition or identification or classification. It differs from detection in that the crucial question is which signal was sent, not simply was a signal sent. When there are only two signals in the ensemble, however, the difference disappears. Tanner (1956) has described the extension of TSG to recognition in a two-alternative situation. Moreover, he has pointed out the applicability of some of Birdsall's results on the case of m-orthogonal alternatives to the recognition of speech sounds [see 32].

Detection is usually thought of as confined to the realm of weak signals, or of signals comparable in level to the noise. However, the extension of the theory to include recognition, identification, or classification automatically brings large signals into the picture. If alternative signals $\mathcal{S}_1$ and $\mathcal{S}_2$ are close enough together in signal space, it may take a high signal-noise ratio to permit high-probability identification of $\mathcal{S}_1$. Experimental work on problems suggested by this extension is now under way in the Engineering Research Institute at Michigan.

INTERRELATIONS WITH OTHER FORMULATIONS. TSG is very closely related to the less formal application of ideas of statistical-decision theory by Smith and Wilson (1953) and to the more tutorial exposition of the ideas by Marill (1956). The three developments are so similar that they may be lumped together under the heading, "statistical-decision theories of auditory detection."

Also very closely related are models of the auditory process, or parts of it, which do not assume an ideal decision process, but which are nonetheless statistical. These have followed approximately the pattern described earlier as an example of a threshold mechanism not subject to the criticisms directed against the limited conception of threshold. Simple models of that kind have been described, for example, by Schafer, Gales, Shewmaker, and Thompson, (1950) and by Sherwin, Kodman, Kovaly, Prothe, and Melrose (1956). These models are in one sense supplementary to TSG, for they are specific in detail about the parts of the process $\mathcal{F}$ and $\mathfrak{N}''$ that TSG leaves open. On the other hand, they do not assume maximum likelihood decision, and in that respect differ fundamentally.

Considerably further away is the quantum hypothesis of sensory discrimination (Stevens, 1951). The quantum hypothesis assumes internal fluctuations of the sort that might be referred to as neural noise, and it holds that those fluctuations are continually taking the measure of signal strength up and down the scale past the critical, or quantal, levels at which it is marked. Passing a single quantal level is, therefore, not significant of a change in stimulation, but passing two quantal levels almost simultaneously is significant, for the fluctuations practically never move the measure very far in a short interval. The quantum theory does not go into detail about the spectrum of the fluctuations or about other intervening processes. Like TSG, it provides a recipe for, or a guide to, experimental investigation of important parameters. However, the important parameters of the two theories are quite different. That serves to insulate the theories from each other. Further insulation is imposed by the fact that the experimental procedures specified or suggested by the theorists are in some respects essentially incompatible. The sensory quantum theorists have argued for and have used a procedure in which the listener knows when the signal was presented and reports whether or not he heard it. This is completely contrary to the spirit of the statistical-decision theorists who, if they were serving as subjects, would say "I hear it" each time the signal was due. For them, the subject's obligation is not to give an accurate account of his sensory state but to maximize his payoff. It is unfortunate that the two theories are not in closer contact with each other. Perhaps they may be brought into contact despite the insulation.

Finally, there is the rigid sensory threshold theory that supports "correction for chance guessing." The statistical-decision theories collide vigorously with it. Happily, the collision is on a point susceptible to empirical test.

HISTORY OF INTERACTION WITH RESEARCH

EXPERIMENTS RELATED TO THE THEORY. The experiments of Smith and Wilson (1953) showed clearly that listeners can adjust their "thresholds" in response to the experimenter's verbal instructions concerning the relative costs of misses and false alarms. Tanner and Swets (1954*a*,

1954*b*), in a visual experiment, actually used a monetary payoff matrix, changes in which markedly affected the experimental estimates of $P_s(S)$ and $P_{\bar{s}}(S)$. They showed that application of corrections for chance led to "thresholds" that depended upon the false-alarm rate, thereby revealing the inconsistency in the rigid threshold concept. Then Tanner, Swets, and Green (1956) demonstrated that the same applies to hearing.

The equality of the values of d' determined in yes-no and in multi-location forced-choice trials was demonstrated in vision (Tanner and Swets, 1954*a*; Tanner and Swets, 1954*b*) and then in hearing (Tanner and Norman, 1954; Tanner, Swets, and Green, 1956). This must be regarded as a real accomplishment for the theory and a break in the trend that has been developing—to regard the results of a psychophysical test as meaningless except in relation to the procedure of the test.

The experimental results to date indicate that the curve of the function relating $P_s(S)$ to $P_{\bar{s}}(S)$ for constant stimulus conditions and varying payoff matrix is indeed approximately a curve of constant d'. That is the same as saying that the curve is approximately linear when the probabilities are plotted on normal probability paper. The finding is itself one with important practical application.

The extension to the study of recognition of one or the other of two tones differing in frequency involved the assumption that the recognition axis (the decision axis on which the cut is made between "higher" and "lower") is the axis of the resultant of two vectors. One vector is a value of $\mathfrak{L}$ on the detection decision axis for the higher tone and the other is a value of $\mathfrak{L}$ on the detection decision axis for the lower tone. From his data, Tanner (1956) estimated the angle between the two detection decision axes. Zero corresponded to identity of the two axes; 90° corresponded to complete independence of the two component decisions. Tanner estimated the angle for various intervals of separation in frequency between the two tones, and it turned out that the separation required for effective independence, i.e., about 70°, was about the same as the critical bandwidth determined by Fletcher (1938, 1940) and by Schafer et al. (1950). That amounts to a demonstration that the theory can handle an important substantive problem. In the isolated instance, it offers no clear advantage over other formulations (Fletcher and Schafer et al. determined "thresholds"), but it holds out the promise of handling other problems within the same framework. Providing a common framework for the study of a variety of auditory problems would constitute an important contribution.

Apparently in an effort to develop such a role for the theory, the Michigan group has focused its attention during the last year on a series of substantive auditory problems. Until the results of these and still further studies are available, we cannot see how successful the theory is in its "framework" role. In one instance, however, there is a preliminary report (Green, personal communication), and also a simultaneous and independent study for comparison, a study made outside the specific framework of TSG but within the framework of statistical-decision theory (Marill, 1956).

Using the forced-choice procedure, Green and Marill studied the problem of "summation." If two segments of sinusoid $\mathfrak{S}_1$ and $\mathfrak{S}_2$ are equally detectable—have the same probability of correct response in forced-choice trials—how detectable is their sum $\mathfrak{S}_3 = \mathfrak{S}_1 + \mathfrak{S}_2$? Both Green and Marill asked that question for pairs of frequencies within the interval of a critical bandwidth and also for pairs of frequencies more widely separated. Green used binaural (diotic) presentation, applying the same waveform to both ears of his listeners, whereas Marill used monaural presentation. When the two frequencies were within the critical bandwidth, there was summation in both experiments: $\mathfrak{S}_3$ was detected more often than $\mathfrak{S}_1$ or $\mathfrak{S}_2$. But with widely spaced frequencies, Green found summation and Marill did not. That called for a careful investigation of all possibilities, which Green is now making with Marill's apparatus, and with both monaural and binaural (diotic) presentation. Thus far, Green's data are supporting the conclusion that there is more two-frequency summation with two ears than with one. Tanner (personal communication) is therefore doing an experiment with three frequencies.

On the basis of the summary of research just given, it is obvious that it is too early to judge the theory on the basis of evidence pro and con. Thus far, there is no strong contrary evidence, but neither is there evidence capable of destroying all the alternatives. Actually, because of the nature of the theory, it is unlikely that it will be proved or disproved. Certainly parts of it will change, and new parts will be added. Despite its surface formality, the theory is flexible enough to adapt.

The most vulnerable point appears to me to be the "sweepable filter." It is a formulation, in the terms used by electronic and communication engineers, of a conception that is perhaps as accurately described in the very different terms of the searchlight analogy of attention. The searchlight sweeps back and forth across the data display surface, but it cannot illuminate the entire surface at once. A critical test of this notion in the auditory context would have to be made with signals that constitute better Gestalten than do the compounds of sinusoids used in the experiments. The problem is to determine whether or not two widely separated components of the external signal can contribute simultaneously to the signal in internal signal space, and thereby to the measure on the decision axis. It might be possible to design a critical test by momentarily eliminating one narrow frequency band and then another of a random noise. The eliminations could be made of such short duration that a sweeping filter of the postulated bandwidth and sweep speed would miss some of them. The question would then be, of course, whether or not a listener would fail to notice some of them, too. My guess is that he would be embarrassingly sensitive to such changes in the noise spectrum. On the other hand, the theory may protect itself even here through its flexibility. The theory is not committed to any assumption of fixed bandwidth. Perhaps the filter would just broaden itself instead of sweeping.

THE FUTURE OF THE THEORY

Early experiments mentioned in the preceding section were set up to test either the statistical-decision theory or a rival formulation. The later experiments were part of a program to bring within the framework of the theory various substantive parts of the field of hearing. We shall doubtless have more of both kinds. We shall also have experiments less directly, but nonetheless clearly, influenced by statistical-decision theory. They will employ payoff matrixes or the forced-choice procedure, but they will probably not assume maximum likelihood estimation.

The part of the program aimed at testing the theory will probably focus on the question of internal consistency: Do various procedures yield the same value of d'? It may prove possible to discriminate experimentally between TSG and formulations involving fluctuating thresholds. If so, there is sure to be activity along that line.

The part of the program aimed at unifying a considerable area of psychoacoustics within the statistical-decision framework will continue, if present plans are followed, with experiments on the detection of signals not specified exactly to the listener, on the recognition of signals selected from various numbers of alternatives, and on the progressive increase in detection probability with repeated presentation of the same signal. These experiments will get at such questions as the extent to which phase information is used by the auditory system, the precision with which frequency information is transmitted, the usefulness of the detection theory concepts in the realm of strong signals, and the properties of the neural noise.

Finally, the broader influence of statistical-decision theory, extending beyond the specific formulation we have discussed, will almost surely encompass most of psychoacoustics. More and more, workers in the field are growing dissatisfied with the classical psychophysical techniques, particularly with the method of "adjustment" or "production" that lets the listener attend to the stimulus for an unspecified length of time before deciding that he can "just hear it" and with the methods of "limits" and "constants" (in their usual forms) that ask the listener to report "present" or "absent" when he already knows "present." It is widely felt that the "thresholds" yielded by these procedures are on such an insecure semantic basis that they cannot serve as good building blocks for a quantitative science. That means that practically the whole of classical auditory psychophysics needs to be redone with payoff matrixes or forced choices among alternative locations. With the old areas to be resurveyed and with new horizons opening up, it may be a busy time.

ACKNOWLEDGMENTS

This is a part of an article entitled "Three Auditory Theories" which appeared in S. Koch (Ed.), Psychology: A Study of Science, Vol. 1. New York: McGraw-Hill, 1959, pp. 41–144.

References

- Fletcher, H. The mechanism of hearing as revealed through experiment on the masking effect of thermal noise. *Proc. Nat. Acad. Sci.,* 1938, **24,** 265–276.
- Fletcher, H. Auditory patterns. *Rev. Modern Phys.,* 1940, **12,** 47–65.
- Fox, W. C. Signal detectability: a unified description of statistical methods employing fixed and sequential observation processes. University of Michigan: Electronic Defense Group, 1953, Technical Report No. 19.
- Marill, T. Detection theory and psychophysics. Massachusetts Institute of Technology: Research Laboratory of Electronics, 1956, Technical Report No. 319.
- Peterson, W. W., and Birdsall, T. G. The theory of signal detectability. University of Michigan: Electronic Defense Group, 1953, Technical Report No. 13.
- Peterson, W. W., Birdsall, T. G., and Fox, W. C. The theory of signal detectability. *Trans. IRE Professional Group on Information Theory,* 1954, **PGIT-4,** 171–212.
- Schafer, T. H., Gales, R. S., Shewmaker, C. A., and Thompson, P. O. The frequency selectivity of the ear as determined by masking experiments. *J. acoust. Soc. Am.,* 1950, **22,** 490–496.
- Shannon, C. E. *The mathematical theory of communication.* Urbana, Ill.: University of Illinois Press, 1949.
- Sherwin, C. W., Kodman, F., Jr., Kovaly, J. J., Prothe, W. C., and Melrose, J. Detection of signals in noise: a comparison between the human detector and an electronic detector. *J. acoust. Soc. Am.,* 1956, **28,** 617–622.
- Smith, M., and Wilson, E. A. A model of the auditory threshold and its application to the problem of the multiple observer. *Psychol. Monogr.,* 1953, **67,** No. 9, Whole No. 359.

- Stevens, S. S. Mathematics, measurement, and psychophysics. In S. S. Stevens (Ed.), *Handbook of experimental psychology*. New York: Wiley, 1951, Chapter 1.
- Tanner, W. P., Jr. Theory of recognition. *J. acoust. Soc. Am.*, 1956, **28,** 882–888. [19]
- Tanner, W. P., Jr., and Norman, R. Z. The human use of information, II: Signal detection for the case of an unknown signal parameter. *Trans. IRE Professional Group on Information Theory*, 1954, **PGIT-4,** 222–227.
- Tanner, W. P., Jr., and Swets, J. A. A new theory of visual detection. University of Michigan: Electronic Defense Group, 1954*a*, Technical Report No. 18.
- Tanner, W. P., Jr., and Swets, J. A. The human use of information, I: Signal detection for the case of the signal known exactly. *IRE Trans. Professional Group on Information Theory*, 1954*b*, **PGIT-4,** 213–221.
- Tanner, W. P., Jr., and Swets, J. A. Psychophysical application of the theory of signal detectability. University of Michigan: Engineering Research Institute, 1954*c*. Reprinted from Minutes of Armed Forces-NRC Vision Committee, Nov. 13, 1953.
- Tanner, W. P., Jr., Swets, J. A., and Green, D. M. Some general properties of the hearing mechanism. University of Michigan: Electronic Defense Group, 1956, Technical Report No. 30.

4

Is There a Sensory Threshold?

John A. Swets

One hundred years ago, at the inception of an experimental psychology of the senses, G. T. Fechner focused attention on the concept of a sensory threshold, a limit on sensitivity. His *Elemente der Psychophysik* (1860) described three methods—the methods of adjustment, of limits, and of constants—for estimating the threshold value of a stimulus. The concept and the methods have been in active service since. Students of sensory processes have continued to measure the energy required for a stimulus to be just detectable, or the difference between two stimuli necessary for the two to be just noticeably different. Very recently there has arisen reasonable doubt that sensory thresholds exist.

The threshold thought to be characteristic of sensory systems has been regarded in the root sense of that word as a barrier that must be overcome. It is analogous to the threshold discovered by physiologists in single neurons. Just as a nervous impulse either occurs or does not occur, so it has been thought that when a weak stimulus is presented we either detect it or we do not, with no shades in between. The analogy with the neuron's all-or-none action, of course, was never meant to be complete; it was plain that at some point above the threshold sensations come in various sizes.

From the start the triggering mechanism of the sensory systems was regarded as inherently unstable. The first experiments disclosed that a given stimulus did not produce a consistent "yes" ("I detect it") response or a consistent "no" ("I do not detect it") response. Plots of the "psychometric function"—the proportion of "yes" responses as a function of the stimulus energy—were in the form of ogives, which suggested an underlying bell-shaped distribution of threshold levels. Abundant evidence for continuous physiological change in large numbers of receptive and nervous elements in the various sensory systems made this picture eminently reasonable. Thus, the threshold value of a stimulus had to be specified in statistical terms. Fechner's experimental methods were designed to obtain good estimates of the mean and the variance of the threshold distribution.

It was also assumed from the beginning that the observer's attitude affects the threshold estimate. The use of ascending and descending series of stimulus energies in the method of limits, to take one example, is intended to counterbalance the errors of "habituation" and "anticipation"—errors to which the observer is subject for extrasensory reasons. Typically, investigators have not been satisfied with experimental observers who were merely well motivated; they have felt the need for elite observers. They have attempted, by selection or training, to obtain observers who could maintain a reasonably constant criterion for a "yes" response.

The classical methods for measuring the threshold, however, do not provide a measure of the observer's response criterion that is independent of the threshold measure. As an example, we may note that a difference between two threshold estimates obtained with the method of limits can be attributed to a criterion change only if it is assumed that sensitivity has remained constant, or to a sensitivity change only if it is assumed that the criterion has remained constant. So, although the observer's response criterion affects the estimate of the threshold, the classical procedures do not permit calibration of the observer with respect to his response criterion.

Within the past 10 years methods have become available that provide a reliable, quantitative specification of the response criterion. These methods permit isolation of the effects of the criterion, so that a relatively pure measure of sensitivity remains. Interestingly, the data collected with these methods give us good reason to question the existence of sensory thresholds, to wonder whether anything more than a response criterion is involved in the dichotomy of "yes" and "no" responses. There is now reason to believe that sensory excitation varies continuously and that an apparent threshold cut in the continuum results simply from restricting the observer to two categories of response.

The methods that permit separating the criterion and sensitivity measures, and a psychophysical theory that incorporates the results obtained with these methods, stem directly from the modern approach taken by engineers to the general problem of signal detection. The psychophysical "detection theory," like the more general theory, has two parts. One part is a literal translation of the theory of testing statistical hypotheses, or statistical decision theory. It is this part of the theory that provides a solution to the criterion estimation problem and deals with sensitivity as a continuous variable. The second part is a theory of ideal observers. It specifies the mathematically ideal detection performance—the upper limit on detection performance that is imposed by the environment—in terms of measurable parameters of the signal and of the masking noise.[1]

We shall turn in a moment to a description of the theory and to samples of the supporting data. Before proceeding any further, however, we must note that, although Fechner started the study of sensory functions along lines we are now questioning, he also anticipated the present line of attack in both of its major aspects. For one thing, he regarded Bernoulli's ideas on statistical decision as highly relevant to psychophysical theory (Boring, 1950, p. 284). More important, while advancing the concept of a threshold, he spoke also of what he called "negative sensations"—that is, of a grading of sensory excitation below the threshold. That subsequent workers in the field of psychophysics have shown little interest in negative sensations is apparent from the fact that, 75 years after Fechner's work, Boring could write: "So also a sensation either occurs from stimulation or it does not. If it does not, it has no demonstrable intensity. Fechner talked about negative (subliminal) degrees of intensity, but that is not good psychology today. Above the limen we can sense degrees of intensity, but introspection cannot directly measure these degrees. We are forced to comparison, and there again we meet an all-or-none principle. Either we can observe a difference or we cannot. Introspection as to the amount of difference is not quantitatively reliable" (Boring, 1933).

DECISION ASPECTS OF SIGNAL DETECTION

How detection theory succeeds in estimating the response criterion may be described in terms of "the fundamental detection problem." The experimenter defines an interval of time for the observer, and the observer must decide whether or not a signal is present during the interval. It is assumed that every interval contains some random interference, or noise—noise that is inherent in

[1] The general theory of signal detectability is presented in Peterson, Birdsall, and Fox (1954). Psychophysical theories similar to it have been suggested by Smith and Wilson (1953) and Munson and Karlin (1954). The first application of detection theory in psychophysics is described in Tanner and Swets (1954).

the environment, or is produced inadvertently by the experimenter's equipment for generating signals, or is deliberately introduced by the experimenter, or is simply a property of the sensory system. Some intervals contain a specified signal in addition to the background of noise. The observer's report is limited to these two classes of stimulus events—he says either "yes" (a signal was present) or "no" (only noise was present). Note that he does not say whether or not he *saw* (or *heard*) the signal; he says whether, under the particular circumstances, he prefers the decision that it was present or the decision that it was absent.

There is presumably, coinciding with the observation interval, some neural activity in the relevant sensory system. This activity forms the sensory basis—a part of the total basis—for the observer's report. This "sensory excitation," as we shall call it, may be in fact either simple or complex; it may have many dimensions or few; it may be qualitative or quantitative; it may be anything. The exact, or even the general, nature of the actual sensory excitation is of no concern to the application of the theory.

Only two assumptions are made about the sensory excitation. One is that it is continually varying; because of the ever-present noise, it varies over time in the absence of any signal, as well as from one presentation to the next of what is nominally the same signal. The other is that the sensory excitation, insofar as it affects the observer's report, may be represented as a unidimensional variable. In theory, the observer is aware of the probability that each possible excitatory state will occur during an observation interval containing noise alone and also during an observation interval containing a signal in addition to the noise, and he bases his report on the ratio of these two quantities, the likelihood ratio. The likelihood ratio derived from any observation interval is a real, nonzero number and hence may be represented along a single dimension.

THE LIKELIHOOD-RATIO CRITERION. The observer's report after an observation interval is supposed to depend upon whether or not the likelihood ratio measured in that interval exceeds some critical value of the likelihood ratio, a response criterion. The criterion is presumed to be established by the observer in accordance with his detection goal and the relevant situational parameters. If he wishes to maximize the number of correct responses, his criterion will depend upon the a priori probability that a signal will occur in a given interval. If he chooses to maximize the total payoff, his criterion will depend on this probability and also on the values and costs associated with the four possible outcomes of a decision. Several other detection goals can be defined; the way in which each of them determines the criterion has been described elsewhere (Swets, Tanner, and Birdsall, 1955). In any case, the criterion employed by the observer can be expressed as a value of the likelihood ratio. Thus, the observer's decision about an interval is based not only on the sensory information he obtains in that interval but also on advance information of various kinds and on his motivation.

Next, consider a probability defined on the variable likelihood ratio—in particular, the probability that each value of likelihood ratio will occur with each of the classes of possible stimulus events: noise alone and signal plus noise. There are, then, two probability distributions. The one associated with signal plus noise will have a greater mean. (Indeed, its mean is assumed to increase monotoncially with increases in the signal strength; but for the moment we are considering a particular signal.) Now, if the observer follows the procedure we have described—that is, if he reports that the signal is present whenever the likelihood ratio exceeds a certain criterion and that noise alone is present whenever the likelihood ratio is less than this criterion—then, from the fourfold stimulus-response matrix that results, one can extract two independent measures: a measure of the observer's response criterion and a measure of his sensitivity.

THE OPERATING CHARACTERISTIC. The extraction of these two measures depends upon an analysis in terms of the operating characteristic. If we induce the observer to change his criterion from one set of trials to another, and if, for each criterion, we plot the proportion of "yes" reports made when the signal is present (the proportion of hits, or p_1) against the proportion of "yes" reports made when noise alone is present (the proportion of false alarms, or p_0), then, as the criterion varies, a single curve is traced (running from 0 to 1.0 on both coordinates) that shows the proportion of hits to be a nondecreasing function of the proportion of false alarms. This operating-characteristic curve describes completely the successive stimulus-response matrices that are obtained, since the complements of these two proportions are the proportions that belong in the other two cells of the matrix. The particular curve generated in this way depends upon the signal and noise parameters and upon the observer's sensitivity; the point on this curve that corresponds to any given stimulus-response matrix represents the criterion employed by the observer in producing that matrix.

It has been found that, to a good approximation, the operating-characteristic curves produced by human observers correspond to theoretical curves based on normal probability distributions. These curves can be characterized by a single parameter: the difference between the means of the signal-plus-noise and noise-alone distributions divided by the standard deviation of the noise distribution. This parameter has been called d'. Moreover, the slope of the curve at any point is equal to the value of the likelihood-ratio criterion that produces that point.

THE YES-NO EXPERIMENT. The procedure employed in the fundamental detection problem is often referred to as the "yes-no procedure," and we shall adopt this terminology. Two operating-characteristic curves resulting from this procedure are shown in Fig. 1. The data points were obtained in an auditory experiment in which the observers attempted to detect a tone burst in a background of white noise. The curves are the theoretical curves that fit the data best. The inserts at lower right in the two graphs show the normal probability distributions underlying the curves and the five criteria corresponding to the data points. In this particular experiment the observers changed their criteria from one set of trials to another as the experimenter changed the a priori probability of the occurrence of the signal. The distance between the means of the two distributions is shown as 0.85 for observer No. 1 and as 1.40 for observer No. 2; this distance is equal to d' under the convention that the standard deviation of the noise distribution is unity.

We may note that the curve fitted to the data of the first observer is symmetrical about the negative diagonal, and that the curve fitted to the data of the second observer is not. Both types of curves are seen frequently; the second curve is especially characteristic of data collected in visual experiments. Theoretically, the curve shown in the graph at left will result if the observer knows the signal exactly—that is, if he knows its frequency, amplitude, starting time, duration, and phase. A theoretical curve like the one shown in the graph at right results if the observer has inadequate information about frequency and phase, or, as is the case when the signal is a white light, if there is no frequency and phase information. The probability distributions that are shown in the inserts reflect this difference between the operating-characteristic curves.

Both of the curves shown are based on the assumption that sensory excitation is continuous, that the observer can order values of sensory excitation throughout its range. Two other experiments have been employed to test the validity of this assumption: one involves a variant of the forced-choice procedure; the other involves a rating procedure. We shall consider these experiments in turn.

THE SECOND-CHOICE EXPERIMENT. In the forced-choice procedure, four temporal intervals were defined on each trial, exactly one of which contained the signal. The signal was a small spot of light projected

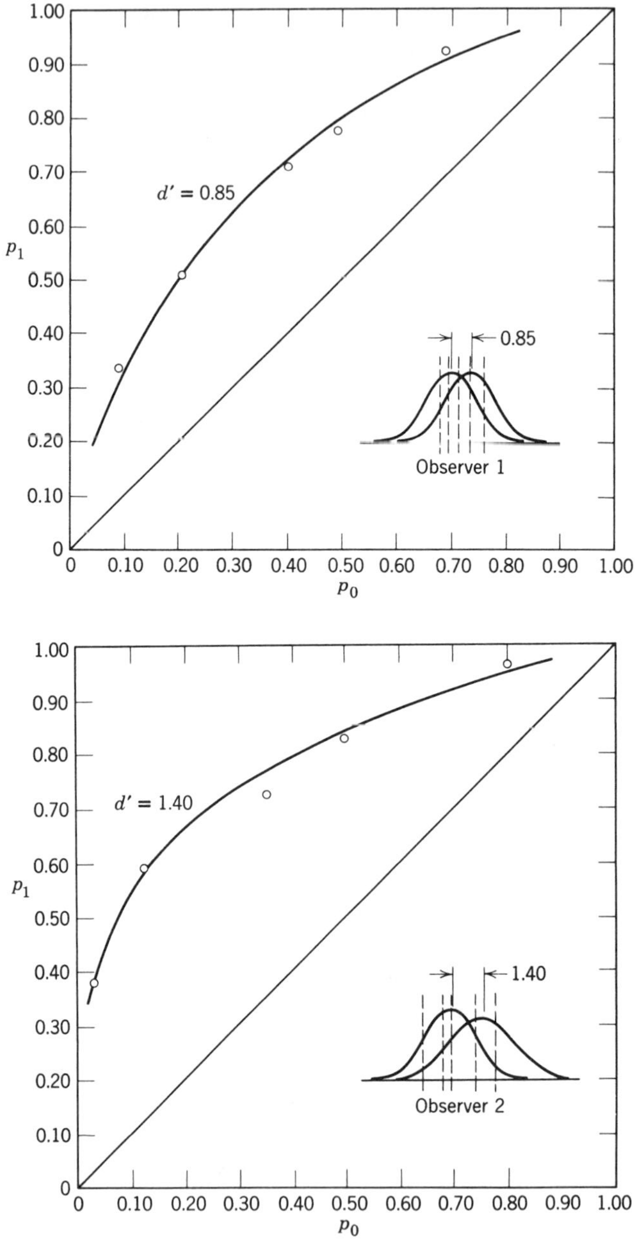

FIG. 1. Two theoretical operating-characteristic curves, with data from a yes-no experiment.

briefly on a large, uniformly illuminated background. Ordinarily, the observer simply chooses the interval he believes most likely to have contained the signal. In this experiment the observer made a second choice as well as a first.

The results are shown in Fig. 2. The top curve is the theoretical function relating the proportion of correct first choices to d'; the lower curve is the theoretical relation of the proportion of correct second choices to d'. The points on the graph represent the proportions of correct second choices obtained by experiment. They are plotted at the value of d' corresponding to the observed proportion of correct first choices.

It may be seen that the data points are fitted well by the theoretical curve. The rather considerable variability can be attributed to the fact that each point is based on less than 100 observations. In spite of the variability, it is clear that the points deviate significantly from the horizontal dashed line. The dashed line may be taken as a baseline; it assumes a sensory threshold such that it is exceeded on only a negligible proportion of the trials when noise alone is presented. Should such a threshold exist, the second choice would be correct only by chance. The data indicate that the observer is capable of ordering values of sensory excitation well below this point. Two sensory thresholds are shown in the insert at lower right in Fig. 2. The threshold on the right, at three

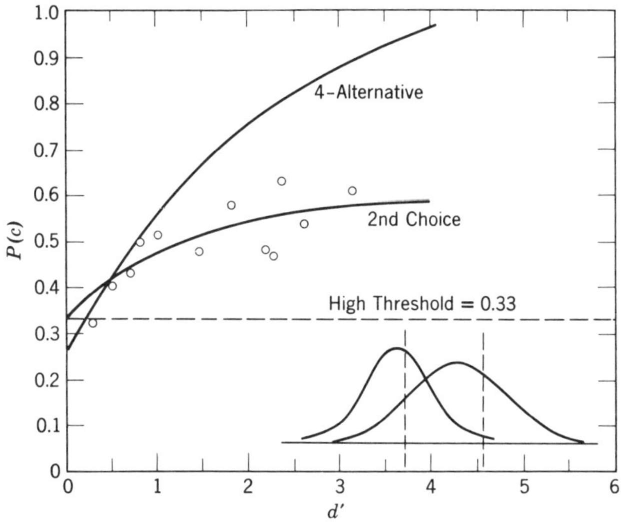

FIG. 2. The results obtained in a second-choice experiment, shown with the prediction from detection theory. Data from Swets, Tanner, and Birdsall (1955).

standard deviations from the mean of the noise distribution, corresponds to the horizontal dashed line in the upper part of the figure. The data indicate that, were a threshold to exist, it would have to be at least as low as the left-hand threshold, at approximately the mean of the noise distribution.

THE RATING EXPERIMENT. In the rating procedure, as in the yes-no procedure, a signal is either presented or not presented in a single observation interval. The observer's task is to reflect gradations in the sensory excitation by assigning each observation to one of several categories of likelihood of occurrence of a signal in the interval.

The results of a visual experiment are displayed in Fig. 3. The abscissa represents a six-point scale of certainty concerning the occurrence of a signal. The six categories were also defined in terms of the a posteriori probability of occurrence, but, for our purpose, only the property of order need be assumed. The ordinate shows the proportion of the observations placed in each category that resulted from the presentation of the signal.

Five curves are shown in Fig. 3. Four of them correspond to the four observers; the fifth, marked by ×'s, represents the average. It may be seen that the curves for three of the four observers increase monotoni-

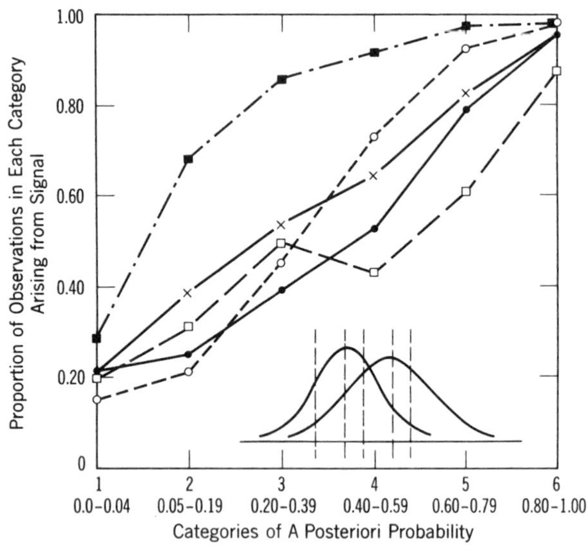

FIG. 3. The results of a rating experiment. Data from Swets, Tanner, and Birdsall (1955).

cally, while that for the fourth has a single reversal. The implication is that the human observer can distinguish at least six categories of sensory excitation.

It is possible to compute operating-characteristic curves from these data, by regarding the category boundaries successively as criteria. The curves (not shown here) are very similar in appearance to those obtained with the yes-no procedure (Swets, Tanner, and Birdsall, 1955). By way of illustration, the five criteria used by one of the observers (the one represented by solid circles) are shown in the insert at lower right in Fig. 3.

THE EXPERIMENTAL INVARIANCE OF d'. It has been found experimentally, in vision (Swets, Tanner, and Birdsall, 1955) and in audition (Tanner, Swets, and Green, 1956), that the sensitivity measure d' remains relatively constant with changes in the response criterion. Thus, detection theory provides a measure of sensitivity that is practically uncontaminated by the factors that might be expected to affect the observer's attitude.

It has also been found that the measure d' remains relatively invariant with different experimental procedures. For vision (Tanner and Swets, 1954) and audition (Swets, 1959) the estimates of d' from the yes-no procedure and from the four-interval, forced-choice procedure are very nearly the same. Again, consistent estimates are obtained from forced-choice procedures with 2, 3, 4, 6, and 8 intervals (Swets, 1959). Finally, the rating procedure yields estimates of d' indistinguishable from those obtained with the yes-no procedure (Egan, Schulman, and Greenberg, 1959).

Thus, the psychophysical detection theory has passed some rather severe tests—the quantity that is supposed to remain invariant does remain invariant. This finding may be contrasted with the well-known fact that estimates of the threshold depend heavily on the particular procedure used.

THEORY OF IDEAL OBSERVERS

Detection theory states, for several types of signal and noise, the maximum possible detectability as a function of the parameters of the signal and the noise. Given certain assumptions, this relationship can be stated very precisely. The case of the "signal specified exactly" (in which everything about the signal is known, including its frequency, phase, starting time, duration, and amplitude) appears to be a useful standard in audition experiments. In this case, the maximum d' is equal to the quantity $(2E/N_0)^{1/2}$, in which E is the signal energy and N_0 is the noise power in a one-cycle band. An ideal observer for visual signals has also been defined (Tanner and Jones, 1959).

It can be argued that a theory of ideal performance is a good starting point in working toward a descriptive theory. Ideal theories involve few variables, and these are simply described. Experiments can be used to uncover whatever additional variables may be needed to describe the performance of real observers. Alternatively, experiments can be used to indicate how the ideal theory may be degraded—that is, to identify those functions of which the ideal detection device must be deprived—in order to accurately describe real behavior.

Given a normative theory, it is possible to describe the real observer's efficiency. In the present instance, the efficiency measure η has been defined as the ratio of the observed to the ideal $(d')^2$. It seems likely that substantive problems will be illuminated by the computation of η for different types of signals and for different parameters of a given type of signal. The observed variation of this measure should be helpful in determining the range over which the human observer can adjust the parameters of his sensory system to match different signal parameters (he is, after all, quite proficient in detecting a surprisingly large number of different signals), and in determining which parameters of a signal the observer is not using, or not using precisely, in his detection process (Tanner and Birdsall, 1958).

The human observer, of course, performs less well than does the ideal observer in the great majority of detection tasks, if not in all. The interesting question concerns not the amount but the nature of the discrepancy that is observed.

The human observer performs less well than the ideal observer defined for the case of the "signal specified exactly." That is to say, the human observer's psychometric function is shifted to the right. More important, the slope of the human observer's function is greater than that of the ideal function for this particular case—a result sometimes referred to as "low-signal suppression." Let us consider three possible reasons for these discrepancies.

First, the human observer may well have a noisy decision process, whereas the ideal decision process is noiseless. For example, the human observer's response criterion may be unstable. If he vacillates between two criteria, the resulting point on his operating-characteristic curve will be on a straight line connecting the points corresponding to the two criteria; this average point falls below the curve (a curve with smoothly decreasing slope) on which the two criteria are located. Again, the observer's decision axis may not be continuous. It may be, as far as we know, divided into a relatively small number of categories—say, into seven.

A second likely cause of deviation from the ideal is the noise inherent in the human sensory systems. Consistent results are obtained from estimating the amount of "internal noise" (that is, noise in the decision process and noise in the sensory system) in two ways: by examining the decisions of an observer over several presentations of the same signal and noise (on tape) and by examining the correlation among the responses of several observers to a single presentation (Swets, Shipley, McKey, and Green, 1959).

A third, and favored, possibility is faulty memory. This explanation is favored because it accounts not only for the shift of the human observer's psychometric function but also for the greater slope of his function. The reasoning proceeds as follows: If the detection process involves some sort of tuning of the receptive apparatus, and if the observer's memory of the characteristics of the incoming signal is faulty, then the observer is essentially confronted with a signal not specified exactly but specified only statistically. He has some uncertainty about the incoming signal.

If uncertainty is introduced into the calculations of the psychometric function of the ideal detector, it is found that performance falls off as uncertainty increases, and that this decline in performance is greater for weak signals than for strong ones (Peterson, Birdsall, and Fox, 1954). That is, a family of theoretical uncertainty curves shows progressively steeper slopes coinciding with progressive shifts to the right. This is what one would expect; the accuracy of knowledge about signal characteristics is less critical for strong signals, since strong signals carry with them more information about these characteristics.

It has been observed that visual data (Tanner and Jones, 1959) and auditory data (Green, 1960) are fitted well, with respect to slope, by the theoretical curve that corresponds to uncertainty among approximately 100 orthogonal signal alternatives. It is not difficult to imagine that the product of the uncertainties about the time, location, and frequency of the signals used in these experiments could be as high as 100.

It is possible to obtain empirical corroboration of this theoretical analysis of uncertainty in terms of faulty memory. This is achieved by providing various aids to memory within the experimental procedure. In such experiments, memory for frequency is made unnecessary by introducing a continuous tone or light (a "carrier") of the same frequency as the signal, so that the signal to be detected is an increment in the carrier. This procedure also eliminates the need for phase memory in audition and location memory in vision. In further experiments a pulsed carrier is used in order to make unnecessary memory for starting time and for duration. In all of these experiments a forced-choice procedure is used, so that memory for amplitude beyond a single trial can also be considered irrelevant. In this way, all of the information thought to be relevant may be contained in the immediate situation. Experimentally, we find that the human observer's psychometric functions show progressively flatter slopes as more and more memory aids are introduced. In fact, when all of the aids just mentioned are used, the observer's slope parallels that for the ideal observer without uncertainty, and it deviates as little as 3 db from the ideal curve in absolute value (Green, 1960).

RELATIONSHIP OF THE DATA TO VARIOUS THRESHOLD THEORIES

Although there is a limit on detection performance, even ideally, and although the human observer falls short of the limit, these facts do not imply a sensory threshold. We have just seen that the human observer's performance can be analyzed in terms of memory, and, conceivably, additional memory aids could bring his performance closer to the ideal. Moreover, consideration of ideal observers concerns an upper rather than a lower limit. The human observer, while falling short of the ideal, can still detect signals at a high rate. Ideally, any displacement of the signal-plus-noise distribution from the noise-alone distribution will lead to a detection rate greater than chance. Although it is difficult to obtain data near the chance point, the theoretical curves that fit the plots of d' against signal energy for human observers go through zero on the energy scale.

This last-mentioned result, of course, based as it is on extrapolation, cannot stand by itself as conclusive argument against the existence of a threshold. The result also depends on a measure of performance that is specific to detection theory. So we shall not be concerned with it further. It is possible, however, to relate the various threshold theories that have been proposed to the experimental results discussed earlier—results obtained with the yes-no, second-choice, and rating procedures, as shown in Figs. 1, 2, and 3. We shall examine these results in relation to threshold theories proposed by Blackwell (1953), Luce (1960), Green (personal communication), Swets, Tanner, and Birdsall (1955), and Stevens (1961*a*, *b*).

BLACKWELL'S HIGH-THRESHOLD THEORY. Blackwell's theory assumes that, whereas the observer may be led to say "yes" when noise alone is presented, only very infrequently is his threshold exceeded by the sensory excitation arising from noise—so infrequently, in fact, that these instances can be ignored. There is a "true" value of p_0—call it p_0'—that for all practical purposes is equal to zero. Corresponding to p_0', there is some true p_1', the value of which depends on the signal strength. Since the observer is unable to order values of sensory excitation below $p_0' \approx 0$, if he says "yes" in response to such a value he is merely guessing and will be correct on a chance basis. The operating-characteristic curve (for a given signal strength) that results from this theory is that of Fig. 4. It is a straight line from (p_0', p_1') through $(p_0 = 1.00,\ p_1 = 1.00)$. The insert at lower right shows the location of the threshold. The data of observer 1 shown in Fig. 1 are reproduced for comparison.

This theoretical curve is described by the equation

$$p_1 = p_1' + p_0(1 - p_1') \tag{1}$$

The observed proportion of "yes" responses to a signal (p_1) equals the proportion of true "yes" responses (p_1') plus a guessing factor (p_0)

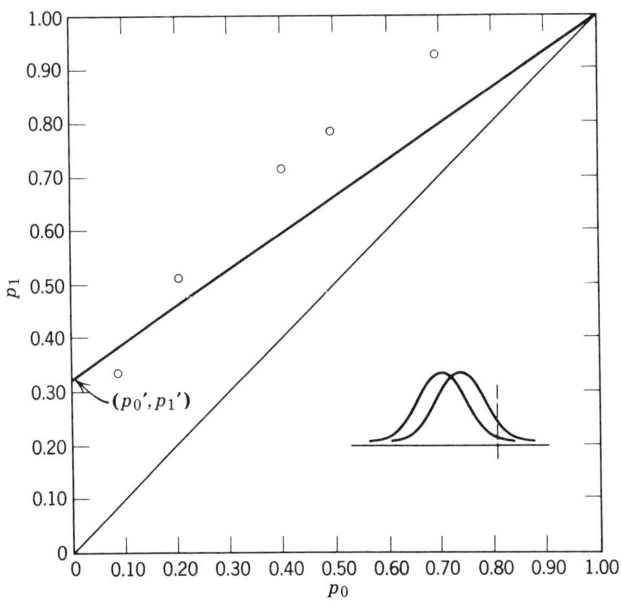

FIG. 4. The results of a yes-no experiment and a theoretical function from Blackwell's high-threshold theory.

modified by the opportunity for guessing $(1 - p_1')$. The beauty of this high-threshold theory is that, if it is correct, the influence of spurious "yes" responses can be eliminated, the proportion of true "yes" responses being left. The familiar correction for chance success

$$p_1' = \frac{p_1 - p_0}{1 - p_0} \tag{2}$$

is a rearrangement of Equation (1). The correction serves to normalize psychometric function so that, whatever the observer's tendency to the guess, the stimulus threshold can be taken as the signal energy corresponding to $p_1' = 0.50$.

However, the theory does not agree with the data. The empirical curve shown in Fig. 4, like the great majority of operating-characteristic curves that have been obtained, is not adequately fitted by a straight line. The horizontal line in Fig. 2, which follows from this theory, does not fit the second-choice data shown there. The rating data of Fig. 3 also indicate ordering of values of sensory excitation below a p_0 of approximately zero. Further, yes-no and forced-choice thresholds calculated from this theory are not consistent with each other (Blackwell, 1953).

LUCE'S LOW-THRESHOLD THEORY. Luce has suggested that a sensory threshold may exist at a somewhat lower level relative to the distribution of noise—that is, that p_0' may be substantial. Apart from this, the low-threshold theory is like the high-threshold theory, only twice so. Whereas Blackwell's theory permits the observer to say "yes" without discrimination when the sensory excitation fails to exceed the threshold, Luce's theory also permits the observer to say "no" without discrimination when the sensory excitation does exceed the threshold. Thus the operating-characteristic curve of this theory contains two linear segments, as shown in Fig. 5. Again, the data for observer 1 in Fig. 1 are shown for comparison. The location of the threshold indicated by these data is shown in the insert at lower right.

It may be seen that the two-line curve fits the yes-no data reasonably well, perhaps as well as the nonlinear curve of detection theory. Although the calculations have not been performed, it seems probable that this theory will also be in fairly good agreement with the second-choice data of Fig. 2. It provides for two categories of sensory excitation, and two categories would seem sufficient to produce a proportion of correct second choices significantly above the chance proportion. However, on the face of it, a two-category theory is inconsistent with the six categories of sensory excitation indicated by the rating data of Fig. 3.

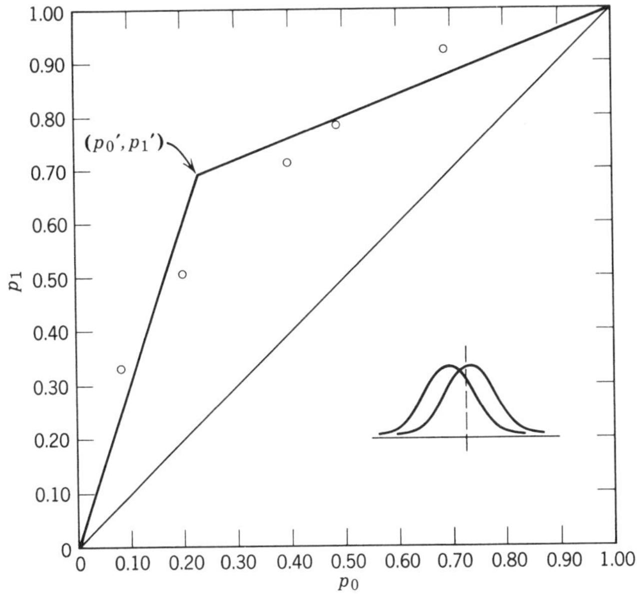

FIG. 5. The results of a yes-no experiment and a theoretical function from Luce's low-threshold theory.

(We may note in passing that the theory raises the interesting question of how another threshold, the one above which a more complete ordering exists, might be measured.)

GREEN'S TWO-THRESHOLD THEORY. Green has observed that operating-characteristic data, perhaps adequately fitted by Luce's curve of two segments, are certainly better fitted by a curve with three linear segments. This curve, shown in Fig. 6, corresponds to a theory that includes a range of uncertainty between a lower threshold, below which lies true rejection, and an upper threshold, above which lies true detection. The insert at lower right shows the location of the two thresholds.

As is evident from Fig. 6, the curve of three line segments fits the yes-no data at least as well as the nonlinear curve of detection theory. Again, the calculations have not been performed, but it seems very likely that a three-category theory can account for the second-choice data. Even a three-category theory, however, is inconsistent with the six categories of sensory excitation indicated by the rating data.

There is, of course, no need to stop at two thresholds and three categories. A five-threshold theory, with a curve of six line segments,

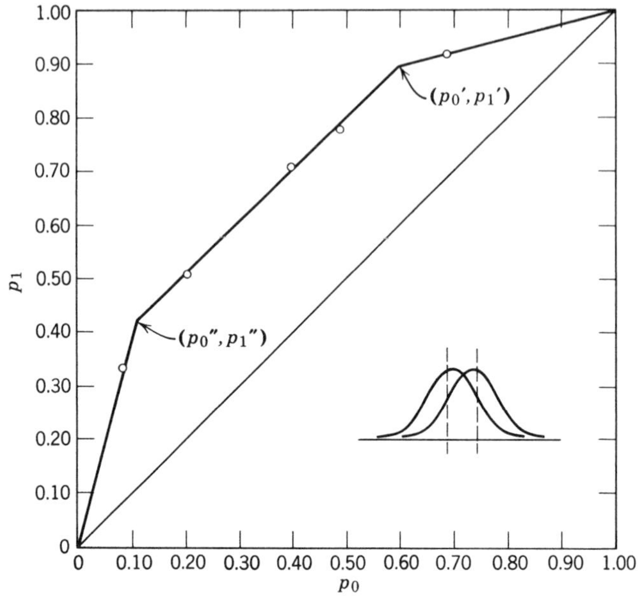

FIG. 6. The results of a yes-no experiment, and a theoretical function from Green's two-threshold theory.

would fit any operating-characteristic data very well indeed and would also be entirely consistent with the second-choice and rating results. However, such a theory is irrelevant to the question under consideration. It is hardly a threshold theory in any important sense. It may be recalled that we considered it earlier as a variant of detection theory.

SWETS, TANNER, AND BIRDSALL'S LOW-THRESHOLD THEORY. Tanner, Birdsall, and I proposed a threshold theory that may be described as combining some of the features of Blackwell's and Luce's theories. This theory permits ordering of values of sensory excitation above the threshold but locates the threshold well within the noise distribution. The corresponding operating-characteristic curve is composed of a linear segment above some substantial value of p_0 (say, 0.30 to 0.50) and a curvilinear segment below this value. Inspection of Fig. 1 shows that such a curve fits yes-no data rather well. It is evident that the second-choice data, and rating data exhibiting six categories, could also be obtained without ordering below this threshold.

STEVENS' QUANTAL-THRESHOLD THEORY. The quantal-threshold theory advocated by Stevens cannot be treated on the same terms as the other threshold theories. The data of Figs. 1, 2, and 3 are not directly relevant to it. The reason is that, whereas the other threshold theories give a prominent place to noise, collection of data in accordance with the quantal theory requires a serious attempt to eliminate all noise, or at least enough of it to allow the discontinuities of neural action to manifest themselves.

We may doubt, a priori, that noise can in fact be reduced sufficiently to reveal the "grain" of the action of a sensory system. Although the other theories we have examined apply to experiments in which the noise is considerable and, as a matter of fact, are typically applied to experiments in which noise (a background of some kind) is added deliberately, they are not generally viewed as restricted to such experiments. In adding noise we acknowledge its universality. The assumption is that the irreducible minimum of ambient noise, equipment noise, and noise inside the observer is enough to obscure the all-or-none quality of individual nervous elements in a psychological experiment. Noise is added in order to bring the total, or at least that part of it external to the observer, to a relatively constant level, and to a level at which it can be measured.

A recent article reviewing the experiments that have sought to demonstrate a quantal threshold has questioned whether any of the experiments suffices as a demonstration (Corso, 1956). Even if we ignore some technical questions concerning curve-fitting procedures and grant that some experiments have produced data in agreement with the quantal-threshold theory, we must observe that obtaining such data evidently depends upon the circumstance of having elite experimenters as well as elite observers (Stevens, 1961*a*). A relatively large amount of negative evidence exists; several other experimenters have attempted to reproduce the conditions of the successful experiments without success (Corso, 1956).

A striking feature of the quantal-theory experiments, in the present context, is the stimulus-presentation procedure employed. Although not contingent upon anything in the theory, the recommended procedure is to present signals of the same magnitude on all the trials of a series and to make known to the observer that this is the case. This procedure provides an unfortunate protection for the theory; if the observer is likely to make noise-determined "yes" responses, the fact will not be disclosed by the experiment. Licklider (1959) has expressed aptly the growing discomfiture over this procedure: "More and more, workers in the field are growing dissatisfied with the classical psychophysical techniques, particularly with the [methods that ask the observer] to report 'present' or 'absent' when he already knows 'present.' It is widely felt that the 'thresholds' yielded by these procedures are on such an insecure semantic basis that they cannot serve as good building blocks for a quantitative science.'' Although the original intent behind the use of this procedure in the quantal-theory experiments was to make the task as easy as possible for the observer, from the point of view of detection theory the procedure presents a very difficult task—it requires that the observer try to establish the response criterion that he would establish if he did not know that the signal was present on every trial.

Thus the advocates of the quantal theory specify a procedure that makes detection theory inapplicable. The result is that, as things stand, the conflict between the two theories cannot be resolved to the satisfaction of all concerned, as it conceivably could be if both theories could be confronted with the same set of data. However, there is reason to hope —since the quantal-theory procedure is not intrinsic to the theory but rests rather on a sense of experimental propriety, which is a relatively labile matter—that such a confrontation will some day be possible.

IS THERE A SENSORY THRESHOLD?

We have considered the data of three experiments—the yes-no, second-choice, and rating experiments—in relation to five competing theories concerning the processes underlying these data. The three sets of data are in agreement with detection theory, a theory that denies the existence of a sensory threshold, and also with the version of a low-threshold theory proposed by Tanner, Birdsall, and me. Blackwell's high-threshold theory is inconsistent with all three sets of results. Luce's low-threshold theory is consistent with the first, perhaps consistent with the second, and inconsistent with the third. Green's two-threshold theory fits the first two sets of results but not the last. We also considered the only other explicit threshold theory available—the quantal theory, to which the three experiments are not directly relevant.

The outcome is that, as far as we know, there may be a sensory threshold. The possibility of a quantal threshold cannot be discounted, and certainly not on the basis of data at hand. On another level of analysis, there may be what we have termed a low threshold, somewhere in the vicinity of the mean of the noise distribution. The low-threshold theory proposed by Tanner, Birdsall, and me fits all of the data we examined. If the rating experiment can be dismissed (there is now no apparent reason for giving it less than full status), then Luce's and Green's theories, which involve a low threshold, fit the remaining data.

On the other hand, the existence of a sensory threshold has not been demonstrated. Data consistent with the quantal theory are, at best, here today and gone tomorrow, and the theory has yet to be tested through an objective procedure. With respect to a low threshold, we may ask whether demonstration of such a threshold is even conceivable.

It is apparent that it will be difficult to measure a low threshold. Consider the low-threshold theory that permits complete ordering above the threshold in connection with the forced-choice experiment. The observer conveys less information about his ordering than he is capable of conveying if only a first choice is required. We saw in the preceding discussion that the second choice conveys a significant amount of information. Another experiment, in which the observer tried to be incorrect, indicated that he can order four choices (Tanner, Swets, and Green, 1956). Thus it is difficult to determine when enough information has been extracted to yield a valid estimate of a low threshold.

Again, it is difficult to imagine how one might determine the signal energy corresponding to the thresholds of Luce's and Green's theories. The determination is made especially difficult by the fact that, in general, empirical operating-characteristic curves for various signal energies are fitted well by the theoretical curves of detection theory. Consequently, the line-segment curves that best fit the data have lines intersecting at a value of p_0 that depends on the signal energy. The implication is that the location of the threshold depends on the signal energy that is being presented.

IMPLICATIONS FOR PRACTICE

We have, then, the possibility of a threshold, but it is no more than a possibility, and we must observe that since it is practically unmeasurable it will not be a very useful concept in experimental practice. Moreover, even if the low threshold proposed by Tanner, Birdsall, and me did exist, and were measurable, it would not restrict the application of detection theory. We may note that yes-no data resulting from a suprathreshold criterion depend upon the criterion but are completely independent of the threshold value. The same limitation applies to the quantal threshold. It appears that a compelling demonstration of this concept will be difficult to achieve, so that in practice a theory and a method that deal with noise will be required.

Accordingly, with any attempt to measure sensitivity by means of "yes" and "no" responses, a measure of the observer's response criterion should be obtained. The only way known to obtain this measure is to use catch trials—randomly chosen trials that do not contain a signal. The methods of adjustment, limits, and constants in their usual forms, in which the observer knows that the signal is present on every trial, are inappropriate.

A large number of catch trials should be presented. It is not sufficient to employ a few catch trials, enough to monitor the observer, and then to remind him to avoid "false-positive" responses each time he makes one. This procedure merely forces the criterion up to a point where it cannot be measured, and it can be shown that the calculated threshold varies by as much as 6 db as the criterion varies in this unmeasurable range (Swets, Tanner, and Birdsall, 1955). Precision is also sacrificed when, because highly trained observers are employed, the untestable assumption is made that they do maintain a constant high criterion. Even if all laboratories should be fortunate enough to have such observers, we would have to expect a range of variation of 6 db among "constant criterion" observers in different laboratories. To be sure, for some problems, this amount of variability is not bothersome; for others it is.

The presentation of a large number of catch trials—enough to provide a good estimate of the probability of a "yes" response on such a trial—is still inadequate if this estimate is then used to correct the proportion of "yes" responses to the signal for chance success. The validity of the correction for chance depends upon the existence of a high threshold that is inconsistent with all of the data that we examined. It should be noted that the common procedure of taking the proportion of correct responses that is halfway between chance and perfect performance as corresponding to the threshold value of the signal is entirely equivalent to using the chance correction.

In summary, in measuring sensitivity it is desirable to manipulate the response criterion so that it lies in a range where it can be measured, to include enough catch trials to obtain a good estimate of this response criterion, and to use a method of analysis that yields independent measures of sensitivity and the response criterion. One qualification should be added: We can forego estimating the response criterion in a forced-choice experiment. Under the forced-choice procedure, few observers show a bias in their responses large enough to affect the sensitivity index d' appreciably. Those who do show such a bias initially can overcome it with little difficulty. As a result, the observer can be viewed as choosing the interval most likely to contain a signal, without regard to any criterion. For this reason, the forced-choice procedure may be used to advantage in studies having an emphasis on sensory, rather than on motivational or response, processes.

ACKNOWLEDGMENTS

This article is adapted from an address delivered at a centennial symposium honoring Fechner, sponsored by the American Psychological Association and the Psychometric Society, held in Chicago in September, 1960. The preparation of this article was supported by the U. S. Army Signal Corps, the Air Force (Office of Scientific Research and Operational Applications Laboratory), and the Office of Naval Research, under contracts administered by the Research Laboratory of Electronics, Massachusetts Institute of Technology. This article appeared as Tech. Rept. No. AFCCDD-TR-61-10, and in Science, *1961,* **134,** *168–177.*

References

- Blackwell, H. R. *Threshold psychophysical measurements.* Unpublished. See also Psychophysical thresholds: Experimental studies of methods of measurement. University of Michigan: Engineering Research Institute, 1953, Bulletin No. 36.
- Boring, E. G. *The physical dimensions of consciousness.* New York: Century, 1933.
- Boring, E. G. *A history of experimental psychology.* (2nd ed.) New York: Appleton-Century-Crofts, 1950.
- Corso, J. F. The neural quantum theory of sensory discrimination. *Psychol. Bull.,* 1956. **53,** 371–393.
- Egan, J. P., Schulman, A. I., and Greenberg, G. Z. Operating characteristics determined by binary decisions and by ratings. *J. acoust. Soc. Am.,* 1959, **31,** 768–773. [7]
- Fechner, G. T., *Elemente der Psychophysik.* 1860.
- Green, D. M. Psychoacoustics and detection theory. *J. acoust. Soc. Am.,* 1960, **32,** 1189–1203. [2]
- Licklider, J. C. R. Three auditory theories. In S. Koch (Ed.), *Psychology: A study of a science.* Vol. I. New York: McGraw-Hill, 1959. [3]
- Luce, R. D. Detection thresholds: a problem reconsidered. *Science,* 1960, **132,** 1495.
- Munson, W. A., and Karlin, J. E. The measurement of human channel transmission characteristics. *J. acoust. Soc. Am.,* 1954, **26,** 542–553.
- Peterson, W. W., Birdsall, T. G., and Fox, W. C. The theory of signal detectability. *Trans. IRE Professional Group on Information Theory.* 1954, **PGIT-4,** 171–212.
- Smith, M., and Wilson, E. A. A model of the auditory threshold and its application to the problem of the multiple observer, *Psychol. Monogr.,* 1953, **67,** No. 9, Whole No. 359.
- Stevens, S. S. Is there a quantal threshold? In W. A. Rosenblith (Ed.), *Sensory communication.* New York: Technology Press and Wiley, 1961*a*.
- Stevens, S. S. To honor Fechner and repeal his law. *Science,* 1961*b*, **133,** 80–86.
- Swets, J. A. Indices of signal detectability obtained with various psychophysical procedures. *J. acoust. Soc. Am.,* 1959, **31,** 511–513. [6]

- Swets, J. A., Shipley, E. F., McKey, M. J., and Green, D. M. Multiple observations of signals in noise. *J. acoust. Soc. Am.*, 1959, **31,** 514–521. [9]
- Swets, J. A., Tanner, W. P., Jr., and Birdsall, T. G. The evidence for decision-making theory of visual detection. University of Michigan: Electronic Defense Group, 1955, Technical Report No. 40. This material also appears as: Decision processes in perception. *Psychol. Rev.*, 1961, **68,** 301–340. [1]
- Tanner, W. P., Jr., and Birdsall, T. G. Definitions of d' and η as psychophysical measures. *J. acoust. Soc. Am.*, 1958, **30,** 922–928. [5]
- Tanner, W. P., Jr., and Jones, R. C. The ideal sensor system as approached through statistical decision theory and the theory of signal detectability. Proceedings of the Armed Forces-NRC Vision Committee meeting, Washington, D. C., 1959.
- Tanner, W. P., Jr., and Swets, J. A. A decision-making theory of visual detection. *Psychol. Rev.*, 1954, **61,** 401–409.
- Tanner, W. P., Jr., Swets, J. A., and Green, D. M. Some general properties of the hearing mechanism. University of Michigan: Electronic Defense Group, 1956, Technical Report No. 30.

section two

MEASUREMENT

The articles in this section present detailed definitions of the dependent variables stipulated by detection theory, and supply evidence that the sensitivity measure d′ *consistently reflects the effective signal-to-noise ratio in several different experimental procedures.*

Tanner and Birdsall in "Definitions of d′ *and* η *as Psychophysical Measures" [5] derive the measure* d′ *for forced-choice and yes-no response procedures for the ideal observer, and show how the ideal result may be used as a standard of comparison for real observers by means of the efficiency measure* η. *Swets compares "Indices of Signal Detectability Obtained with Various Psychophysical Procedures" [6], in particular the yes-no procedure and the forced-choice procedure with two to eight alternatives, and finds that the value of* d′ *for a given observer and a given signal level is practically invariant. Egan, Schulman, and Greenberg in "Operating Characteristics Determined by Binary Decisions and by Ratings" [7] also obtain an invariance of* d′ *when comparing the values obtained from the yes-no procedure and the values obtained using a rating scale. In "Auditory Detection of an Unspecified Signal" [8], Gundy demonstrates another aspect of the stability of* d′*; he shows that, under ordinary experimental conditions, practice effects are small and of short duration.*

5

Definitions of d' and η as Psychophysical Measures

Wilson P. Tanner, Jr., and Theodore G. Birdsall

The theory of signal detectability (Peterson, Birdsall, and Fox, 1954; Van Meter and Middleton, 1954) has provided a model useful to the study of psychophysical phenomena. Smith and Wilson (1953) and Munson and Karlin (1954) report data suggestive of this application in psychoacoustics. Tanner and Swets (1954) present a more formal treatment of the application of the model to visual experiments, and this formal application is extended to psychoacoustics for both detection and recognition studies (Tanner and Norman, 1954; Tanner, Swets, and Green, 1956; Green, Birdsall, and Tanner, 1957; Tanner, 1956; Swets and Birdsall, 1956). Marill (1956) demonstrated the symmetry of the two-alternative forced-choice experimental technique. FitzHugh (1957) used the model in studies of the physiology of vision employing microelectrode techniques. Egan and his associates find the model useful in the study of voice communication channels (Egan, 1957; Egan, Clarke, and Carterette, 1956; Egan and Clarke, 1956).

The purpose of this report is to clarify the definitions of d' and η as used in the studies of the authors and their co-workers, and to clarify the reasons for employing these variables in psychoacoustical experiments.

Both of these variables are defined within the framework of the theory of signal detectability (Peterson, Birdsall, and Fox, 1954; Van Meter and Middleton, 1954). The word "detectability" is used, rather than

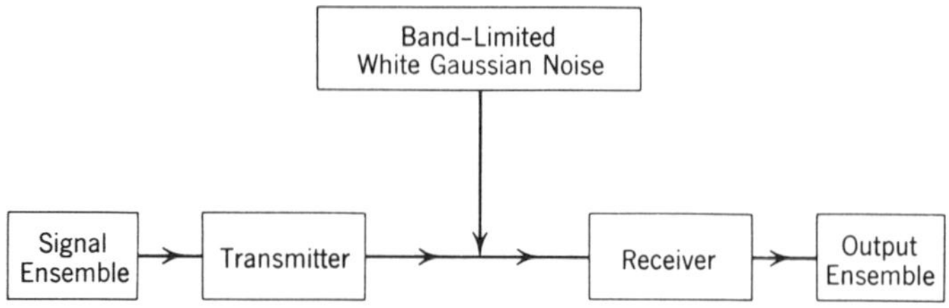

FIG. 1. Basic psychophysical experiment in block diagram form.

the word "detection," because the theory is one describing the limits placed on the performance of a receiver by the signal energy and noise energy of the channel. It is like the limitations on measurement imposed by nature, in this case the channel.

The fundamental problem considered in the theory of signal detectability is illustrated in the block diagram of Fig. 1. A signal from an ensemble of signals is transmitted with a fixed probability over a channel in which noise is added. The receiver is permitted to observe during a fixed observation interval in time, at the end of which it must state whether the observation was one of noise alone or signal plus noise.

The particular case upon which this discussion is based is that of an ensemble containing only one signal. That one is a signal known exactly: its voltage, point-for-point in time during the observation interval, is known to the receiver. It is not known that the signal exists during the interval. The signal is transmitted over a channel in which band-limited white Gaussian noise is added. By employing a sampling theorem (Peterson, Birdsall, and Fox, 1954), it is shown that the detectability of this signal in this channel can be described by the ratio $(2E/N_0)^{1/2}$, in which E is the signal energy and N_0 is the noise power per unit bandwidth.[1]

The meaning of this ratio, or detectability index, can be illustrated by the diagram in Fig. 2. Any finite waveform can be expressed by the instantaneous values at $2WT$ independent sampling points where T is the duration of the waveform in seconds and W is its bandwidth. Thus every waveform can be expressed as a point in a space with $2WT$ dimensions. There is associated with each point the likelihood, or probability density, that this point would occur, given each of the alternatives to be tested. In the signal detection task there are only two alternatives: noise alone and signal plus noise. All of the information relevant to the

[1] The ratio $2E/N_0$ can be expressed in the form $2WT\ S/N$, where S is the signal power and N is the noise power, if the noise is white over the band of the signal. ST is the signal energy and N/W is the noise power per unit bandwidth.

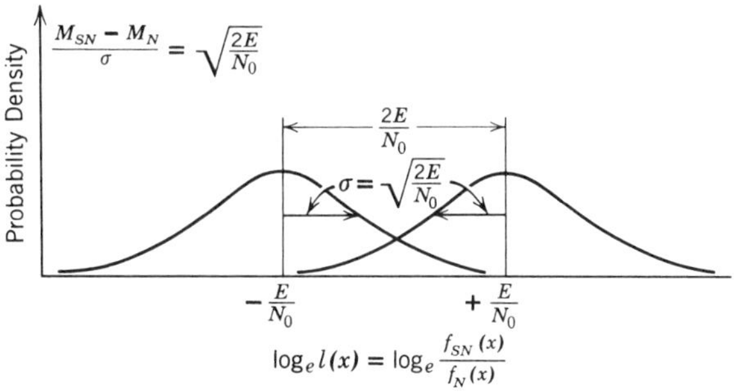

FIG. 2. Probability densities for $\log_e l(X)$ conditional on noise alone and on signal plus noise.

signal detection task can be expressed as a single-number likelihood ratio. This is the ratio of the likelihood that the point or observed waveform occurs, if signal plus noise is present, to the likelihood of the occurrence of the point, if noise alone exists. Thus, the observations in any given signal detection task can be plotted on a unidimensional axis on which the measure is likelihood ratio. Any variable which is a monotonic transformation of likelihood ratio is equally useful in the signal detection task. In this case the natural logarithm of likelihood ratio leads to convenient statistics. Therefore, it is used as the variable and is plotted on the abscissa in Fig. 2. This is called the decision axis. The ordinate of Fig. 2 is the probability density of the natural logarithm of likelihood ratio.

There are two distributions shown in Fig. 2. One is conditional upon the existence of noise alone, the other conditional upon the existence of signal plus noise. Peterson, Birdsall, and Fox (1954) show that, for the case in point these distributions both are normal and have equal variance. The mean of the distribution for noise alone is $-E/N_0$ and for signal plus noise is $+E/N_0$. The difference of the means is $2E/N_0$. The standard deviation of each of the distributions is $(2E/N_0)^{1/2}$. Thus the, difference in the means divided by the standard deviation is the detectability index $(2E/N_0)^{1/2}$.

The way in which a measure such as that illustrated in Fig. 2 is a statement of capacity is illustrated in Figs. 3*a* and 3*b*. Figure 3*a* is an ROC (receiver operating characteristic) curve as defined by Peterson, Birdsall, and Fox. Plotted on the abscissa is the probability that, if noise alone exists, the receiver says that the signal exists. On the ordinate is plotted the probability that, if signal plus noise exists, the receiver will accept the observation as arising from signal plus noise. An ROC

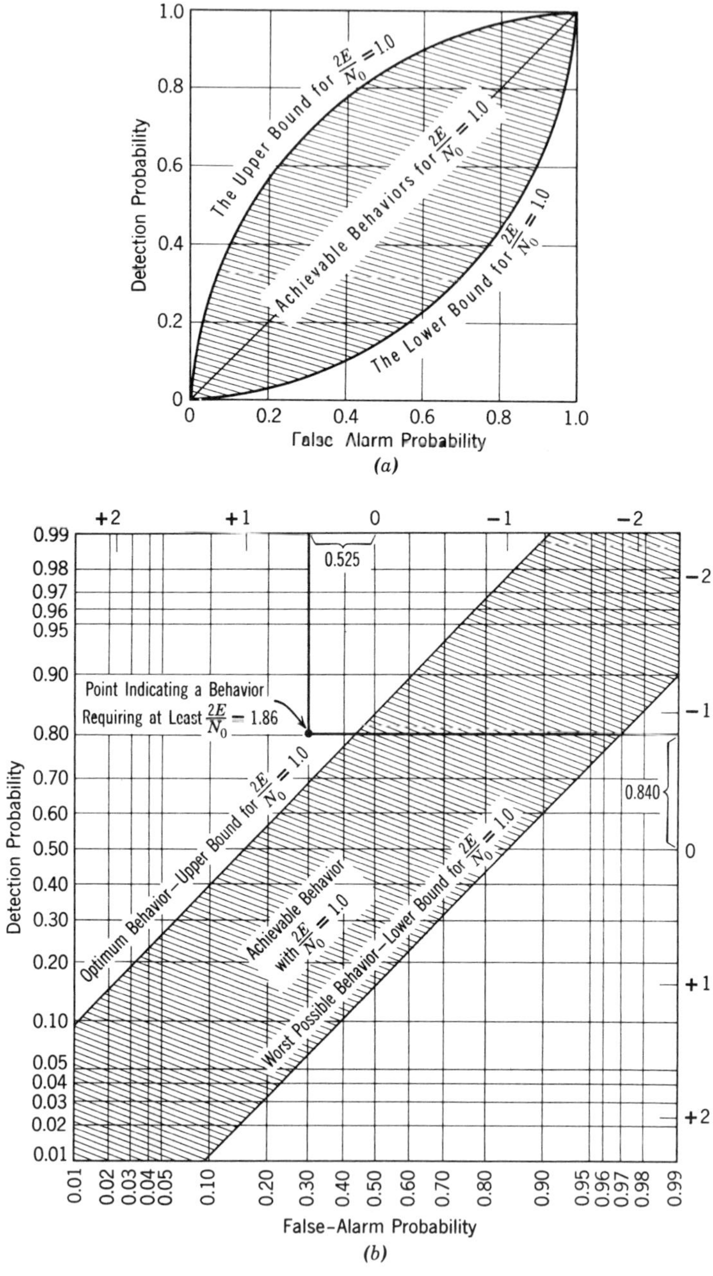

FIG. 3. (*a*) Receiver operating characteristic (ROC) for the ideal receiver when $2E/N_0 = 1.00$. (*b*) Transformation to double probability paper.

curve thus shows the detection probability as a function of the false-alarm probability.

An ROC curve is constructed from the probability distributions of Fig. 2. In an experiment involving a choice between two alternatives there is a critical number. Whenever the likelihood ratio is greater than this number, one alternative is chosen. The natural logarithm of the critical number is a point on the abscissa of Fig. 2. The area under the curve for noise alone to the right of the point is the probability that if noise alone exists the receiver will say that signal plus noise exists, whereas the area under the curve for signal plus noise to the right of the point is the probability that if signal plus noise exists the receiver will say that signal plus noise exists. These two areas define the location of a point on an ROC curve. The first of the areas defines the location of the point on the abscissa and the second defines the location on the ordinate. The procedure can then be repeated for other values which the critical number can assume, each value defining a point on an ROC curve. The ROC curve is the collection of all such points, each arising from a critical number.

The exact location of the points of an ROC curve depends on the separation of the two probability density curves of Fig. 2. For the ideal receiver, there is an ROC curve for each value of $(2E/N_0)^{1/2}$. This curve represents the set of all performances utilizing all of the information. The ROC curve is thus an upper bound on performance.

The mirror image of the ROC curve contains the set of points illustrating the worst possible behavior; i.e., the highest possible miss probability as a function of false-alarm probability. The shaded area between the curves contains all achievable operating points, whereas the bounds of this area are behaviors using the capacities of the signals to be detected. The exact location of the curves and the amount of shaded area depend on the value of $(2E/N_0)^{1/2}$, the separation between the statistical hypotheses.

The same ROC curve is plotted in Fig. 3*b* with a transformation of the axes from linear to probability scales. Since this transformation scales standard deviations linearly, and since the distributions of noise alone and signal plus noise have equal standard deviations for the signal known exactly, the ROC curve for the ideal case is a straight line with slope 1. The vertical and horizontal scales to the right and above the graph show this linear scaling.

In an experiment, the false-alarm rate and the detection rate can be used as estimates of the probabilities necessary to define a point on an ROC curve. If, in Fig. 3*b*, one reads the coordinates of this point on the scales to the right and above, the distances of the critical value from the two means in standard units are obtained. The difference between these distances is the minimum value of $(2E/N_0)^{1/2}$ necessary to lead to this performance; i.e., the particular detection probability when the particular false alarm probability exists.

BASIC DEFINITIONS OF d' AND η

Consider now the experimental arrangement illustrated in Fig. 4. The particular experiment being performed is defined by the positions of switches 1 and 2.

A channel includes the transmitter and the receiver. The block diagrams of Figs. 4 and 5 illustrate this use. In Fig. 4 there are two possible types of transmitters and two possible types of receivers. The positions of the two switches determine those which are actually in the channel. The switch positions are used as subscripts to specify the channel.

C_{11} is the channel in which the signal transmitted is one known exactly and the receiver is an ideal receiver designed to operate on the particular signal specified (Fig. 5*A*).

C_{12} is the channel in which the signal transmitted is one known exactly and the receiver is the one under study (Fig. 5*B*).

C_{21} is the channel in which the signal transmitted is one known statistically and the receiver is an ideal receiver designed to operate on a particular statistical ensemble of signals. The receiver is designed only with reference to a particular statistical ensemble (Fig. 5*C*).

C_{22} is the channel in which the signal transmitted is one known statistically and the receiver is the one under study (Fig. 5*D*).

In each of these channels Fourier-series, band-limited white Gaussian noise is added.

The following symbols are also defined.

η_r is the efficiency of the receiver in the channel C_{12}. Since all other components in that channel are ideal, the difference between the performance of channels C_{12} and C_{11} is attributable entirely to the receiver.

η_t is the efficiency of the transmitter in channel C_{21}, since all other components in that channel are ideal.

η_{tr} is the efficiency of channel C_{22}.

E_{ij} is the energy required of channel C_{ij} to achieve a given level of performance. The subscript i refers to the position of the first switch and the subscript j, to the position of the second switch.

First, an experiment is performed in which a signal known exactly of energy E_{12} is transmitted over the channel C_{12} with band-limited white Gaussian noise, of noise power per cycle N_0, added. The output is presented to the receiver under study, either a human observer or "black

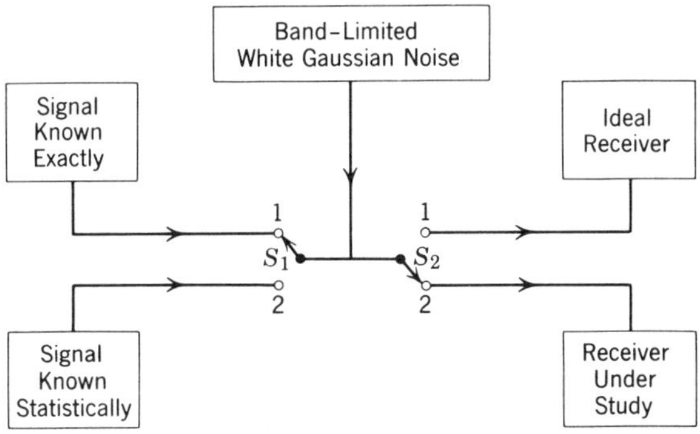

FIG. 4. Composite block diagram of channels for psychophysical experiment.

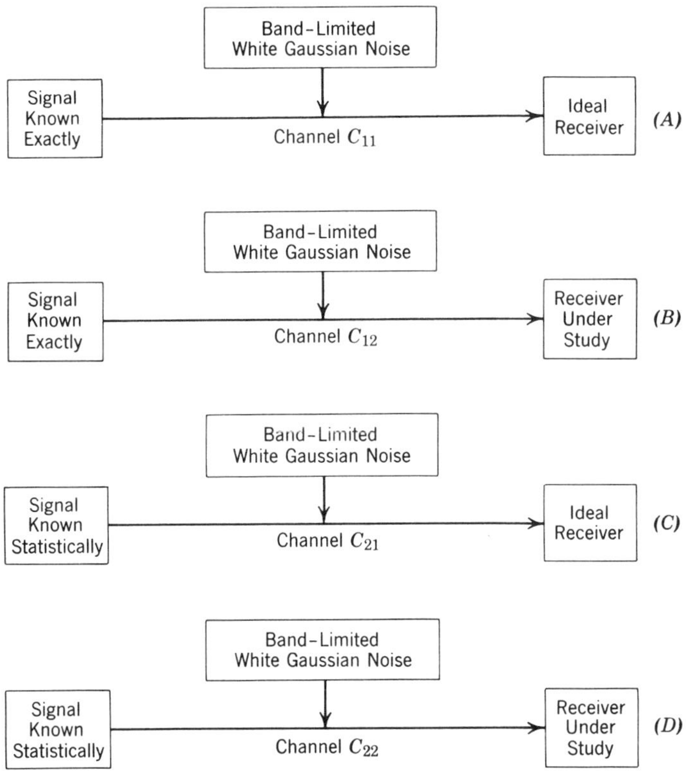

FIG. 5. Individual block diagrams of channels for psychophysical experiment.

box." The task of the receiver is to observe a specified waveform and to determine whether or not that waveform contains a signal. If the question is asked a large number of times, both when the signal is present and when the signal is not present, the data necessary for estimating the false-alarm probability $P_N(A)$ and the detection probability $P_{SN}(A)$ are obtained.

The next experiment (a mathematical calculation) performed is the same, except that the ideal receiver is substituted for the receiver under study. In this experiment the energy of the signal is "attenuated" at the transmitter (N_0 is the same as in the previous experiment) until the performance obtained in the previous experiment is matched. The energy (E_{11}) leading to the matched performance is then determined. The efficiency of the receiver is defined as

$$\eta_r = E_{11}/E_{12} \tag{1}$$

and the measure d' is defined by the equation

$$(d')^2 = \eta_r(2E_{12}/N_0) = 2E_{11}/N_0 \tag{2}$$

Thus $(d')^2$ is that value of $2E/N_0$ required to lead to the receiver's performance if an ideal receiver were employed in its place.

This second experiment is not performed in the laboratory, since the problem has a mathematical solution (Peterson, Birdsall, and Fox, 1954). The procedure outlined in the previous section is followed. One takes the performance of the receiver under study and plots the point on the graph paper of Fig. 3*b*. The coordinates of this point are read on the axis to the right and the axis above. The difference of the distances in standard value units is $(2E_{11}/N_0)^{1/2}$. The value $2E_{12}/N_0$ is measured physically. Since N_0 is assumed constant,

$$\eta_r = \frac{2E_{11}/N_0}{2E_{12}/N_0} = \frac{E_{11}}{E_{12}} \tag{3}$$

The measure d' is illustrated in Fig. 6. Figure 6*a* contains the probability distributions of Fig. 2. Figure 6*b* is a transformation of the variable to a new variable

$$X = \frac{\log_e l(x) + (E/N_0)}{(2E/N_0)^{1/2}} \tag{4}$$

This new variable is distributed normally. The mean of the probability density distribution for noise alone is 0 and the variance, unity. The mean of the signal plus noise distribution is $(2E/N_0)^{1/2}$ and the variance, unity.

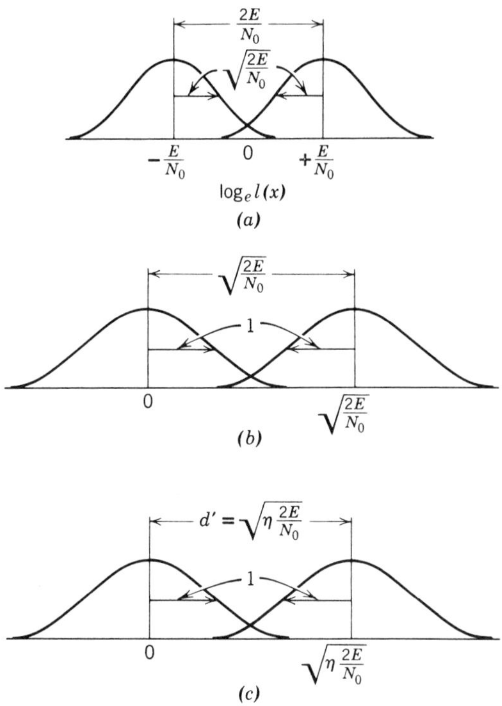

FIG. 6. Relation between d' and $(2E/N_0)^{1/2}$.

Figure 6*c* is the distribution of the variable upon which an ideal receiver would be operating if it were to match the performance of the receiver under study. The mean of the noise distribution is 0, and the mean of the signal plus noise distribution is $d' = (\eta 2E/N_0)^{1/2}$. The variances are again unity.

Both the measure of d' and η are specific to a particular performance in terms of false-alarm rate and detection rate. If a different experiment were performed employing the same signal and noise conditions, and permitting a different false-alarm rate and, consequently, a different detection rate, both d' and η might assume different values. This would be the case if something happened in the receiver to upset the equal-variance condition for noise alone and signal plus noise. However, an examination of the specific cases studied in the theory of signal detectability suggests that there are a large number of cases in which this departure, though it exists, is not important. That is, the departure over the range likely to be investigated experimentally is not sufficient to lead to significant changes in d' and η.

Next, consider a mathematical experiment in which a signal known statistically (SKS) is transmitted over the channel to an ideal receiver for that statistical ensemble. Again, the energy E_{21} is employed, and performance is measured. Furthermore, a second mathematical experiment is performed transmitting a signal known exactly (SKE) to the ideal receiver, determining the E_{11} necessary to give the same performance. This permits calculation of η_t, the efficiency of a transmitter with that statistical ensemble. Both of these experiments are mathematical calculations.

A THEOREM FOR EXPERIMENTAL INTERPRETATION

When $\eta_t = \eta_r$, each referring to the case in which the signal is known exactly, it can be said that the amount of uncertainty represented by the statistical parameters of the transmitter ensemble SKS is reflected to the receiver when SKE is transmitted. This is the same thing as saying that knowledge which the receiver cannot use might as well not be available. If the receiver under study has no provisions built into it for the use of phase information, but all other knowledge can be utilized optimally, then the channel C_{12} is expected to lead to the same performance as the channel C_{21} when the signal is known except for phase.

Actually, it is not the specific uncertainty, but rather the degree of uncertainty which is matched when $\eta_t = \eta_r$. A signal known except for phase is one in which all phases are equally likely. Measurement is required in two orthogonal dimensions (Peterson, Birdsall, and Fox, 1954). If the uncertainty were one of frequency such that any frequency within a band were equally likely, and if this band is such that again measurement in two orthogonal dimensions is sufficient, then this leads to the same change in performance as does the uncertainty of phase. The parameter, m, is defined as the number of orthogonal dimensions over which the statistical uncertainty exists. It is now possible to state a theorem leading to inference about the receiver based on the measurement of η.

> If $\eta_r = \eta_t$, then the receiver, through its inability to use knowledge contained in SKE, introduces an equal statistical uncertainty, m, to that of the transmitter, SKS. If the channel SKS to the receiver under study is then established and η_{tr} equals η_r equals η_t, then the receiver with SKE has introduced exactly that uncertainty existing in SKS.

The first part of the theorem states that if

$$\eta_r = E_{11}/E_{12} = \eta_t = E_{11}/E_{21}$$

then the receiver has introduced the same amount of uncertainty into the channel C_{12} as the transmitter into the channel C_{21} for that statistical ensemble. Essentially, this means that if the efficiency is less than one, there is uncertainty due to something other than white Gaussian noise which was added in the channel. Since in one case the transmitter is ideal, this uncertainty must be introduced by the receiver. In the other case, the receiver is ideal, and the uncertainty must be introduced by the transmitter. The usefulness of the theorem arises from the fact that the amount of uncertainty introduced by SKS can be stated quantitatively.

The second part of the theorem states that if

$$\eta_{tr} = E_{11}/E_{22} = \eta_t = E_{11}/E_{21} = \eta_r = E_{11}/E_{12}$$

then the exact uncertainties are introduced in the receiver in one case, and in the transmitter in the other case. If particular information, such as the phase of the signal, is not used by the receiver, then the introduction of phase uncertainty into the transmitter will not degrade the receiver's performance. The concepts may be thought of as a procedure for determining what aspects of the signal the receiver cannot utilize in detection.

If the theory of signal detectability is applicable, then η is the variable which contains the information necessary to modify the ideal receiver to match the receiver under study.

GENERALIZED DEFINITION OF d'

So far the discussion of d' has been entirely in reference to the detectability of signals. The measure can also be applied to the ability of two signals to lead to recognition.

First consider the two-alternative forced-choice experiment, in which a signal known exactly is presented in one of two positions in time. The receiver is asked to state in which of the two positions in time the signal did, in fact, occur. This is essentially a recognition experiment. The question asked the receiver is whether the signal is a 01 or a 10.

An ideal receiver can test each position for the existence of the 1. The position more likely to contain the signal is the one that he chooses. The information upon which he bases his decision is the difference between the two measures. The distribution of the difference is illustrated in Fig. 7, a normal distribution with mean d' and standard deviation $\sqrt{2}$. If the two signals are equally likely, then the shaded area represents the probability of a correct choice.

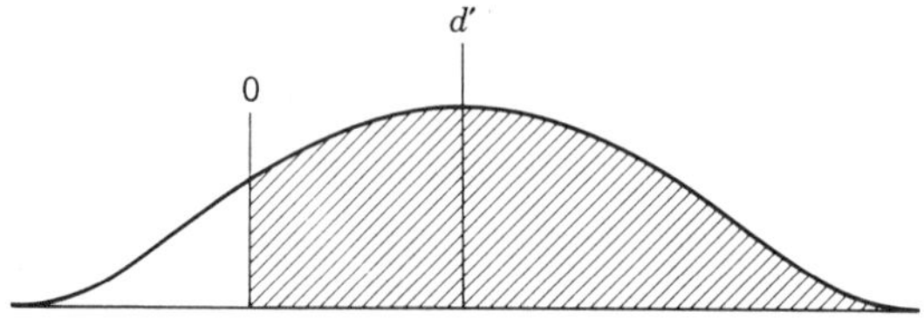

FIG. 7. Distribution of the difference between two variables for the two-alternative forced-choice experiment.

Another way of looking at this type of experiment is to treat the task as one of recognition as illustrated in Fig. 8. In this case, the signal shown in line 1 can be subtracted from the observed input, which contains either the signal of line 1 plus additive noise or the signal of line 2 plus additive noise. The subtraction leaves noise alone if the signal of line 1 was present, or the signal of line 3 plus noise, if the signal of line 2 was present. Now the receiver can test for the presence of the signal in line 3 in the noise. If the measure is sufficient to state that the signal of line 3 was present, he chooses the signal of line 2. Otherwise, he chooses the signal of line 1. This experiment is like a detection experiment with twice the energy.

A third way of looking at this experiment is illustrated in Fig. 9, taken from an earlier paper (Tanner, 1956). The two signals are orthogonal; that is, the angle θ is 90°. If $(2E_1/N_0)^{1/2}$ and $(2E_2/N_0)^{1/2}$ are equal, then the recognition decision axis is $(4E/N_0)^{1/2}$, consistent with the result of the previous two views.

Now, in the two-alternative forced-choice experiments in which the alternatives have equal energy, one could measure either (1) the dis-

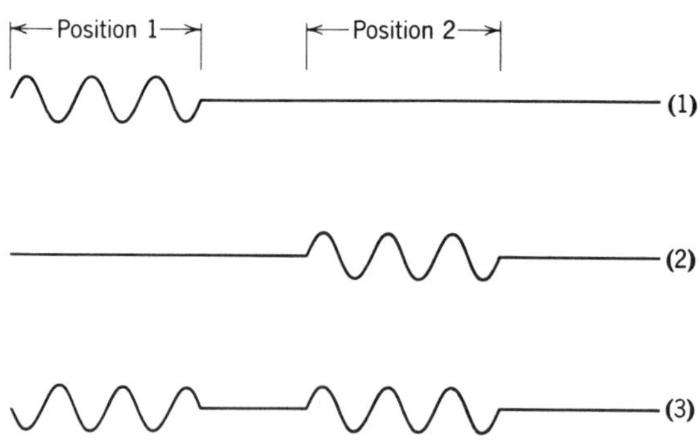

FIG. 8. Difference signal for the two-alternative forced-choice experiment.

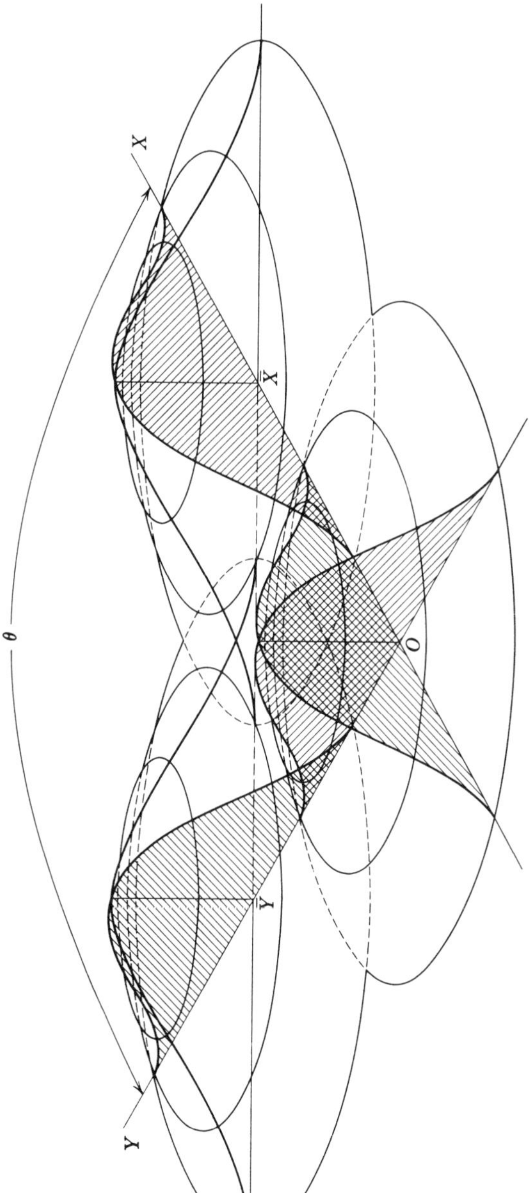

FIG. 9. Illustration of recognition space for definition of θ.

tance $(\eta 4E/N_0)^{1/2}$, (2) the recognition $d'_{1,2}$, or (3) the distance $(\eta 2E/N_0)^{1/2}$ (the detection d' for the signal which is presented in one of the two positions in time). Since in forced-choice experiments involving more than two alternatives, with each containing equal energy, a single number permitting analysis is the detection d', the authors and their colleagues have been using this measure. Thus, when a d' is presented without a subscript, or with a single subscript, it is a measure of the difference between two hypotheses, one of which is noise alone. Whenever the d' is intended to indicate the difference between two signals, each is indicated by a subscript. In Fig. 9, d'_1 refers to the distance 0 to $\bar{X}$, d'_2 to the distance 0 to $\bar{Y}$, and $d'_{1,2}$ to the distance $\bar{X}$ to $\bar{Y}$.

If a two-alternative forced-choice experiment is found to lead to a percentage of correct choices, this can be used as an estimate of the probability of a correct choice. This estimate is the data necessary to enter the graph in Fig. 3*b*. The point to be plotted projects on the ordinate at $P(c)$ and on the abscissa at $1 - P(c)$. The sum of the standard units is $d'_{1,2}$ and $\sqrt{2}d'_1$, if $d'_1 = d'_2$.

Now, let us consider a more general case illustrated in Fig. 10. In this case the angle θ can assume any value and the energies of the two signals, S_1 and S_2, are not necessarily equal. If an experiment is now performed in which one or the other of the two signals is presented at a fixed position in time, and the receiver is asked to state which one, again the data are furnished for entering the graph of Fig. 3*b*. The estimated probabilities required are $P_{S_1}(A_1)$, the probability that if S_1 is presented the receiver is correct, and $1 - P_{S_2}(A_2)$, the probability that if S_2 is presented the receiver is incorrect. The d' so estimated is $d'_{S_1,S_2} = (\eta 2E_\Delta/N_0)^{1/2}$ where E_Δ is the energy of the difference signal. This can be referred to a shifted point of origin 0′ with reference to which these

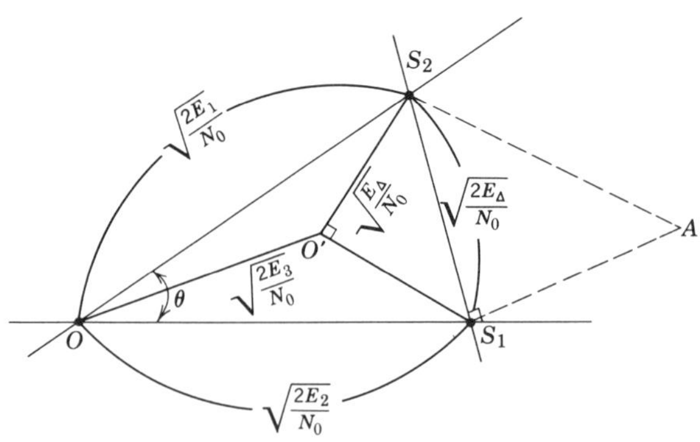

FIG. 10. Recognition space for large signals.

signals are orthogonal. The distance from $0'$ to each of the signals is $(\eta E_{\Delta}/N_0)^{1/2}$. The energy required to shift the point of origin from 0 to $0'$ is redundant energy. It may be useful in phasing the receiver or bringing it on frequency. It does not, however, contribute to the capacity of the signals to lead to a decision.

If S_1 and S_2 are now presented in random order and the receiver is asked to state the order, again the data necessary to enter the graph of Fig. 3*b* is available. In this case, the pairs can be considered orthogonal to each other. Thus, the measure is now $d'_{S_1, A} = \sqrt{2}d'_{S_1S_2}$.

The theory of signal detectability deals only with signals for which the space for any set of signals in a given noise background is Euclidean. Distances in this space are linearly related to the square root of the energy of the difference signal represented by two points. The unit of measure is the square root of one-half the noise power per unit bandwidth, $(N_0/2)^{1/2}$.

CONCLUSIONS

From the preceding discussion it is obvious that, in psychoacoustics at least, d' is a voltage-type variable. Ideally, d' is linearly related to the square root of the energy of the information carrying component of the signal, not to its power. In studies in which a receiver's response to an incremental stimulus is investigated, the incremental stimulus should be stated in terms of added voltage, not added energy. If one's measure is that quantity leading to a constant d', as would be the case if one measured a "difference limen," then this constant d' would be expected to result when there is a constant voltage difference between the two signals, rather than a constant energy difference. This should be the case whenever there is enough redundant energy to remove the statistical uncertainty of the signal.

In some cases, where there is an uncertainty which cannot be removed, as in the case of the signal which is a sample of white Gaussian noise, the energy of the signal is the basis for a good approximation of the detectability.

On the other hand, η is an energy ratio, since efficiency is commonly measured in terms of energy. This term is useful in inferring the properties of the receiver under study.

SUMMARY

Because studies employing d' and η are based on the theory of signal detectability, the theory is reviewed in sufficient detail for the purposes of definition. The efficiency, η, is defined as the ratio of the energy required by an ideal receiver to the energy required by a receiver under study when the performance of the two is the same. The measure d' is that value of $(2E/N_0)^{1/2}$ necessary for the ideal receiver to match the performance of the receiver under study, where E is the energy of the signal, and N_0 is the noise power per unit bandwidth. The measure is extended to include the recognizability of two signals. Every set of signals is described by a Euclidean space in which distances are the square roots of the energy of the difference signal, $(E_\Delta)^{1/2}$. The unit of measure is the square root of one-half of the noise power per unit bandwidth $(N_0/2)^{1/2}$.

ACKNOWLEDGMENTS

This article was prepared in the laboratories of the Electronic Defense Group of the University of Michigan with support from the Operational Applications Laboratory of the U. S. Air Force. It appeared as Tech. Rept. No. AFCRC-TR-57-57, and in J. acoust. Soc. Am., *1958,* **30,** *922–928.*

References

- Egan, J. P. Message repetition, operating characteristics, and confusion matrices in speech communication. Indiana University: Hearing and Communication Laboratory, 1957, Technical Report No. AFCRC-TR-57-50.
- Egan, J. P., and Clarke, F. R. Source and receiver behavior in the use of a criterion. *J. acoust. Soc. Am.,* 1956, **28,** 1267–1269. [30]
- Egan, J. P., Clarke, F. R., and Carterette, E. C. On the transmission and confirmation of messages in noise. *J. acoust. Soc. Am.,* 1956, **28,** 536–550.
- FitzHugh, R. The statistical detection of threshold signals in the retina. *J. gen. Physiol.,* 1957, **40,** 925–948. [17]
- Green, D. M., Birdsall, T. G., and Tanner, W. P., Jr. Signal detection as a function of signal intensity and duration. *J. acoust. Soc. Am.,* 1957, **29,** 523–531. [11]
- Marill, T. Detection theory and psychophysics. Massachusetts Institute of Technology: Research Laboratory of Electronics, 1956, Technical Report No. 319.
- Munson, W. A., and Karlin, J. E. The measurement of human channel transmission characteristics. *J. acoust. Soc. Am.,* 1954, **26,** 542–553.
- Peterson, W. W., Birdsall, T. G., and Fox, W. C. The theory of signal detectability. *Trans. IRE Professional Group on Information Theory,* 1954, **PGIT-4,** 171–212.
- Smith, M., and Wilson, E. A. A model of the auditory threshold and its application to the problem of the multiple observer. *Psychol. Monogr.* 1953, **67,** No. 9, Whole No. 359.

- Swets, J. A., and Birdsall, T. G. The human use of information: III. Decision making in signal detection and recognition situations involving multiple alternatives. *Trans. IRE Professional Group on Information Theory*, 1956, **IT-2,** 138–165.
- Tanner, W. P., Jr. Theory of recognition. *J. acoust. Soc. Am.*, 1956, **28,** 882–888. [19]
- Tanner, W. P., Jr., and Norman, R. Z. The human use of information: II. Signal detection for the case of an unknown signal parameter. *Trans. IRE Professional Group on Information Theory*, 1954, **PGIT-4,** 222–227.
- Tanner, W. P., Jr., and Swets, J. A. The human use of information: I. Signal detection for the case of the signal known exactly. *Trans. IRE Professional Group on Information Theory*, 1954, **PGIT-4,** 213–221.
- Tanner, W. P., Jr., Swets, J. A., and Green, D. M. Some general properties of the hearing mechanism. University of Michigan: Electronic Defense Group, 1956, Technical Report No. 30.
- Van Meter, D., and Middleton, D. Modern statistical approaches to reception in communication theory. *Trans. IRE Professional Group on Information Theory*, 1954, **PGIT-4,** 119–145.

6

Indices of Signal Detectability Obtained with Various Psychophysical Procedures

John A. Swets

The emergence, in recent years, of the theory of statistical decision as an appropriate model in the study of psychophysical phenomena has led to the current usage of the measure d' as an index of signal detectability. The definition of d', the manner in which it is estimated from data collected with various psychophysical methods, and a variety of studies in which it has been employed, have recently been summarized by Tanner and Birdsall (1958).

According to decision theory, a given signal-to-noise ratio should yield a particular value of d', irrespective of the procedure by which the data are collected. The experiments presented in this paper were designed to provide an empirical test of this presumed comparability of the estimates of d', as obtained from the forced-choice (FC) method with different numbers of alternatives, and from the yes-no (YN) method. Data from two studies are presented. In the first study, experiments were conducted employing the FC method with two and with four alternatives, and the YN method, in every case with the same four levels of signal energy. In the second study, estimates of d' for one signal energy were obtained from FC experiments which involved two, three, four, six, or eight alternatives. The alternatives in the FC experiments were, in each instance, alternative positions in time. The observers knew that one of the N temporal intervals presented on each trial contained the signal. In the YN experiment, the decision on each trial was based on a single observation interval, this interval containing a signal on half of the trials.

The signal used in these experiments was a pulsed tone, presented in a background of white noise. A less extensive test of the comparability of estimates of d', employing a visual signal, has been reported previously by Tanner and Swets (1954). In the visual experiment, the near equivalence of estimates of d' obtained from the YN method and from the four-alternative FC method was demonstrated.

THRESHOLD ESTIMATIONS

It is a commonplace that the procedure for calculating the threshold value of the signal does not provide a detectability index that is general to the various procedures of data collection. (See, for example, Osgood, 1952.) To select a single example from the literature that is especially pertinent to the present study, it has been shown that thresholds obtained with the FC method are lower than those obtained with the YN method (Blackwell, 1953). The second study reported in this chapter shows the estimated threshold to vary with the number of alternatives used in an FC experiment.

In both cases, the threshold was defined by assuming that a signal is detected when some hypothetical variable exceeds some critical (threshold) value, and by assuming, further, that this variable rarely exceeds the critical value when no signal is presented. Then the probability of a correct detection, $P(c)$, is given by

$$P(c) = p + c(1 - p) \tag{1}$$

where p is the probability that a signal will cause the threshold to be exceeded, or the true probability of detection. The second term of the equation is the probability of a correct guess c weighted by the opportunity for guessing, namely $(1 - p)$, the probability that the threshold will not be exceeded. With the YN method, the observed proportion of "yes" responses made on trials when no signal is presented is taken as an estimate of c; with the FC method, c is equal to $1/N$, where N is the number of alternatives presented.

Given this conception of the mechanism of detection, the threshold may be calculated by applying the correction for chance success to the obtained values of $P(c)$ corresponding to various signal energies. This correction

$$p = \frac{P(c) - c}{1 - c} \tag{2}$$

is simply a rearrangement of Equation (1). The threshold value of the signal is then taken as the signal energy corresponding to $p = 0.5$. Thus, a finding that different psychophysical procedures yield different values for the threshold is equivalent to the statement that a given signal-to-noise ratio does not lead to the same value of p with one procedure that it does with another. It should be noted in this connection that a frequently used computational procedure does not use the chance correction in the estimation of p or of the threshold, but is nevertheless equivalent; this method takes as the FC threshold the signal energy corresponding to a value of $P(c)$ lying halfway between $1/N$ and 1.0.

The finding that thresholds obtained with the FC method are lower than those obtained with the YN method is accounted for, in terms of decision theory, by the fact that the calculated threshold varies monotonically with c—with high thresholds corresponding to low values of c such as were obtained in these YN experiments. The theoretical relationship between c and the signal energy required to yield a $p = 0.5$ is shown in Fig. 1. Since d' is approximately proportional to signal power (Green, Birdsall, and Tanner, 1957), a change in c from, say, 0.2 to 0.001 will result in an increase of approximately 5 db in the threshold. An experimental demonstration of the dependency of the calculated threshold on c, in the visual YN case, has been described by Swets, Tanner, and Birdsall (1955).

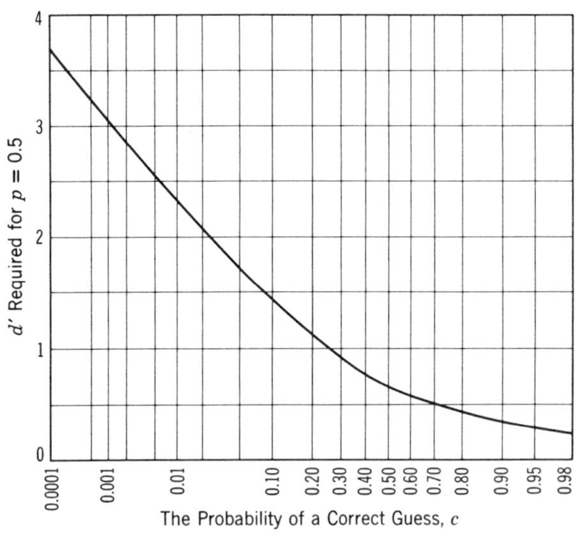

FIG. 1. The relationship between d' and the probability of a correct guess c at threshold. From Birdsall (1955).

EXPERIMENTAL PROCEDURE

Throughout both of the studies reported, the signal was a tone of 1000 cps, with a duration of 0.1 sec. The first study was conducted at the Psychophysical Laboratory, Electronic Defense Group, University of Michigan. The basic apparatus and procedure have been described elsewhere (Green, Birdsall, and Tanner, 1957). The noise spectrum level was approximately 50 db *re* 0.0002 d/cm^2; the four signal energies, in terms of 10 log E/N_0, were 9.7, 10.7, 11.6, and 12.2 db. E is the signal energy or time integral of power, and N_0 is the noise power per unit bandwidth. Three students, observing two hours a day, made 500 observations at each signal energy, under each of three procedures: YN, two-alternative FC (2AFC), and four-alternative FC (4AFC). The observers had had several weeks of practice prior to these experiments.

The second study was conducted at the Massachusetts Institute of Technology under comparable conditions. The noise spectrum level was again approximately 50 db *re* 0.0002 d/cm^2; the signal energy (10 log E/N_0) was 13.5 db. Again, three students with considerable practice served as observers. The number of observations made in each of the NAFC experiments varied with the number of alternatives as follows: 2AFC—300, 3AFC—500, 4AFC—600, 6AFC—900, and 8AFC—1200. Each of the alternatives was 0.1 sec in duration, separated by spacing intervals lasting 0.6 sec; on each trial the warning light lasted 0.3 sec, the answer period 0.8 sec, and the period in which the observers were informed of the correct answer lasted 0.3 sec. In both studies, the various conditions were counterbalanced so that all conditions were represented on each day.

RESULTS

The results of the first study are presented in Fig. 2. The value of d' is plotted vs. the signal energy E/N_0. The estimates may be seen to be quite comparable. The estimates from the 2AFC and 4AFC experiments are nearly identical; the YN estimates are very similar though more variable. No systematic bias in the various estimates is apparent. As referred to earlier, d' varies approximately linearly with signal power. Given this last-mentioned result, we may note that the three estimates of d' at each signal level fall within a range of 1 db.

Thresholds have not been calculated for comparison in this first study, in part because of the prior result that YN thresholds depend upon c and in part because the second study, to be described in what follows,

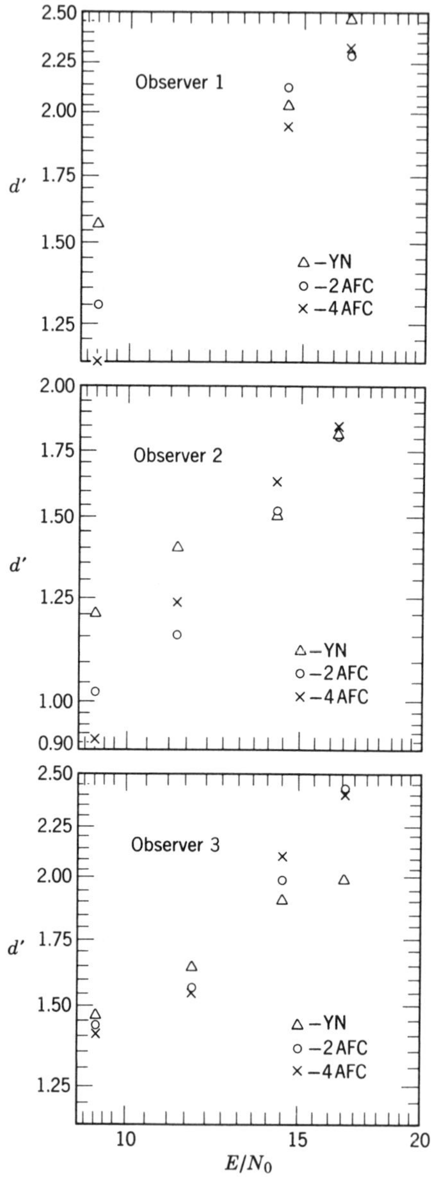

FIG. 2. The estimate of d' plotted versus the signal power E/N_0 for three observers in YN, 2AFC, and 4AFC experiments.

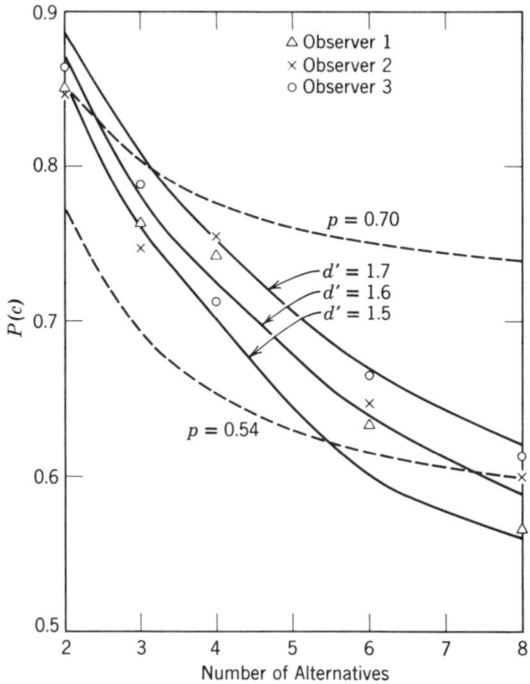

FIG. 3. The obtained values of $P(c)$ plotted versus the number of alternatives in various FC experiments. The solid curves are theoretical curves of $P(c)$ for constant d'; the dashed curves are theoretical curves of $P(c)$ for constant p.

offers a wider range with respect to the number of alternatives used with the FC method.

The results of the second study are displayed in Fig. 3. $P(c)$ is plotted vs. the number of alternatives. The solid curves show the predicted values of $P(c)$ for constant d'.[1] The dashed curves show the predicted values of $P(c)$ for constant p. The data follow the trend of the theoretical curves of constant d'. They are fitted very well by the curve of $P(c)$ for $d' = 1.60$. As a matter of fact, the curves for $d' = 1.50$ and 1.70 shown in Fig. 3 are within 0.5 db of each other, a difference that is within the range of experimental error. The theoretical curve of constant p that is extrapolated from the 2AFC data ($p = 0.70$) is not well fitted by the 4, 6, and 8AFC data; similarly, the curve for $P(c)$ for $p = 0.54$ that is

[1]W. W. Peterson and T. G. Birdsall, "The probability of a correct choice among m alternatives" (unpublished). These calculations are reproduced in Green and Birdsall (1958).

extrapolated from the 8AFC data does not fit the data with fewer alternatives.

That the various procedures in this second study yield essentially the same value of d' means that the observers are operating with the same "efficiency" (see Tanner and Birdsall, 1958), irrespective of the number of alternatives. Said another way, since the calculation of d' assumes perfect memory, these results imply that the observers are as capable of storing, and selecting among, the eight measures they obtain in an 8AFC experiment as they are when a smaller number of alternatives is offered. From the standpoint of theory construction, it is encouraging to find that the results of FC experiments with as many as eight temporal alternatives can be predicted from 2AFC experiments, without incorporating into the prediction an empirical constant representing the decay of memory.

SUMMARY

The index of detectability d' was estimated from data collected with various psychophysical procedures, specifically, the forced-choice method with different numbers of alternatives and the yes-no method. The estimates were, in all instances, quite comparable. This result is comforting in view of the fact that none of the other indices extant provide a unification of data collected with different procedures. This result is also somewhat surprising in view of the fact that the calculation of d' assumes perfect memory, and forced-choice experiments were conducted with as many as eight temporal alternatives.

ACKNOWLEDGMENTS

The various contributions to this study made by Ann Mills, Elizabeth F. Shipley, Mary J. McKey, Susan Sewall, and Arthur Wasserman are gratefully acknowledged.

This article was prepared in the Research Laboratory of Electronics of the Massachusetts Institute of Technology with support from the Operational Applications Laboratory of the U. S. Air Force. It appeared as Tech. Rept. AFCRC-TN-58-74, and in J. acoust. Soc. Am., *1959,* **31,** *511–513.*

References

- Birdsall, T. G. The theory of signal detectability. In H. Quastler (Ed.), *Information theory in psychology.* Glencoe, Ill.: Free Press, 1955, pp. 391–402.
- Blackwell, H. R. Psychophysical thresholds: experimental studies of methods of measurement. University of Michigan: Engineering Research Institute, 1953, Bulletin No. 36.

- Green, D. M., and Birdsall, T. G. The effect of vocabulary size on articulation score. University of Michigan: Electronic Defense Group, 1958, Technical Memorandum No. 81. [32]
- Green, D. M., Birdsall, T. G., and Tanner, W. P., Jr. Signal detection as a function of signal intensity and duration. *J. acoust. Soc. Am.*, 1957, **29,** 523–531. [11]
- Osgood, C. E. *Method and theory in experimental psychology.* New York: Oxford University Press, 1952.
- Swets, J. A., Tanner, W. P., Jr., and Birdsall, T. G. The evidence for a decision-making theory of visual detection. University of Michigan: Electronic Defense Group, 1955, Technical Report No. 40. [See 1]
- Tanner, W. P., Jr., and Birdsall, T. G. Definitions of d' and η as psychophysical measures. *J. acoust. Soc. Am.*, 1958, **30,** 922–928. [5]
- Tanner, W. P., Jr., and Swets, J. A. A decision-making theory of visual detection. *Psychol. Rev.*, 1954., **61,** 401–409.

7

Operating Characteristics Determined by Binary Decisions and by Ratings

James P. Egan, Arthur I. Schulman, and Gordon Z. Greenberg

The theory of signal detectability provides a framework for the study of the detectability of a signal by the human listener (Peterson and Birdsall, 1953; Smith and Wilson, 1953; Tanner and Swets, 1954; Tanner, 1956; Marill, 1956; Green, Birdsall, and Tanner, 1957; Egan, 1957; Pollack and Decker, 1958; Egan, 1958, see also Licklider and Pollack, 1948; Tanner and Birdsall, 1958). Within this framework, it is possible to derive a measure of performance which is relatively independent of the particular procedure employed (Swets, 1959). This measure of performance is d', and, unlike the threshold as it is usually measured, the value of d' is largely unaffected by those circumstances that may influence the criterion adopted by the listener.

One of the procedures that has been developed within the framework of the theory of signal detectability has been called the "fixed-interval observation experiment." For each observation by the listener, a single temporal interval is well defined. These intervals consist of two types: (1) those that contain the signal plus Gaussian noise, and (2) those that contain noise alone. Thus, there are two stimulus situations, and there is no longer any special meaning intuitively ascribed to the presentation of a "stimulus." After each interval, the listener responds with *yes* or *no*. Each of these decisions is made according to some fixed arbitrary criterion adopted by the listener. The two types of intervals, *SN* and *N*, and the two responses, y and n, result in four stimulus-response conjunctions. The important descriptive probabilities are as follows: $p(SN) + p(N) = 1.0$, $p(y|SN) + p(n|SN) = 1.0$, and $p(y|N) + p(n|N) = 1.0$. By empirical tests, it turns out that the three formally independent probabilities $p(y|SN)$, $p(y|N)$, and $p(SN)$ give a comprehensive description of the behavior of the real listener in the detection of a signal in noise.

For fixed average conditions of signal and noise, the two conditional probabilities $p(y|SN)$ and $p(y|N)$ are determined for several different criteria, and the relation between these two criterial probabilities is termed the *operating characteristic*. From the operating characteristic, the measure of detectability d' is derived.

Actually, for the determination of d', a temporal forced-choice procedure (with two or more observation intervals per trial) is more economical than the procedure that uses a single fixed interval for an observation. However, for certain purposes, the nature of the problem may demand that a single interval for observation be employed. In such cases, the basic procedure requires that the subject make a binary decision. According to this binary-decision procedure, the listener adopts one criterion for a series of observation intervals. He then adopts a different criterion for the next series of intervals, and this process is continued until a sufficient number of pairs of values of the two criterial probabilities is obtained. Now, if the listener adopts a given criterion for a long series of observation intervals, many of his yes-no decisions are well within and many well outside that criterion. Consequently, the listener should be able to order his yes-no decisions and thereby assign ratings to each of his responses. The rating method utilizes the fact that, during a single series of observation intervals, the human listener is capable of adopting multiple criteria. For comparable reliability, the rating method with four categories should require about one-third the number of trials as that used for the binary-decision procedure, provided the listener can in fact maintain several criteria during a single series of observation intervals. If it can be shown that nearly the same value of d' is obtained by the rating method as is obtained by the binary-decision procedure, then a very considerable saving will result in future determinations of d'.

The relation between the binary-decision procedure and the rating method is as follows. In the rating method, the assignment of 1 represents a "yes" under a strict criterion. If the observation interval in fact contains the signal, then $p(r_1|SN)$ is equivalent to $p(y|SN)$, where r_1 is the assigned rating 1. Similarly, for the noise-alone intervals, $p(r_1|N) = p(y|N)$.

Next, the conditional probability of the assignment of 2 to an *SN* interval is computed. The reasonable assumption is then made that all "1's" would fall within the criterion designated by the assignment of "2's." More generally speaking, the assumption is the following: observation intervals that are accepted as containing the signal under a given criterion will also be accepted under a less strict criterion.[1] Therefore, the second value of $p(y|SN)$ is $p(r_1|SN) + p(r_2|SN)$. Thus, the value of $p(y|SN)$ corresponding to the criterion established by the rating c is the cumulative probability

$$p(y|SN) = \sum_{i=1}^{c} p(r_i|SN)$$

For the same criterion, the corresponding value of $p(y|N)$ is

$$p(y|N) = \sum_{i=1}^{c} p(r_i|N)$$

Computation of $p(y|SN)$ and $p(y|N)$ over the entire rating scale, $i = 1, 2, \cdots, r$, generates the operating characteristic.

The following two experiments were conducted in order to compare the values of d' and (σ_{SN}/σ_N) as they are obtained by two methods, the binary-decision procedure and the rating method.

GENERAL PROCEDURE

A "fixed-interval observation experiment" is one in which (1) the listener knows that a signal, if presented, will occur in a well-delimited interval of time, and in which (2) a decision of some sort is required after each observation. A single temporal interval for observation by the listener is the principal part of a *trial*, and Fig. 1 diagrams the sequence of events. In the experiments, a trial began with a white light (W) which served as a warning signal and which remained on for 1.5 sec. The last 0.5 sec of W was the fixed interval for observation, and was marked by the presence of a red light (R). The signal, when presented, also had a duration of 0.5 sec with its onset and offset synchronous with the onset and offset of R. The response interval was 5 sec, and the listener responded with a binary decision or with a rating, as the case might be, by

[1] The rating scale as here applied is assumed to have only ordinal properties; no assumption is made with regard to the numerical properties of the rating scale other than that of order.

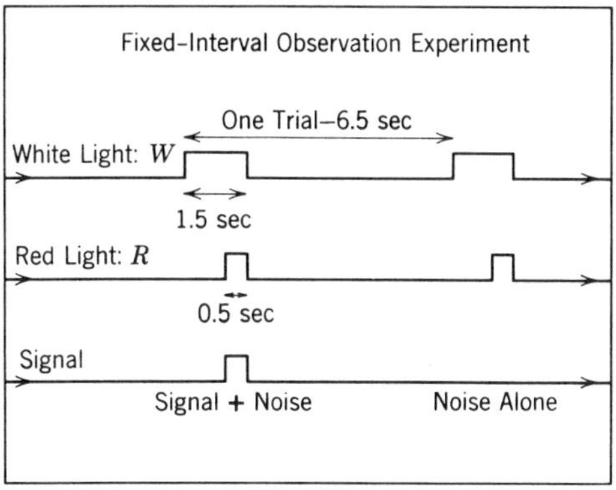

FIG. 1. Schema showing the sequence of events in each trial. The red light (R) marked the interval for observation, and the signal of 1000 cps was presented with a probability of 0.5. The listener responded by pressing the appropriate key after the termination of W and R. Although the white noise is not represented, it was on continuously throughout the session.

pressing the appropriate key during the early part of this interval. The subject was not informed whether his decision was correct or incorrect.

The signal was a "pure tone" of 1000 cps. The signal voltage was turned on without regard for phase and without the use of special devices, so that the (negligible) transients were determined by the response of the earphone (Permoflux Corporation, PDR-10). In both experiments, the a priori probability of the signal $p(SN)$ was 0.5, and the listener knew this fact. The white noise was generated by a 6D4 tube (Noise Generator, Model 455-B, Grason-Stadler Company). The over-all sound pressure level of the noise was about 65 db *re* 0.0002 μbar, and it was held constant for all tests at this comfortable level for listening. The signal and the noise were mixed electrically and then presented over a binaural headset with the two earphones wired in parallel and in phase. The noise was present continuously throughout the session.

The primary environmental condition will be specified in the present experiments by the value of E/N_0, in which E is the signal energy, or the time integral of power, and N_0 is the noise power per unit bandwidth.

Experiment I

In separate sessions, data were obtained by the binary-decision procedure and by the rating method. In order to obtain a quite different criterion from one series of trials to the next for the binary-decision procedure, the listeners were first trained to adopt three different criteria which were specified as "strict," "medium," and "lax." For purposes of instructing the listener during the experiment proper, the following conditions were chosen: (1) *strict*, $0.05 \leq p(y|N) \leq 0.10$; (2) *medium*, $p(y|SN) + p(y|N) = 1.00 \pm 0.07$; (3) *lax*, $0.90 \leq p(y|SN) \leq 0.95$. After each block of 240 trials, all at a given criterion, the experimenter calculated the conditional probabilities of a "yes." If the obtained value(s) fell within the appropriate range indicated in the foregoing, the listener was told that his performance was "good." If the value(s) fell outside the specified range, the listener was told that he had been "too strict" or "too lax," as the case might be. These remarks were repeated to the listener the next time he used that criterion in an effort to induce him to operate within the desired range. For the rating method, a similar instructional procedure was used. The listener divided his responses into four categories. On this scale, a "1" was meant to correspond approximately to a "yes" given as a response when the listener was making binary decisions under a strict criterion; a "2" corresponded to a "yes" with a medium criterion; a "3" to a "yes" with a lax criterion; and a "4" to a "no" with a lax criterion. No other instructions were given. The listener was not informed of the *level* of his performance at any time during the experiment.[2]

Nine daily sessions were administered individually to three listeners. On days 1–3 and 7–9 the listener used binary decisions. On day 4 the listener was given practice on the rating method, and on days 5 and 6 he was tested on the rating method. Each daily session consisted of 9 test periods of 80 trials each, separated by short rest intervals. In order to reinforce the listener's memory for the signal frequency, an extra trial was given before each test period with the signal intensity increased by 10 db over its normal level.

For each binary-decision session, three consecutive periods, giving a

---

[2] The measure d' depends upon how well the listener *partitions* each of his response categories between the two stimuli, *SN* and *N*. In situations that require a binary decision, the response probabilities are simply $p(y) + p(n) = 1.0$; the corresponding probabilities for the rating method are: $p(r_1) + \cdots + p(r_4) = 1.0$. These probabilities are easily manipulated by a host of variables, including the instructions given to the listener. Some psychologists are concerned with the social, motivational, and learning variables which affect these response probabilities. However, it should be clear by now that, in the study of signal detection, the great virtue of d' is its independence from such sociopsychological factors.

total of 240 trials, were devoted to each of the 3 criteria. Over the 6 sessions, each listener was presented once with each of the 6 ways of ordering the 3 criteria. All told, 4320 test trials under the binary-decision procedure were administered to each listener. Each of these same listeners rated 1440 test trials. The computation of each pair of criterial probabilities was based upon the 240 trials that occurred in 3 consecutive periods. In about one-half of these 240 trials, the observation interval contained the signal. Perhaps it should be pointed out that, in the binary-decision procedure, only one point for the operating characteristic was provided by 240 trials; on the other hand, in the rating method, 3 points were available from 240 trials.

All tests for this experiment were conducted with $E/N_0 = 15.8$; expressed in decibels this value is

$$10 \log(E/N_0) = 12 \text{ db}$$

The results for each listener are shown separately as operating characteristics in Figs. 2 to 4. The data obtained by the binary-decision procedure and by the rating method are shown, respectively, in the upper and the lower graphs of each figure. The data for each operating characteristic are plotted on normal-normal coordinates. For this purpose, each probability scale, $p(y|SN)$ and $p(y|N)$, is so transformed that the corresponding normal deviates (z scores) are linearly spaced. In the figures, these z-score axes are referred to as $z(y|SN)$ and $z(y|N)$.

In effect, a curve was fitted to the data by passing the criterion cut through two normal curves of equal area plotted on a common decision axis. When the operating characteristic is generated in this way, it is linear on a z-score plot. Two parameters, based upon these two normal curves, were then adjusted to give a least-squares fit to the data. One of these parameters is the difference between the means of the two normal curves, expressed as follows: $d' = (M_{SN} - M_N)/\sigma_N$. The other independent parameter is σ_{SN}/σ_N.

Actually, a straight line was fitted to the data by that method of least squares which minimizes the sum of the squared perpendicular distances between the data points and the straight line. The two constants of this straight line determine the two parameters required to specify the two normal curves referred to previously. For purposes of simplicity, the value of d' will be taken as the "x intercept," that is to say, d' is here defined as the coordinate $z(y|N)$ for the point at which the operating characteristic intersects the horizontal line, $z(y|SN) = 0$. The ratio

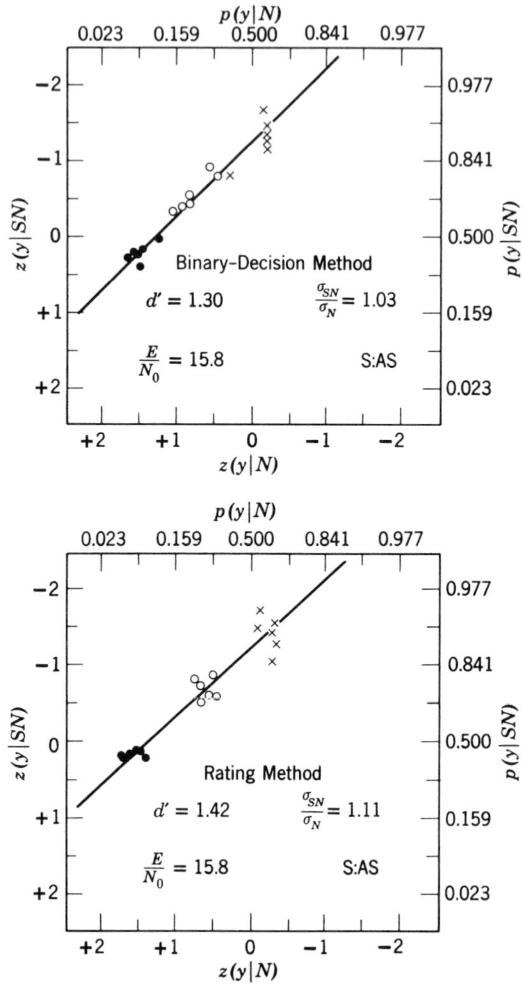

FIG. 2. To obtain these operating characteristics, a single listener made decisions concerning the presence of the signal in a series of observation intervals. The two criterial probabilities associated with each point, $p(y \mid SN)$ and $p(y \mid N)$, were transformed to normal deviates, and a straight line was fitted to the data with respect to the z-score axes. The two parameters of this line define d' and (σ_{SN}/σ_N). For each point of the upper graph, the listener adopted a fixed criterion for 240 trials, and the three symbols are associated with the three criteria of strict, medium, and lax. For the lower graph, each series of 240 trials resulted in three points, corresponding to these same three criteria.

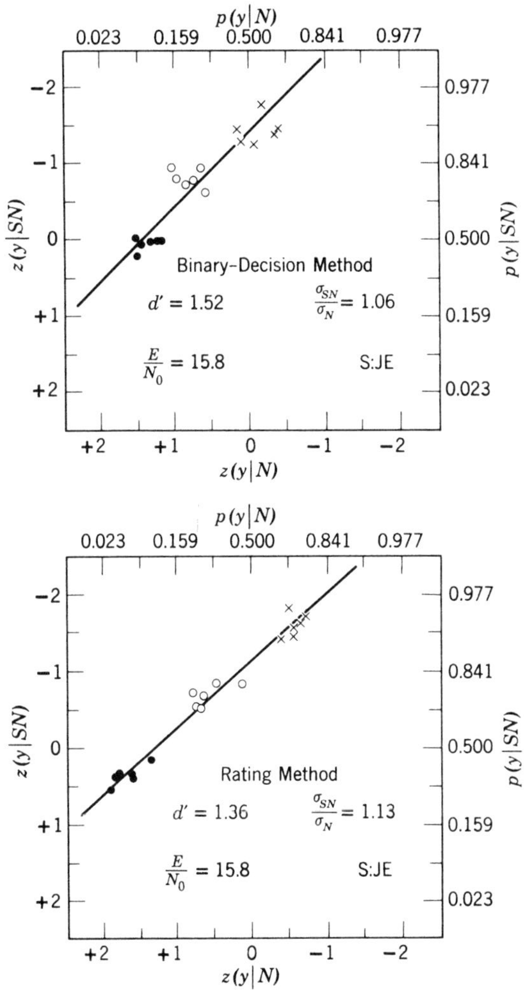

FIG. 3. These operating characteristics were obtained with a second listener under the same conditions as those for Fig. 2.

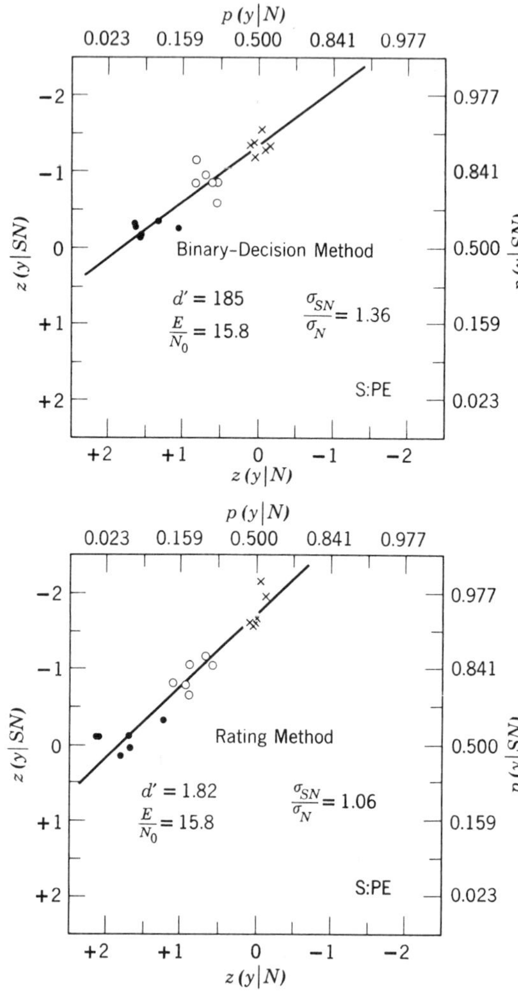

FIG. 4. These operating characteristics were obtained with a third listener under the same conditions as those for Fig. 2.

σ_{SN}/σ_N is given by the reciprocal of the slope of the straight line with respect to the z-score axes.[3]

It is fairly obvious from an inspection of Figs. 2 to 4 that the data fall along a straight line. Of course, the obtained proportions plotted in Figs. 2 to 4 are subject to random sampling errors. The scatter of each set of points is well within the limits expected on the basis of chance fluctuations.

Each operating characteristic shown in Figs. 2 to 4 has a value of d' and of σ_{SN}/σ_N. These values are also presented in Table I for comparative purposes. It is clear that the trained listener can perform as well when he adopts the multiple criteria necessary for the rating method as when he adopts the single criterion required by the binary-decision procedure.

The theory of signal detectability makes it possible to set an exact upper bound upon the detectability of the signal. Therefore, the efficiency of the real listener may be expressed in terms of the performance of an ideal observer (Tanner and Birdsall, 1958). The amplitude of the signal used for the listener is attenuated until the performance of the ideal observer is the same as that of the listener. The ratio of the corresponding signal energies defines the efficiency η of the listener.[4] On the basis of the average d' for the three listeners (Table I), the value of η is 0.076, or -11 db.

---

[3] Strictly speaking, we are taking the value of d' at which $p(y|SN)$ is 0.5. When the slope of the straight line of best fit is not one, d', as defined by Tanner and Birdsall (1958), becomes a function of the criterion adopted. Nevertheless, the two values, the "x intercept" and the reciprocal of the slope, are two constants that give a comprehensive description of the listener's behavior. In a personal communication, Clarke, Birdsall, and Tanner have recently defined a measure of performance which they denote by $\sqrt{d_e}$. The value of $\sqrt{d_e}$ is computed as follows. The coordinates with respect to the z-score axes of the *point of intersection* between the ROC curve and the negative diagonal are determined. The ordinate minus the abscissa of this point of intersection is the value of $\sqrt{d_e}$. In Experiment I, the mean value of $\sqrt{d_e}$ for the binary-decision procedure is 1.45, and the corresponding value for the rating method is 1.46.

In Egan (1958), the advantages of specifying performance in terms of the coordinates of the point of intersection are discussed. When the a priori probabilities of the two types of intervals are equal, then, at the point of intersection, (1) one-half of the intervals are in the criterion of acceptance, and (2) the rate of correct acceptance is equal to the rate of correct rejection.

[4] In this computation, it is assumed that the signal is known exactly. If the phase at the onset of the signal had been known to the listener, he almost certainly could not have used this information in the situation being studied here. Therefore, part of the inefficiency of the listener, relative to the ideal observer, is his inability to use phase information.

Experiment II

In the second experiment, only the rating method was used to determine the relation between d' and E/N_0. The same three listeners were employed. For two of the listeners (JE and AS), operating characteristics were determined at each of the following values of E/N_0: 7.9, 15.8, and 31.6. For the other listener (PE), the three E/N_0's were: 6.3, 12.6, and 25.1. Each subject was run for 6 sessions, 2 at each of the three E/N_0's. A session consisted of 9 periods of 80 trials each. The first 3 periods of each session were "practice," and, on the basis of these 240 trials, the subject was informed whether or not he had adopted the appropriate criteria for each of the rating categories. These criteria corresponded to those established for the binary-decision procedure in Experiment I. The criterial probabilities for the operating characteristic were estimated from the 480 test trials given in the last 6 periods of each session. As in Experiment I, the probability that a signal would be presented was 0.5, so that each criterial probability is based upon about 240 test trials.

The sequence of warning signals and the corresponding temporal intervals were the same as those shown in Fig. 1.

Figures 5 to 7 display the results as operating characteristics on normal-normal coordinates. The straight line passing through the data

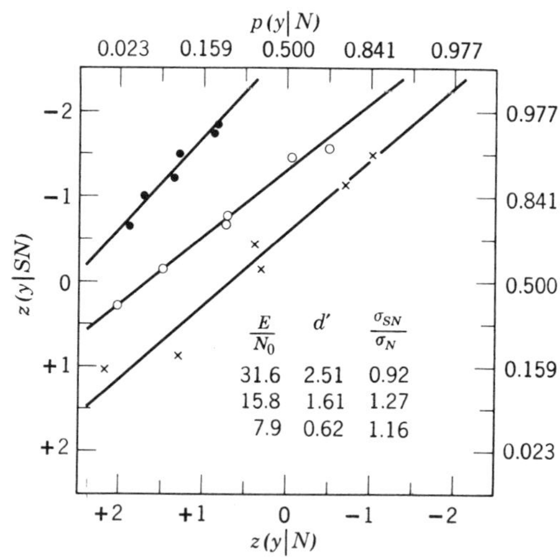

FIG. 5. Operating characteristics obtained by the rating method. At each of two sessions, 480 test trials were conducted at a given value of E/N_0. These 480 test trials resulted in three points for a given operating characteristic. A straight line was fitted to the data with respect to the z-score axes, and the two parameters of this line define d' and σ_{SN}/σ_N.

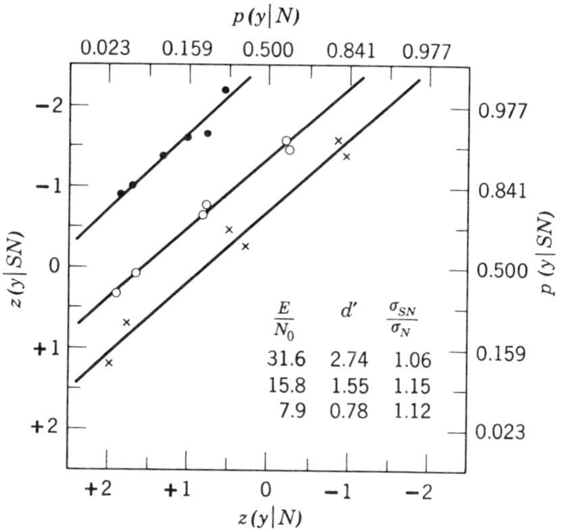

FIG. 6. Operating characteristics obtained with a second listener under the same conditions as those for Fig. 5.

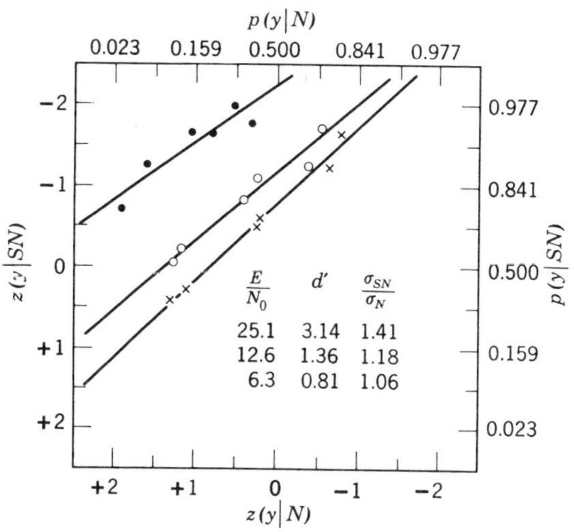

FIG. 7. Operating characteristics obtained with a third listener under the same conditions as those for Fig. 5.

TABLE I. COMPARISON OF VALUES OF d' AND OF VALUES OF σ_{SN}/σ_N AS OBTAINED BY THE BINARY-DECISION METHOD (BD) AND BY THE RATING METHOD (R). THE DATA ARE TAKEN FROM FIGS. 2–4 IN WHICH $E/N_0 = 15.8$.

Subject	d'		(σ_{SN}/σ_N)	
	BD	R	BD	R
AS	1.30	1.42	1.03	1.11
JE	1.52	1.36	1.06	1.13
PE	1.85	1.82	1.36	1.06
Mean	1.56	1.53	1.15	1.10

points was fitted by the same method of least squares as that used in Experiment I. The constants, d' and σ_{SN}/σ_N, associated with each operating characteristic, are also shown. For two of the listeners, JE and AS, one of the values of E/N_0, 15.8, was used in Experiment II as well as in Experiment I. Both listeners showed a small improvement in performance from the first to the second experiment.

The values of d' taken from Figs. 5 to 7 are plotted as a function of E/N_0 in Fig. 8. A straight line, constrained to pass through the origin, was fitted to the data by the standard method of least squares. The equation of this line is $d' = 0.095(E/N_0)$. The constant, 0.095, differs

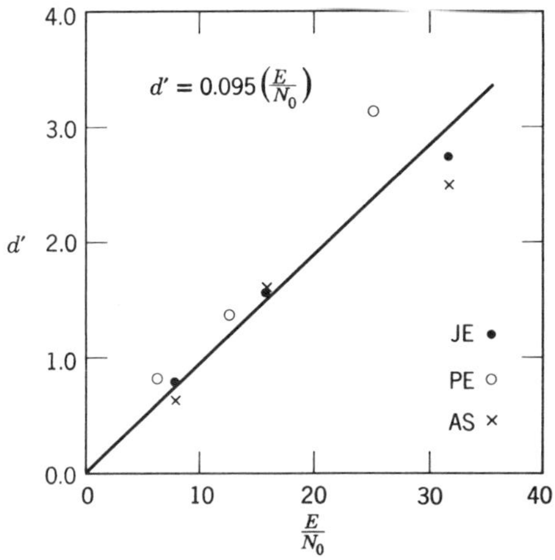

FIG. 8. Data based on the operating characteristics of Figs. 5 to 7. The derived measure d' is plotted against E/N_0, and, for $d' \leq 3.0$, the resulting function may conveniently be considered as linear.

from that obtained in other laboratories by the equivalent of about 1 db in the value of E/N_0. On the basis of all available data, this constant appears to be about 0.08.

On the basis of the foregoing experiments, it is concluded that the rating method (4 categories) is superior to the binary-decision procedure for the following reasons. (1) Nearly the same measures of performance are obtained by the two methods. (2) Although only one-third as many trials were administered for the rating method as for the binary-decision procedure, these two methods provide about the same reliability.

SUMMARY

With the theory of signal detectability as a framework, two psychophysical experiments were conducted in which each observation interval was well defined for the listener. Each interval contained noise, and it either did or did not ($p = 0.5$) contain a signal (1000 cps, 0.5 sec in duration). In separate sessions of the first experiment, either the listener gave a yes-no decision or he responded with a rating (1 to 4) after each observation interval. Operating characteristics were obtained with E/N_0 equal to 15.8. It is clear from the data that the trained listener can perform as well when he adopts the multiple criteria necessary for the rating method as when he adopts the single criterion required by the binary-decision procedure. In the second experiment, only the rating method was used to determine the relation between d' and E/N_0. The resulting function, for $d' \leq 3.0$, approximates a straight line which passes through the origin and which has nearly the same slope as that obtained in other laboratories.

ACKNOWLEDGMENTS

The writers are indebted to Dr. James D. Miller and to Mr. Charles S. Watson for their assistance in the design and construction of Audiac, a flexible assembly of components for the investigation of the detection of signals presented at fixed or at random times.

This research was conducted in the Hearing and Communication Laboratory of Indiana University with support from the Operational Applications Laboratory of the U. S. Air Force. It appeared as Tech. Rept. No. AFCRC-TN-59-50, and in J. acoust. Soc. Am., *1959,* **31,** *768–773.*

References

• Egan, J. P. Message repetition, operating characteristics, and confusion matrices in speech communication. Indiana University: Hearing and Communication Laboratory, 1957, Technical Report No. AFCRC-TR-57-50.

- Egan, J. P. Recognition memory and the operating characteristic. Indiana University: Hearing and Communication Laboratory, 1958, Technical Note AFCRC–TN-58-51.
- Green, D. M., Birdsall, T. G., and Tanner, W. P., Jr. Signal detection as a function of signal intensity and duration. *J. acoust. Soc. Am.*, 1957, **29,** 523–531. [11]
- Licklider, J. C. R., and Pollack, I. Effects of differentiation, integration, and infinite peak clipping upon the intelligibility of speech. *J. acoust. Soc. Am.*, 1948, **20,** 42–51.
- Marill, T. Detection theory and psychophysics. Massachusetts Institute of Technology: Research Laboratory of Electronics, 1956, Technical Report No. 319.
- Peterson, W. W., and Birdsall, T. G. The theory of signal detectability. University of Michigan: Electronic Defense Group, 1953, Technical Report No. 13.
- Pollack, I., and Decker, L. R. Confidence ratings, message reception and the receiver operating characteristic. *J. acoust. Soc. Am.*, 1958, **30,** 286–292. [31]
- Smith, M., and Wilson, E. A. A model for the auditory threshold and its application to the problem of the multiple observer. *Psychol. Monogr.* 1953, **67,** No. 9, Whole No. 359.
- Swets, J. A. Indices of signal detectability obtained with various psychophysical procedures. *J. acoust. Soc. Am.*, 1959, **31,** 511–513. [6]
- Tanner, W. P., Jr. Theory of recognition. *J. acoust. Soc. Am.*, 1956, **28,** 882–888. [19]
- Tanner, W. P., Jr., and Birdsall, T. G. Definitions of d' and η as psychophysical measures. *J. acoust. Soc. Am.*, 1958, **30,** 922–928. [5]
- Tanner, W. P., Jr., and Swets, J. A. A decision-making theory of visual detection. *Psychol. Rev.*, 1954, **61,** 401–409.

8

Auditory Detection of an Unspecified Signal

Richard F. Gundy

Virtually all studies of auditory detection within the framework of the theory of signal detectability have dealt with signals that are specified to the subject at the beginning of the experimental session. That is, the subject is usually given an opportunity to hear the signal or signals to be added to the noise on subsequent trials, and he is told the relative frequency of occurrence of the noise and signal-plus-noise. Experimenters in this area have not been particularly concerned with the learning aspects of the detection situation. More investigations of auditory discrimination learning have come from research involving the measurement of the quiet absolute threshold.

Although most of these audiometric studies have treated learning effects by discussing ways of designing them out of the experiment, a recent paper by Zwislocki, Maire, Feldman, and Rubin (1958) considers the effects of "practice and motivation" as the central topic of investigation. In their study, five experiments were conducted with naive subjects listening to pure tones under quiet conditions. Thresholds seemed to decrease with repeated testing sessions, one week apart. The introduction of reinforcement accentuated the effect. Essentially similar results were observed in the five experiments and these in turn agreed well with previous findings (Zwislocki, 1955). To these authors the results suggest that "the threshold of audibility . . . [is] determined by discrimination against the background of physiological noise and . . . during the practice period more sensitive cues are learned."

The present study was undertaken to investigate further some aspects of auditory discrimination learning within the framework of the theory of signal detectability. This context seemed particularly suitable because the theory has dictated measures of detectability which are relatively invariant over a wide variety of conditions (Clarke, Birdsall, and Tanner, 1959; Swets, 1959; Tanner and Birdsall, 1958). In this investigation, human detection of a pure-tone signal against a background of noise was studied for possible changes in performance over a series of trials. The effects of giving the listener (*a*) prior specification of the signal, and/or (*b*) feedback on each trial, were examined, with the ratio of signal energy to noise power per unit cycle entering as a parameter.

METHOD

One hundred and twenty experimentally naive subjects, students at Indiana University, participated in this experiment. During the experiment, the subject was seated in front of a panel on which were mounted three pilot lamps: a *ready* light, a *trial* light, and a *feedback* light. Four telegraph keys, numbered from 1 to 4, were mounted on the writing arm of the subject's chair.

Noise and signal were mixed electrically and delivered to the subject through a pair of Permoflux PDR-10 earphones. The signal, a 1000-cps tone, was presented without regard to phase for a duration of approximately 0.25 sec. The output of a noise generator was presented continuously at an overall level of 65 db *re* 0.0002 microbar.

Certain basic conditions were the same for all subjects. Trials were indicated by the appearance of the pilot lights on the panel in front of the subject; the sequence of events defined by these lights coincided with what has been called a fixed-interval observation experiment by Tanner and Swets (1954) and by Egan, Schulman, and Greenberg (1959). A cam timer operated the sequence of lights that defined a trial. Approximately one-half sec after the onset of the ready light, the trial light appeared. If a signal was to be delivered on the trial, the onset of the signal followed the appearance of the trial light by approximately 0.1 sec. After the signal had appeared for 0.25 sec, it was terminated; about 0.1 sec later, the ready and trial lights disappeared simultaneously. Approximately 4 sec later, the ready light appeared to indicate the beginning of another trial. All subjects were permitted to observe the light sequence for two trials at the beginning of the session.

The subject was instructed to decide whether or not he heard the signal, and to rate his confidence in the decision by pressing one of the four telegraph keys in front of him. (For a discussion of this rating procedure, see Egan, 1958.) The time allotted for his decision was approximately 4 sec, the intertrial interval quoted previously.

Each subject served in one experimental session which was approximately 1 hour long. The session consisted of four 100-trial periods with a 2-min rest between periods. At the beginning of each trial, presentation of signal-plus-noise or noise alone was determined by the experimenter by means of a table of random numbers. For each subject, a block of 400 random digits was drawn, corresponding to the 400 trials of the experimental session, and for every even digit in the block, a signal trial was presented.

Eight experimental groups were distinguished as follows. Subjects were first classified on the basis of the signal intensity used within the experimental session. The ratio E/N_0 of the signal energy E to the noise power per unit cycle N_0 was chosen as the measure of the stimulus. Half the subjects were run at a "low" value of E/N_0, the other half at a "high" E/N_0. For the "high" group, denoted henceforth by H, the value of E/N_0 was 25.1; for the "low" group, denoted henceforth by L, it was 15.8. The difference in E/N_0 for the two groups was obtained by attenuating the signal amplitude by 2 db, while the noise was maintained at a fixed level, as described.

The L and H groups were each divided in half to form the "feedback" F and "no feedback" NF groups. Subjects in the F group were told after each trial whether or not a signal was sent. When, in fact, a signal had been sent, the subject's response was followed by the appearance of the feedback light. On the other hand, the subjects in the *NF* group were never told whether or not a signal had been presented.

Each of the groups was further subdivided into "specification" S and "no specification" NS groups. The subjects in the S group were treated as follows. After the instructions were given, but before the regular series of trials began, the subject was given an opportunity to hear the tone. For the first three presentations of the tone, the amplitude of the signal was presented 10 db above the level to be used in the main series of trials. The ready and trial lights appeared in a typical sequence, and the signal was presented on each of three consecutive trials. After the third presentation, the signal was attenuated by 10 db, and the presentations were continued in succession until the subject twice reported hearing the tone. The demonstration of the signal was repeated exactly as described after every block of 100 trials.

The NS group received no demonstration *until* the beginning of the fourth period, that is, before the last 100 trials. Specifically, these subjects were given the following variation on the basic instructions.

"Now about the signal. I cannot tell you what 'the signal' is. You will probably discover what it is as the trials progress and consequently do a better job at detecting it. But don't be discouraged at the beginning if the task is difficult. We will run a few blocks of trials, then I will tell you what the signal is, let you hear it clearly, then run another block of trials to finish the session."

Each subject can be classified by his status with regard to: (1) E/N_0 level (L or H), (2) feedback or no feedback (F or NF), and (3) specification or no specification (S or NS). Sixty subjects were used in each of the L and H groups. The L and H groups were, in turn, divided in half to form the two feedback conditions, F and NF. These two subdivisions yielded four groups of 30 subjects each. From each of these four groups, 10 subjects were chosen to be given prior information about the signal, as described above. The remaining 20 were given no opportunity to hear the signal until the beginning of the fourth period. These successive subdivisions created eight distinct and independent groups, denoted by the initials used above. These groups are listed, with the number of subjects composing each one, in Table I.

TABLE I. Number of Subjects within Each of the Eight Experimental Groups

Group	No. of subjects
NFNS-H	20
NFNS-L	20
FNS-H	20
FNS-L	20
NFS-H	10
NFS-L	10
FS-H	10
FS-L	10
Total	120

RESULTS AND DISCUSSION

As described, each subject furnished 400 confidence-rating responses. It should be recalled that, as far as the subject was concerned, the experimental session was divided into *four* periods of 100 trials each. In the analysis of the data, however, the relevant sub-divisions were *not* these periods, but the *two 50-trial blocks* within each period, yielding 8 consecutive blocks. Within each of the 8 blocks, it was possible to determine how the subject allocated his ratings on signal and noise trials, and therefore, to obtain an operating characteristic for each block.

The procedure for obtaining an operating characteristic from the subject's protocol has been described in detail elsewhere (Clarke, Birdsall, and Tanner, 1959; Egan, 1958; Pollack, 1959). The index of detectability, here referred to as d_s (Pollack, 1959), was obtained by doubling the absolute value of the abscissa of the point of intersection of the ROC curve with the diagonal line drawn from the upper left to the lower right-hand corner of the normal-normal grid.

In the course of the analysis, a number of "pathologies" appeared, most of them due to the very small number of responses used to determine each ROC curve. It was sometimes impossible to harvest three points for the ROC curve from a 50-trial block because the subject failed to use one or more of the available rating categories. To a large extent, this was obviated by phrasing the instructions to emphasize the importance of distributing responses in all categories. However, the instructions failed on occasion, and in various degrees. At one extreme, some subjects confined their responses to a single key to indicate that they heard no signal. In these instances, no coordinates exist for the normal-normal plot; consequently, the operating characteristics could not be determined by the usual technique. On these occasions, the index of detectability was taken to be zero.

One-point records resulted when the subject restricted his responses to two of the four available keys. Usually this happened when the detectability was high, or very low. To estimate an index of detectability in these cases, the pair of proportions was plotted on the normal-normal grid, and a line with a unit slope was drawn through the plotted point. This line was defined as the ROC curve for the block and the d_s was calculated as described above. No gross inconsistencies appeared as a result of these conventions; the indices defined in this manner were in close agreement with the values derived from adjacent blocks where no such device was required.

Somewhat more often, subjects failed to respond on one of the four keys. Such behavior produced records from which only two points could be obtained. The rule in these cases was simply to connect these two points; the line so described was taken to be the ROC curve for the block.

Typically, three points were obtained from a block of 50 trials to determine an ROC curve; the one- and two-point records were relatively infrequent. Of all 960 ROC curves obtained, 89 per cent were plotted on the basis of three points, 9 per cent on the basis of two points, and 2 per cent on the basis of one point.

When three points were available, the straight edge was placed on the extreme points. Maintaining the angle determined by the line connecting the two extreme points, the straight edge was moved laterally until it was approximately equidistant from the middle and extreme points, a line was drawn, and the index of detectability was recorded, always to the nearest tenth of one standard deviation unit.

Mean learning curves: d_s vs. blocks of fifty trials

The eight values of d_s computed for each subject permitted examination of detectability as a function of consecutive blocks of 50 trials. Within each group, the values of d_s were averaged over subjects at each of the eight blocks, and the results plotted in Figs. 1 and 2. Figure 1 exhibits the results for the four combinations of prior information and trial-by-trial feedback, at the low (L) level of E/N_0. Figure 2 illustrates the same conditions at the high (H) level of E/N_0. The curves in both figures are discontinued after the sixth block to indicate the point at which all subjects were allowed to hear the tone, before the beginning of the last 100 trials.

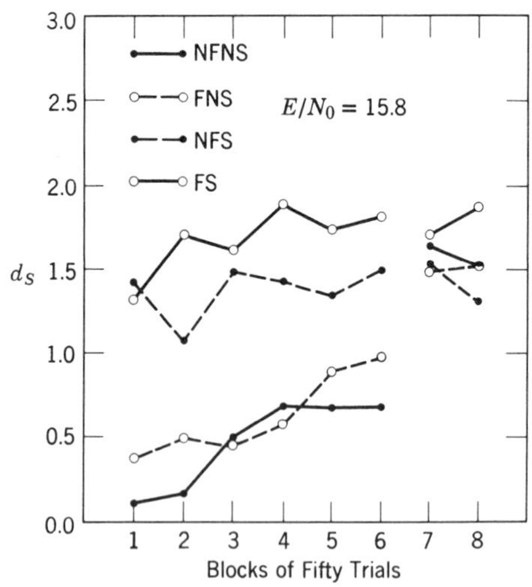

FIG. 1. Mean d_s as a function of successive blocks of 50 trials for low (L) group.

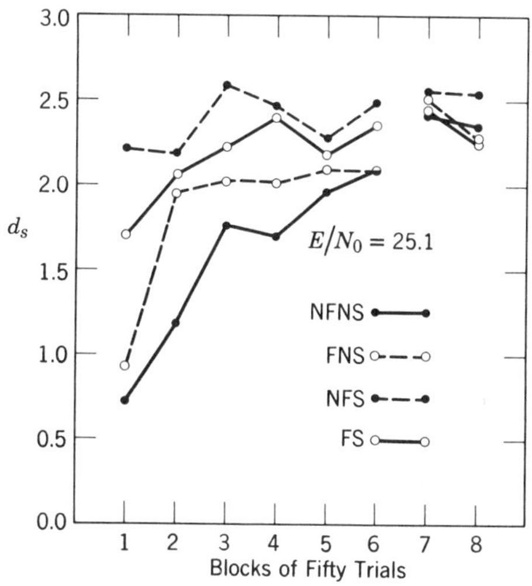

FIG. 2. Mean d_s as a function of successive blocks of 50 trials for high (H) group.

Specification of signal

The effect of giving the subject an opportunity to hear the signal before the session began (S vs. NS) can best be evaluated by examining the data from the first block alone—before learning effects became pronounced. From Figs. 1 and 2, it can be seen that at both E/N_0 levels, the difference between the S groups and the NS groups was marked. Giving prior specification of the signal resulted in asymptotic or near-asymptotic performance at the end of the first 50 trials. A Kruskal-Wallis test was performed at each E/N_0 level to test the hypothesis that the four treatments (NFNS, NFS, FNS, and FS) had no differential effect on detectability. Both results were significant beyond the 0.01 level.

Figure 3 shows the inter-subject standard deviations for the S and NS groups; i.e., the distinctions between the feedback conditions and the two E/N_0 levels were disregarded, and subjects were separated on the S and NS classifications only.

In the group that had no opportunity to hear the signal before the session began (NS), the inter-subject variability tended to increase as the session progressed from trial 1 through trial 300. No such tendency was noted in the group that received prior information about the signal (S); the variability remained fairly uniform throughout the session. A Mann-Whitney statistic was computed from the inter-subject standard deviations on blocks one to six. The difference between the S and NS groups was significant at beyond the 0.0001 level. The increasing vari-

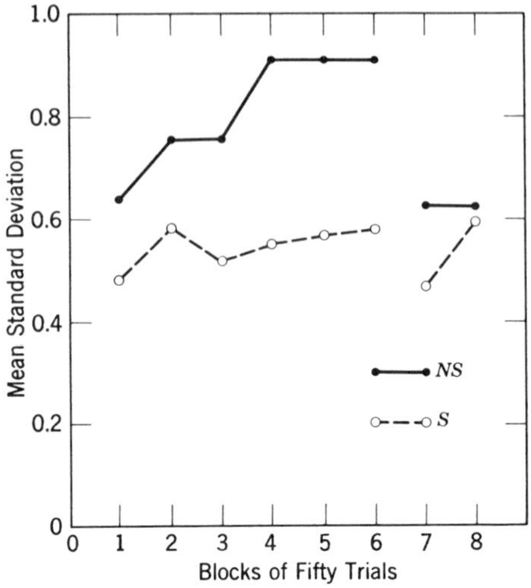

FIG. 3. Inter-subject variability for the S and NS groups as a function of blocks of 50 trials.

ability shown in the NS curve from blocks one to six illustrates an aspect of the data which cannot be seen in Figs. 1 and 2. This increase in variability is due to the fact that when information about the signal was withheld, some subjects failed to improve as the session progressed, others improved slightly, and still others reached asymptotic level by the fifth or sixth block. Though this indicates that performance was not entirely uniform within each experimental group, the mean curves do not seem to misrepresent the individual data.

Feedback

As indicated in Fig. 1, at the low E/N_0 level, feedback had little effect. The mean curve for the group that received feedback on each trial, plus information about the signal before the session began (FS), is slightly above the curve for the group which received prior information but no feedback (NFS). However, the maximum difference between the two curves is just less than 0.6 of a d_s unit, approximately equal to the average of the inter-subject standard deviation for the two groups.

The order of the corresponding curves in Fig. 2 is reversed from Fig. 1; the NFS curve is slightly above the FS curve. The maximum difference between the curves is about half of a d_s unit, again comparable to the inter-subject standard deviation. Taken together, the results at both levels seem to indicate that giving the subject trial-by-trial feedback has little effect, provided the subject has been given an opportunity to hear the tone before the beginning of the session.

When no prior specification about the signal was given, again feedback seemed to have little effect at the low E/N_0 level, as illustrated in the two lower curves of Fig. 1. At the higher E/N_0 level, the mean curve for the NFNS group is below the FNS curve at every block except the last. This may indicate that feedback facilitated improvement, shown as an increase in d_s as the session progressed. However, again, any inference should be somewhat guarded, since the variability at each block is about as large as the largest difference between groups.

On blocks seven and eight, just after the subjects in *all* groups were allowed to hear the signal, almost identical behavior was exhibited by the NS and S groups, as shown by the measure d_s (see Figs. 1 and 2). Further, the inter-subject variability in the NS group decreased to the level found in the S group (see Fig. 3). The homogeneity of *both* means and standard deviations, when conditions were similar for all subjects, seems to be a noteworthy comment on the reliability of the measure of detectability d_s.

Index of detectability as a function of E/N_0

For a tone of 1000 cps with a duration of 0.25 sec, Egan, Greenberg, and Schulman (1959) found that the measure of d_s was approximately described by a linear function of E/N_0 with slope 0.137 and intercept zero. For the same stimulus, the asymptotic values of d_s obtained in the present experiment plotted against E/N_0 can be fitted well with a straight line passing through the origin, with a slope of 0.094.

Two estimates of d_s

A check for artifacts due to the scoring conventions was made in the following way. Since 50-trial blocks represent arbitrary and very small segments of behavior from which to compute ROC curves, d_s was computed in two ways for a large portion of the data. For blocks seven and eight, when all subjects were treated alike, an estimate of the typical value of d_s was computed for each level of E/N_0 by *averaging all of the d_s values taken from blocks seven and eight* within each of the L and H groups. The values obtained by this method were 1.52 for the L group and 2.37 for the H group. An ROC curve was also plotted on the basis of the *100 trials formed from the last two 50-trial blocks of each session.* The values of d_s, taken from this new ROC curve, yielded another set of estimates.

When these estimates were averaged at each level of E/N_0, the obtained values were 1.56 and 2.36 for the L and H groups, respectively.

If the same computations are performed on the data from earlier trials, the average values are no longer meaningful since the experimental treatments are quite dissimilar. However, it is possible to compute *absolute differences* between the two values of d_s obtained as described, then to average these differences over subjects. This computation was performed on the data from blocks two and three, for each subject; the average absolute difference between the two measures of d_s over all subjects was 0.10. The corresponding average for blocks seven and eight was 0.07. Since values of d_s were read only to the nearest tenth, the agreement seems surprisingly good.

CONCLUSIONS

Strictly speaking, most of these data cannot be analyzed in terms of efficiency relative to an "ideal observer" as suggested by the theory of signal detectability: the absence of any advance signal specification for some of the listeners places their decision problem beyond the boundary of the problems discussed by Peterson and Birdsall (1953), Birdsall (1960), and Gundy (1961). However, the results of these experiments may provide information about situations in which such an analysis is appropriate.

When the efficiency of a subject's performance is evaluated relative to the optimum procedure for an idealized experiment, assumptions must be made concerning the amount of initial information given the decision maker in order to guarantee the existence of a solution for the optimization problem. In fact, the "ideal observer" of the theory of signal detectability requires complete specification of all parameters as an initial condition. Analogously, this initial condition is met in the actual experiment by providing the listener with an estimate of the relative frequency of signal and noise trials, and an opportunity to hear both signal and noise before the beginning of the session. With highly trained listeners, it is assumed that this kind of signal specification is sufficient to eliminate systematic changes in performance as the trials progress. To some extent, the effectiveness of this procedure is revealed by the results of this investigation.

That signal demonstrations do, in fact, eliminate large changes in performance as trials progress is shown in the groups given an opportunity to hear the signal before each 100 trials. On the other hand, when no demonstrations are given, initial performance is noticeably poorer.

At the higher signal intensity, there is a gradual improvement as the session progresses, until, at the end of the 300 trials, the level of performance is close to the level of the group given signal demonstrations. At the lower signal intensity, some improvement occurs. However, after the introduction of a signal demonstration at the beginning of the final 100 trials, all groups performed at the same level.

Additional information in the form of feedback cues given on every trial had no effect in the groups given the signal demonstrations, and in the groups which received no demonstration, the effect of feedback was only slightly discernible at the higher signal intensity.

Finally, it should be noted that the requirements of this investigation demand an analysis of very small segments of the performance of experimentally naive subjects—conditions somewhat alien to the tradition of psychophysical experimentation. Under these circumstances, the results were surprisingly stable: both the average level of detectability and the variability around this average remained roughly constant throughout the experiment, and no essential change in these results appeared when the data were pooled for analysis in larger segments.

SUMMARY

Listeners were required to detect an auditory signal against a background of "white noise." The effects (1) of giving trial-by-trial information as to whether or not a signal was delivered, and (2) of giving the subject an opportunity to hear the signal before the test sequence began, were studied at two levels of signal energy. The results were analyzed within the context of the theory of signal detectability. Subjects who were given an opportunity to hear the signal before the test sequence began maintained a stable level of performance throughout the experimental session. On the other hand, subjects who were given no opportunity to hear the signal performed near chance level at the beginning of the session but showed gradual improvement as trials progressed. The effect of trial-by-trial feedback was surprisingly small in all groups. Near the end of the session, the signal was demonstrated to all subjects and the differences between the groups vanished.

ACKNOWLEDGMENTS

This research was conducted in the Hearing and Communication Laboratory of Indiana University with support from the Operational Applications Laboratory of the U. S. Air Force. It appeared as Tech. Rept. No. AFCCDD-TR-61-1, and in J. acoust. Soc. Am., *1961,* **33,** *1008–1012.*

References

- Birdsall, T. G. Detection of a signal specified exactly with a noisy stored reference signal. *J. acoust. Soc. Am.*, 1960, **32,** 1038–1045.
- Clarke, F. R., Birdsall, T. G., and Tanner, W. P., Jr. Two types of ROC curves and definitions of parameters. *J. acoust. Soc. Am.*, 1959, **31,** 629–630.
- Egan, J. P. Recognition memory and the operating characteristic. Indiana University: Hearing and Communication Laboratory, 1958, Technical Note AFCRC–TN-58-51.
- Egan, J. P., Greenberg, G. Z., and Schulman, A. I. Operating characteristics, signal detectability, and the method of free response. Indiana University: Hearing and Communication Laboratory, 1959, Technical Report No. AFCRC–TR-59-58. [See **15**]
- Egan, J. P., Schulman, A. I., and Greenberg, G. Z. Operating characteristics determined by binary decisions and by ratings. *J. acoust. Soc. Am.*, 1959, **31,** 768–773. [7]
- Gundy, R. F. Remarks on Birdsall's "Detection of a signal specified exactly with a noisy stored reference signal." *J. acoust. Soc. Am.*, 1961, **33,** 696.
- Peterson, W. W., and Birdsall, T. G. The theory of signal detectability. University of Michigan: Electronic Defense Group, 1953, Technical Report No. 13.
- Pollack, I. On indices of signal and response discriminability. *J. acoust. Soc. Am.*, 1959, **31,** 1031.
- Swets, J. A. Indices of signal detectability obtained with various psychophysical procedures. *J. acoust. Soc. Am.*, 1959, **31,** 511–513. [6]
- Tanner, W. P., Jr., and Birdsall, T. G. Definitions of d' and η as psychophysical measures. *J. acoust. Soc. Am.*, 1958, **30,** 922–928. [5]
- Tanner, W. P., Jr., and Swets, J. A. A decision-making theory of visual detection. *Psychol. Rev.* 1954, **61,** 401–409.
- Zwislocki, J. Design and testing of earmuffs. *J. acoust. Soc. Am.*, 1955, **27,** 1154–1163.
- Zwislocki, J., Maire, F., Feldman, A. S., and Rubin, H. On the effect of practice and motivation on the threshold of audibility. *J. acoust. Soc. Am.*, 1958, **30,** 254–262.

section three

EXPANDED OBSERVATIONS

The simple detection tasks emphasized in the preceding sections can be expanded in several ways. One can increase the duration of the signal, the number of signal components, the number of observations preceding a decision, or the number of observers contributing to each decision. According to statistical theory and the theory of signal detectability, the variable d′ *will increase as the square roots of the signal duration and of the number of signal components, observations, or observers. The prediction has been confirmed in each case. Studies of signal duration and of the number of observations are reported in this section; studies of multiple signal components are included in Section 6 [24, 25], for they are an integral part of the theory of frequency analysis; the studies of multiple observers have not been published.*

One can also expand the interval in which a signal of fixed duration is presented, or leave the observation interval almost completely undefined. The theory predicts the effect of specified amounts of temporal uncertainty; it must be imaginatively elaborated to deal with the flexible and realistic "vigilance" or "free-response" task.

In "Multiple Observations of Signals in Noise" [9], Swets, Shipley, McKey, and Green show d′ *to increase as the square root of the number of observations when the successive samples of masking noise are independent. Repetition of the signal in the same sample of noise allows them to make inferences about the magnitude of the noise internal to the observer. They also use the procedure of multiple presentations as an approach to the problem of auditory frequency selectivity. In each of these cases, the number of observations was determined by the experimenter. Alternatively, the observer may determine the number of observations; after each observation in a given noise or signal-plus-noise sequence he can report "Yes," "No," or "Continue." This problem of deferred decision is considered by Swets and Green in "Sequential Observations by Human Observers of Signals in Noise" [10]. The results are in qualitative agreement with statistical theory—the observed error rates, and the observed average number of observations preceding a terminal decision, change appropriately with changes in signal probability, signal intensity, and decision values and costs.*

In "Signal Detection as a Function of Signal Intensity and Duration" [11], Green, Birdsall, and Tanner examine the improvement in d′ *with increasing signal duration, and the trading relationship between intensity and duration. The square-root improvement is obtained within a specified range of durations. Creelman, in "Human Discrimination of Auditory Duration" [12], describes the observer's ability to detect temporal differences between two signals.*

In a set of three articles, Egan, Schulman, and Greenberg report the results of progressive deteriorations in the observer's knowledge of the time of signal occurrence. In the study entitled "Interval of Time Uncertainty in Auditory Detection" [13], the signal could occur anywhere in a defined interval substantially longer than the signal. In the study of "Memory for Waveform and Time Uncertainty in Auditory Detection" [14], the observation interval was defined a specified time after it occurred. In the article entitled "Operating Characteristics, Signal Detectability, and the Method of Free Response" [15], they show how a detection probability and a false-alarm probability, and thus an estimate of d′, *can be determined when the signal is presented several times at random, unspecified intervals in a relatively long observation period.*

9

Multiple Observations of Signals in Noise

John A. Swets, Elizabeth F. Shipley, Mary J. McKey, and David M. Green

The problem of how much the detectability of a signal will be enhanced by additional observations is a familiar one, commonly referred to as the "multiple-look" problem. Although it is generally recognized that the amount of improvement to be obtained by additional observations will depend upon the nature of the signal, and upon the nature of the noise in which it is embedded, no extensive parametric studies have been reported in the case of audition. The experiments on multiple observation that are reported here employed a variety of signals and two types of noise. Their concern lay, however, not with establishing the amount of improvement to be expected with several signals and noises that are frequently encountered, but rather with the ability to infer certain general properties of the hearing process from the relative rates of gain in detectability of some special types of signals and noise.

The effect of multiple observations of auditory signals in noise has been investigated previously by Schafer and Shewmaker (1953), and by Schreitmueller (1952). Schafer and Shewmaker's observers were required to locate an 800-cps pulse, of 5 and 45 msec in two different experiments, which could appear anywhere within a period of noise of approximately 3 sec. Ten observations of each signal were offered. The proportion of correct responses was determined for each observation for various signal-to-noise ratios. The signal-to-noise ratio yielding a 0.5 proportion of correct responses was determined by interpolation. This signal-to-noise power ratio declined as the square root of the number of observations.

In Schreitmueller's study, the signal consisted of an 800-cps pulse, 0.16 sec in duration. Each trial consisted of an 8-sec period of noise, which was subdivided into eight intervals of 1 sec for the observer. On a given trial, either one, two, four, six, or eight intervals contained a signal. The observer's task was to report whether or not at least one signal was present after listening to all eight intervals. In one condition the sample of noise in each interval was the same for all eight intervals of a trial. In another condition, the samples of noise in the eight intervals were statistically independent of one another. The proportion of correct detections of the signal increased as the number of signals increased, when independent samples of noise were used. When the eight samples of noise were identical, detection was at a maximum when only two signals were presented, and declined steadily as more signals were presented.

The experiments reported here employed procedures that differed in certain respects from those used in the two studies just reviewed. A *trial*, as we shall use the term, consisted of five *observations;* each observation consisted of a fixed number of temporal intervals, one of which contained the signal. The observer responded after each observation by specifying the interval which he believed to contain the signal; that is, a temporal forced-choice procedure was used. The observer knew that the signal would occur in the same interval in all of the five observations of a given trial; he was asked to consider all of the observations he had made previously within the trial in making each decision. In the first set of experiments, as in Schreitmueller's study, both *variable noise,* or noise that is statistically independent from one observation to another, and *constant noise,* or noise that is identical on each of the five observations comprising a trial, were used. In these experiments, the signal was a 1000-cps pulse; a four-alternative, forced-choice procedure was used. In a second set of experiments, with only variable noise, the signal was either one of 2 frequencies in one case, any one of 16 widely spaced frequencies in another case, and all 16 of these frequencies in a third. These experiments employed a two-alternative, forced-choice procedure. In all the experiments, the signal was of 0.1-sec duration, and the background noise was white.

SIGNAL OF KNOWN FREQUENCY, CONSTANT AND VARIABLE NOISE

Procedure and apparatus

Before each observation a cue signal was presented at the same frequency, duration, and intensity as the signal to be detected, but with no noise present. The onset of noise followed the cue signal by 0.4 sec, and the signal occurred 0.33, 1.08, 1.82, or 2.58 sec after the onset of the noise. The duration of the noise on each observation was 3 sec. After each observation, the observers had 1 sec in which to make a response. The observers were told which interval was correct following their response to the fifth observation.

The signal and noise were presented by magnetic tape. Variable-noise tapes were constructed by gating the signal and the noise through telephone relays and recording the signal on one channel and the noise on the other channel of an Ampex model 350 tape recorder. Constant-noise tapes were constructed by recording the same cue tone, noise, and signal five times on a second two-channel Ampex recorder. Two minutes of noise and two minutes of tone were recorded on each tape to enable measurement of the signal and noise levels presented to the observers.

In presenting the signal to the observers, a voice key, triggered by the cue signal, activated a series of timer relays which gave the observers a warning signal and defined the signal intervals and the answer period by means of lights on each observer's answer box. A teletype reader, programmed in accord with the magnetic tape, supplied the observers with the correct answer by means of a light after the answer to the fifth observation. The observers gave answers after every observation by pressing keys on their answer boxes. The observers were given their cumulative scores of the number of correct answers on each observation after each experimental session.

Signal and noise could be attenuated separately by two attenuators which received the output from the signal and noise channels separately. From a mixer, signal and noise were fed to an amplifier, and through an attenuator, to the earphones and a Ballantine model 320 true-RMS voltmeter. The noise was measured through a band-pass filter of 200 cps centered at the signal frequency. PDR-8 earphones were used.

Three undergraduates at MIT served as observers for two hours a day, four days a week. After training on single observations, experiments were conducted with variable noise and constant noise on alternate days until 600 trials (1 trial = 5 observations) with variable noise and 520 trials with constant noise were presented. The noise spectrum level in these experiments was approximately 35 db *re* 0.0002 d/cm^2; the signal level, in terms of $10 \log E/N_0$, was 12.5 db. E is the signal energy, or time integral of power, and N_0 is the noise power per unit bandwidth.

Derivation of the detectability index d′

The procedures used in the analysis of the data are those suggested by a theory of detectability modeled after the theory of statistical decision (Tanner and Swets, 1954). In the following paragraphs, this theory of detectability (usually referred to as "decision theory" when the context makes the reference clear) is briefly characterized, and its predictions for these experiments are derived.

Decision theory assumes, in this case, two distributions of a hypothetical variable X, one resulting from presentations of noise alone and a second (with a larger mean) resulting from presentations of signal plus noise. In the specific form of decision theory discussed here, the distributions are assumed to be normal and to have the same variance. When the distinction is convenient, X_{S+N} will designate the variable resulting from signal plus noise, and X_N, the variable resulting from noise alone.

On a given observation under the forced-choice procedure, the observer is assumed to obtain a value of X from each interval, and to use these values to decide which interval contained the signal. It is assumed that he selects the interval having the largest value associated with it. A correct choice is made when the value resulting from the signal plus noise is greater than the value(s) resulting from noise alone. The probability of a correct response in a forced-choice procedure is given by

$$P(c) = \int_{-\infty}^{+\infty} F(X)^{M-1} g(X) dX \qquad (1)$$

where $F(X)$ is the area from minus infinity to X of the distribution resulting from noise alone, and $g(X)$ is the ordinate of the signal-plus-noise distribution at X. M is the number of alternatives, one of which the observer must select.

Since the distributions are assumed to be normal, X_N has the normal density function $\Phi[(X - 0)/\sigma]$ with mean zero and standard deviation σ, i.e., $E(X_N) = 0$, $D^2(X_N) = \sigma^2$. X_{S+N} has the normal density function $\phi[(X - m)/\sigma]$ with mean m and standard deviation σ, i.e., $E(X_{S+N}) = m$, $D^2(X_{S+N}) = \sigma^2$. Therefore Eq. (1) can be written

$$P(c) = \int_{-\infty}^{+\infty} \Phi\left(\frac{X - 0}{\sigma}\right)^{M-1} \phi\left(\frac{X - m}{\sigma}\right) dX \qquad (2)$$

Let d' designate the normalized difference between the means of the X_N and the X_{S+N} distributions, that is,

$$d' = (m - 0)/\sigma \tag{3}$$

The value of d' can be determined given $P(c)$ without specifying the values of m and σ. A table relating $P(c)$ to d' for four alternatives has been published previously (Green, Birdsall, and Tanner, 1957).

Value of d′ as a function of the number of observations

When the observer is permitted multiple observations of the signal, it is assumed that he sums the values obtained from each of the intervals constituting a forced-choice observation, and that after each observation he selects the interval with the largest sum. The probability of a correct response on the nth observation is the probability that the sum for the interval containing the signal is greater than the sum(s) for the interval(s) containing noise alone.

From statistical theory it is known that the distribution of the sum of n random variables has a mean equal to the sum of the means and a variance equal to the sum of the variances. Thus, the value of d' following the nth observation, under variable noise, is related to the value of d' after the first observation as follows:

$$d_n' = \frac{n(m - 0)}{\sigma(n)^{1/2}} = n^{1/2} \cdot \frac{m}{\sigma} = n^{1/2} d_1' \tag{4}$$

Hence, according to decision theory, when variable noise is used, d_n' will increase over multiple observations as $n^{1/2}$.

Results obtained with variable noise

Table I displays the results obtained in the experiment employing variable noise. Each value of $P(c)$, and hence each value of d', is based upon 600 observations. The ratio d_n'/d_1' for each value of n, obtained from each of the three observers, should be compared with the values of d_n'/d_1' predicted by decision theory, as shown in the right-most column. To facilitate this comparison, these data are shown graphically in Fig. 1. It should be noted that the solid line in Fig. 1—the predicted change in d' with additional observations—has been made to intercept the vertical axis at the value of d' corresponding to $n = 1$, and is, therefore, not necessarily the best-fitting line, with a slope of ½, to the obtained points. Clearly, the data obtained from the second observer would

TABLE I. THE PROBABILITY OF A CORRECT RESPONSE, $P(c)$, AND THE DETECTABILITY INDEX, d', FOR EACH OF FIVE OBSERVATIONS, USING VARIABLE NOISE

	Observer 1			Observer 2			Observer 3			Prediction
n	$P(c)$	d'	d_n'/d_1'	$P(c)$	d'	d_n'/d_1'	$P(c)$	d'	d_n'/d_1'	d_n'/d_1' (based on $n^{1/2}$)
1	0.81	1.93	1.00	0.80	1.87	1.00	0.82	1.98	1.00	1.00
2	0.92	2.66	1.38	0.89	2.33	1.25	0.95	2.97	1.50	1.41
3	0.97	3.30	1.71	0.95	2.86	1.53	0.97	3.39	1.71	1.73
4	0.99	3.92	2.03	0.96	3.15	1.68	0.98	3.51	1.77	2.00
5	0.99	3.92	2.03	0.98	3.54	1.89	0.99	4.12	2.08	2.24

be better fitted by the predicted line if this restriction had not been made.

It is of interest to note, in relation to another paper (Swets, McKey, and Green, 1958), that if d' does not increase with repeated observations, the theory of sequential decision would be of no value in describing the behavior of human observers. In experiments involving sequential decisions, as opposed to experiments involving trials with a fixed number of observations as discussed here, the observer determines the number of observations he makes of each signal.

It may be observed in Table I that improvement continues over four observations for Observer 1, and over the five observations for Observers 2 and 3. Since d' is approximately proportional to signal power (Tanner, Swets, and Green, 1956), the improvement obtained over five observations is equivalent to approximately 3 db.

Results obtained with constant noise

Table II shows the results obtained in the experiment employing constant noise. $P(c)$ and d', here based on 520 presentations at each observation stage, may be seen to increase over additional observations, but considerably less than under variable noise. Whereas the values of $P(c)_1$ are comparable for the two different noises, $P(c)_5$ is approximately 0.86 under constant noise, as opposed to 0.99 under variable noise. Similarly, d_5'/d_1' under constant noise is approximately 1.20, as compared with 2.0 under variable noise.

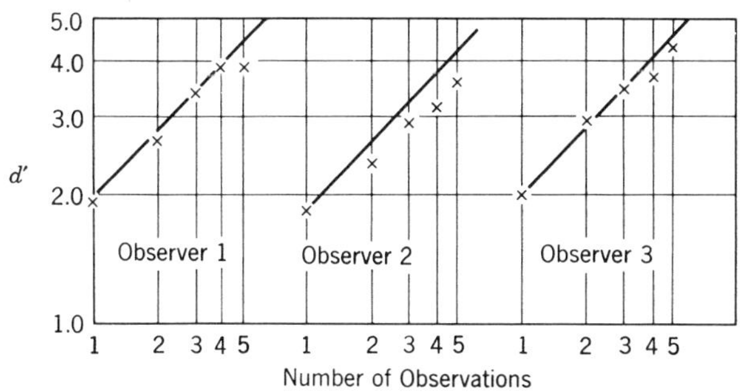

FIG. 1. The increase in detectability over five successive observations of a signal presented in variable noise. The line represents the $n^{1/2}$ prediction for the increase in d'; this line has been forced through the obtained value of d' at $n = 1$. Since the scale on the ordinate is twice the scale on the abscissa, a slope of ½ appears as a slope of 1.

TABLE II. THE PROBABILITY OF A CORRECT RESPONSE, $P(c)$, AND THE DETECTABILITY INDEX, d', FOR EACH OF FIVE OBSERVATIONS, USING CONSTANT NOISE

	Observer 1			Observer 2			Observer 3		
n	$P(c)$	d'	d_n'/d_1'	$P(c)$	d'	d_n'/d_1'	$P(c)$	d'	d_n'/d_1'
1	0.80	1.89	1.00	0.74	1.65	1.00	0.82	1.98	1.00
2	0.84	2.08	1.10	0.80	1.89	1.14	0.86	2.18	1.10
3	0.86	2.18	1.15	0.83	2.03	1.23	0.87	2.24	1.13
4	0.86	2.18	1.15	0.85	2.13	1.29	0.89	2.36	1.19
5	0.86	2.18	1.15	0.85	2.13	1.29	0.88	2.29	1.16

Estimate of the magnitude of internal noise

When the same external noise is presented on each observation, the observer is again assumed to make his choice on the basis of the sums of the values of the variable X obtained from the different intervals. In this case, however, the variability of the values from one observation to another for a given interval is determined only by internal variability, or internal noise. That is to say, any improvement in detectability under constant noise results from integrating over internal noise only. Let x represent the contribution of external noise, y represent the contribution of internal noise, and m represent the contribution of the signal to the variable X. Let the subscript E refer to external noise and the subscript I to internal noise. Then

$$X_N = x + y,$$

$$X_{S+N} = x + y + m,$$

$$E(x) = 0, \quad D^2(x) = \sigma_E^2,$$

$$E(y) = 0, \quad D^2(y) = \sigma_I^2,$$

$$E(X_N) = E(x + y) = 0, \quad D^2(X_N) = D^2(x + y) = \sigma_E^2 + \sigma_I^2,$$

$$E(X_{S+N}) = E(x + y + m) = m, \quad D^2(X_{S+N}) = \sigma_E^2 + \sigma_I^2 \text{ and}$$

$$d_1' = \frac{m}{(\sigma_E^2 + \sigma_I^2)^{1/2}} \tag{5}$$

Consider the sums of the values of the variable for n observations when the external noise is constant: for signal plus noise

$$\sum_{i=1}^{n} (X_{S+N_i}) = n \cdot x + n \cdot m + y_1 + y_2 \cdots + y_n$$

and for noise alone,

$$\sum_{i=1}^{n} (X_{N_i}) = n \cdot x + y_1 + y_2 \cdots + y^n$$

Further,

$$E[\sum_{i=1}^{n} (X_{S+N_i})] = n \cdot m$$

and

$$E[\sum_{i=1}^{n} (X_{N_i})] = 0$$

Considering the variance:

$$\begin{aligned} D^2[\sum_{i=1}^{n} (X_{S+N_i})] \\ &= E[\sum_{i=1}^{n} (X_{S+N_i})]^2 - E[\sum_{i=1}^{n} (X_{S+N_i})]^2 \\ &= E(nx + nm + y_1 \cdots + yn)^2 - n^2m^2 \\ &= E(n^2x^2 + n^2m^2 + y_1^2 \cdots + y_n^2 + 2n^2xm + 2nxy_1 \cdots \\ &\quad + 2nxy_n + 2nmy_1 \cdots + 2nmy_n + 2y_1y_2 \cdots + 2y_{n-1}y_n) - n^2m^2 \end{aligned}$$

However,

$$E(n^2m^2) = n^2m^2;\ E(n^2x^2) = n^2\sigma_E^2;\ E(y_i^2) = \sigma_1^2;\ E(x) = 0;$$
$$E(y_i) = 0;\ E(xy_i) = 0; \quad \text{and} \quad E(y_iy_j) = 0, \quad i \neq j$$

Therefore,

$$D^2[\sum_{i=1}^{n} (X_{S+N_i})] = n^2\sigma_E^2 + n\sigma_I^2$$

and, similarly,

$$D^2[\sum_{i=1}^{n} (X_{N_i})] = n^2\sigma_E^2 + n\sigma_I^2$$

Thus,

$$d_n' = \frac{n \cdot m}{(n^2\sigma_E^2 + n\sigma_I^2)^{1/2}} \tag{6}$$

Using Eqs. (5) and (6), we have

$$\frac{d_n'}{d_1} = \frac{n \cdot m/(n^2\sigma_E^2 + n\sigma_I^2)^{1/2}}{m/(\sigma_E^2 + \sigma_I^2)^{1/2}} = \frac{[1 + (\sigma_I^2/\sigma_E^2)]^{1/2}}{[1 + (\sigma_I^2/\sigma_E^2)\ (1/n)]^{1/2}}$$

Let $k = \sigma_I^2/\sigma_E^2$; then

$$\frac{d_n'}{d_1'} = \frac{(1 + k)^{1/2}}{(1 + k/n)^{1/2}} \tag{7}$$

Thus, by plotting calculated values of d_n'/d_1' against n for various assumed values of k, the obtained value of k (the ratio of internal to external noise) can be estimated from the best fit to the obtained values of d_n'/d_1'. The data of Table II are plotted in this fashion in Fig. 2. The estimates of k range from 0.5 to 1.0. In other words, the internal noise is approximately equal to the external noise at the level of external noise used in the experiment.

Consistency check on the estimate of internal noise

If the parameters of the internal noise are independent of the external noise, then with smaller values of external noise the estimated value of k should be larger. That is, internal noise would then constitute a larger proportion of the total noise affecting the detection process. To test this, another experiment was conducted, like the previous one in all respects except that the noise was attenuated by approximately 20 db. The noise spectrum level was approximately 17 db *re* 0.0002 d/cm²; 10 logE/N_0 was 13 db.

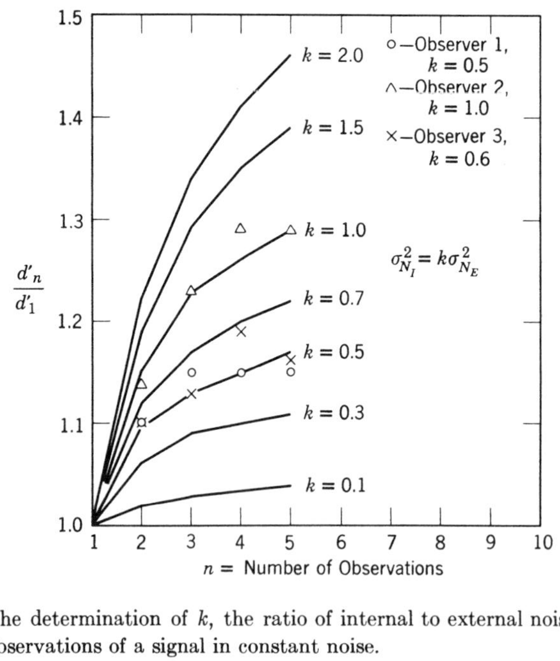

FIG. 2. The determination of k, the ratio of internal to external noise, using five successive observations of a signal in constant noise.

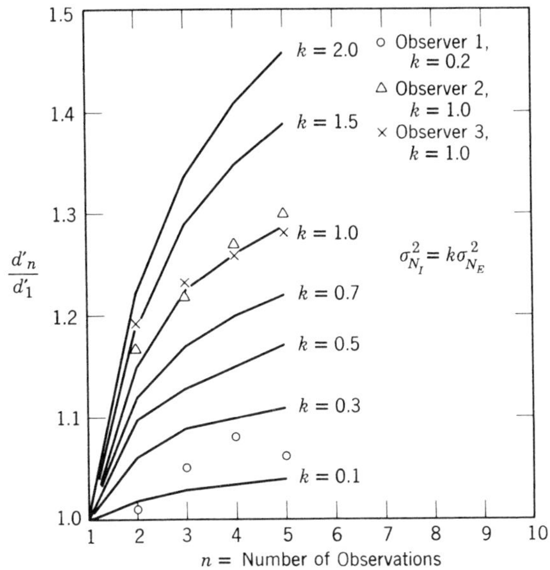

FIG. 3. The determination of k, the ratio of internal to external noise, at a lower level of external noise.

The results are presented in Fig. 3. The assumption that internal noise is independent of external noise would lead us to expect values of k of approximately 50 to 100, since the external noise had been attenuated by a factor of 100. Instead, the values of k are very similar to those obtained in the previous experiment. This result is consistent with a previous study by Green (unpublished) which employed multiple observers rather than multiple observations. Green found the correlation between observers to be independent of the level of the external noise; for several levels of external noise the inter-observer correlation was approximately 0.75, equivalent to a k of unity. Apparently, the parameters of the internal noise are not independent of the external noise.

Several alternatives are open to us in attempting to deal with these data. We may, for example, accept at face value the data indicating a correlation of internal and external noise. We may, on the other hand, speculate about the existence of a nonlinear device, such as an automatic volume control on external noise. Or we may be led to question the validity of the assumptions underlying the derivation of k.

Relationship of the data to results previously reported

The data obtained using variable noise are consistent with the results of Schafer and Shewmaker that are described in the foregoing. These investigators found that the signal power required to yield a given detectability decreased as $n^{1/2}$; we find d' to increase as $n^{1/2}$. Since d' is approximately proportional to signal power, the two results are equivalent.

Unlike Schreitmueller, we find detectability to improve beyond the second observation when constant noise is used. As he suggests, his results may be attributed to the procedure he used. Although the noise was the same in each of the eight intervals of a trial, the number of signals presented varied. It is conceivable that his observers listened for a difference between successive intervals of a trial, and that this comparison became increasingly difficult as more of the intervals contained a signal.

A prediction for improvement with additional observations that is frequently quoted is $P(c)_n = 1 - [1 - P(c)_1]^n$. This prediction is based upon the assumptions that the sensory input must reach a certain value (threshold) for detection to occur, and that successive observations are independent. Hence the probability that detection will not occur on any of n observations is equal to the product of the respective probabilities that detection will not occur on a given observation. Taking into account the chance success that this assumption implies in the forced-choice procedure, a value of $P(c)_1 = 0.80$ will lead to values of $P(c)_2 = 0.95$ and $P(c)_3 = 0.99$. Although the value of $P(c)_1 = 0.80$, as obtained in the experiment reported, is too high for a sensitive test of this prediction, it may be seen from Table I that this prediction does not fit the data as well as the prediction that d' is proportional to $n^{1/2}$.

SIGNALS OF UNKNOWN FREQUENCY OR OF SEVERAL FREQUENCIES

A second set of experiments was conducted using different types of signals. These experiments were exploratory in nature; they were conducted to determine whether the rate of improvement over successive observations of some special signals would aid in distinguishing among alternative models of the process of frequency analysis. In one experiment, the signal was one of 2 frequencies; in a second experiment, the signal was one of 16 widely spaced frequencies; and, in a third, the signal was composed of all 16 of these frequencies. These are detection, not recognition, experiments. The observer was asked to state only which interval contained the signal; he was not asked to state which frequency had been presented.

Previous studies (Tanner, Swets, and Green, 1956) have shown that when the observer is uncertain of the frequency of a signal, his detection performance is poorer than in the case where the signal frequency is known and, further, that the size of decrement resulting from uncertainty increases with increasing separation of the signal frequencies. These data have been interpreted by two different models: a narrow-band scanning model (Tanner, Swets, and Green, 1956) and a multiband model (Green, 1958).

The former model assumes that the observer is sensitive to only a narrow band of the frequency continuum at a given instance, and that, although the center of the band can vary in time, its speed is restricted so that two widely separated frequencies cannot both be observed during a brief observation interval. The observed decrement with frequency uncertainty is assumed to result from the fact that the band is not always centered at the signal frequency that is presented. The probability of a correct detection of one of two equally likely signals that are widely separated can be predicted if an assumption is made about the probability of the band being centered on the correct frequency, and if $P(c)$ is known for the case where the signal frequency is known to the observer.

The multiband model assumes that the observer can select the number and center frequency of the bands to which he listens. The distribution of the variable X, when noise alone is presented and the observer listens to s bands, is the sum of the s noise distributions corresponding to the s bands. Assuming that the noise in each band is independent of the noise in any other band, $E(X_N) = 0$, and $D^2(X_N) = s\sigma^2$, where σ^2 is the variance of the noise in a single band. The distribution corresponding to a signal of a single frequency, when the observer is listening to s bands, is the sum of the $s - 1$ distributions corresponding to noise alone and the one distribution corresponding to signal plus noise. In this case, $E(X_{S+N}) = m$ and $D^2(X_{S+N}) = s\sigma^2$. Thus, when the observer listens to s bands, $d_s' = m/\sigma s^{1/2} = d'/s^{1/2}$, where d' is the obtained d' when a single frequency is presented, and the observer listens to a single band.

Consider these two models for the process of frequency analysis with respect to multiple observations and uncertain signal frequency. If the observer listens to bands centered on all possible signal frequencies, the predicted improvement with additional exposures is the same as when the signal frequency is known. However, if the observer listens to a single frequency at a time, the rate of improvement with additional observations will depend upon which frequency is listened to on each presentation. For a signal that is composed of several frequencies, all equally detectable, both models make the $n^{1/2}$ prediction.

Procedure

Variable noise was used with a two-alternative, forced-choice procedure.[1] The detectability of a signal for five observations was determined with a signal equally likely to be 500 cps or 1100 cps on a given trial. The observers were not told which frequency was presented. The detectability for a single observation, with the frequency of the signal known by the observer, i.e., 500 cps in one case and 1100 cps in another, was also determined. The three conditions were run in a counterbalanced order. On a given day, series of trials were run under each condition; in total, 500 trials were presented for each of the signals of known frequency, and 480 trials (each containing five observations) were presented of the signal of unknown frequency.

The detectability over five observations was also determined with a two-alternative, forced-choice procedure for a 16-component signal consisting of frequencies which were multiples of 250 cps, and for a signal whose frequency was equally likely to be any one of the 16, with the frequency not known to the observer. In both cases, 480 trials were presented. The 16 frequencies were equated for detectability on the basis of the results of a different experiment[2] (Green, McKey, and Licklider, 1959).

The details of apparatus and procedure were the same in this set of experiments as in those described in the foregoing, except that no cue signal was given. The duration of the noise was again 3 sec, with signal onset 1.22 sec or 1.76 sec after the onset of noise. The noise spectrum level was approximately 50 db *re* 0.0002 d/cm^2; 10 $\log E/N_0$ was 12.6 db for the signal at 1100 cps, 10.6 db for the signal at 500 cps, and 14.7 db for the 16-component signal. Different observers were used in these experiments; they were also MIT students.

---

[1] The value of d' corresponding to a $P(c)$ obtained with a two-alternative, forced-choice procedure may be obtained by referring to a table of area under the normal curve.

[2] We would like to express our appreciation to Dr. J. C. R. Licklider for the use of these tapes.

Results

The results of the experiment in which the signal was either of two frequencies are shown in Table III. Shown along the top of the table are the values of $P(c)$ obtained when the signal frequency was known; the

TABLE III. THE PROBABILITY OF A CORRECT RESPONSE FOR EACH OF FIVE OBSERVATIONS WHEN THE SIGNAL IS KNOWN TO BE EITHER OF TWO FREQUENCIES

		Observer 1		Observer 2		Observer 3	
Signal known	500 cps	0.76		0.72		0.79	
exactly			0.75		0.74		0.80
	1100 cps	0.74		0.76		0.81	
5 observations of 1	1	0.62		0.63		0.72	
of 2 signals	2	0.64		0.69		0.72	
	3	0.75		0.70		0.79	
	4	0.78		0.75		0.82	
	5	0.81		0.77		0.86	
Scanning prediction		0.63		0.62		0.65	
Multiband prediction		0.68		0.68		0.72	

average values are 0.75, 0.74, and 0.80, respectively, for the three observers. The middle of the table displays the values of $P(c)$ for each of five observations when the signal frequency was unknown. On the first observation of an unknown frequency, $P(c)$ drops to 0.62, 0.63, and 0.72, respectively. At the bottom are listed the values of $P(c)_1$ that are predicted for the case of unknown frequency by the scanning and multiband models.

The scanning prediction is made on the assumption that the observer listens to the frequency that is presented on one half of the trials, and that, when he listens to the frequency presented, his probability of being correct is equal to that when the frequency is known; on the other half of the trials, when he listens to the wrong frequency, chance determines the probability of a correct detection. Thus, $P'(c) = 0.5P(c) + 0.5(0.5)$, where $P(c)$ is the average probability of a correct detection when the frequency is known, and $P'(c)$ is the predicted probability when the signal is either of two equally likely frequencies. Recall that a two-alternative, forced-choice procedure was used. The multiband prediction is based upon the assumption that the observer is listening at once to both of the frequency bands that contain signal frequencies; then, as noted earlier, d_1' with frequency uncertain equals the d' for known frequency divided by $\sqrt{2}$. This value of d' has been converted to $P(c)$ for inclusion in the table.

It may be seen that the data of Observers 1 and 2 are well fitted by the scanning prediction, whereas Observer 3 matches the multiband prediction. If one assumes binomial statistics, the standard deviation of these proportions is approximately 0.02. Then, for every observer, the obtained proportion is less than 0.3σ from one of the predicted proportions, and from 2.5σ to 3.0σ from the other. These data are similar to the data obtained in the earlier experiment by Tanner, Swets, and Green (1956). In that experiment, which employed two observers at each of two signal durations, the obtained proportions were between 0.3σ and 1.0σ from the scanning prediction and between 3.0σ and 6.0σ from the multiband prediction, in three cases, and 4.0σ from the scanning prediction and 1.3σ from the multiband prediction, in the fourth case.

Consider now the improvement over successive observations of the signal that is either of two frequencies. The multiband model predicts $n^{1/2}$ improvement. No simple prediction follows from the scanning model, since the observer can, under its terms, adopt any of a number of strategies in choosing which frequency band to listen to on successive observations. Making exact predictions is practicable only for extreme and unlikely strategies, such as listening to the same frequency band over five observations, or alternating frequency bands from one observation to another.

The results that are shown in Table III are displayed graphically in Fig. 4 to facilitate comparison with the $n^{1/2}$ prediction. The first impression is that these data are not simply described by the multiband, or $n^{1/2}$, prediction, since there is considerably more scatter about the predicted

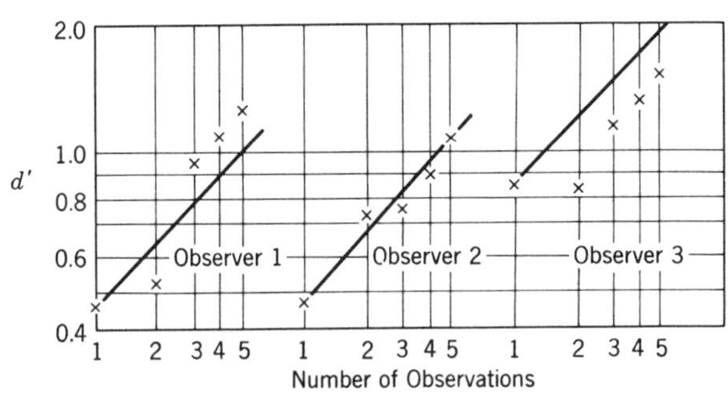

FIG. 4. The detectability of a signal that is either one of two frequencies, expressed in d', on five successive observations. The line represents the $n^{1/2}$ prediction for the increase in d'.

line here than is evidenced for a single frequency, as exemplified in Fig. 1. However, it should be noted that the experimental points are at a much lower value of d' in Fig. 4, where the logarithmic scale magnifies the apparent variance.

This experiment was undertaken, in part, because, if the scanning model is correct in assuming that the decrement with uncertainty, as evidenced by a single observation, results from the observer being incorrectly tuned on half of the trials, this fact should be made more apparent by the observer's behavior when given an additional observation. For the trials on which the observer is correctly tuned on the first observation, if he continues to observe at that frequency, $P(c)_2$ will be greater than the $P(c)$ obtained on one presentation when the frequency is known. For the trials on which he is incorrectly tuned on the first presentation, if he shifts frequency, $P(c)_2$ will equal the (Pc) obtained on a single presentation when the frequency is known. Considering both types of trials, since the observer is more likely than not to know whether he was tuned correctly after an observation, $P(c)_2$ should be at least as large as the $P(c)$ on a single presentation for a signal known in frequency. Certainly, if the observer routinely listens at one frequency on the first presentation and at the other on the second presentation, $P(c)_2$ will closely approximate, if he is capable of retaining the value of X associated with each interval, the $P(c)$ for a signal of known frequency after a single observation. Such an improvement from the first observation to the second is greater than $n^{1/2}$. We may see in Table III, however, that the observers do not attain by the second presentation the $P(c)$ that is obtained when the signal's frequency is known. Observers 1 and 3 reach this $P(c)$ on the third presentation, whereas Observer 2 reaches it only on the fourth presentation. Observers 1 and 3 show less than $n^{1/2}$ improvement from $n = 1$ to $n = 2$. It is as if the observers use the first two presentations solely to determine which frequency is being presented, by listening regularly to one frequency on the first presentation and to the other on the second presentation, and do not retain information concerning which interval is most likely to contain the signal.

Additional analysis of these data, in particular a contingency analysis, supports the scanning model. The probability of a correct response after the first observation on a given trial was determined separately for the four conditions which held after the last observation on the previous trial: (*a*) same frequency, correct, (*b*) same frequency, incorrect, (*c*) different frequency, correct, and (*d*) different frequency, incorrect. These data are shown in Table IV. They suggest strongly that the observer, at a given point in time, is differentially sensitive to the two frequencies—in

TABLE IV. Signal One of Two Possible Frequencies: The Proportions of Correct Responses on the First Observation, for the Four Conditions of the Last Observation of the Previous Trial, and, in Parentheses, the Number of Observations on Which They Are Based

Last observation, previous trial	Observer 1		Observer 2		Observer 3	
Same frequency, correct	0.70	(193)	0.66	(182)	0.71	(205)
Same frequency, incorrect	0.52	(42)	0.60	(52)	0.67	(27)
Different frequency, correct	0.62	(208)	0.62	(196)	0.71	(218)
Different frequency, incorrect	0.72	(50)	0.75	(63)	0.84	(43)

particular, that on the first observation of a trial he tends to listen to the same frequency he listened to on the last observation of the previous trial.

When the signal is one of 16 frequencies, the improvement is regular, but definitely less than $n^{1/2}$, for all three observers, as shown in Fig. 5. This suggests that the observer is not listening to the correct frequency on all presentations, and to that extent these data are consistent with the scanning model. The failure of these data to follow the $n^{1/2}$ prediction makes them inconsistent with a multiband model that asserts the observer listens to all possible frequency bands. One could, of course, assume that several bands are listened to simultaneously, but that the number of bands is less than 16.

When a signal consisting of 16 frequencies is presented, the data are not unlike the $n^{1/2}$ prediction, as shown in Fig. 6. They are thus consistent with both of the models under discussion. Here again, however, the individual differences are striking. Although the three observers show nearly equal detectability in the one-of-16 case, they differ widely in this case. The better performance of Observer 3 suggests that he is listening to more bands than are the other two observers; this is the observer who

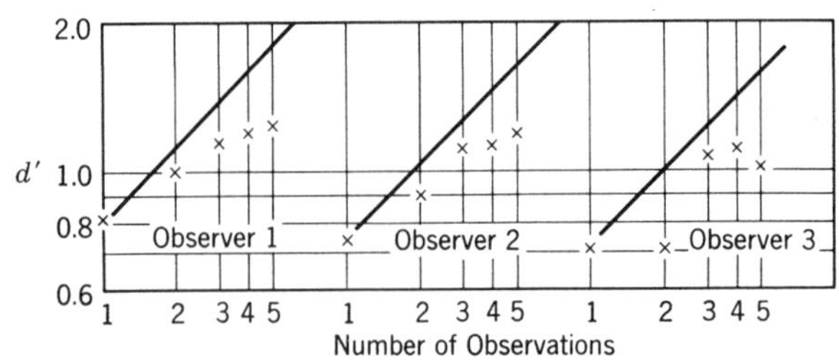

Fig. 5. The detectability of a signal that is any one of 16 frequencies, expressed in d', for five successive observations. The line represents the $n^{1/2}$ prediction for the increase in d'.

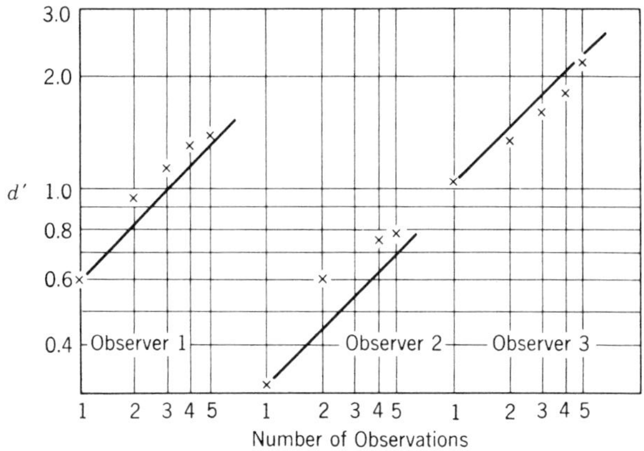

FIG. 6. The detectability, on five successive observations, of a signal consisting of 16 frequencies. The line is the $n^{1/2}$ prediction for the increase in d′.

performed as if listening to both bands in the experiment involving either of two frequencies.

In summary, although the results of these experiments do not enable us to decide unequivocally between the two models of frequency analysis, they should contribute to the final evaluation of these models by presenting negative instances for each of them. In short, these results suggest that neither of the models may be found to apply to all observers under all experimental conditions. They suggest that the observers are capable of adopting strategies consistent with either the scanning model or the multiband model, and that, when the relative efficacy of the two is not clear, observers will differ in their choice of a strategy.

SUMMARY

The use of repeated presentations of a given signal event as an experimental technique in psychoacoustic studies provides information about several general properties of the hearing process. From the relationship between the gain in detectability that results from additional observations and the type of signal and noise employed, inferences can be made about: (1) the observer's ability to integrate over time, (2) the amount of noise generated by the auditory system, (3) the nature of the process of frequency analysis, and (4) the observer's mode of dealing with uncertainty as to signal frequency. The first set of experiments permitted five observations of each signal where the signal consisted of a pulsed tone, of known frequency, in noise. Both variable noise, i.e., noise that is statistically independent from one presentation to another, and constant noise, i.e., noise that is exactly the same on each of the five presentations, were used. With variable noise, the detectability index d' improves, as predicted, as the square root of the number of observations. The use of constant noise, which results in less improvement, provides an estimate of the portion of the total noise affecting detection that is of internal origin. The results under different levels of external noise indicate that internal noise is proportional to external noise. A second set of experiments employed signals whose frequencies were unknown to the observers, and signals comprising several widely spaced frequencies. Their results are discussed in relation to three alternative models of the process of frequency analysis.

ACKNOWLEDGMENTS

This research was conducted in the Research Laboratory of Electronics of the Massachusetts Institute of Technology with support from the Operational Applications Laboratory of the U. S. Air Force. Green held a fellowship from the National Science Foundation. This article appeared as Tech. Rept. No. AFCRC-TN-58-72, and in J. acoust. Soc. Am., *1959,* **31,** *514–521.*

References

• Green, D. M. Detection of multiple component signals in noise. *J. acoust. Soc. Am.,* 1958, **30**, 904–911. [25]

• Green, D. M., Birdsall, T. G., and Tanner, W. P., Jr. Signal detection as a function of signal intensity and duration. *J. acoust. Soc. Am.,* 1957, **29,** 523–531. [11]

• Green, D. M., McKey, M. J., and Licklider, J. C. R. Detection of a pulsed sinusoid in noise as a function of frequency. *J. acoust. Soc. Am.,* 1959, **31,** 1446–1452. [26]

• Schafer, T. H., and Shewmaker, C. A. A comparative study of the audio, visual and audio-visual recognition differentials for pulses masked by random noise. Naval Electronics Laboratory, 1953, Report 372.

• Schreitmueller, R. F. Effect of repeated presentations on the detection of signals in noise. Unpublished M.S. thesis, Massachusetts Institute of Technology, 1952.

• Swets, J. A., McKey, M. J., and Green, D. M. On sequential decisions by human observers in a signal detection problem. *J. acoust. Soc. Am.,* 1958, **30,** 673. (Abstract) [See 10]

• Tanner, W. P., Jr., and Swets, J. A. A decision-making theory of visual detection. *Psychol. Rev.,* 1954, **61**, 401–409.

• Tanner, W. P., Jr., Swets, J. A., and Green, D. M. Some general properties of the hearing mechanism. University of Michigan: Electronic Defense Group, 1956, Technical Report No. 30.

10

Sequential Observations by Human Observers of Signals in Noise

John A. Swets and David M. Green

The principal measures in the study of behavior are the *time* that is required to perform a certain act and the *errors* that are committed during the performance. Most studies employ one of these measures to the exclusion of the other. In the field of mental testing, for example, we speak of 'speed' tests and 'power' tests. Similarly, in sensory testing we typically fix the time allowed for the response, as well as the duration of the stimulus, and then observe the error rate; or we arrange conditions so that errors will be negligible and record the reaction time. In the less frequent instances in which both measures are used, it is usually expected that they will vary together, and, in so doing, corroborate each other. Thus, the experimenter may manipulate the signal strength or the number of alternatives in a sensory task and observe that both errors and reaction time increase as the task becomes more difficult. In studies of conditioning, or of the learning of motor skills, or of verbal learning, the number of errors and the time taken by the response decrease together as practice makes the task progressively less difficult.

It seems strange that very few behavioral studies have attempted to examine the trading relationship that so commonly exists between time and error. A striking aspect of many of the motor and intellectual tasks we perform is that we must choose either to proceed with care and thereby reduce the likelihood of a mistake, or to buy time at the expense of error. The necessity of making this choice is perhaps less obvious, but no less a fact, in those sensory tasks in which time can be traded for more information or more information processing. Indeed, in almost any perceptual task that comes to mind, ranging from the most simple to the most complex, the observer possesses the ability to balance time and accuracy.

In this paper we report the results of a preliminary investigation of the trading relationship between time and error in a very simple perceptual task, specifically, in a signal detection task. The observer must decide whether or not a signal exists in a background of noise—he is allowed to make as many observations as he chooses before making this decision.

We speak as if a report of the presence or absence of a signal represents a decision made by the observer. We do so advisedly. The present study follows several others which have shown that the theory of statistical decision provides a quite accurate description of the behavior of human observers in a detection task. Almost all of the previous studies have required a decision from the observer shortly after a single observation of fixed duration. They have shown that the observer is capable of adjusting his decision criterion—the criterion that must be met by the sensory information in order for him to report that a signal was present—and that he does so accordingly as changes are made in the a priori probability of signal existence, in the values associated with the four possible outcomes of a decision, and in the signal strength (Swets, Tanner, and Birdsall, 1961). An important aspect of the application of statistical-decision theory to psychophysical problems is that it permits indexing the observer's sensitivity independently of changes in his decision criterion.

In one study that was a direct forerunner to the present one (Swets, Shipley, McKey, and Green, 1959), each of the observer's decisions was based on several observations. In that study we were concerned simply with determining how detectability improves with additional observations when the number of observations entering a decision is determined, and fixed in advance, by the experimenter. We found that the rate of decrease in error with additional observations agreed with that predicted from statistical theory. As we have indicated, our present interest is in a task in which the observer is an active participant in the trade between time and error. We shall now describe this task explicitly.

In this experiment the observer is allowed to make as many observations as he chooses before deciding whether the signal is present or absent. In particular, each observation is made during some specified interval in time called an *observation interval.* All of the observation intervals *in a given sequence* of such intervals either do or do not contain a specified signal, and the observer's decision is based on all of the intervals in the immediate sequence. That is to say, following each observation interval, the observer makes one of three responses: *Yes* (i.e. the signal is present in this sequence of intervals), *No* (i.e. the signal is not present in this sequence of intervals), or *Continue* (i.e. I would like to make another observation before saying *Yes* or *No*). It will be noted that this is essentially the familiar *yes–no–doubtful*, or three-category, psychophysical procedure—with the modification that if the response is *doubtful* the presentation, signal or no signal as the case may be, is repeated. If the presentation is repeated, it is an *independent* presentation. By this it is meant that the noise is independent. Whether or not the sequence of intervals contains a signal, the sample of noise presented in any interval is independent of that in any other interval in the sequence. Once a terminal decision is made, either *Yes* or *No*, a new sequence of observation intervals begins, and continues until the observer makes a terminal decision. This new sequence either contains a signal throughout or does not, depending upon a priori probabilities fixed by the experimenter and known by the observer.

Wald (1947) has developed an extension of statistical-decision theory (the theory of sequential analysis) to deal with a problem in statistics that is analogous to the psychophysical task just described. We shall consider the theory of sequential analysis as a model for the observer's behavior in this task. We shall present the theory in more detail shortly, but since the qualitative predictions that follow from it will be in close agreement with the reader's intuition, they can be simply summarized now. The theory leads to the prediction that, for a given signal strength, the error rate and average number of observations preceding a terminal decision will vary inversely. If we elaborate the theory, as we shall, to represent a situation in which values are associated with the four possible outcomes of a terminal decision (positive values with the correct outcomes and negative values with the incorrect outcomes), and in which a price must be paid for making each additional observation, the prediction follows that the average number of observations per sequence will increase and the error rate will decrease as the values of the decision outcomes increase relative to the cost of an additional observation. Another prediction of the theory of sequential analysis is that sequential tests, that is, those tests in which the observer determines the number of observations, will be more efficient than tests of fixed length. That is to say, sequential tests will require fewer observations on the average than tests of fixed length to yield the same error rates. This again is intuitively plausible, for sequential tests may take advantage of sequences in which the evidence happens to be very persuasive at an early stage of observation. We shall compare our experimental data with these predictions from the sequential model.

Following the presentation of these data we shall turn to the question of the behavioral process that lies behind them. Interestingly enough, it is quite possible for our data to agree closely with the predictions that we have listed and yet, upon re-analysis, to be shown to be inconsistent with the process assumed by the sequential model. In fact, it is possible for the data to agree with the predictions described above and, at the same time, to be consistent with a very different process, one for which another model exists. The basic question is this: does the observer integrate the information obtained from the successive observations in a sequence, or does he treat the observations independently? Stated otherwise: does the observer make a terminal decision when the combined evidence from all of the intervals in the sequence is sufficiently persuasive, or does he make a terminal decision only when the evidence from a single observation is sufficiently persuasive, independent of the preceding evidence? The assumption of integration is central to the theory of sequential analysis. We have found that it provides a good explanation of the data obtained in the earlier study of tests of fixed length (Swets, Shipley, McKey, and Green, 1959). The assumption of independence, on the other hand, has been associated with sensory theory for a long time. The independence model (in particular, the formula $1 - (1 - p)^n$, in which p is the probability that a correct detection will result from any observation and n is the number of observations) has been applied frequently to multiple observers as well as to multiple observations. This model has recently been reported by Egan (1957) to describe the results of his experiments on the repetition of items in a word-articulation test.

We shall now describe briefly the statistical-decision model and its extension for the sequential case, and then present the results of our experiments. We should first point out, however, that we are not concerned, in this initial attempt to apply decision theory to a very flexible psychophysical procedure, with a detailed, quantitative comparison of the theory and the experimental results. The flexibility of the procedure would make this difficult, at best. Furthermore, the quantities estimated in the theory are quite unreliable for such small average numbers of observations as we shall be considering in the psychophysical task. Rather, our interest in this study is in certain qualitative comparisons, and in demonstrating some techniques for investigating the processes underlying the trade of error for time.

THE SEQUENTIAL MODEL

In our formal analysis of the observer's behavior in a sequential detection problem, we shall begin by reviewing the simpler yes–no, or two-category, problem and then extend the analysis to the sequential problem. We shall present the qualitative relationships among the variables that are necessarily involved in a sequential observation task.

The essential feature of the simple yes–no situation is a set of two events or hypotheses—either a signal is presented by adding it to the noise (denoted SN), or only the noise is presented (denoted N). These events occur during a specified observation interval. Following the observation interval the observer responds by accepting one or other of the hypotheses. For the purpose of the model, we assume that the information the observer obtains during the observation interval can be represented by a value of a hypothetical decision variable, say, x. (We shall henceforth use the term *observation* to refer to the sensory datum, x, as well as to the process by which x is obtained.) Since noise is always present, we would expect different values of x for different observations, and, in fact, we assume the existence of a population of values of x. Each observation is viewed as an instance or sample from this population. The probability density function for the samples of noise alone is labeled $f_N(x)$ in Fig. 1. The effect of the presentation of the signal during the observation interval is interpreted simply as a shift in the density function for noise alone. The distribution resulting from the occurrence of the signal is represented by the density function $f_{SN}(x)$ in Fig. 1. It has been shown previously that, to a good approximation, we can assume the density functions to be normal in form and to have approximately the same variance. The mean of the noise distribution can be chosen arbitrarily, since only the shift in the mean that is caused by the signal is relevant. Thus any particular signal can be characterized by a single normalized number, namely, the difference in the means of the two distributions divided by the standard deviation. This normalized variable has been called d'. If we consider the density functions to have unit variance, then d' is simply the difference between the means of the two distributions, as shown in Fig. 1.

In the simple yes–no case it is assumed, for the purpose of analysis, that the observer establishes a cut-off point, or criterion, along the variable x. In other words, he divides the continuum of observations into two mutually exclusive and exhaustive *critical regions*. If a particular observation exceeds the criterion, he states that a signal is present. If the observation falls below the criterion, he states that no signal is

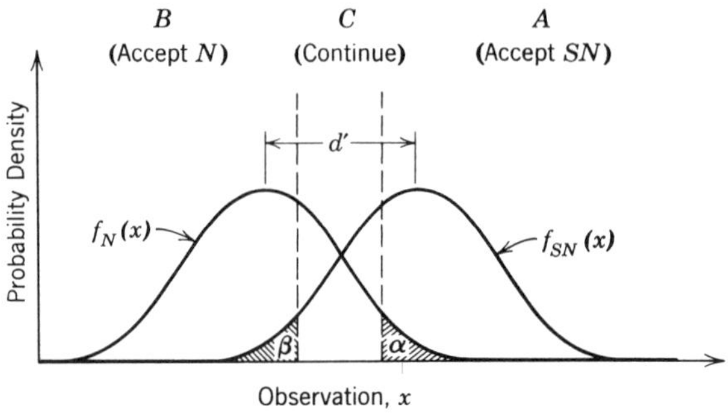

FIG. 1. A representation of the sequential decision problem.

present. In the sequential task on the other hand, the observer is assumed to adopt two criteria, or three critical regions. These regions, at least those pertaining to the first observation, are represented as A, B and C in Fig. 1. If the first observation falls in A the observer says *Yes*, if it falls in B he says *No*, and if it falls in C he says *Continue*.

As we have indicated, the theory of sequential analysis assumes that the successive observations are integrated and that the integrated value is compared with the three critical regions at each observation stage. Thus, it is assumed in the theory that a terminal decision is made whenever the combined evidence for one or the other of the two hypotheses is sufficiently persuasive. Whether the human observer will integrate the successive observations is, of course, an empirical question. We have expressed our belief that it is an important question, and we shall examine it in a later section of the paper.

The selection of the three critical regions determines the four dependent variables of the sequential task. These variables are:

(1) The number of observations needed, on the average, to make a terminal decision, given the event N.

(2) Similarly, the average number of observations preceding a terminal decision, given the event SN.

(3) The conditional probability of an incorrect terminal decision, given N.

(4) The conditional probability of an incorrect terminal decision, given SN.

Thus, there is a pair of numbers corresponding to each type of observation sequence. We shall take the average number of observations preceding a terminal decision to be simply the mean number and denote this quantity $E_N(n)$ or $E_{SN}(n)$. We shall estimate the conditional probability of an incorrect terminal decision under N from the obtained proportions of such decisions, and denote it α. This quantity may be referred to as the *false-alarm* probability. We shall similarly estimate the conditional *miss* probability, denoted β. A graphic representation of α and β is given in Fig. 1.

The first problem encountered in sequential analysis is to determine exactly how α, β, $E_N(n)$ and $E_{SN}(n)$ are related. This problem is a difficult one for the reason that the relationship of the critical regions to the density functions of N and SN is not known beyond the first observation. It will be apparent that the relationship depicted in Fig. 1 holds only for the first observation in a sequence. A second observation is required only if the first falls in the intermediate region, C. The combination of the first and second observations, therefore, will not be normally distributed, for it results from the addition of a normal variable and a normal variable with both tails missing. Although Wald (1947) has provided approximations to the various equations of interest, these approximations are unreliable for small numbers of observations.[1] Unfortunately, in the detection problem we are concerned with small numbers. We shall content ourselves, in this paper, with the qualitative result that the error probabilities and the expected number of observations will vary inversely as the critical regions are varied.

We shall now define the variables that determine the observer's particular choice of the critical regions—the independent variables in the sequential detection task. It may be noted that we could simply instruct the observers to be more or less conservative and, in that way, manipulate the critical regions and hence α, β, and the expected number of observations. We preferred, however, to cast the problem in the framework of a game. Specifically, we assigned various values to the four possible outcomes of a terminal decision and assessed a fixed cost for each additional observation. We actually paid the observers a bonus in accordance with the assigned values, in addition to their regular wage. It was our intention, with this procedure, to emphasize for the observer the trading relationship between time and error. Under this scheme, he considers whether another observation will be worthwhile in order to add more certainty to his terminal decision, with the realization that each additional observation reduces the profit that he will gain from a correct terminal decision. The balance he adopts between time and error is thus made a matter of direct consequence to him.

We should mention that there are two additional determinants of the critical regions in such a game, namely, the a priori probabilities of signal

[1] The approximation is related to the so-called 'excess-over-the-boundary' argument. See Wald (1947), pp. 43–48.

plus noise and of noise alone, and the detectability of the signal. In our experiments we fixed the values of these two variables, as well as the cost per observation, and manipulated the critical regions by changing only the values associated with the decision outcomes. If the observer tries to maximize his payoff, then increases in the values of the decision outcomes will result in decreased error probabilities and an increased number of observations.[2]

It will be apparent that the game, as we have described it so far, does not prescribe in detail a particular experimental procedure. One must decide, for example, whether to fix the number of sequences to be presented and allow the observers to determine the total experimental time, or to fix the experimental time and allow the observers to determine the number of sequences presented within that limit. We chose the latter course. A related decision is required by the fact that we wanted to test more than one observer at a time. We had to choose either to present a new sequence only when all the observers had made terminal decisions on the previous sequence, or to establish a truncation in advance. Both of these alternatives represent a compromise, for, under the first, the observer is likely to be influenced by his fellows and, under the second, he is not given completely free rein. We used both of these procedures in different experiments, and noticed no special effects.

Three experiments are reported in this chapter. We shall first examine their results to determine whether the error rates and mean number of observations vary appropriately as the payoff values are changed. We shall then compare the efficiency of sequential tests and tests of fixed length. Following this, we shall determine whether or not the observers combined the information in successive observations.

THE EXPERIMENTAL RESULTS

Throughout the three experiments to be reported, the a priori probability of signal occurrence was fixed at 0.50 and the cost of each additional observation was fixed at 1.0. In each experiment the values asso-

---

[2] The general relationships specified in this model have been investigated in a psychological experiment by Irwin and Smith (1957). In a task in which the subject drew numbered cards from a pack until reaching a decision that the pack's mean was greater or less than zero, they found that the number of cards drawn varied in the expected direction with changes in the values of the decision outcomes, the cost per observation, and the mean number of the pack. The psychological application of some other aspects of the theory of sequential analysis has been investigated by Becker (1958).

ciated with the terminal decision outcomes were varied systematically. Four or five different sets of values were used in an experiment, with a given set being in effect for approximately 500 sequences of observations. The payoff matrices were in every case symmetrical, that is, the four possible decision outcomes always had equal values, though the values were positive for correct decisions and negative for incorrect decisions. The various sets of values were presented in a random order.

The three experiments differed slightly from one another with respect to the particular payoff values used and also with respect to the strength of the signal. In the first two experiments, a new sequence was begun as soon as all of the observers had made terminal decisions; in the third, a fixed number of observation intervals was presented in every sequence, the number being chosen on the basis of preliminary trials such that less than 1 per cent of the sequences would be forcibly terminated. The third experiment also differed in that tests of fixed length were conducted along with the sequential tests.

In each experiment the sequential tests were preceded by a simpler test whose purpose was to provide an index of the detectability of the signal in terms of the variable d' as defined above. This was either a yes–no or a forced-choice test. We have already described the procedure of the yes–no test. In the forced-choice test, the signal is presented in one of two temporal intervals and the observer states in which interval he believed the signal occurred. The method of calculating d' from the data obtained with each of these procedures has been presented elsewhere (Swets, Tanner, and Birdsall, 1961). In brief, in the yes–no test the proportion of correct detections and the proportion of false-alarm responses are used in conjunction with a table of the normal integral to obtain an estimate of d' that is independent of the observer's criterion; in the forced-choice test one simply enters the table with the proportion of correct responses under the assumption that no preference exists for one of the temporal intervals. These two procedures have been shown previously (Swets, 1959) to yield comparable estimates of d'. In the second and third experiments, such a test was also conducted at the conclusion of the sequential tests to provide an index of the stability of the experimental equipment and of the observers throughout the experiment.

The general procedures and the basic apparatus used in the experiments have been described in the earlier report of the results of tests of fixed length (Swets, Shipley, McKey, and Green, 1959). In all of the experiments, the signal was a pulsed tone of 1,000 cps with a duration of 0.1 second. It was presented in a continuous background of white noise; the noise spectrum level was approximately 50 db *re* 0·0002 dyne/cm². The signal levels for the three experiments were 8.5 db, 11.0 db and 10.5 db, respectively. These signal levels are expressed in terms of 10 log E/N_0, where E is the signal energy, or time integral of power, and N_0 is the noise power in a one-cycle band. The observers were college students with previous observing experience. They observed for two hours a day, five days a week.

The trade of time and error

The results of the first experiment are shown in Table I. It may be seen that the signal level used led to a value of d' of approximately 0.55 for both observers in the preliminary tests. In the column headed V are listed the values associated with the terminal decisions in the four separate conditions of the sequential tests. (Recall that the matrix of values is symmetrical, and the cost per observation is unity.) The

TABLE I. THE RESULTS OF EXPERIMENT I

	Observer 1				Observer 2			
I. Forced choice								
$P(c)$*	0.65				0.65			
d'	0.55				0.55			
					(1,200 observations)			
II. Yes–No								
α	0.47				0.41			
β	0.29				0.37			
d'	0.63				0.56			
					(1,800 observations)			
III. Sequential decision								
V	α	β	$E_N(n)$	$E_{SN}(n)$	α	β	$E_N(n)$	$E_{SN}(n)$
15	0.40	0.34	1.6	1.5	0.35	0.38	2.0	1.8
30	0.39	0.30	2.4	2.2	0.38	0.36	2.8	2.7
80	0.34	0.21	4.0	3.0	0.32	0.24	4.3	3.5
200	0.23	0.16	7.0	5.3	0.35	0.26	5.7	4.6
					(500 sequences of observations in each of the four conditions)			

* $P(c)$ = proportion of correct responses.

primary data—the error rates, α and β, and the mean numbers of observations, $E_N(n)$ and $E_{SN}(n)$—are listed for each condition. Note that, as the values increase, the error rates tend to decrease and the mean numbers of observations tend to increase; this is consistent with the model. These quantities are rank-ordered perfectly in the case of the first observer, whereas the data of the second observer show reversals only in the error rates.

The second experiment was conducted, in part, to determine whether or not the same correlation would be observed if a smaller range of values was used. We were also concerned about the level of motivation in the first experiment, since we had used a very low signal level. The signal level used in the second experiment yielded a value for d' of approximately 1.30 in the preliminary test. This can be seen in Table II. Another determination of d' at the close of the experiment (bottom of Table II) indicates good stability of both equipment and observers. Given a prior empirical result that d' is approximately proportional to

TABLE II. THE RESULTS OF EXPERIMENT II

	Observer 1				Observer 2			
I. Forced choice								
$P(c)$	0.83				0.81			
d'	1.33				1.23			
					(800 observations)			
II. Sequential decision								
V	α	β	$E_N(n)$	$E_{SN}(n)$	α	β	$E_N(n)$	$E_{SN}(n)$
5	0.22	0.22	1.2	1.1	0.30	0.29	1.0	1.0
10	0.16	0.17	1.7	1.4	0.22	0.20	1.9	1.6
15	0.18	0.19	1.8	1.5	0.26	0.17	2.1	1.7
25	0.17	0.13	2.2	1.6	0.22	0.27	2.0	1.5
60	0.11	0.11	4.3	3.0	0.11	0.13	3.8	2.4
					(400 sequences of observations in each of the four conditions)			
III. Forced choice								
$P(c)$	0.83				0.82			
d'	1.33				1.31			
					(600 observations)			

signal power (Green, Birdsall, and Tanner, 1957), the initial and final estimates of d' are within 0.25 db of each other.

The results of the sequential tests in the second experiment conform to those of the first experiment. We may note, however, that *both* the error rates and the mean numbers of observations are generally smaller, and that this is consistent with the fact that the detectability of the signal is greater, and that the values of the decision outcomes are smaller, than were the case in the first experiment.

Both sequential tests and tests of fixed length were conducted in the third experiment. The results are shown in Table III. Note first that both yes–no and forced-choice tests were employed at the beginning and at the end of the experiment. The values of d' estimated from these tests tend to be greater for the yes–no than for the forced-choice tests, and greater for the final than for the initial tests. The discrepancies, however, are not great; a very small minority of the twelve possible comparisons between tests exhibit a difference greater than one decibel. The performance in the sequential tests is very similar to that observed previously; the mean numbers of observations rank exactly as expected, and the error rates show only two reversals in the expected rank.

Table III also shows the results of the fixed-length tests. In these tests, each sequence contained six observation intervals. The observer made a 'yes' or 'no' decision *after each interval* with respect to the entire sequence. This permits us to analyse the results of the single test of six intervals in length to indicate the results that would be obtained with tests containing fewer intervals in a sequence. In these tests, as in the sequential tests, the a priori probability of signal occurrence was 0.50, and the decision outcomes were valued equally.

As shown in the previous paper (Swets, Shipley, McKey, and Green, 1959), the statistical model leads to the prediction that, in fixed-length tests, d' will increase as the square root of the number of observations. This is analogous to the familiar result in statistics that the standard deviation of the estimate of a population mean decreases as the square root of the number of samples. To facilitate the comparison of the present results with this prediction, they are presented graphically in Fig. 2. The lines in the figure represent the $n^{1/2}$ increase in d'. They are not the best-fitting lines with a slope of $\frac{1}{2}$; rather, they are drawn through the value of d' obtained at $n = 1$. There appears to be slightly less than the $n^{1/2}$ improvement obtained in the earlier study.

Figure 3 shows the error rates corresponding to different numbers of observations in both the sequential and fixed-length tests. It is apparent that the error rates obtained in the sequential tests are generally lower

TABLE III. THE RESULTS OF EXPERIMENT III

I. Forced choice

	Observer 1		Observer 2		Observer 3	
	Initial	Final	Initial	Final	Initial	Final
$P(c)$	0.69	0.77	0.69	0.73	0.66	0.75
d'	0.71	1.02	0.71	0.85	0.59	0.93
					(500 observations)	

II. Yes–No

	Observer 1		Observer 2		Observer 3	
	Initial	Final	Initial	Final	Initial	Final
α	0.29	0.18	0.32	0.42	0.28	0.33
β	0.37	0.39	0.34	0.25	0.39	0.29
d'	0.90	1.17	0.91	0.89	0.87	1.03
					(500 observations)	

III. Sequential decision

	Observer 1				Observer 2				Observer 3			
V	α	β	$E_N(n)$	$E_{SN}(n)$	α	β	$E_N(n)$	$E_{SN}(n)$	α	β	$E_N(s)$	$E_{SN}(n)$
5	—	—	—	—	0.29	0.26	1.8	1.6	0.23	0.45	0.3	1.2
10	0.09	0.37	2.6	2.5	0.18	0.30	2.7	2.6	0.12	0.30	2.5	2.3
25	0.05	0.31	4.1	4.3	0.07	0.21	4.4	3.8	0.10	0.24	4.2	4.3
50	—	—	—	—	0.10	0.06	6.4	5.0	0.10	0.17	5.3	5.1
									(300 sequences of observations in each of the four conditions)			

IV. Fixed length

	Observer 1			Observer 2			Observer 3		
n	α	β	d'	α	β	d'	α	β	d'
1	0.15	0.54	0.92	0.21	0.48	0.86	0.30	0.41	0.76
2	0.16	0.45	1.14	0.19	0.39	1.16	0.26	0.37	0.98
3	0.13	0.40	1.40	0.16	0.28	1.56	0.26	0.34	1.05
4	0.10	0.32	1.74	0.15	0.28	1.61	0.25	0.31	1.20
5	0.11	0.29	1.79	0.15	0.26	1.70	0.22	0.31	1.30
6	0.13	0.25	1.83	0.15	0.22	1.80	0.22	0.26	1.43
							(375 observations at each stage)		

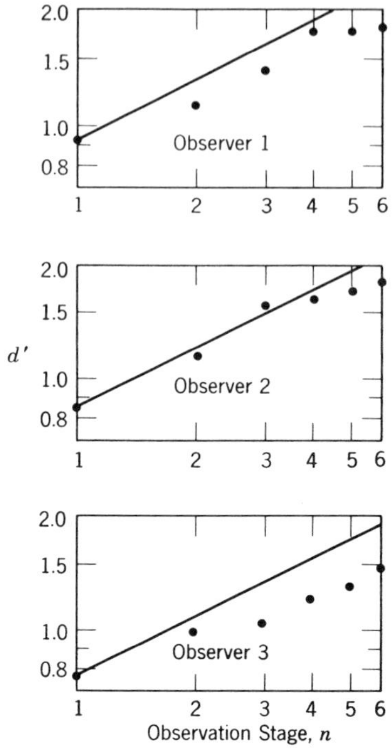

FIG. 2. Plot of d' against n in the tests of fixed length.

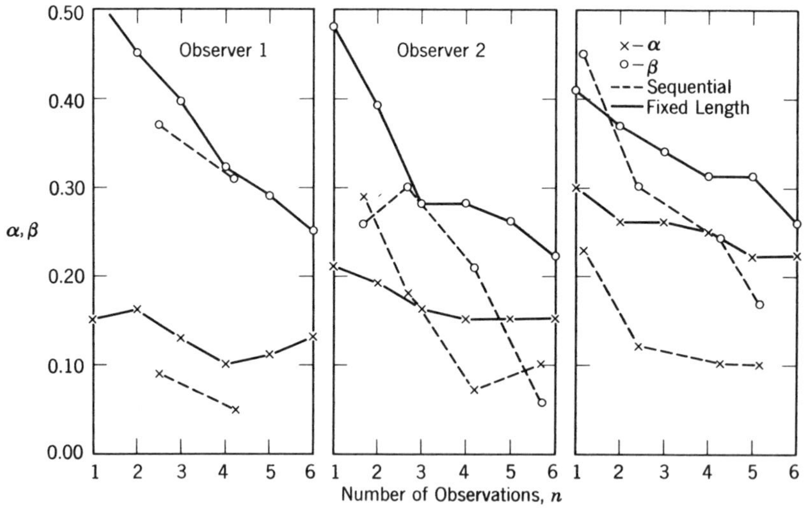

FIG. 3. The observed error rates as a function of the number of observations, in sequential tests and tests of fixed length, for three observers.

than those obtained in the tests of fixed length. If, however, we attempt to determine the ratio of the number of observations in sequential tests to the number of observations in fixed-length tests, for various error rates, we find no simple generalization to describe the data. We might, in a bold moment, describe the saving effected by sequential tests as approximately 25 per cent for the first two observers, and as more than 50 per cent for the third. Whatever the percentage, the reliable result is that sequential detection tests yield a saving even with small numbers of observations.

The question of integration

We have stated that there are two fundamental problems involved in sequential observation. One concerns the factors that determine a termination of the sequence of observations, specifically, the relationship that exists between the number of observations and the error rates, and between these two variables and the payoff values. The second problem concerns the way in which the observer uses the information obtained in successive observations, in particular, whether or not the observer integrates the successive observations. Thus far, we have considered only the experimental results relevant to the former. We have found that the error rates and the mean numbers of observations vary with each other and, in addition, vary with the payoff values, in accordance with the model we have described. The three experiments are in agreement on this point, showing rank-order correlations that are consistently near unity. Thus, on a general level, the sequential model provides a good description of the behavior of human observers. A further prediction, that sequential tests are more efficient than fixed-length tests, is also supported. Let us return now to the three experiments and consider them from the point of view of the integration problem. This will involve an investigation of the observer's performance, stage by stage, within a given value condition.

First of all, we are interested in the number of terminal decisions made at each observation stage. This analysis of the data of the first experiment is presented in Fig. 4. Similar plots of the data of the second and third experiments show essentially the same result, the only difference worthy of note being that the tendency of the peak of the function to be displaced to a value of $n > 1$ (the tendency that is observed in Fig. 4 for the higher value conditions) is seen also in the data of the lower value conditions in the third experiment.

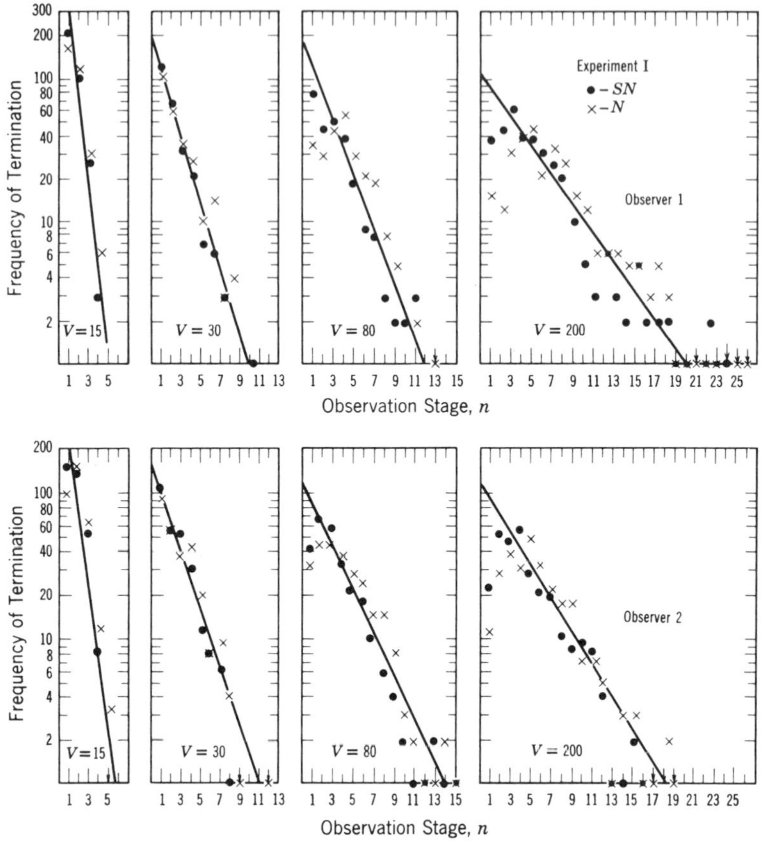

FIG. 4. The number of terminal decisions made at each observation stage by the two observers in Experiment I.

The exponential form of this function is provocative. It suggests that on a finer level the data may not support the sequential model we have described, for this is the function that would result if the observer failed to integrate the successive observations, that is, if he set constant criteria and made a terminal decision when, and only when, a criterion was exceeded by a single observation. This is equivalent to ignoring, if an observation falls in the critical region C, just where in that region it falls. Thus our data are consistent with what may be termed the 'independence' model, or the 'amnesic-observer' model, of the process underlying successive observations. It is an open question whether or not the exponential form is also consistent with an integration of the successive observations, a question we shall turn to in a moment.

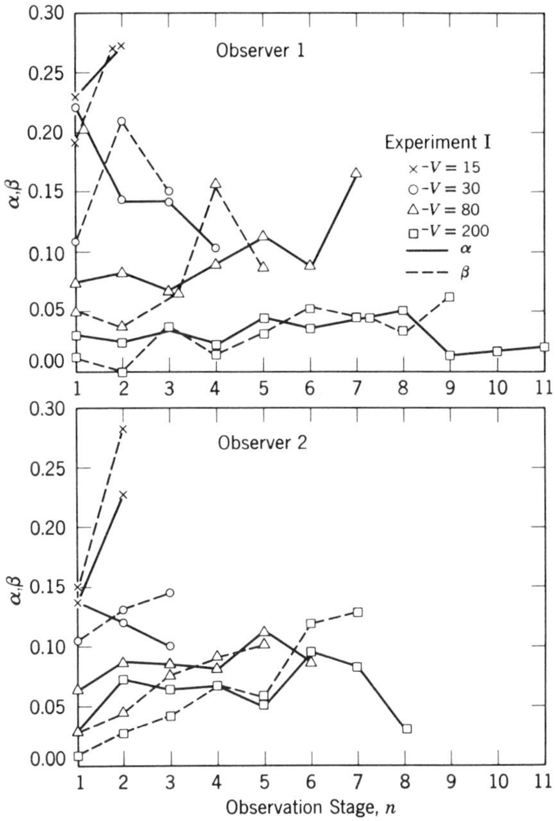

FIG. 5. The error rates α and β as a function of the observation stage in Experiment I. Two observers.

Before we do so, let us ask whether the observer maintains constant criteria over the successive observations in a given value condition. The answer will not distinguish between the two models, for this procedure is assumed by the sequential model and it is also consistent, as we have just noted, with the simpler model that is suggested by the stage-by-stage analysis of the data. Nevertheless, the result is of some interest. Our indices of the criteria chosen by the observer are given by the error probabilities α and β. Figure 5 shows the obtained values of α and β as a function of n for the first experiment. The points shown are those in each value condition that are based on more than 50 observations. When sampling error is considered, plus the fact that several of the points are based on only slightly more than 50 observations, it is clear that the best assumption is that the observer does maintain relatively constant criteria. No other trend is apparent. The results of the second and third experiments are very similar.

Let us return now to the question of whether or not the form of the function that relates the number of terminal decisions to the observation stage is consistent with both of the models we have described. In particular, let us ask whether or not the data require that we accept the amnesic-observer model and reject the sequential model for the process underlying successive observations. We may answer this question by the technique of predicting the number of terminations at each stage from the observed error rates at each stage, under the assumption that d' remains constant over successive observations. If we can predict the data by this technique we must accept the amnesic-observer model of the process in preference to the sequential model.

Returning to the situation of Fig. 1, it should be apparent that the proportion of terminations at each stage is determined by four probabilities: the probabilities that an observation will fall in region A, given either the existence of noise alone or of signal plus noise, and the probabilities that an observation will fall in region B, given either alternative. We can test the validity of the two models by extracting two of these probabilities from the data, and by using these along with an assumed constant value of d' to predict the other two probabilities, and hence the total probability of termination under each of the alternatives at each observation stage.

To illustrate this technique, let us suppose that we are predicting the number of N and SN presentations terminated at the second stage of observation for a given value condition. Suppose also that d' has been established in a preliminary test. Of the N presentations reaching the second stage, the observer responds *Yes* to some and thus provides an estimate of α; of the SN presentations reaching the second stage, he responds *No* to some, yielding an estimate of β. The probability α determines the distance of the upper criterion from the mean of $f_N(x)$. Since the distance between the means of $f_N(x)$ and $f_{SN}(x)$ is assumed to be d', the distance from the mean of $f_{SN}(x)$ to the upper criterion is determinable. The probability that the observer will make a terminal decision to an SN presentation is the probability that the upper criterion will be exceeded by an observation of SN, plus the probability that he will respond *No* to an SN presentation, β. Similarly for the N presentations, β determines the distance of the lower criterion from the mean of $f_{SN}(x)$.

Subtracting d' yields the distance of the lower criterion from the mean of $f_N(x)$. The probability that an observation will fall below this criterion is the probability of saying *No* to an N presentation. This probability, plus the probability of saying *Yes* to an N presentation, or α, is the total probability of terminating an N presentation.

The value of d' assumed for each observer in our calculations is that determined by the preliminary yes–no test in the first and third experiments, and since a yes–no test was not conducted in the second experiment, by a preliminary forced-choice test in that experiment. Since the data of the observers within a given experiment are practically identical for the present purpose, they have been combined on a single graph. Figure 6a shows one plot of obtained against predicted numbers of terminal decisions for both observers and for all value conditions in the first experiment; Fig. 6b shows a similar plot for these observers in the second experiment. The terminal decisions under noise alone and under signal plus noise have not been differentiated since the patterns are not noticeably different. The logarithmic scales are used to make evident the points at the lower numbers; the hatched square at the lower left corner is meant to indicate a large cluster of points at coordinates 1, 1.

This analysis leaves little doubt that, for the first two experiments, the assumption of no integration over successive observations is a good one; it permits prediction of the number of terminal decisions at each stage. In sampling various value conditions, we find coefficients of correlation between predicted and obtained values of the order of 0.90.

With these data from the first two experiments in hand, the third experiment was conducted with explicit instructions to the observers to attempt to integrate over successive observations. Thus, in the third experiment, we were asking not whether human observers in a sequential detection problem would integrate if left to their own devices, but whether they could integrate if encouraged to do so. Figure 7 shows the results of the attempt to predict the number of terminal decisions in the third experiment under the assumption of no integration. The data of the three observers for all value conditions are again combined in the one graph. The existence of more terminations than would result from no integration is apparent. Approximately 80 per cent of the points fall above the diagonal line, whereas in the first and second experiments, 54 per cent and 50 per cent, respectively, fall above the diagonal. The evidence, then, indicates that human observers are indeed capable of integrating the information in successive observations.

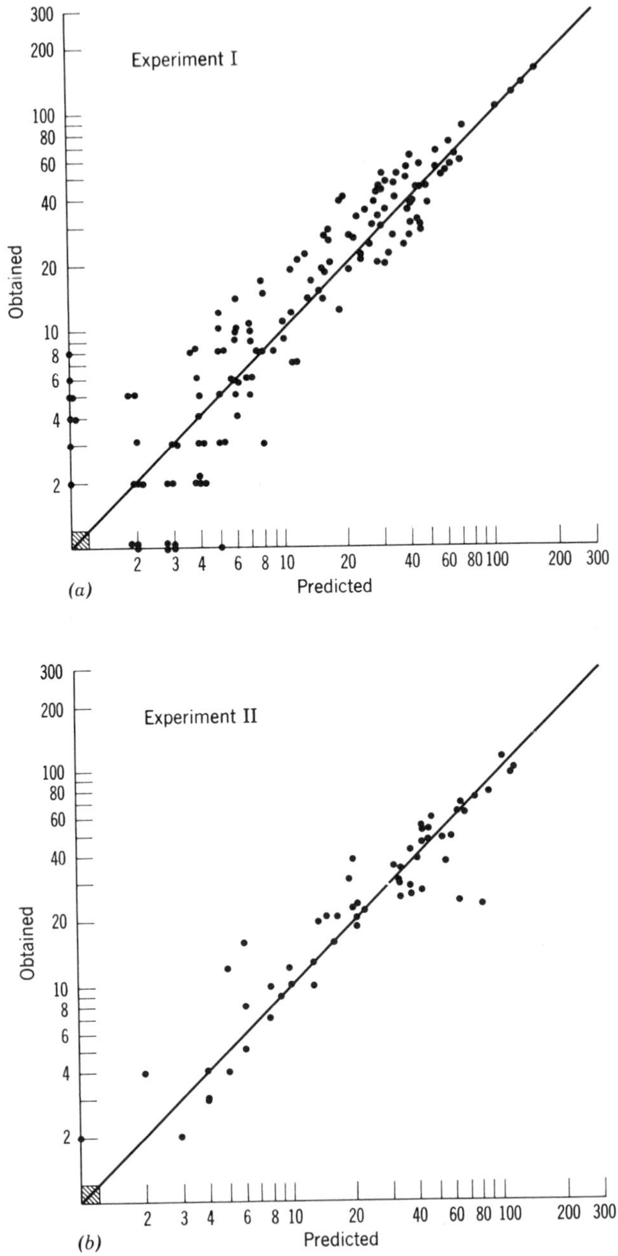

FIG. 6. The predicted and obtained numbers of terminal decisions at each observation stage in Experiment I (*a*) and Experiment II (*b*).

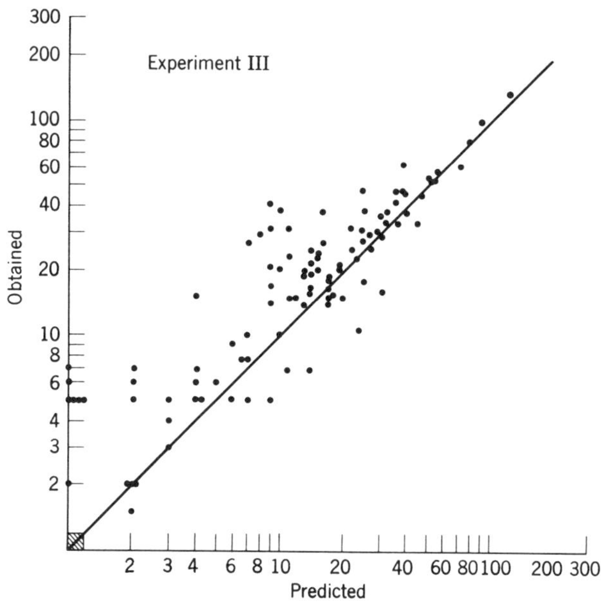

FIG. 7. The predicted and obtained numbers of terminal decisions at each observation stage in Experiment III.

ACKNOWLEDGMENTS

We gratefully acknowledge the valuable assistance of Miss Mary J. McKey and Mrs. Susan T. Sewall in collecting and analyzing the data of these experiments, and of Mr. Arthur Wasserman in the design of the experimental equipment.

This research was conducted in the Research Laboratory of Electronics, Massachusetts Institute of Technology, with support from the U. S. Army Signal Corps, the Air Force (Operational Applications Laboratory and Office of Scientific Research), and the Office of Naval Research. This article appeared as Tech. Rept. No. AFCCDD-TR-60-21, and in C. Cherry (Ed.), Information theory, *London: Butterworths, 1961, pp. 177–195.*

References

- Becker, G. M. Sequential decision making; Wald's models and estimates of parameters. *J. exp. Psychol.*, 1958, **55,** 628–636.
- Egan, J. P. Message repetition, operating characteristics, and confusion matrices in speech communication. Indiana University: Hearing and Communication Laboratory, 1957, Technical Report No. AFCRC-TR-57-50.
- Green, D. M., Birdsall, T. G., and Tanner, W. P., Jr. Signal detection as a function of signal intensity and duration. *J. acoust. Soc. Am.*, 1957, **29,** 523–531. [11]

- Irwin, F. W., and Smith, W. A. S. Value, cost and information as determiners of decision. *J. exp. Psychol.,* 1957, **54,** 229–232.
- Swets, J. A. Indices of signal detectability obtained with various psychophysical procedures. *J. acoust. Soc. Am.,* 1959, **31,** 511–513. [6]
- Swets, J. A., Shipley, E. F., McKey, M. J., and Green, D. M. Multiple observations of signals in noise. *J. acoust. Soc. Am.,* 1959, **31,** 514–521. [9]
- Swets, J. A., Tanner, W. P., Jr., and Birdsall, T. G. Decision processes in perception. *Psychol. Rev.,* 1961, **68,** 301–340. [1]
- Wald, A. *Sequential analysis.* New York: Wiley, 1947.

11

Signal Detection as a Function of Signal Intensity and Duration

David M. Green, Theodore G. Birdsall, and Wilson P. Tanner, Jr.

In attempts to establish a theory or model of how a human observer detects auditory signals, many parameters of the signal may be varied which will provide information as to how the mechanism operates. Until recently, comparatively little research has been devoted to a study of one of these parameters, the duration of the signal. All of the recent studies in this area have had a common approach, which was to determine the duration and intensity of the signal necessary for the observer to report he heard the tone. Looking at these studies in another way, one might say the research was designed to determine the signal intensity and duration necessary to produce a constant detectability. In essence, then, these studies varied signal intensity and duration with detectability held constant. The results of such studies are usually reported in terms of the familiar time-intensity graph. An example of such is shown in Fig. 1, which is taken from Garner (1947).

This study employs a slightly different procedure which will supplement the data previously gathered. The major change in this study was to allow detectability to vary. Thus this study could be considered an attempt to investigate the surface of detectability in the space defined by signal duration, intensity, and detectability. To accomplish this purpose three experiments were conducted with the same observers throughout. The manner in which each experiment was conducted is discussed later in this chapter.

Previous research

Hughes (1946) presented some data using pure tones (of six different durations, ranging from 63 to 739 msec) and employing five frequencies. He obtained the intensity of the signal necessary for the subject to report that he heard the signal for each duration under absolute threshold conditions. He suggested that the following equation closely fitted his data:

$$I/I_0 = b + a/t \tag{1}$$

where I is intensity, I_0 is a constant intensity, b and a are constants, with t signifying signal duration. If this equation holds as duration approaches infinity, then $b = I_\infty/I_0$, where I_∞ is the intensity used with an extremely long signal. Substituting this value in Eq. (1), we find

$$t(I - I_\infty) = aI_0 = C \tag{1a}$$

where C is some constant.

Investigating the masked tonal threshold, Garner and Miller (1947) employed eight durations ranging from 12.5 to 2000 msec. They used four frequencies and six noise levels ranging from 20 to 110 db sound pressure levels. They presented what Licklider (1951) has called the "diverted input hypothesis." This hypothesis maintains that a certain portion I_0 of the stimulus intensity is not an effective stimulus for the ear. All the stimulus energy above this value is integrated linearly with time.

Mathematically, this hypothesis can be expressed as follows:

$$t(I - I_\infty) = C \tag{1b}$$

where I_∞ is the value of intensity necessary for the detection of an extremely long signal and C is a constant.

This equation, which is identical with Hughes' equation, also fits with reasonable accuracy the data presented by Garner and Miller. In their paper they go on to point out that these data are not inconsistent with Crozier's statistical theory, although the latter theory requires one more degree of freedom.

Thus for the range of durations from about 12.5 to 2000 msec it is apparent that Eq. (1) provides a fairly good approximation to the form of the data.

Garner, in a paper concerned with very short duration, has extended knowledge in this area. Using pure tones with durations ranging from 1 to 100 msec he obtained the data presented in Fig. 1. Considering the

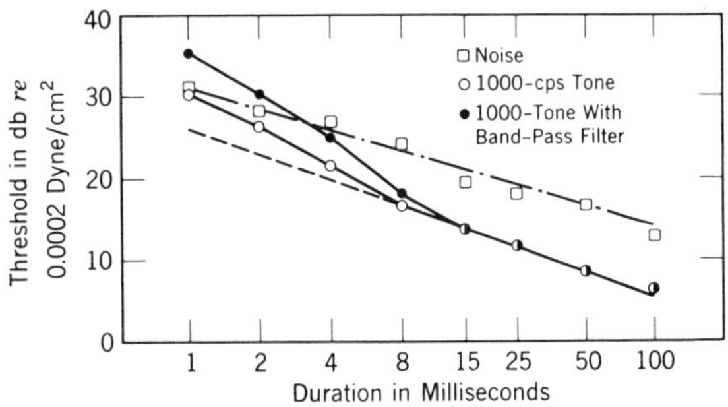

FIG. 1. The signal intensity and duration necessary to maintain some constant detectability (from Garner, 1947).

power spectrum of short tones he advanced the hypothesis: "The rate of temporal integration of energy in the ear is dependent on the width of the frequency band of the energy to be integrated." The higher detectability of the pure-tone signal as compared with the noise signal, until very brief durations are reached, supports this hypothesis, since at very short durations the power spectrum of the gated sine wave closely resembles that of the noise power spectrum.

If this hypothesis is correct, then the concept of critical bands (Fletcher, 1940) may be employed to explain time and intensity results. This suggestion will be pursued further in a later section.

Mechanisms responsible for time-intensity results

Although partial explanations have been suggested for some of the previous results, no consistent model has been suggested to explain the results over the entire range of duration investigated.

In particular the diverted input hypothesis for very short duration, Eq. (1), would be closely approximated by the following equation:

$$It = C \tag{1c}$$

As Garner's work demonstrates, this does not hold. This is presumably explained by the spectrum characteristics of very short gated sine waves, as discussed previously. Nevertheless no suggestion of why the diverted input hypothesis should approximate the data has been advanced, or why some minimal intensity should not be an effective stimulus for the ear.

MEASURE OF DETECTABILITY

Since, in the present research, the detectability of the signal will be allowed to vary rather than being held constant, the major problem to be met is that of determining a measure of detectability. Certainly, there are several reasonable ways to accomplish this task. There are, however, certain properties of the measure which would seem desirable to everyone. Consider a test situation where the signal is presented in one of four time intervals. The observer's job is to specify in which time interval he thinks the signal occurred. He is forced to choose one of the four intervals. This situation will be called a *forced-choice situation*, and since there are four alternatives it is specifically a *four-alternative forced-choice* test. It appears obvious that the more correct identifications the observer can make of a particular signal in this situation, the more detectable this signal is. This is certainly one necessary property of the measure. For reasons of generality it would also be advantageous to obtain a measure of detectability which would yield approximately the same number for some fixed situation whether two, four, or more alternatives are used in a forced-choice test. Also, the measure should be applicable to a test situation where there is only one time interval and the subject gives a yes or no response. That is, the measure should make possible comparison over different test situations. The only variable which seems to accomplish this task is the index d' suggested by Tanner and Swets (1954). Tanner, Swets, and Green (1956) have demonstrated that this index, d', yields approximately the same value in a forced-choice as in a yes-no test situation if the same physical parameters are employed.

Definition of the detectability index

The general conception of signal detection is available elsewhere (Tanner and Swets, 1954; Tanner, Swets, and Green, 1956). Since a four-alternative forced-choice method was used in the research, d' will simply be defined by the transform of the probability of a correct detection as given by Table I. This table is derived from the following formula:

$$P(c) = \int_{-\infty}^{+\infty} \Phi^3(x)\phi(x - d')dx \tag{2}$$

where $P(c)$ is the probability of a correct detection, $\Phi(x)$ is a normal distribution function with some mean and unit standard deviation, and $\phi(x - d')$ is a normal density function with mean d' above the other mean and the same variance.

TABLE I. Probability of a Correct Detection in a Four-Alternative Forced-Choice Test as a Function of d'

Probability of a correct detection	d'	Probability of a correct detection	d'
0.25	0.0	0.63	1.26
0.26	0.04	0.64	1.29
0.27	0.08	0.65	1.32
0.28	0.12	0.66	1.35
0.29	0.16	0.67	1.38
0.30	0.20	0.68	1.42
0.31	0.24	0.69	1.46
0.32	0.27	0.70	1.50
0.33	0.30	0.71	1.53
0.34	0.34	0.72	1.57
0.35	0.37	0.73	1.61
0.36	0.41	0.74	1.65
0.37	0.43	0.75	1.69
0.38	0.47	0.76	1.73
0.39	0.50	0.77	1.77
0.40	0.52	0.78	1.80
0.41	0.56	0.79	1.85
0.42	0.58	0.80	1.89
0.43	0.61	0.81	1.93
0.44	0.64	0.82	1.98
0.45	0.68	0.83	2.03
0.46	0.71	0.84	2.08
0.47	0.74	0.85	2.13
0.48	0.77	0.86	2.18
0.49	0.81	0.87	2.24
0.50	0.84	0.88	2.29
0.51	0.87	0.89	2.36
0.52	0.91	0.90	2.42
0.53	0.94	0.91	2.50
0.54	0.97	0.92	2.60
0.55	1.00	0.93	2.70
0.56	1.03	0.94	2.80
0.57	1.06	0.95	2.92
0.58	1.09	0.96	3.02
0.59	1.12	0.97	3.14
0.60	1.16	0.98	3.25
0.61	1.19	0.99	
0.62	1.22		

The formula expresses the probability that if four random samples are drawn, three from a certain normal distribution, the fourth from a distribution with a mean d' higher than the others, the highest sample value will be associated with this fourth distribution. Throughout this paper the obtained percentage of correct detection is used as an estimate of the probability of being correct and the corresponding estimate of d' is obtained by means of this formula.

EXPERIMENTAL APPARATUS

Audio channel

Figure 2 shows, in block diagram form, the relevant aspects of the audio channel. The headphones, used binaurally, in phase, were PDR-8's. The frequency of the tone was 1000 cps throughout all the experiments. Gaussian noise, provided by a General Radio noise source, was used to mask the signal. The signal gate turned on the sine wave only at a positive-going zero crossing and permitted only an integral number of cycles to pass.

Audio measurements

Two voltmeters, of the average-reading full-wave-rectifier type and calibrated in sine wave rms, were used to measure the signal and noise. Both meters showed a systematic error at low scale readings; therefore, graphs were obtained using a voltage divider procedure to convert the

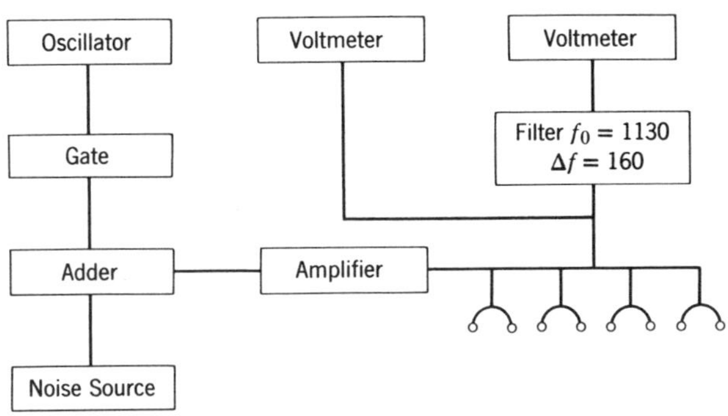

FIG. 2. A block diagram of the apparatus used in the experiment. The oscillator was a Hewlett-Packard type 200-I. The noise source was a General Radio type 1390-A. Both voltmeters were Hewlett-Packard model 400-D. Further details are included in the text.

"scale" readings to the "true" voltage. The resistance box used in the voltage divider procedure had an accuracy of 0.1 per cent. One meter served for the wide band, and the other read the output of a single-tuned circuit. This filter was centered at 1130 cps and had a band pass of about 160 cps. The comparison of the two meters provided an indication of any change in the noise spectrum level. No such change was noted in the course of the experiment. The duration calibration was accomplished by displaying the signal on a DuMont model 329 oscilloscope. Three complete checks of the calibration of the signal circuit were made at different times in the experiment, and on over one-half of the durations a check was made immediately before this duration was used in the experiment. The noise level employed in all experiments was about 60 db (*re* 0.0002 dyne/cm^2 per cycle). This measurement was made at the output of the headsets with a 6-cc coupler and a Western Electric condenser microphone, type 640-AA.

The results are presented in terms of E/N_0. E is signal energy, acoustic power multiplied by duration, and N_0 is the noise spectrum level, that is, the power in a certain frequency band divided by the equivalent square bandwidth. Since bandwidth has the dimensions of cycles per second, N_0 has the dimensions of energy. E/N_0 is thus a dimensionless quantity. In the third experiment the signal amplitude was held constant, as was N_0, while signal duration was varied. The quantity P/N_0 is presented in the results. This quantity has the dimension of reciprocal time (in seconds). To obtain the correct E/N_0 multiply the appropriate signal duration (in seconds) by the quantity P/N_0.

Programming of the experiment

Throughout the experiments a four-alternative forced-choice procedure was used. Four subjects observed simultaneously in a sound-treated room. The subjects were warned that a trial was to begin by a flash of a green light. A white light blinked four times in coincidence with the beginning of the four temporal intervals in which the signal could occur. A red light then signaled the observer that a choice must be registered by pressing one of four buttons. This choice was then automatically recorded. Only one choice was possible and this choice could be recorded only during the "record" interval. At the end of the "record" interval the subject was notified (by means of another light) which answer was correct. The next trial then began. The masking noise was present in the subjects' earphones through a trial period.

The length of the four intervals was adjusted in accordance with the duration of the signal. For the longest signal duration used (a 3-sec signal)

4 sec was allowed for each interval, making a total of 16 sec to complete all four intervals. For signals shorter than about 0.5 sec, 0.75 sec was used for each interval, making a total of about 3 sec for the four intervals. All subjects agreed that the faster the cycling went the less bored they became in making their judgments. The experimenter on several occasions insisted on a slower speed but could find no significant differences between this procedure and a more rapid one. Thus, the experimenter yielded to the complaints of the subjects and adjusted the interval to that which the subjects judged to be a convenient speed.

The programming of the experiment was accomplished electronically. A device called N. P. Psytar (*N*oise *P*rogramed *Psy*chophysical *T*ester *a*nd *R*ecorder) accomplished this task. The selection of the interval in which the signal is to be presented is of considerable importance in forced-choice experiments. N. P. Psytar samples the output of a noise tube in order to determine which interval will be selected on each trial. Thus, it is believed, an essentially random process governs the selection. Tests have been conducted to determine the randomness of this procedure, and the null hypothesis could not be rejected.

One male and three female subjects were used throughout all of the experiments. All were students at the University of Michigan. All subjects were in their late teens or early twenties. All subjects were trained for at least two hours a day for twenty days before any data reported in this paper were taken. Three of the four had participated in a previous experiment lasting about four months.

Each cycle during which four intervals are presented and a choice obtained is defined as a trial. One-hundred trials constitute a single session. At most durations six or seven sessions were run per day. This required about seventy minutes of actual running time. The subjects took about two hours with rests between each session to conduct the six or seven sessions. The results of the experiment were obtained in about three months.

For the longer durations, for example, with the 3-sec signal duration, only fifty trials were conducted each session. Each session, therefore, took about 16 min to run. The subjects found the long duration signals very tedious and consequently were given longer rest periods.

RESULTS OF THE EXPERIMENTS

Experiment I

In this experiment the independent variable was the intensity, or power, of the signal. The dependent variable was the percentage of correct responses by the observer. The per cent correct was converted to the corresponding d' by means of Eq. (2) and was used as the abscissa of the graph. The parameter was the signal duration which was held constant at three values: 5, 50, and 500 msec. The results of Experiment I are given in Fig. 3. Several of the points displayed on the graphs were not actually obtained from Experiment I. These points were obtained in other experiments using the same observer where the physical parameters were the same as they were for this experiment but were taken at a later date. They are labeled and the experiment in which they were obtained may be determined by the key. These points were obtained one to two months later than the majority of the points shown on the graph. The high degree to which they correspond to the remaining points displays the long-term stability of both equipment and observers. The line drawn through the data points is of the general form $d' = K(E/N_0)$ where K is a function of signal duration. A more complete discussion of the authors' attempt to fit the data will be given later.

Experiment II

Pairs of values for signal power and duration were selected so that a constant energy signal was presented to the observer. The per cent correct detection was obtained for each pair of values. The per cent correct detection was converted to d' and plotted with signal duration as the independent variable. The data obtained in Experiment II are plotted in Fig. 4. The middle, flat, section of each graph reflects an area where detection remains constant for a constant energy signal. This is the only period of time when the ear is able to integrate acoustic power linearly with time. For short durations the data are fairly well approximated by a curve of the type $d' = C(E/N_0)t^{\frac{1}{2}}$ where C is a constant. For longer durations the data are approximated by a curve of the type $d' = C(E/N_0)t^{-\frac{1}{2}}$. The line fitted to the data is determined by an equation, the parameters of which are determined from the first experiment. This will be discussed more completely in the following pages.

Experiment III

In this experiment the independent variable was the signal duration. The dependent variable was the per cent correct detections, which has been converted to d', the detectability index. The parameter was sig-

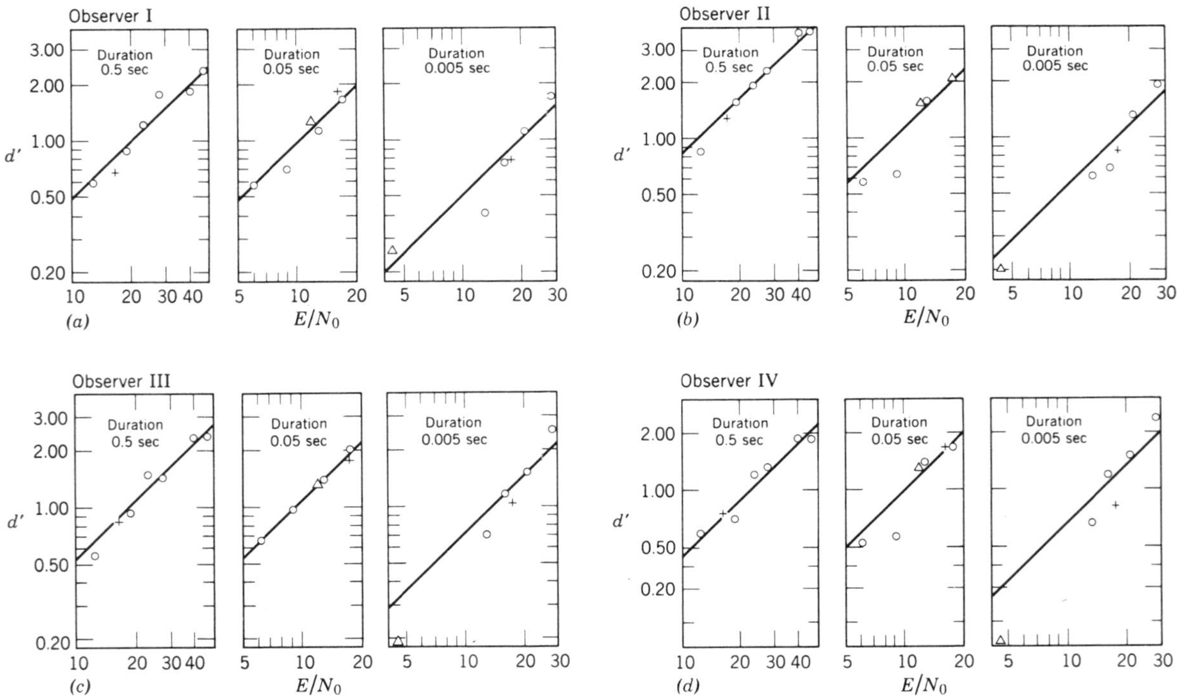

FIG. 3. The detectability of the signal as a function of E/N_0 for three signal durations. The points marked by open circles were obtained in the first experiment; the plus signs were obtained in Experiment II; the triangles in Experiment III. The slope of the line is 1.

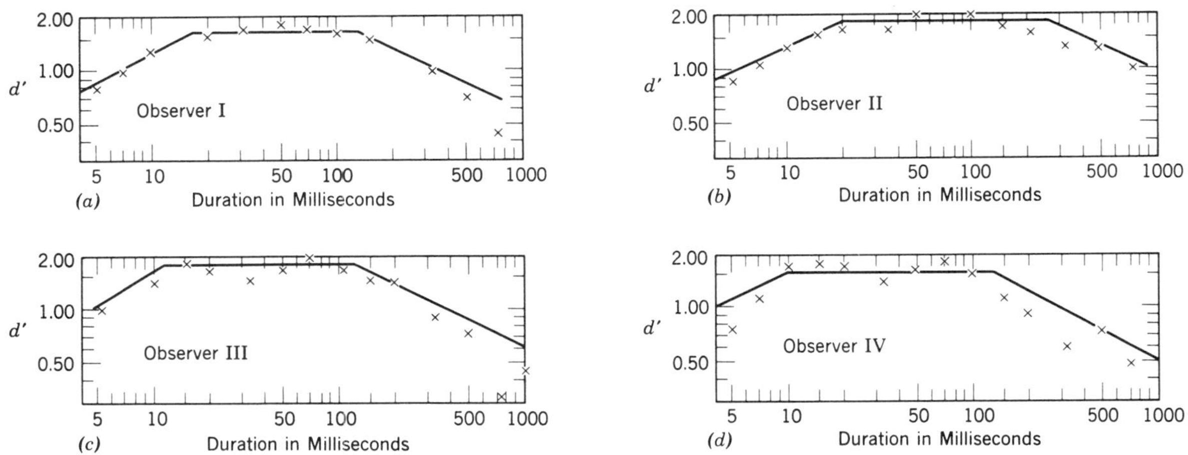

FIG. 4. Detectability of a constant energy signal as a function of signal duration. The breaks in the line represent the durations T_1 and T_2. $E/N_0 = 16.9$ for all four observers.

nal power. The results for the four observers are plotted in Fig. 5. Three functions were fitted to the data, one for each region of signal duration. For short durations, $d' = Kt^{3/2}$ where K is a function of signal power and noise level. For medium durations, $d' = Kt$. Finally, for long durations, $d' = Kt^{1/2}$. The reader is referred to a later section for a discussion of how the solid line was fitted to the data.

A rather surprising finding was the continued increase in detectability of the signal that resulted from extending the duration from 250 to 1000 to 3000 msec while signal power was held constant. It is usually believed that for some long durations detection will be independent of signal duration and completely dependent on signal amplitude and noise level. At least for the durations investigated, this long duration has not been reached. For all four observers, the per cent correct increased as the duration was extended. The average increase from the 1-second to the 3-second signal was almost 10 per cent in per cent correct detections. On the assumption that this is a binomial process, the standard deviation of the difference would be about 4 per cent, which means that the null hypothesis (no increase) could be rejected at better than the 5 per cent level.

EMPIRICAL FIT TO DATA

After the data had been collected, the following set of equations appeared to fit the data with reasonable accuracy.

$$d' = k(E/N_0)(t/T_1)^{1/2} \quad \text{for } t < T_1 \tag{3}$$

$$d' = k(E/N_0) \quad \text{for } T_1 < t < T_2 \tag{4}$$

$$d' = k(E/N_0)(T_2/t)^{1/2} \quad \text{for } T_2 < t \tag{5}$$

where E is the signal energy, t is signal duration, T_1 and T_2 are individual constants having the dimensions of time, k is some numerical constant reflecting an individual observer constant, and N_0 is the noise spectrum level. It may be noted again that d', the detectability index, is dimensionless.

The equations just presented suggest functions which are discontinuous at the durations T_1 and T_2. The authors do not believe that such discontinuities are in fact present in the hearing mechanism. These equations are advanced in the nature of asymptotic approximations. These simple functions appear to express these relations well enough for present purposes. As a matter of fact, the fit to the data is surprisingly good even at the discontinuities of the function, as shown in a later section.

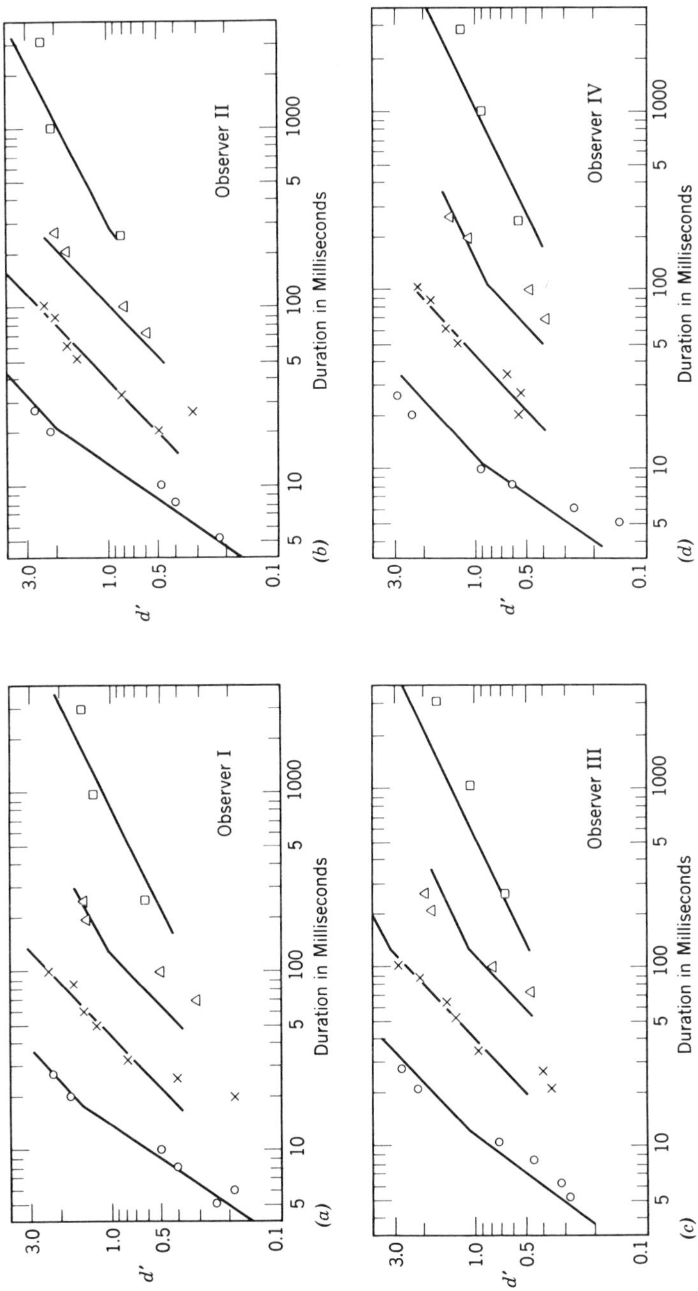

FIG. 5. The detectability of the signal as a function of duration at four intensities. For the circles the P/N_0 values are 867.4; for the X's, 243.4; for the triangles, 87.6; and for the squares, 33.7.

A related point concerns the region where detection is claimed to be proportional to energy. Whether such a region actually exists is almost impossible to determine with existing psychophysical procedures. If any finite error is allowed one can find some finite range of time where this approximation seems justifiable.

A third point to be made concerns the visual impression of the extent to which the data fit the functions. The equations suggested above were arrived at after considering all three experiments and all four observers. Certain changes could be made in the function for any single experiment or observer which would improve the fit. Usually, such changes considerably weaken the fit in the other experiments.

Estimation of the parameters

As can be seen from the preceding section, the parameters k, T_1, and T_2 must be estimated in order to fit the data obtained in this study. In order to fit the data the following procedure was adopted. On the basis of the data obtained in the first experiment, it was apparent that the three signal durations fell in the three different regions of time for all the observers; 5 msec for $< T_1$, 50 msec between T_1 and T_2, and 500 msec for $> T_2$. Hence, considering only the data in Experiment I, all three parameters could be obtained. The 50-msec signal duration provided six points, and a least-squares technique was used to provide an estimate of k. From the 5-msec data, a least-squares technique provided a value of $k(T_1)^{-1/2}$. Since k had been estimated from the 50-msec curve, T_1 could be determined. Likewise, the parameter $k(T_2)^{1/2}$ could be estimated from the 500-msec experiment.

In summary, the data from the first experiment provided, by a least-squares technique, the estimates of the three parameters associated with each observer. Table II lists these parameters for each observer.

Table II shows sizeable individual differences in the three parameters, especially those having to do with the times T_1 and T_2. The ratio of mean to standard deviation of these four observers is about 3 for the two time parameters. Thus, to average data in experiments of this type appears hazardous. As an extreme example, consider the plot in Fig. 4*b* giving the results obtained with the second observer when signal energy was held constant. Had one assumed that T_2 was about 120 msec, which is the average T_2 for the other three observers, the average error for the longer times would have been approximately 6 db. A far more serious consequence of the averaging procedure would have been to obscure the form of the data.

TABLE II. PARAMETERS AS ESTIMATED FROM EXPERIMENT I

Observers	k	T_1 msec	T_2 msec
I	0.10	18	132
II	0.11	20	276
III	0.11	12	122
IV	0.09	10	108

Since the constants listed in the table were obtained from the data in the first experiment, the data obtained in the second and third experiment were "predicted." The curves shown in Figs. 3 through 5 are those which would be obtained using the constants estimated and the equations listed above. As can be seen, the fit is fairly good.

Test of goodness of fit

To measure the goodness of fit, two procedures were used. The first procedure is of theoretical interest. It was assumed that the per cent correct obtained in each experiment resulted from a binomial process. The standard deviation could thus be estimated from the equation $(pq/n)^{1/2}$, where p is the probability of a correct detection, $q = (1 - p)$, and n is the number of observations used to estimate the point. Since the expected d' could be obtained from the equations, this leads to some expected per cent correct. The sum of the squared differences between the expected and obtained per cent correct divided by the standard deviation of expected p should be distributed as chi square if the difference between the predicted and obtained points is simply the result of binomial variation. The number of degrees of freedom would be the number of differences evaluated in this manner minus three, since three parameters are estimated from the data. A chi-square value was obtained from each observer's data. The associated probability values were of such a magnitude that this hypothesis could easily be rejected (e.g., $P = 10^{-5}$). Hence either the theoretical curve is incorrect or the observed per cent correct is not simply a binomial process. Both alternatives appear likely.

A second procedure of more practical interest was to evaluate the average error in terms of the decibel error; that is, to evaluate how much one would have to change the signal power on the average to obtain a perfect fit of the data. This was computed by evaluating the average absolute deviation between the expected d' and the obtained d' divided by the expected d'. This average per cent deviation was then reflected to signal power since d' and signal power are approximately linearly related (see Fig. 3). This average deviation varied between 13 per cent and 16 per cent. This would indicate an average error in terms of signal power of at most 0.8 db.

Comparison of the obtained equations and previous data

The comparison of the results of this study and previous data is difficult because in some other studies average data were presented. That is, the data were averaged over subjects. It will be assumed that the subjects were similar enough so that no untoward results are to be expected. Rewriting the equation presented previously so as to allow a direct comparison with the equation found to fit data collected under the conventional threshold procedure, one finds

$$It^{3/2} = C_1 \qquad t < T_1$$

where

$$C_1 = [(d'N_0)T_1^{\frac{1}{2}}]/k \tag{6}$$

$$It = C_2 \qquad T_1 < t < T_2$$

$$C_2 = (d'N_0)/k \tag{7}$$

$$It^{1/2} = C_3 \qquad T_2 < t$$

$$C_3 = (d'N_0)/kT^{\frac{1}{2}}) \tag{8}$$

where I is the intensity or power of the signal.

For the middle range of duration there is essentially no disagreement because the diverted input equation approximates this form at short signal durations. For the very short duration Eq. (6) is precisely the form of the relation obtained in Garner's (1947) study. Equation (6) predicts a decrease in signal strength (as time is increased) of 4.5 db per octave. Figure 1 taken from Garner shows this relation for the 1000-cps tone. The value of T_1 as obtained from Garner's data is about 10 msec. This value is only 5 msec different from the average value of T_1 obtained from the observers in this study (Table II), and is the same as the value obtained from one observer used in this study.

For the longer duration the results obtained in these experiments indicate that to hold detectability constant one must decrease signal amplitude 1.5 db per octave. About the only other study which covered the range of signal duration necessary to test this relation is that of Garner and Miller (1947). They determined signal powers necessary to obtain a constant detectability for the durations 200, 500, 1000, 2000 msec and a "very long" duration at four signal frequencies.

The decreases found were about 1 db per octave or less, depending on the signal frequency. The fact that the "very long" duration did not indicate a much smaller signal power is at variance with Eq. (8). The most probable conclusion is that the present study did not extend signal duration far enough to obtain this result. That is, the 3-sec duration was not "very long."

A point may be made concerning the use of extremely long duration signals. If the duration is much longer than about 1 or 2 sec a very good procedure would be to make a decision every second or so, i.e., make a decision that the signal is either present or not present. Assume that one could then remember the previous decision and simply add up the number of "yes" decisions. The result would be a binomial process with some fixed mean, depending on signal strength, and a variance which would decrease linearly with the number of decisions, and hence linearly with signal duration. That is, the variance of the mean, where the mean is based on n samples, is n times better than the variance of a single sample. This argument leads to the conclusion that d' should increase at the rate of the square root of duration if signal power is held constant. Whether or not such a model is reasonable is, of course, an empirical question. The data obtained in this study are consistent with this interpretation.

DISCUSSION

One of the main objectives in conducting the present experiments was to compare the results obtained from the observers with a model obtained from the work on signal detectability by Peterson and Birdsall (1953). Specifically, the experiments conducted provided a direct comparison with the model designated "signal-known-exactly." This model supposes the receiver has an exact copy of the signal to be detected or, equivalently, has a filter constructed on the basis of exact knowledge of the signal. It also knows the exact starting time of the signal as well as its frequency, and the exact statistical characteristics of the masking noise. Although both a priori grounds and empirical data suggest that the model is an inadequate conceptualization of the way in which the human observer behaves, no empirical comparisons have been made concerning the effects of signal duration.

Analysis from a signal-to-noise ratio standpoint has shown that the effects of signal duration and receiver bandwidth are closely linked. The optimum procedure for detecting a signal of known duration is to adjust the receiver bandwidth to approximately the reciprocal of the signal duration. Lawson and Ulhenbeck (1950) show this result for a variety of receivers. Peterson and Birdsall (1953) have also demonstrated this result. The effects of mismatching the receiver bandwidth and the reciprocal of signal duration is also known, i.e., adjusting the filter either too wide or too narrow. Considering the product of bandwidth times pulse duration, the effect of mismatching is approximately 3 db signal-to-noise ratio loss per octave mismatch, when the noise spectrum level and signal energy are held constant.

There are several ways one may understand this result. One way to consider the phenomenon is to realize that the bandwidth determines the rise time of output of the filter. If the filter is too narrow for the signal duration it acts as an integrator for the entire duration of the signal, but the signal terminates before the maximum rise of the filter has been reached. If the filter is too wide the signal reaches the maximum and continues at that level until the signal terminates. However, it allows more interfering noise into the receiver than is necessary. The optimum condition is obtained when the signal duration is about the reciprocal of the receiver's bandwidth; then the output of the filter reaches its maximum rise just as the signal terminates. (For a more complete discussion of this problem see Lawson and Uhlenbeck, 1950, especially Fig. 8.10, page 104).

Garner (1947) has suggested another way to understand the result which is obtained when the receiver's bandwidth is too narrow for the signal duration. He considered the Fourier energy spectrum of a short duration signal. As the signal duration decreases, if the receiver's bandwidth is fixed, more and more of the signal energy falls in a frequency range outside the receiver's bandwidth. This analysis is exactly equivalent to the preceding.

Returning to the discussion of the detection model (Peterson and Birdsall, 1953, 1955) for the signal-known-exactly, the following equations will hold, depending on the relation of the receiver's bandwidth and signal duration:

$$d' = (2E/N_0)^{1/2}(t/T_1)^{1/2} \qquad t < T_1 \tag{9}$$

where the receiver bandwidth (w) is fixed at $T_1 = 1/w$ and is the maximum bandwidth of the receiver,

$$d' = (2E/N_0)^{1/2} \qquad T_1 < t < T_2 \tag{10}$$

where the receiver bandwidth (w) is $w = 1/t$ and is adjusted for each signal duration,

$$d'(2E/N_0)^{1/2}(T_2/t)^{1/2} \qquad T_2 < t \tag{11}$$

where the receiver bandwidth (w) is fixed at $T_2 = 1/w$ and is the minimum bandwidth of the receiver,

and where d' yields the same per cent correct detection in the experiment considered as that expressed in Table I.

Only Eq. (10) is true for the signal-known-exactly *ideal* receiver. Equations (9) and (11) are true for less than ideal models, i.e., the ideal receiver with bandwidth mismatching. These equations are not precisely correct at durations near T_1 and T_2. They are the asymptotic approximations to the actual equations and are presented in this form to facilitate comparison with the empirical equations (3), (4), and (5).

The equations provided by the model and those fitted to the data differ in two important respects. For the observer, d' appears to vary linearly with signal power. The model indicates that d' should be linear with the square root of signal power. Secondly, each equation obtained from the model must be multiplied by the square root of duration in order to obtain the same relation between d' and duration as those obtained from the observer. If, however, signal *energy* is held constant the equations predicted by the model and those obtained from the human observer exactly coincide, except for an attenuation factor. That is, if one considers only the results of the second experiment the data and the predictions of this model are completely consistent except for an attenuation factor. It is this peculiar counterbalancing of error that makes it difficult to devise a model which will yield predictions consistent with the human's behavior. Once signal power or duration is independently varied, serious disagreement between data and theory becomes apparent. In either situation the signal-known-exactly model makes predictions which differ from the empirical equations by a factor of the square root of signal energy.

The failure of the signal-known-exactly model is not surprising. It seems highly unlikely that the human observer can adjust, or in any case maintain, the parameters of the hearing mechanism to the degree required by the model. Nevertheless, the failure of this model to handle the effects of variation in duration and intensity is instructive.

Since the signal-known-exactly model appears to be inadequate, one might think another model, assuming some uncertainty in the signal or noise parameters, might provide a more favorable comparison between prediction and data. If a new model were considered, some new relation would be obtained between the physical parameters of the signal and noise and the detection index as defined in this paper. For the purposes of discussion let us view this new model as changing the definition of d' and maintaining the same relation between the physical variables and the new d' as the signal-known-exactly model. In short, all the change may be considered as having been reflected to the relation between d' and the percentage of correct detections.

To obtain agreement between the new model's predictions and the observer's performance is not difficult. A new model which yields a detection index of about the square root of the present index for the same per cent correct detection will provide consistent relationships in an experiment such as the first or third of this chapter.

Models of this type are not difficult to find. Any one of a number of uncertainties concerning the signal parameters will yield approximately this relation, at least for small signal-to-noise ratios like those used in this study. Such a redefinition, however, accomplishes nothing, for the results of the second experiment are inconsistent. If the change previously suggested is adopted, then the second experiment will be different by a factor of the fourth root of signal duration for all but the middle range of duration.

In general, if one remembers that Experiments I and III are inconsistent, while Experiment II is consistent, with the signal-known-exactly analysis, then in order to make all of the experiments consistent clearly requires more than a redefinition of the detection index.

The crux of the difficulty in the model lies with the filter analogy. Any number of simple linear filters show 3 db per octave relations. The shape of the band pass affects parameters in the equation, but the 3 db per octave variation is the same. Thus any simple linear filter model seems at best to provide a qualitative analysis of the problem and predict the direction of change. The filter model, in this simple form, is not an adequate model to account, in a quantitative manner, for the effects of signal duration upon detection.

The final point to be made is of a more encouraging nature. For the range of durations investigated, one finds that detection varies as some function of the signal power times some function of the signal duration. Thus, if either physical variable is held constant, the relation between the logarithm of detection and the logarithm of the physical variable is the same for some intercept factor. Another way to express this result is to say that signal duration and intensity do not interact if the logarithms of these quantities are taken. Such a relation indicates that the study of time-intensity data from the standpoint of some constant detectability is acceptable as long as one can be sure that this constant is maintained for all conditions of the experiment.

The question of how duration affects the hearing mechanism is an important and challenging one. Few theories deal with this question either implicitly or explicitly. The present paper and previous papers provide a fairly consistent body of measurement concerning how duration affects the hearing mechanism. A rational theory is still badly needed which will explain why these or similar relationships exist.[1]

SUMMARY

The object of this study was to determine how signal amplitude and duration affect the detectability of a pure tone partially masked by random noise. With signal duration and amplitude considered as two dimensions in a space, the study attempted to determine the surface of detectability in this space. To accomplish this task three experiments were conducted with the same observers in each experiment. In the first experiment signal duration was held constant while amplitude was varied. In the second experiment signal energy was held constant while various pairs of values of signal duration and amplitude were tested. In the third, signal amplitude was held constant and signal duration varied. A three-parameter equation was determined which provided a reasonable fit to this surface of detectability in the plane of signal amplitude and duration. The equations are consistent with the data of previous research in this area. Finally, a comparison of the results and the predictions generated by a simple filter model is discussed.

ACKNOWLEDGMENTS

This research was conducted in the laboratories of the Electronic Defense Group of the University of Michigan with support from the U. S. Army Signal Corps. D. M. Green held a fellowship from the National Science Foundation. This article appeared as Tech. Rept. No. 42 of the Electronic Defense Group and in J. acoust. Soc. Am., *1957,* **29,** *523–531.*

References

- Fletcher, H. Auditory patterns, *Revs. modern Phys.,* 1940, **12,** 47–65.
- Garner, W. R. The effect of frequency spectrum on temporal integration of energy in the ear. *J. acoust. Soc. Am.,* 1947, **19,** 808–815.
- Garner, W. R., and Miller, G. A. The masked threshold of pure tones as a function of duration. *J. exp. Psychol.,* 1947, **37,** 293–303.

---

[1] The data of this study are on record in tabular form at the American Documentation Institute, 1719 N Street N.W., Washington 6, D. C.

- Hughes, J. W. The threshold of audition for short periods of stimulation. *Proc. Roy. Soc. (London),* 1946, **133** B, 486–490.
- Lawson, J. L., and Uhlenbeck, G. E. *Threshold signals.* New York: McGraw-Hill, 1950.
- Licklider, J. C. R. Basic correlates of the auditory stimulus. In S. S. Stevens (Ed.), *Handbook of experimental psychology.* New York: Wiley, 1951, p. 1021.
- Peterson, W. W., and Birdsall, T. G. Theory of signal detectability, Parts I and II. University of Michigan: Electronic Defense Group, 1953, Technical Report No. 13. Also summarized in 1954 Symposium on Information Theory, *Trans. IRE,* 1954, **PGIT-4,** 171–212.
- Peterson, W. W., and Birdsall, T. G. Signal detection with a panoramic receiver. University of Michigan: Electronic Defense Group, 1955, Technical Report No. 38.
- Tanner, W. P., Jr., and Swets, J. A. A decision-making theory of visual detection. *Psychol Rev.,* 1954, **61,** 401–409.
- Tanner, W. P., Jr., Swets, J. A., and Green, D. M. Some general properties of the hearing mechanism. University of Michigan: Electronic Defense Group, 1956, Technical Report No. 30.

12

Human Discrimination of Auditory Duration

C. Douglas Creelman

These experiments measured the ability of human observers to discriminate differences in duration between short auditory signals. An understanding of time judgment is important for theories of signal detection, since detection depends on attention during the time of the signal, and only during that time. A practical problem related to temporal discrimination arises in speech perception, where cues to linguistic meaning in some languages, and cues to stress and inflection in English, seem to depend on relative duration (cf. Peterson and Lehiste, 1960). A quantitative theory of temporal discrimination is developed to account for discrimination in the range ordinarily covered by speech sounds and the signals used in psychoacoustic experiments.

The study of time discrimination is a poor stepchild of the growth of psychophysical research. Titchener (1905) characterized the area as a "microcosm, perfect to the last detail," exemplifying in miniature the course of development to that time of psychophysical methods, concepts, and empirical knowledge. Study of temporal discrimination, and the estimation of time, has remained a microcosm, somewhat isolated from the main stream of empirical research on sensory capacities.

A reason for this neglect was pointed out by Nichols (1891) in an early scholarly and historical review of the philosophy and psychology of time. This was the problematic status of the "time sense" as an independent psychic faculty, aside from the content of sensory input. The question has not yet been resolved, and continues to haunt the researches and theoretical efforts of psychologists.

Reviews of the experimental literature after Nichols were presented by Dunlap (1911, 1912, 1914, 1916), Axel (1925), Weber (1933), Gilliland et al. (1946), and most recently by Wallace and Rabin (1960). Chapters on time perception were offered by Tichener (1905), by Boring (1942), and by Woodrow (1951). With all this activity, we still find that there is ". . . as yet no generally accepted view as to how we perceive or estimate time" (Gilliland et al., 1946), and fourteen years later we find ourselves still on the trail of the "hitherto elusive 'time sense' " (Wallace and Rabin, 1960).

Although an experiment by Stott (1935) was primarily concerned with the analysis of "time errors," enough data were reported to draw some conclusions about the temporal sensitivity of his observers. The observations were made in a group setting, and the data were averaged over subjects, a questionable practice in the light of the large individual differences found in such experiments (e.g., Nakajima, 1958). An experiment by Henry (1948) was a latter-day attempt to check the validity of Weber's law in the discrimination of auditory duration. The data were reported in terms of the Weber ratio $\Delta T/T$ where ΔT was the increment necessary to give an average performance of 75 per cent positive identifications when added to a "base" duration T.

Small and Campbell (unpublished) have recently redone and expanded these experiments, using more precise control of signal duration. Their signals were gated electronically, as opposed to the mechanical shutters used by Stott and the electrical switches used by Henry. The Small and Campbell study is the latest one of many to find no systematic effect of order of presentation on the accuracy of the judgment of duration differences. Their experimental design was like the earlier studies, in that for each fixed duration a range of increments was presented, and a psychometric function constructed. The data from Stott, Henry, and Small and Campbell will be compared to those from the present experiments in the discussion section to follow.

The question remains whether a duration can be judged independently of the sensory events which occur during that duration. On the side of a negative answer to the question is the considerable weight of the opinion of William James (1890) and, in more modern times, of Fraisse (1957), the author of a text on the psychology of time written mostly from a phenomenalistic point of view. Time seems to pass faster when we are occupied, and by the same token temporal intervals would be expected to seem to pass faster if they were filled by continuing stimuli than if they were simply marked off by clicks. However, there seems to be no reason to expect the two situations to be the same. Fortunately some data are available on the question.

Clausen (1950) compared the estimation of filled and unfilled intervals of 5, 10, and 15 sec. The results showed no difference in performance between the two procedures. Another deduction from the assumption of dependence of temporal judgment is that accuracy should depend on the intensity of the signals. Henry found no effect of auditory intensity on the accuracy of judgment. Oléron (1952) and Lifshitz (1935–1936), on the other hand, reported studies which did show dependence of time judgment on the intensity of the signal.

The studies of Chistovich (1959) used short clicks to delimit the stimuli. A duration was marked off, and then another duration followed, both bounded by clicks. The task of the observers was to state whether the second was equal to the first or differed from it by ΔT. It was not stated explicitly, but we may safely assume that 50 per cent of the trials actually had the longer duration as the second of the pair. This method is subject to the pitfalls of the "yes-no" procedure, and the observers in this experiment were further handicapped by a 10-sec wait between presentations of the two durations to be compared. Data from Chistovich are presented later, along with the data for filled auditory intervals. These data appeared to be much like those from experiments on filled intervals, and the conclusion drawn was that discrimination between open and filled intervals is the same task.

The logical question of the independent status of a sense of duration was considered by Boring (1936). In an argument based on the (then very new) approach of operationism, he attempted to show that the philosophical question disappears as soon as the data are considered in their own right. People were able to give introspective reports involving elapsed durations, and experiments showed subjects able to differentiate sensory events on the basis of duration alone. Boring argued that these data were sufficient for the scientist, if he was an operationist; the existence of the data eliminated any problem. It has become clear since 1936 that the answer is not as simple as it once seemed. More is necessary for understanding processes than the raw data, either in the form of introspective reports or behavioral observations.

Some years ago Hirsh (1952) called for an empirical measure of ability to discriminate temporal events analogous to measures of visual acuity. He pointed out that the lack of such a measure may be in large part the cause of the poor correspondence between experimental measures of auditory abilities and auditory discrimination in everyday experience. The present experiments and the theoretical model which describes the results are a first attempt toward identification of this measure.

APPARATUS AND PROCEDURE

Apparatus

All of the experiments followed the same general procedure, and used the N. P. Psytar apparatus at the Psychophysical Laboratory of the Cooley Electronics Laboratory, the University of Michigan. The general nature of the equipment has been described by Bilger (1959). Figure 1 shows a block diagram.

An oscillator could be connected to one of two gates, which were set to deliver different signal durations. The gates passed a segment of a sine wave which began at a positive-going zero crossing and continued for an integral number of cycles. The oscillator output was always set at a fixed voltage, and any desired signal voltage could be obtained by means of the divider network, constructed of high-precision fixed resistors. The gated signal was mixed with continuous wide-band white noise. The observers' PDR-8 earphones were wired for monaural presentation.

Procedure

The events of a single experimental trial are summarized in Fig. 2. The top line represents the times of occurrence of the observers' signal lights and the bottom line represents the auditory signals. One signal was presented for the duration T, and the other for duration $T + \Delta T$. The order

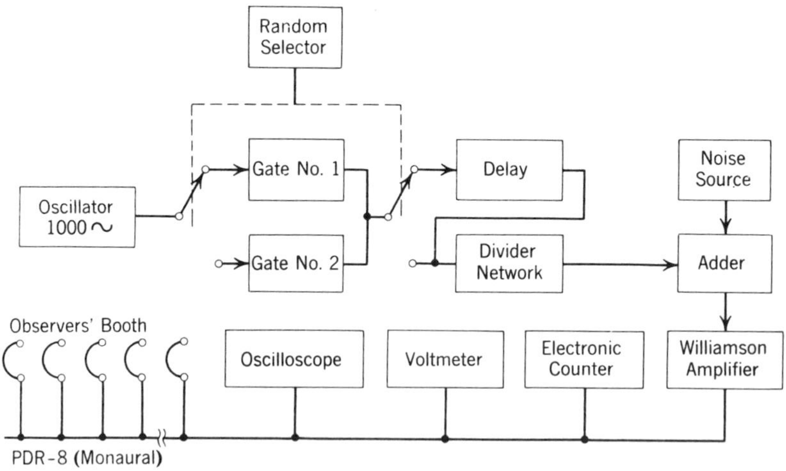

FIG. 1. Block diagram of apparatus.

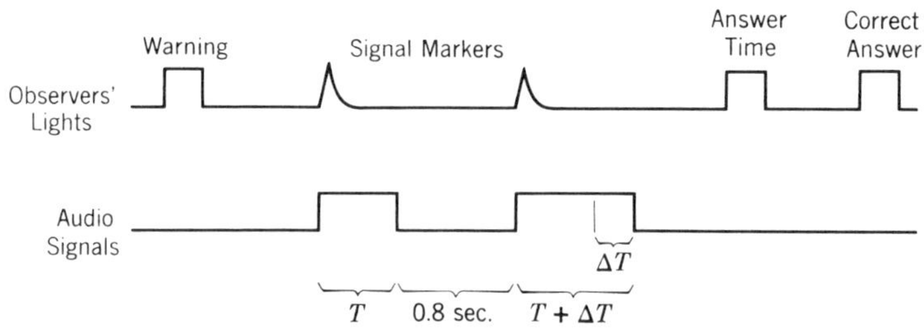

FIG. 2. Sequence of events in an experimental trial.

of presentation was decided by the automatic random selector for each trial, with the long or the short signal equally probable as the first of the pair. The time between the end of the first signal and the start of the second was fixed at 0.8 sec.

The observers were all students, paid at an hourly rate. They worked 2 hours per day, 5 days a week, for the duration of an academic semester or summer session. A bonus of 0.1 cent was paid for each correct answer, with the same amount subtracted for each incorrect answer. The observers were given at least 2 weeks' practice before any data were collected. Before each new experiment was begun, at least a day was spent familiarizing the observers with the new task. In addition, each experimental run was preceded by a series of trials with the masking noise turned off, to make sure that the observers knew the nature of the particular signals being used.

The design of each experiment was roughly the same. Each value of the independent variable was presented for two or three successive experimental runs of 100 trials. Then a new value was selected and used, until all had been presented. The order of selection was random. This procedure was repeated until roughly 1000 observations had been obtained for each value, with a new random order used for each repetition.

Independent variables

The experiments measured the effects on discrimination of three variables: "base" duration T; difference duration ΔT; and signal voltage V_S. In general, while the effects of one variable were being estimated, the others were held fixed at arbitrary constant values. Throughout all the experiments the background noise was held constant at a wide-band reading of 0.01 v rms to the observers' earphones. This corresponds to a noise power density of 3.6×10^{-7} v²/cps. The data reported are from two different sets of observers run at different times, and each group was run using different sets of experimental variables. The results are presented in terms of the detectability measure d' and, to make it easier to follow the presentation, a brief summary of the concepts underlying this measure is presented.

Dependent variable d'

In recent years evidence has accumulated in support of the usefulness of a decision-theoretical model as an interpretive tool for psychophysical data (cf. Creelman, 1960; Green, 1960; Swets, 1961). This approach views the observer as, in essence, a tester of statistical hypotheses.

The use of d' reflects a belief in the statistical nature of the time-discrimination task. If this belief is correct, it should be possible on the basis of the data to arrive at some understanding of the statistical distributions underlying the task. After the data are presented, a model for the decision procedures used in duration discrimination is developed. The end product of this development is a general expression for performance in a duration discrimination experiment.

The calculation of d' depends on the way in which the data are collected, i.e., on the psychophysical method employed. The two-alternative temporal forced-choice procedure was used throughout the present experiments, and only this procedure is described. The number of correct responses when the longer signal was actually presented first, and the number of correct responses when the longer signal was actually presented second, were used to obtain estimates of the probability of being correct under each experimental condition. These probabilities were then used to enter a table of the normal probability integral. The distance in units of standard deviation from the mean of the distribution to a distance sufficient to yield the obtained probability was read from the table. The two deviation values, one representing each presentation interval, were added to give the reported value of d'. If the two obtained scores, corresponding to the two temporal intervals, were equal, d' as defined here would be related to per cent correct as shown in Fig. 3. This may be viewed as an operational definition of the dependent variable.

In order to remain consistent with the previously published study by Tanner (1956), the abscissa of Fig. 3 is labeled $d'_{1,2}$. The present case is identical with Tanner's case of recognizing one of two orthogonal signals. Here the signals were orthogonal in time; it is assumed that the occurrence of one input signal has negligible influence on the observation of another signal presented 0.8 sec after it.

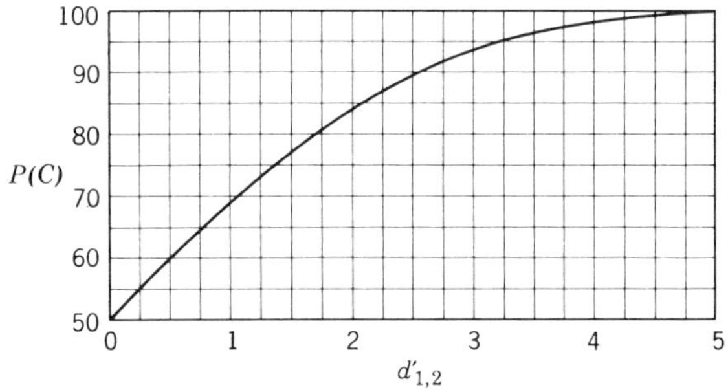

FIG. 3. Per cent correct as a function of $d'_{1,2}$.

When the distributions underlying the detection situation are not of equal variance, the present approach is an alternative to one proposed by Clarke, Birdsall, and Tanner (1959) for the analysis of data collected by the "yes-no" procedure. If the two methods were applied to the same set of data, the prediction is that $d'_{1,2}$ will be larger than $(d_e)^{1/2}$ by a factor of $\sqrt{2}$. This conclusion is supported by data reported by Swets (1959).

The procedure used here to estimate d' allows, since the responses to each of the time intervals are analyzed separately, for the possibility of a degree of response bias, or "time error," on the part of the observers. If such bias is present, transformations which use an average over the two intervals to estimate the probability of correct response underestimate the size of the actual d'.

EXPERIMENTAL RESULTS

As was mentioned, all the experiments were conducted in a continuous background of white masking noise. The problem might be treated by the observers as a signal-detection task, where the signal consists of the energy present during the interval ΔT. If this were the case, we might expect performance to vary with signal voltage in much the same way as signal-detection performance.

Experiment 1: Effects of signal voltage on duration discrimination

In this experiment, T and ΔT were fixed at 0.1 and 0.03 sec, respectively. The two signals to be discriminated were thus 0.10 and 0.13 sec in duration. Both were presented at the same voltage, mixed with the continuous background noise. Signal-voltage values were chosen to cover a wide range of detectability so that a psychometric function could be obtained. The results are shown in Fig. 4 for three observers. In this figure the obtained $d'_{1,2}$ is plotted as a function of signal voltage, on logarithmic axes. Detection of a duration difference increases rapidly with signal voltage, but only at low signal-to-noise ratios; the dependence becomes negligible as the signals are made "loud and clear" above the noise.

These results may be contrasted to the available data on signal detection in noise as a function of signal energy. There is no evidence for any similar leveling off of performance, whether observers attempt to detect signals alone or increments added to signals already present. Recently Green (1960) discussed such detection curves and presented some representative data, which are in no way similar to the curves of Fig. 4. It seems reasonable to conclude that duration discrimination is not treated by human observers simply as a signal detection task, but that some other explanation is necessary.

Experiment 2: Discrimination as a function of "base" duration

For this experiment a signal voltage of 0.084 v was used which, on the basis of the data of Experiment 1, is well above the range where performance is influenced by voltage. The duration of the increment ΔT was held constant at 0.01 sec. Five durations of T, ranging from 0.02 to 0.32 sec, were used. The results for four observers are presented in Fig. 5, where detectability of the duration increment is plotted as a function of base time T. The axes are logarithmic and the solid lines are derived from the model presented later. Detection falls off as the base time is increased. A straight line would show this decrease to be not so great as $1/T$, and

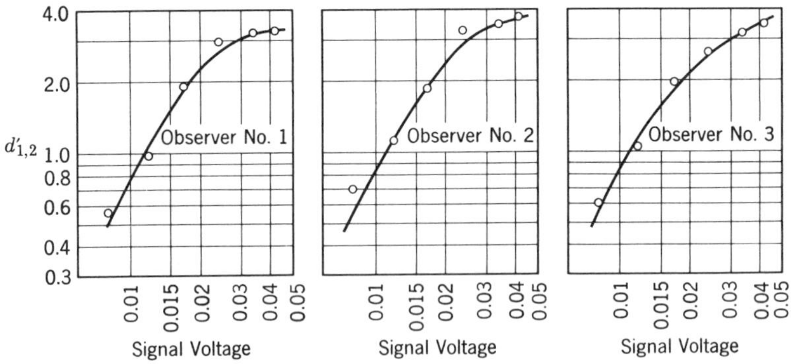

FIG. 4. Duration discrimination as a function of signal voltage. Experiment 1.

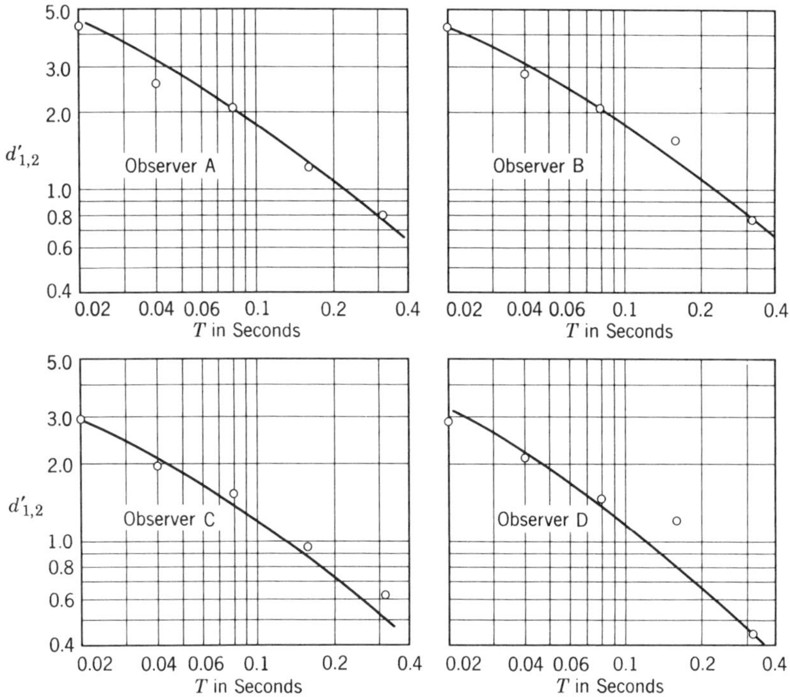

FIG. 5. Duration discrimination as a function of base duration. Experiment 2.

somewhat greater than $1/T^{1/2}$. That is, the slope of these lines lies somewhere between -1 and $-1/2$ on the log-log plot.

Experiment 3: Discrimination as a function of increment duration

In this experiment T was fixed at 0.16 sec, and ΔT was varied. Two signal-voltage values were used, 0.042 and 0.010 v, and the experiment was repeated at each voltage. The results are presented in Fig. 6, with $\log d'_{1,2}$ plotted as a function of $\log \Delta T$. The signal voltage is the parameter. The solid lines, derived from the theoretical model, show detection to be a linear function of the increment duration. Although lower signal voltage tends to depress performance, the shape of the two curves is the same; there is no interaction between the effects of increment duration and signal voltage.

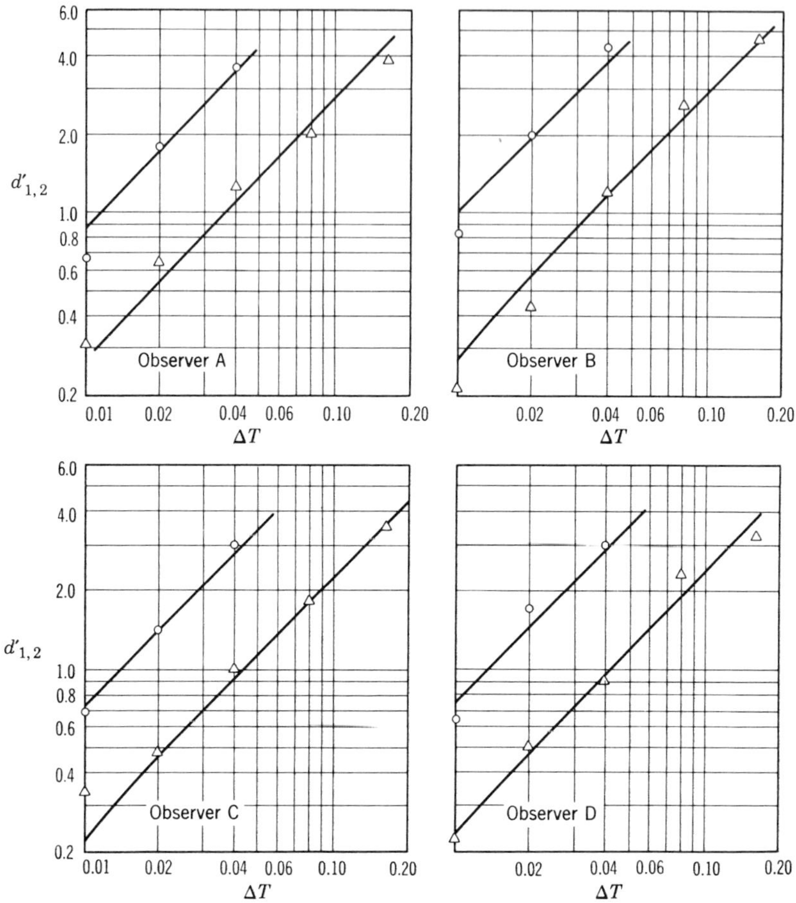

FIG. 6. Duration discrimination as a function of increment duration. Signal voltage is the parameter. $T = 0.16$ sec; circle represents $V_s = 0.042$ v; triangle represents $V_s = 0.010$ v. Experiment 3.

Experiment 4: Discrimination as function of base duration and signal voltage

In a fourth experiment the effect of base time on detection was measured in a situation much like that of Experiment 2. In this case ΔT was 0.04 sec, and the experiment was repeated at two values of signal voltage, 0.042 and 0.010 v, the same as were used in Experiment 3. The results are shown in Fig. 7, where detectability is plotted as a function of T on log axes, and signal voltage is the parameter. The solid lines are predic-

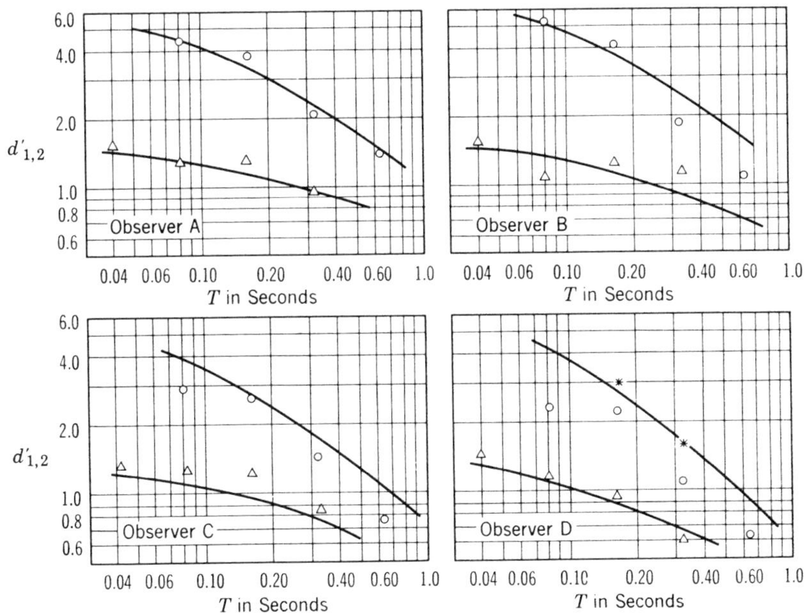

FIG. 7. Duration discrimination as a function of base duration. Signal voltage is the parameter. $\Delta T = 0.04$ sec; circles represent $V_s = 0.042$ v; triangles represent $V_s = 0.010$ v. Experiment 4.

tions from the model on the basis of constants estimated from the results of the previous two experiments.

The data from Observer D for the higher voltage were collected after he had had insufficient practice. He began observing only a few days before this experiment was begun, while the other three observers had been working at this sort of task for over two weeks. The points marked by stars represent data collected in a later experiment in which the same signal values were used. It is probable that the lower performance of Observer D represents a lack of familiarity with the experimental situation. This was also shown by the excessive number of trials on which he did not respond. In general, performance of observers is remarkably constant over time. Comparisons of data taken at different times during the course of the semester showed no large deviations, except for this one instance.

In this experiment, as opposed to Experiment 3, there is an interaction between signal voltage and the base duration in their effects on discrimination. Not only does an increase in the voltage of the signals raise the curve of detection as a function of T, but it also seems to make it steeper; or more likely, a decrease in the signal voltage makes the curve less steep.

The experiment was repeated using the observers of Experiment 1, with ΔT of 0.03 sec. With these observers, values of T of 0.8 sec were run, considerably longer than the longest T in the data just given. The results are shown in Fig. 8. In general, the form of the data is much the same as that for the other observers, with the interaction of T and signal voltage apparent. Here the points represent only 600 observations, and the data show greater variability.

Experiment 5: Discrimination with both $\Delta T/T$ and difference energy constant

In this experiment both T and ΔT were varied together so that the ratio of the two was constant at ⅛. (When ΔT was 0.01 sec, T was 0.08

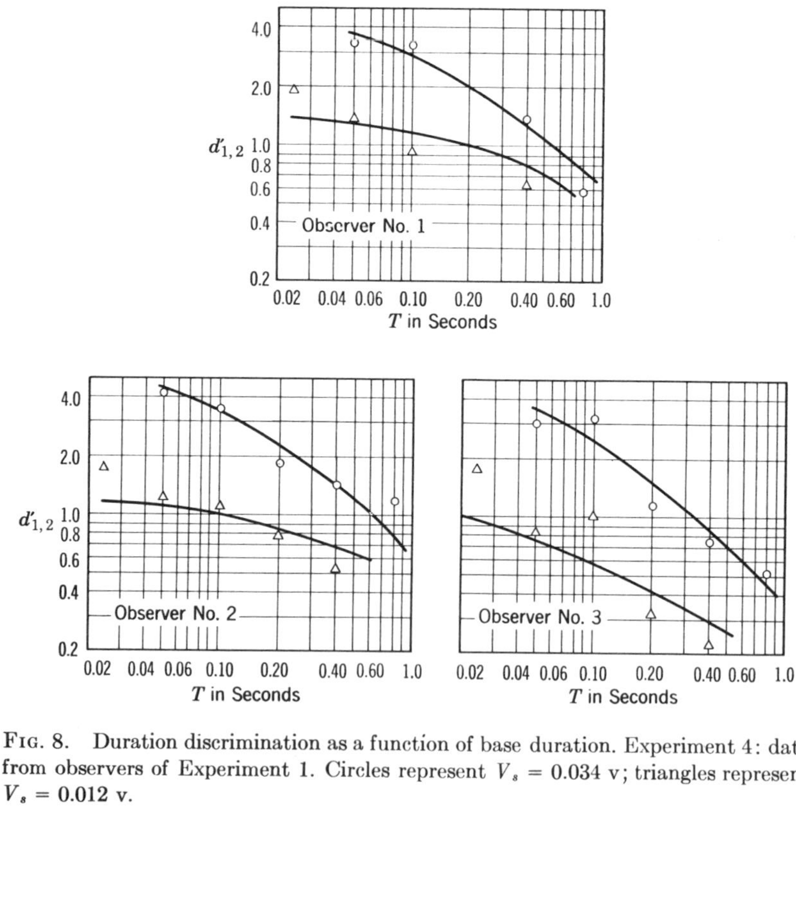

FIG. 8. Duration discrimination as a function of base duration. Experiment 4: data from observers of Experiment 1. Circles represent $V_s = 0.034$ v; triangles represent $V_s = 0.012$ v.

sec, etc.) At the same time, the energy in the increment ΔT was held constant, so that the product $V_S^2 \times \Delta T$ was constant. Thus when ΔT was doubled, V_S was decreased by a factor of $\sqrt{2}$. In this experiment at least 600 observations were collected at each point. Figure 9 shows the results. Log $d'_{1,2}$ is plotted as a function of T. In addition, below each value of T is shown the associated value of ΔT, and below this the two values of signal voltage used. The two sets of signal voltages led to two different values of constant difference energy, and these are the parameters on the graphs, defining two sets of points.

We would expect, on the basis of Experiments 2 and 3, that d' would increase roughly as a function of ΔT, but decrease somewhat as $T^{1/2}$, yielding an overall prediction of increasing performance with a slope of $+\frac{1}{2}$ on a log-log plot. On the other hand, the signal voltage was decreased from left to right, as ΔT was increased, and this would be expected to have an increasing detrimental effect on performance. These notions are given precise form in the theoretical discussion, but for now it is sufficient to note that the overall effect of these influences might be roughly a straight line, i.e., constant detectability for all the experimental conditions. The exact prediction is a pair of shallow curves,

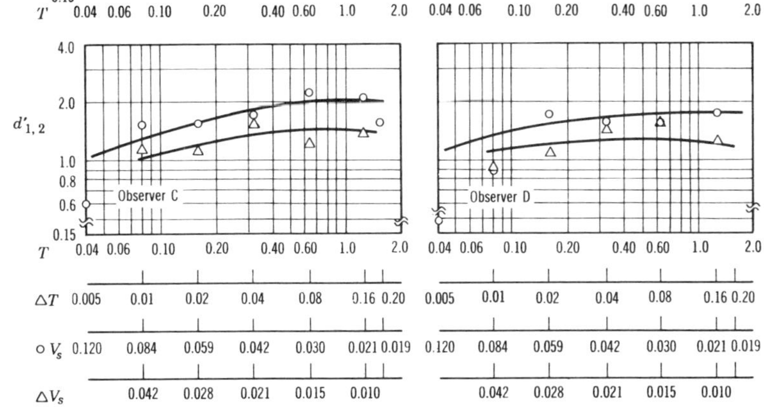

FIG. 9. Duration discrimination as a joint function of three variables. Circles represent $2E/N_0 = 400$; triangles represent $2\ E/N_0 = 100$. Experiment 5.

concave downward, as shown on the plot. Probably because of the smaller number of observations, these data also show more variability. However the trend of the data is clear and is in the predicted direction. Thus, in a sense, Weber's law has been found to hold approximately for duration discrimination, but only in the case of some very special experimental circumstances. An important point is that a fourfold increase in the relevant signal energy resulted in only a slight increase in performance. This is consistent with the finding of Experiment 1, and shows the result to hold over a wide range of experimental conditions.

Experiment 6: Experimental check on procedure

The critical reader probably has noticed an unavoidable flaw in the design of the experiments. Visual information was available, which may have been utilized, regardless of the auditory signals. Two factors were necessary in the presentation of the stimuli; one was that there be a flash of light marking the start of each auditory signal, and the other was that there be a fixed time between the end of the first signal presented in a trial and the beginning of the second. If these two restrictions are met, then there must be a difference in the time between the two light flashes, depending on whether the longer or the shorter of the two signals was presented in the first interval. In the experiments the observers might have been making an absolute judgment as to whether the time between the two flashes of the signal-marking lights was 0.8 sec or $0.8 + \Delta T$ sec in length. The only data presented thus far which could negate such an interpretation were those which showed duration discrimination to be a function of the signal voltage.

In order to test whether visual cues were in fact being used, a bit of deception was resorted to, the only break of faith with the observers in the course of the experiments. This was done during the final few days before the end of the observers' employment, so that danger of contamination of subsequent data would be avoided. In fact they seemed not to suspect that anything untoward was being done. The observers were those of Experiment 1.

The procedure was fairly simple: On trials selected at random, the oscillator was disconnected, so that no signal was present in the continuous noise, while the trial cycle proceeded as usual. The only information present for the observers to use, if they were to perform at better than chance level, was the time between the flashes of the signal lights. When the signals were presented, T was 0.16 sec and ΔT was also 0.16 sec, one of the longest values used in any of the experiments. A signal voltage of

0.004 v was used, and it was almost completely masked by the noise. On one-half the trials, randomly chosen, no signal was presented, and on the other half, two signals were presented in the usual fashion. Since scores under these conditions were very close to 50 per cent, or chance level, runs during which this procedure was used were interspersed with runs in which signals of 0.006 or 0.004 v were presented on every trial. A voltage of 0.004 was sufficient to do better than chance in the experimental conditions, but the observers apparently could not be sure that the signal was not present when in fact it had been turned off. They assumed, when the signal was intermittently turned off, that an even lower signal level was being presented on all trials. In Table I the results for four observers are presented. Only 400 observations defined each d' obtained under the no-signal condition. The standard-deviation figure presented in the table is the theoretical binomial variation around an obtained proportion. Only Observer 1 shows what might be a significant deviation from 50 per cent correct on trials in which no signal was presented. All except Observer 4 showed better than chance performance when the signal voltage was always 0.004, and an improvement when the signal voltage was 0.006.

There is some evidence that one observer may have extracted information from the lights, at least when ΔT was relatively large. In any case the help that the lights gave was negligible, and can be discounted for much smaller values of ΔT. Note that the question the experiment asked

TABLE I. RESULTS OF EXPERIMENT 6

Signal voltage	Number of observations	Observer	Average per cent correct	Expected S.D.
0.06	1000	1	66.91	1.49
		2	71.37	1.43
		3	54.62	1.48
		4	65.83	1.50
0.04	500	1	57.99	2.20
		2	60.31	2.18
		3	53.65	2.23
		4	49.67	2.23
0	400	1	57.66	2.47
		2	49.71	2.50
		3	48.47	2.52
		4	53.51	2.44

was not whether observers can make absolute judgments of empty intervals bounded by flashes of light, but rather whether they tended to do so in the experiments as they were run, when as far as they knew the only available cues were auditory. The author is fairly certain that, given practice in making such discriminatoins and instructions as to what were the relevant cues, the observers' performance would have been considerably higher. With perhaps one exception, the observers in these experiments did not score above chance when no auditory signal was present.

THEORY OF TIME DISCRIMINATION

Derivation

It has been suggested that an observer in a psychophysical experiment can be viewed as a tester of statistical hypotheses. The task now is to fill in the outline for the case of duration discrimination. This involves specification of the basis for judgment, and of the nature of two conditional probability distributions. Without such specifications the model is equivalent to one proposed many years ago by Thurstone (1927). The view of the human observer as rationally testing statistical hypotheses—operating on distributions with precisely specified mathematical properties—characterizes the theory of signal detectability, within the framework of which the present model was derived (cf. Tanner, 1960, for a general discussion of these points).

The model pictures human observers as using a separate and independent mechanism to measure short durations. This mechanism functions by "counting" input pulses during the duration to be judged. It is sufficient for the moment to view the source of pulses as a large number of independent elements whose time of firing is randomly distributed. The performance of such a mechanism in a two-alternative duration discrimination task is derived first, and then two restrictions on the performance of human observers in an actual experiment are discussed.

The basis for decision is the number of pulses which the counting mechanism receives. How many such pulses will arrive at the counter during a duration T? The answer comes from the nature of the assumed source. A large number of elements, each with a fixed probability of firing at any given moment, will produce a total number of pulses over a given time interval whose statistical properties are fairly well understood (Feller, 1957). The probability of n counts occurring in an interval T can be written $P(n) = [(\lambda T)^n/n!][\exp(-\lambda T)]$. The constant λ reflects the probability that a given element in the pulse source will be active at a given time. This is the Poisson distribution, which is closely approximated by the normal distribution when the quantity λT is large. The mean number of counts produced will be λT, and the variance of the number of counts will also equal λT.

In the present experiments two durations were presented, T and $T + \Delta T$. Figure 10 is a representation of the problem. When the duration T is presented, the number of counts will be distributed as the left-hand distribution of Fig. 10, and when the longer duration is presented the number of counts will be distributed as the right-hand distribution. The means and standard deviations of the distributions are shown in the figure. Note that the size of the standard deviation depends on the mean of the distribution. In the two-alternative forced-choice experiment, according to this model, the two observations will produce two numbers, one drawn from each of the distributions of Fig. 10.

In order to approach the best possible score, the decision rule the observer should follow is to indicate as longer the observation which produced the larger number. This strategy will yield the correct response as long as the drawing from the distribution associated with the presentation of $T + \Delta T$ is larger than the drawing from the distribution associated with T, or equivalently, when the difference is greater than zero. The probability density distribution for differences between two such drawings is represented in Fig. 11. Probability of correct response is represented by the area under this curve, to the right of zero. Our measure $d'_{1,2}$ is a constant $\sqrt{2}$ times the distance from zero to the mean of the difference distribution, divided by the standard deviation:

$$\text{(expected) } d'_{1,2} = (2\lambda)^{1/2} \frac{\Delta T}{(2T + \Delta T)^{1/2}} \tag{1}$$

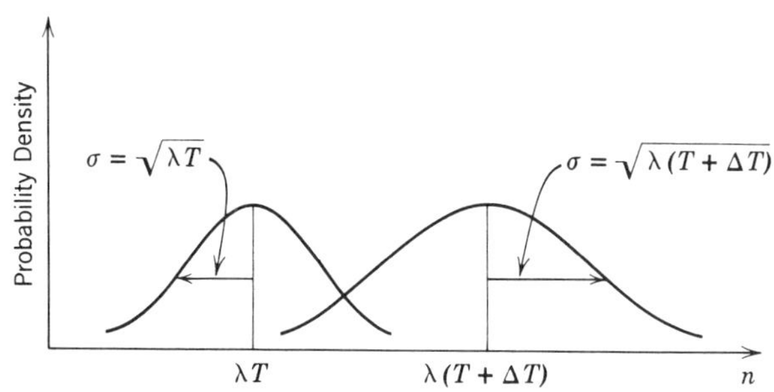

FIG. 10. Probability density distributions of the number of counts from a random source, depending on whether the source is active for T or for $T + \Delta T$.

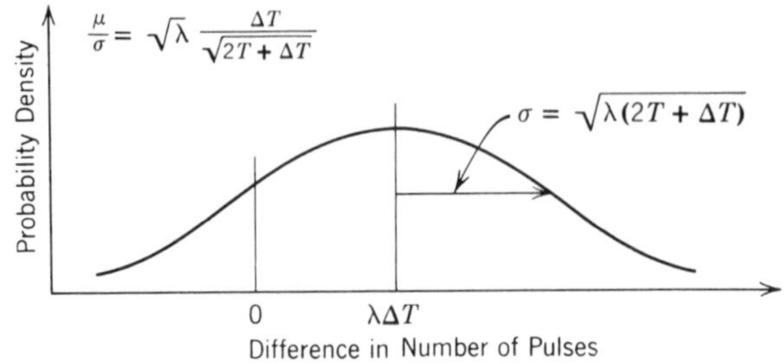

FIG. 11. Probability density distribution for differences in the number of counts, from the distributions of Fig. 10.

Under the counting model this is the basic formula for the detectability of a difference in duration. For performance to meet this expectation, the observer would have to know exactly the starting and ending times of the signal. He would also need perfect memory for the number of counts produced by the first signal until it could be compared with the number produced by the second of the pair. It is reasonable to expect neither of these requirements to be perfectly met by human observers.

That memory over the intersignal interval is not perfect was shown by Creelman and Tanner (unpublished) for frequency discrimination and by Tanner (1959) and Bilger (1960) for amplitude discrimination. Bilger varied both the time between signals and their duration and found that both factors tended to decrease performance. He found that efficiency [proportional to $(d')^2$] varied inversely as $[1 + K(T + \tau)]$, where T was the signal duration, τ was the intersignal interval, and K was a constant characterizing the individual observers. In the present experiments the time between the two stimulus presentations was constant, but the duration was varied. Longer base times would be expected to cause a decrease in performance, and for consistency with the prior findings the basic duration detection formula was modified to yield, when squared to eliminate radicals,

$$\text{(expected) } (d'_{1,2})^2 = \frac{1}{1 + KT}\,\frac{2\lambda\Delta T^2}{2T + \Delta T} \tag{2}$$

where K is again a constant characteristic of the individual observer. The Bilger formula, taking into account the interval between signals, was found not to fit the data adequately. One possible interpretation of this discrepancy is that the problem of memory is insignificant compared to the interference produced in the stored representation of the first signal while the second signal is being presented. The lack of effect due to intersignal interval could also have been due to the use of less than optimal procedures for obtaining such effects. This finding is consistent with the recent study of Small and Campbell.

The duration-counting mechanism must start precisely when the relevant signal begins, and stop precisely at its end. If the signals which mark the beginning and the end of the time intervals are masked by background noise, or are otherwise ambiguous, we expect a larger variance in the number of counts during the observation. This added variance σ_v^2 will be an inverse function of the signal power, or signal-to-noise ratio. The nature of this relation is considered in the following section. The final expression for detectability is then

$$(d'_{1,2})^2 = \frac{1}{1 + KT} \frac{2\lambda\Delta T^2}{2T + \Delta T + \sigma_v^2} \tag{3}$$

The constants λ and K reflect the rate of firing of the pulse source, and the ability to hold in mind the number associated with one signal while listening to another. These were estimated for individual observers, and the nature of the variance due to signal level was ascertained.

Empirical fit to the data

The data of Experiment 1 were fitted by a two-step process. First an asymptote for obtained performance was estimated. For two of the three observers this was not difficult, for they were clearly near it at the largest voltage levels. It was assumed that at the asymptote the variance due to starting time and duration uncertainty was reduced to zero. Then the data were used with Eq. (3) to compute values of σ_v^2 necessary to yield the obtained performance at each signal voltage used. These values were plotted on logarithmic axes, and found to be fitted well by a straight line with the equation $\sigma_v^2 = Av_s^{-b}$, with the exponent somewhat larger than 2 and varying between observers. The curves in Fig. 7 were derived from the straight line relating calculated σ_v^2 to signal voltage.

Experiments 2, 3, and 4 were a related set using the same observers. In Experiment 2 the voltage was large enough to assume that the starting time and duration of the signals were precisely marked. The variance was thus assumed to be negligible, and values of K and λ were chosen by trial and error to fit the data for each observer. In general there was little difficulty in obtaining sets of constants which gave close fits.

The next experiment used two lower values of signal voltage and allowed an estimate of the added variance due to starting time and duration uncertainty at each voltage. The lines shown in Fig. 9 are best fits by eye with the restriction that the slope of the function be nearly unity, as predicted by the theoretical equation.

The estimated values of σ_v^2, together with the estimated constants, were carried over to Experiment 4. These gave the predicted functions shown in Fig. 10. The two signal-voltage levels were retained and a range of values of T was explored with a constant ΔT different from that used in Experiment 2. In general the predicted function is close to the data, and the model is given support from them.

Figure 11 represents a similar set of data from the observers of Experiment 1. Here the constants were estimated from the data themselves with the restriction that the asymptote of Fig. 7 and the obtained values for σ_v^2 remain the same. With the exception of Observer 3, whose data show a tendency toward a steeper slope when the signal voltage is low, the agreement is again good.

Table II lists the constants used to predict the data for Figs. 11 and 12. Note that the number λ is sufficiently large to support the normal approximation assumption used to find d' from per cent correct and, with the exception of Observer 3 again, the number K is relatively small.

The procedure used to predict the results of Experiment 5 was not so precise as those for the other experiments, in that it involved a considerable extrapolation. The two values of σ_v^2 from Table II were plotted on log paper, and a straight line was drawn through them of approximately the right slope on the basis of the data from the first experiment. Values of σ_v^2 were read from this line and used to compute predicted performance at each signal voltage. Although not enough data could be obtained to define the curves precisely, they do show fair agreement with the model. A further reason for the variability is probably that in this experi-

TABLE II. CONSTANTS USED TO FIT THE DATA

Observer	λ	K	σ_{034}^2	σ_{010}^2
1	0.27×10^4	3.0	0.10	1.70
2	0.36×10^4	3.5	0.076	3.17
3	1.0×10^4	20.0	0.40	10.0
Observer	λ	K	σ_{042}^2	σ_{012}^2
A	0.80×10^4	6.06	0.41	7.00
B	0.78×10^4	5.93	0.25	6.50
C	0.35×10^4	5.94	0.15	4.14
D	0.46×10^4	12.35	0.09	4.0

ment all independent variables were changed for each new condition. The observers did not really have sufficient opportunity to "tune in" during the 10 to 20 practice trials given after each such change.

Whatever the inaccuracies involved in the prediction scheme for this final experiment and the variability in the data, two points can be made. Over a fairly wide range of conditions the model predicts the form and level of performance in duration discrimination. However, when ΔT is made as short as 5 msec the model no longer seems to fit; for each observer, performance was far below the prediction. The upper limit on the range over which the model applied could not be tested, for the equipment could only reliably produce signals up to the longest used in this experiment, slightly more than 2 sec.

DISCUSSION

A perceptual theory of the type just advanced must satisfy a number of criteria in addition to being an adequate fit to the data. The mechanisms implied by the mathematical statement must be reasonable and suggestive of possible physiological processes. The model must be not inconsistent with data from related experiments and should have a foundation in available mathematical techniques.

The model suggests neurological processes which could yield the data of these experiments. It does not specify a unique process; a number of possibilities suggest themselves. The "counting mechanism," a simple accumulator, could store neural pulses in reverberatory circuits or, for that matter, store an electrical charge due to a chemical process. The random nature of the source seems possible in terms of either chemical or neural processes.

Let us compare the present data with previous experiments. Earlier work followed the more conventional procedure; ogives were plotted and "thresholds" determined, which were reported in the form of the Weber ratio $\Delta T/T$. For comparison, representative values of the two constants in Table II were chosen, σ_v^2 was assumed negligible, and the Weber ratio was calculated using Eq. (3) to give 75 per cent correct responses. These calculated values are shown by the dotted curve in Fig. 12. Performance was better than the average data from the previous experiments. The present observers were highly trained and motivated, and worked for long periods. The difference between these and the observers of earlier experiments might lie in the "memory factor" of the equation for expected performance. The solid curve in the figure was calculated using

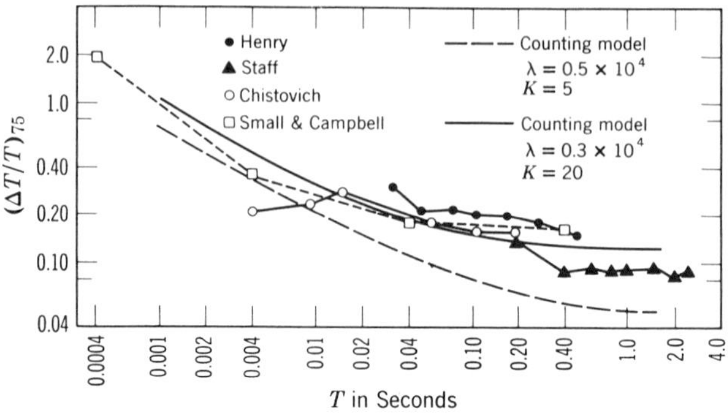

FIG. 12. Comparison with previous data. Smooth curves are from Eq. (3) with representative constants.

a much larger constant, but one which was still within the range obtained. With this correction, the fit of the model to prior data is much improved.

An advantage which the model shares with related studies of signal detectability is that it predicts *performance*, wherever it may lie, and is not concerned with only an arbitrary selected level of performance. The model predicts that if per cent correct is plotted as a function of ΔT, with T as a parameter, the ogive will be positively skewed, with greater skew at short values of T. Woodrow (1951) mentioned this finding, and Small and Campbell noted it in their data as well, with no explanation offered.

The model takes a stand on the old question of whether perception of time is an independent process or is conditional on the nature of the sensory input. If perception is dependent, we might expect loudness to begin to have a determining influence on discrimination at just those levels where this and other studies show the disappearance of any effect. Duration discrimination depends on sufficient intensity to mark the time unambiguously; it depends on detectability but not on loudness.

A model proposed by Stroud (1955) is not inconsistent with these data, or with the mathematical formulation of the counting model. Stroud proposed that subjective time is quantized and that events happening within any one unit interval cannot be differentiated by the human observer. His article brings a great deal of evidence to bear on this hypothesis, but no experimental evidence from the discrimination of durations per se is cited. The mathematical statements of the two models can be made equivalent if: (1) the length of the "psychological moment" is made very short, of the order of microseconds—much shorter than proposed by Stroud; or (2) successive "moments" are perceptually independent, i.e., the decision during one moment as to the existence of the input signal has no effect on the decision with regard to the next "moment." In the former case the practical distinction between the two approaches disappears, and the latter case leads to binomial statistics, and generalizations much like those from the Poisson statistics of the present model.

The model has had nothing to say about the classical area of investigation in this field, time errors. It predicts an increased variance in judgment with elapsed time, which is an entirely different matter. The direction of the "drift" with time is not predicted, and in fact should be random. Nothing is said about systematic "fading" or "enhancement" of an image over time. There was some indication of preference for one interval or the other under some conditions. This was shown by a significantly larger percentage correct in one interval of the two-alternative situation. However, in agreement with Stott and with Woodrow, no systematic effect could be found which was consistent from experiment to experiment for any observer. Evidence of response bias tended to appear when the discrimination task was a difficult one, whether the difficulty was due to low signal voltage, long T, or short ΔT.

Readers will differ in the degree of a priori reasonableness they will grant to the model. It seems clear that no constantly running "internal clock" will account for the data. The model does not insist that the constant λ retain the same value under all circumstances. Studies by Hoagland (1933) and by Hirsh, Bilger, and Deatherage (1956) showed that external factors, such as body temperature and extraneous stimulation, can affect experienced duration. According to Hirsh et al., time seems to "run faster" when, for instance, light signals are presented along with auditory noise. These data suggest that λ reflects a general level of activation, and the duration counter, if it exists anywhere in the nervous system, can receive counting pulses from many different sources.

Mention should be made in closing of implications of the model for psychophysical theory. A signal-detection task requires that the observer know exactly when the signal is to begin and when it will end, and that he consider the auditory input only during that time. Relatively weak signals masked by noise do not carry this information by themselves. To give such information we envision a turnabout for the counting mechanism, controlling the input rather than reacting to it. A recent empirical study on the "time-intensity trade" concept, done by Green, Birdsall, and Tanner (1957), showed decreasing efficiency in detection of long signals. At longer durations constant energy means decreased signal power, and thus, perhaps, greater reliance on the internal clocking mechanism to specify the relevant observation time. Unfortunately, greater time also means, according to the model, greater variance in the specification of duration and thus a lowered detection rate. When an amplitude-discrimination experiment was run on the Green, Birdsall, and Tanner paradigm, the characteristic decrease in detection at long durations was not observed (Creelman, 1961). Presumably the auditory signals were sufficiently detectable to mark the observation interval quite precisely, eliminating the need to rely on the internal timing mechanism.

SUMMARY

A series of experiments measured human ability to discriminate between durations of auditory signals presented in a noise background. Independent variables were the signal voltage, the "base" duration T, and the increment duration ΔT. Separate experiments assessed the effect of each of these on discrimination. A decision-theoretical model is presented, based on a "counting mechanism," which operates on impulses generated over the relevant durations. The source of these impulses is assumed to be random. Limitations on performance come from uncertainty regarding the end points of the time interval and from limited memory. The decision processes underlying the model are presented as a general theory of duration discrimination.

ACKNOWLEDGMENTS

W. P. Tanner provided constant help and encouragement in the course of these experiments, and in the development of the threshold framework. W. Joe Wiesner and Clarence Rivette assisted in the collection of the data. The ever-patient observers served faithfully. I wish to express special gratitude to them all.

The experimental work reported here was supported by contracts between the Cooley Electronics Laboratory and the Communication Sciences Laboratory of the University of Michigan and the U. S. Air Force and the Office of Naval Research. This article is based on a dissertation submitted to the University of Michigan in partial fulfillment of the requirements for the Ph.D. in Psychology. Preparation of the manuscript was supported by a contract between the Office of Naval Research and The Johns Hopkins University. This article appeared as Tech. Rept. No. 114 of the Cooley Electronics Laboratory, and in J. acoust. Soc. Am., *1961,* **34,** *582–593.*

References

- Axel, R. Estimation of time. *Arch. Psychol.,* 1925, **12,** No. 74.
- Bilger, R. C. Laboratory facilities employed in psychophysical memory experiments. University of Michigan: Electronic Defense Group, 1959, Technical Memo. No. 72.
- Bilger, R. C. Amplitude memory as a function of signal duration. Psychonomic Society, Program of First Meeting, 1960, 17. (Abstract)
- Boring, E. G. Temporal perception and operationism. *Am. J. Psychol.,* 1936, **48,** 519–522.
- Boring, E. G. *Sensation and perception in the history of experimental psychology.* New York: Appleton-Century-Crofts, 1942.
- Chistovich, L. A. Perception of time interval between two short sound pulses. *Soviet Physics: Acoustics,* 1959, **5,** 480–484.
- Clarke, F. R., Birdsall, T. G., and Tanner, W. P., Jr. Two types of ROC curves and definitions of parameters. *J. acoust. Soc. Am.,* 1959, **31,** 629–630.
- Clausen, J. An evaluation of experimental methods of time judgment. *J. exp. Psychol.,* 1950, **40,** 756–761.
- Creelman, C. D. Applications of signal detectability theory to psychophysical research: A bibliography. University of Michigan: Electronic Defense Group, 1960, Technical Memo. No. 79.
- Creelman, C. D. Detection of complex signals as a function of signal bandwidth and duration. *J. acoust. Soc. Am.,* 1961, **33,** 89–94.
- Dunlap, K. Rhythm and time I. *Psychol. Bull.,* 1911, **8,** 230–242; II. 1912, **9,** 177–199; III. 1914, **11,** 169–171; IV. 1916, **13,** 206–208.
- Feller, W. *An introduction to probability theory and some of its applications.* 2nd ed. Vol. I. New York: Wiley, 1957, pp. 146ff.
- Fraisse, P. *Psychologie du temps.* Paris: Presses Universitaires de France, 1957.
- Gilliland, A. R., Hofeld, J., and Eckstrand, G. Studies in time perception. *Psychol. Bull.,* 1946, **43,** 162–176.
- Green, D. M. Psychoacoustics and detection theory. *J. acoust. Soc. Am.,* 1960, **32,** 1189–1203. [2]
- Green, D. M., Birdsall, T. G., and Tanner, W. P., Jr. Signal detection as a function of signal intensity and duration. *J. acoust. Soc. Am.,* 1957, **29,** 523–531. [11]
- Henry, F. M. Discrimination of the duration of a sound. *J. exp. Psychol.,* 1948, **38,** 734–742.
- Hirsh, I. J. Certain temporal factors in audition. *Science,* 1952, **116,** 523.
- Hirsh, I. J., Bilger, R. C., and Deatherage, B. H. The effect of auditory and visual background on apparent duration. *Amer. J. Psychol.,* 1956, **69,** 561–574.
- Hoagland, H. The physiological control of judgments of duration: Evidence for a chemical clock. *J. gen. Psychol.,* 1933, **9,** 267–287.
- James, W. *Principles of psychology.* Vol. I. New York: Dover Publications, 1950 (1890), pp. 605–642.

- Lifshitz, S. Apparent duration of sound perception and musical optimum reverberation. *J. acoust. Soc. Am.,* 1935-36, **7,** 213–216.
- Nakajima, S. Time errors in the successive comparison of tonal durations. *Jap. J. Psychol.,* 1958, **29,** 18–27.
- Nichols, H. The psychology of time. *Am. J. Psychol.,* 1891, **3,** 453–529.
- Oléron, G. Influence of the intensity of a sound on its apparent duration. *Année* psychol. 1952, **52,** 382–392.
- Peterson, G. E., and Lehiste, I. Duration of syllable nuclei in English. *J. acoust. Soc. Am.,* 1960, **32,** 693–703.
- Stott, L. H. Time-orders errors in the discrimination of short tonal durations. *J. exp. Psychol.,* 1935, **18,** 741–766.
- Stroud, J. M. The fine structure of psychological time. In H. Quastler (Ed.), *Information theory in psychology.* Glencoe, Illinois: Free Press, 1955.
- Swets, J. A. Indices of signal detectability obtained with various psychophysical procedures. *J. acoust. Soc. Am.,* 1959, **31,** 511–513. [6]
- Swets, J. A. Is there a sensory threshold? *Science,* 1961, **134,** 168–177. [4]
- Tanner, W. P., Jr. Theory of recognition. *J. acoust. Soc. Am.,* 1956, **28,** 882–888. [19]
- Tanner, W. P., Jr. Effect of memory for amplitude on amplitude discrimination. *J. acoust. Soc. Am.,* 1959, **31,** 1575. (Abstract)
- Tanner, W. P., Jr. Theory of signal detectability as an interpretive tool for psychophysical data. *J. acoust. Soc. Am.,* 1960, **32,** 1140–1147.
- Thurstone, L. L. A law of comparative judgment. *Psychol. Rev.,* 1927, **34,** 273–286.
- Titchener, E. B. *Experimental psychology.* Vol. II. New York: Macmillan, 1905.
- Wallace, M., and Rabin, A. I. Temporal experience. *Psychol. Bull.,* 1960, **57,** 216–236.
- Weber, A. O. Estimation of time. *Psychol. Bull.,* 1933, **30,** 233–252.
- Woodrow, H. In S. S. Stevens (Ed.), *Handbook of experimental psychology.* New York: Wiley, 1951, Chapter 32.

13

Interval of Time Uncertainty in Auditory Detection

James P. Egan, Gordon Z. Greenberg, and Arthur I. Schulman

An ideal observer achieves his best performance in the detection of a sinusoid in noise when he has knowledge of the following signal parameters: frequency of the sine wave, amplitude, phase, duration, and starting time. The performance of the human listener is inferior to that of the ideal, and it is important to determine the degree to which each of the five signal parameters listed helps the listener in his decisions as to the presence or absence of the signal (Tanner and Birdsall, 1958). It is known, for example, that uncertainty with respect to the frequency of a sinusoid results in a decrement in performance (Tanner, 1958; Veniar, 1958*a*, 1958*b*; Gundy, 1960). The present series of experiments is concerned with the effect on auditory detection of various amounts of uncertainty with respect to the starting time of the signal (Egan, Greenberg, and Schulman, 1959*b*).

When a listener tries to detect a weak signal in the presence of a continuous noise, he must decide whether his momentary sensory input arose from the signal added to a sample of noise or from a sample of noise alone. Both sensory and nonsensory factors will contribute to his decisions, and the most important of these are listed as follows: sensory input; previous experience and information regarding the properties of the possible sensory inputs, signal and noise parameters; previous experience and information regarding the relative frequencies of occurrence of the possible sensory inputs and regarding their relative importance, a priori probabilities of the alternative stimuli and values and costs of the alternative stimulus-response conjunctions; response alternatives available to the listener (Green, 1960; Tanner, Swets, and Green, 1956; Tanner, 1960). Clearly, in a psychophysical experiment in which the principal interest is in the sensory capacity of the listener, a valid measure of detectability must be largely independent of all non-sensory decision criteria (Swets, 1959).

The experiments to be described were done in the context of the "fixed-interval observation experiment." In such experiments, a single temporal interval for observation by the listener is the principal part of a trial. Two types of intervals are used to make up a series of trials: (1) intervals that contain the signal plus noise, and (2) intervals that contain noise alone. After each interval, the listener indicates, according to some criterion, whether or not the interval contained the signal. The hit rate $p(y|SN)$ is then plotted against the false alarm rate $p(y|N)$, and a measure of detectability may then be derived from the resulting operating characteristic. The rating method was used in securing the data for an operating characteristic, and the ratings were converted to values of $p(y|SN)$ and $p(y|N)$ (Egan, Schulman, and Greenberg, 1959).

A measure of detectability is derived as follows (Egan, 1958; Clarke, Birdsall, and Tanner, 1959; Pollack, 1959). Each probability scale, $p(y|SN)$ and $p(y|N)$, is so transformed that the corresponding normal deviates (z scores) are linearly spaced. These z-score axes are referred to as $z(y|SN)$ and $z(y|N)$. With such a coordinate system the chance line is the locus for which $z(y|SN)$ is equal to $z(y|N)$, and the negative diagonal has the equation, $z(y|SN) = -z(y|N)$. The obtained conditional probabilities are plotted on the normal-normal coordinates and a straight line is fitted to the data. The point at which the operating characteristic intersects the negative diagonal is called the *point of intersection.* The point of intersection associated with a given operating characteristic has certain interesting properties. For example, when the a priori probabilities of the two types of stimuli are equal, then at the point of intersection half of the stimuli are in the criterion of acceptance. A useful measure of detectability may be defined in relation to this point. This measure of detectability d_s is twice the value of the abscissa of the point of intersection.

Figure 1 shows operating characteristics with $p(y|SN)$ plotted against $p(y|N)$. The parameter associated with the family of curves is signal strength (E/N_0). Figure 2 shows one of the operating characteristics of

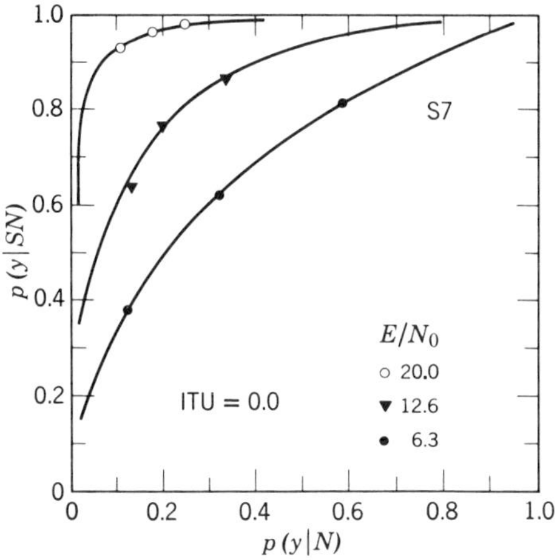

FIG. 1. Three operating characteristics based on a listener's attempt to detect the presence of a sinusoid (1000 cps, 0.25 sec) in noise. The task was defined by the fixed-interval observation experiment; the probability that the signal would occur in a well-defined interval was 0.5, and the listener used a rating scale to indicate his confidence that a signal was present in an observation interval. The parameter of the family of curves is signal strength (E/N_0). The fact that the interval of time uncertainty (ITU) is equal to 0.0 signifies that the listener knew the onset time of the signal. For each curve, a measure of detectability d_s was obtained, as illustrated in Fig. 2. As E/N_0 is increased, these values of d_s are 0.74, 1.52, and 2.76. Each operating characteristic is based upon 510 trials.

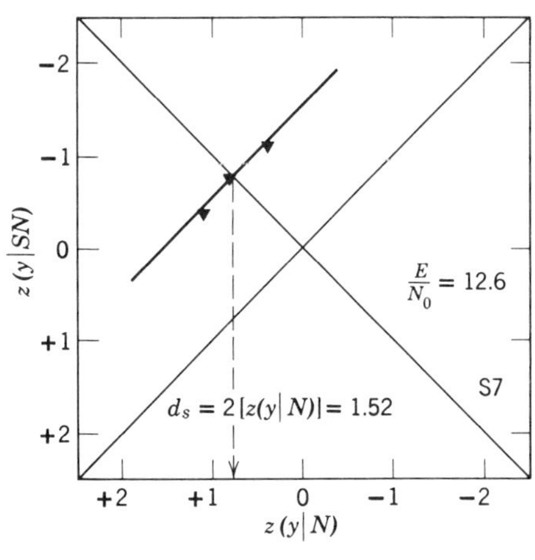

FIG. 2. One of the operating characteristics of Fig. 1, replotted on z-score coordinates, to illustrate the graphical estimation of the detectability index d_s.

Fig. 1 transformed to z-score coordinates, and the graphical computation of the measure of detectability d_s is illustrated.

GENERAL PROCEDURE

In our earlier experiments on signal detection, the onset and duration of the signal were well defined by a light. Figure 3 diagrams the sequence of possible events in the fixed-interval experiment. The upper panel shows the typical situation (Egan, Schulman, and Greenberg, 1959) in which L_1 warns the listener that a trial is about to begin, and L_2 marks off the starting time and the duration of the signal when it is presented. The lower panel also portrays a fixed-interval experiment, but the observation interval (L_2) is considerably longer in duration than the signal. That is to say, the observation interval during which the signal might occur is made longer so that the listener is uncertain of the onset time of the signal. The interval of time uncertainty (ITU) is defined as the interval during which the signal may have its onset. In other words,

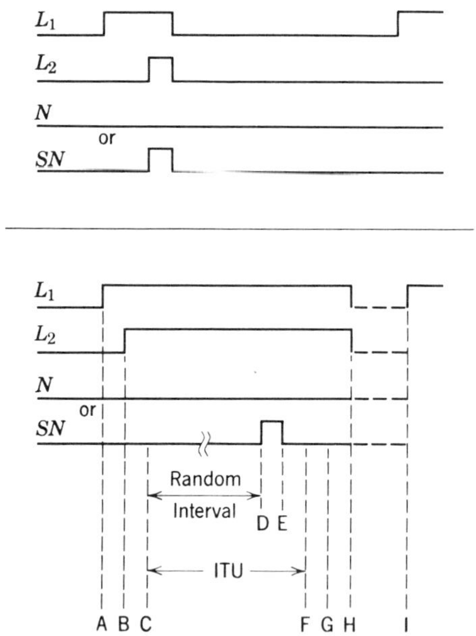

FIG. 3. Schema of the sequence of events during one trial of a fixed-interval observation experiment. The upper panel represents the typical situation, and the lower panel shows how uncertainty about the time of onset of the signal is introduced in the experiments reported here. The important interval is the interval of time uncertainty (ITU), which extends from C to F. Certain other intervals, such as BC and GH, varied slightly from experiment to experiment, as described in the text.

the ITU is the range of possible starting times for the signal. Of course, the signal is presented either only once or not at all in any one observation interval. From trial to trial, the exact temporal position of the signal, if presented, varies randomly. In the present series of experiments, the important interval is CF in Fig. 3, and it is the ITU as defined. The instant C marks the earliest possible onset of the signal, and the instant F marks the latest possible onset. The interval FG is equal to the duration of the signal. The "fringes" BC and GH were included so that random fluctuations in the electronic timers would not alter the duration (and therefore the energy) of the signal, when the earliest or latest possible onset times were sampled. In Experiment I, BC = GH = 0.5 sec; in Experiment II, these intervals were 0.2 sec; in Experiment III, they were 0.1 sec. DE is the duration of the signal. In the three experiments reported here, when a signal was presented with ITU = 0.0, it always fell within the middle portion of the interval BH of Fig. 3.

In all experiments, the a priori probability [$p(SN)$] that the signal occurred exactly once at some time during the observation interval was 0.5, and $p(N)$ was, of course, 0.5. Thus, programming of the trials by the experimenter consisted of two random sampling processes: (1) the determination of whether or not a signal would be presented in the observation interval, and, if the signal was to be presented, (2) the instant within the interval of time uncertainty at which the signal would have its onset.

When the ITU was greater than zero, the position of the signal within ITU was determined randomly before each signal trial. These randomly determined values were 0.1-sec steps on an electronic timer. For the real listener, the steps of 0.1 sec taken in conjunction with the inherent variability of the timer, may be considered small enough to have provided, in effect, a rectangular distribution of random onsets.

The duration of ITU was fixed for any one series of trials, but it was varied systematically from one series of trials to another. The listener was aware of the particular value of ITU being used.

During the response interval (interval HI of Fig. 3), the listener pressed one of four numbered keys which represented a rating scale. On this scale a "1" indicated high confidence that the preceding observation interval had contained a signal, while a "4" indicated low confidence that a signal had been presented. The listener was never informed whether a signal had or had not been presented on a given trial. Each of the four rating categories is assumed to represent a different criterion for acceptance; the relative frequency of occurrence of each rating, conditional on the type of observation interval (SN or N), determines the operating characteristic.

Listeners were advised to use the rating scale in a symmetric manner, employing the "acceptance" end of the scale about as often as the "rejection" portion of the scale. Their performance was monitored on counters and they were regularly told either to alter or to maintain their distributions of responses over the four rating categories. The instructions were based on more or less arbitrary criteria and were read to the listeners at fixed occasions within a session.

The signal and the noise were mixed electrically and then presented over a binaural headset with the two earphones wired in parallel and in phase. For all experiments, the signal was a "pure tone" of 1000 cps. The signal voltage was turned on without regard to phase and without the use of special devices, so that the (negligible) transients were determined by the response of the earphone (Permoflux Corporation, PDR-10). The duration of the signal was 0.5 sec in Experiments I and II, and 0.25 sec in Experiment III. The white noise was generated by a 6D4 tube (noise generator, model 455-B, Grason-Stadler Company). The overall sound pressure level of the noise (50–7000 cps) was about 65 db *re* 0.0002 μbar, and it was held constant for all sessions at this comfortable level of listening. The noise was present continuously throughout a session.

The relation between the signal and the noise will be specified by E/N_0, where E is the signal energy, or the time integral of power, and N_0 is the noise power per unit bandwidth.

Additional procedural details will be mentioned under the individual experiments.

Experiment I

In this first experiment, ITU was systematically varied from 0.0 to 8.0 sec. The intervals in the lower portion of Fig. 3 took on the following values: AB = 1.0 sec, BC = GH = 0.5 sec, DE (duration of signal) = 0.5 sec, and HI = 5.0 sec. All tests were conducted with $E/N_0 =$ 20.0. (Expressed in decibels this value is 10 log (E/N_0) = 13 db.) Two of the authors (GG and AS) served alternately as experimenter and observer; each was run for 12 daily sessions. Only one ITU was used during any one experimental session, which consisted of two practice periods followed by six test periods. Short rest intervals were given between periods. The length of the periods, and consequently of the session, was made nearly independent of ITU by decreasing the number of daily trials as ITU increased. The five durations of ITU were: 0, 1, 2, 4, and 8 sec; the number of trials devoted to each ITU for each listener was: 840, 720, 720, 900, and 648, respectively.

Figures 4 and 5 show the results in the form of operating characteristics

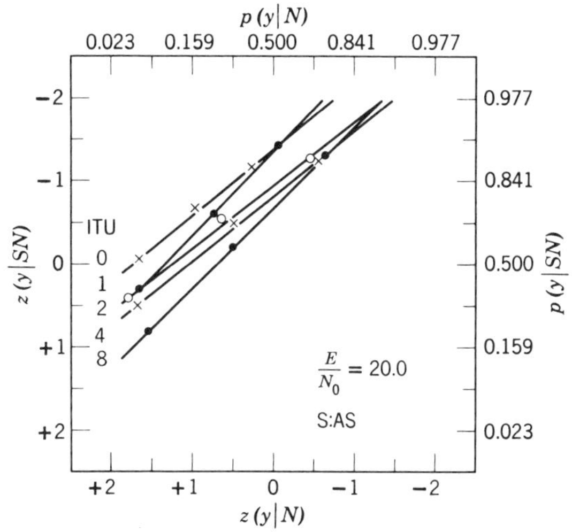

FIG. 4. Five operating characteristics illustrating the progressive decrement in performance that results when the observation interval is lengthened, thus introducing more uncertainty as to the time of onset of a signal within the interval. All these data are from one observer.

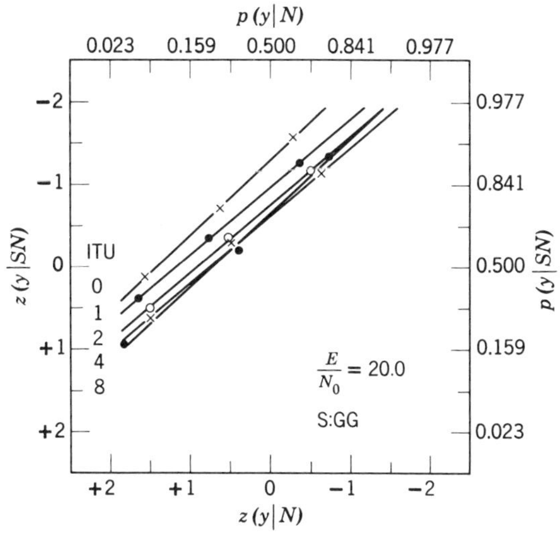

FIG. 5. Five operating characteristics that show, for a second observer, the same relations as those shown in Fig. 4.

on a *z*-score (normal-normal) plot. The parameter associated with each curve is the numerical value of ITU in seconds. In each case, the three points obtained under a given value of ITU fall fairly close to the (least-squares) straight line. The detectability index d_s was determined for each operating characteristic, and Fig. 6 shows the relation obtained between d_s and ITU.

Appendix I describes a control experiment conducted in conjunction with the present experiment.

Experiment II

In Experiment I, only one value of E/N_0 was used. In the second experiment, the relation between d_s and ITU was determined with E/N_0 as the parameter. This experiment was carried out by GG and AS in essentially the same way as the first experiment; the duration of a trial was shortened, however, by reducing intervals BC and GH each to 0.2 sec and also by reducing interval HI to 4 sec (see Fig. 3). Consequently, when ITU was zero, the lower panel of Fig. 3 resembled the upper panel more closely than was the case for Experiment I. The three values of ITU were 0, 1, and 2 sec, and each of these was tested at the following three values of E/N_0: 10.0 (10 db), 20.0 (13 db), and 31.6 (15 db). The duration of the signal, DE of Fig. 3, was again 0.5 sec. Each observer served in two sessions under each of the nine combinations of ITU and E/N_0. The number of trials for each of the 18 sessions ranged from 390 to 400. The experimental conditions were counterbalanced with respect to such variables as practice.

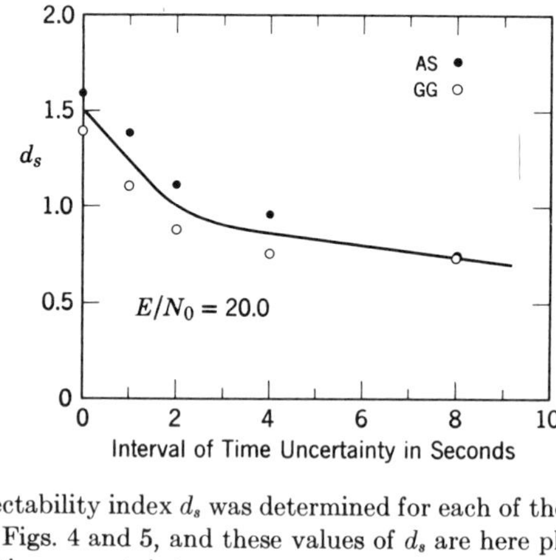

FIG. 6. The detectability index d_s was determined for each of the operating characteristics shown in Figs. 4 and 5, and these values of d_s are here plotted as a function of the interval of time uncertainty.

The results of the second experiment are shown as Fig. 7. Here d_s is plotted against ITU with E/N_0 as the parameter. It is perhaps surprising that the function at the highest signal strength shows as much decrement as it does.

Experiment III

The two exploratory experiments reported above provided a basis for the design of the principal experiment. The procedure was basically the same as that for the two previous studies with the exception of the following details.

The intervals that define the structure of a trial (Fig. 3) were: AB = 0.5 sec, BC = GH = 0.1 sec, DE (duration of signal) = 0.25 sec, and HI = 4.0 sec.

Eight well-practiced listeners, who did not know the purpose of the experiment, were tested in two groups of four listeners each. A description of the training given to these listeners, along with some long-term measures of performance in the detection of signal in noise, are given in Appendix II. The four headsets were wired in parallel so that the instantaneous, as well as the average, signal-to-noise ratio was correlated across a group of four listeners.

For the experiment proper, each listener served for 10 daily sessions with each session lasting about 2 hr. There were 12 combinations of ITU and E/N_0, and these combinations were counterbalanced over sessions.

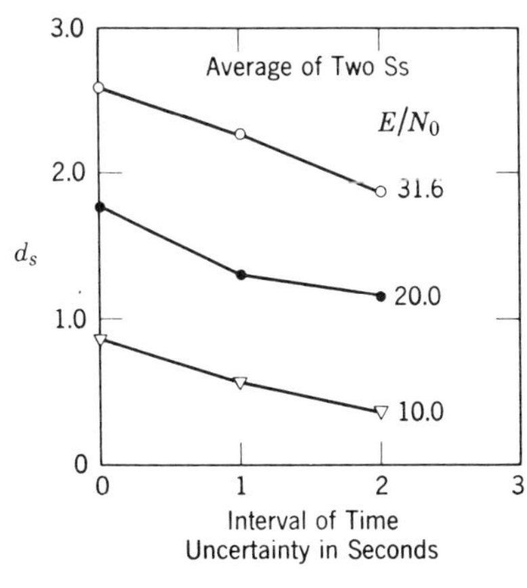

FIG. 7. The detectability index d_s as a function of the interval of time uncertainty with E/N_0 as the parameter. The slope of the middle curve is nearly the same as that of the corresponding portion of the curve of Fig. 6.

A "strong" signal ($E/N_0 = 20.0$) was used with ITU's of 0.0, 0.5, 1.0, 2.0, and 4.0 sec; a "medium" signal ($E/N_0 = 12.6$) with ITU's of 0.0, 0.5, 1.0, and 2.0 sec; and a "weak" signal ($E/N_0 = 6.3$) with ITU's of 0.0, 0.5, and 1.0 sec. In any one session, a single E/N_0 was employed with two or three ITU's. A session consisted of from 7 to 10 test periods, each lasting about 7.5 min. All trials in a given period involved a single value for ITU, and a number of periods were run at one ITU before shifting to another in the course of a given session. The shift, moreover, was always minimal; for example, from an ITU of 1.0 it was permitted to change the ITU to 0.5 or to 2.0, but not to 0.0 or to 4.0. Short rest intervals separated most periods, but a longer rest of 10 min was inserted whenever ITU was changed to a new value. Listeners removed their headsets during all rest intervals. Practice trials were given not only at the beginning of a session but whenever ITU was changed. For each listener, the total number of "data" trials for each combination of ITU and E/N_0 varied from 450 to 510.

The primary results of this experiment consist of 96 operating characteristics (8 listeners × 12 combinations of ITU and E/N_0). The data for each of these 96 operating characteristics were plotted on z-score plots, and a straight line was fitted by eye to the three data points. (In two of the 96 instances, only two points were obtained.) Values of d_s were determined graphically (see Fig. 2). Operating characteristics for three of the eight listeners are shown in Fig. 8. These data were obtained with an E/N_0 of 20.0. The five operating characteristics in a single column represent the results from one listener; ITU increases from the top to the bottom of the panel. (Figure 1 shows additional data drawn from the present experiment.)

The average slope of the 96 operating characteristics obtained in Experiment III was 0.79. There was considerable variability about this mean, as a glance at Fig. 8 will reveal.

Figure 9 shows the effect of time uncertainty upon the detectability of a sinusoid in noise with E/N_0 as the parameter. Each point is based upon the mean of eight values of d_s, one for each listener.

There has been some interest in the shape of the function relating d_s to E/N_0. It seems worthwhile, therefore, to reproduce the data of Fig. 9 in the form shown in Fig. 10. Here, our results seem to demand that a nonlinear, positively accelerated curve be used to fit the data. (See Figs. 11 and 12 for data that satisfy a straight-line relation between d_s and E/N_0 for values of d_s less than 3.0.)

The results shown in Figs. 6, 7, and 9 demonstrate that even a small amount of uncertainty with respect to the time of onset of the signal

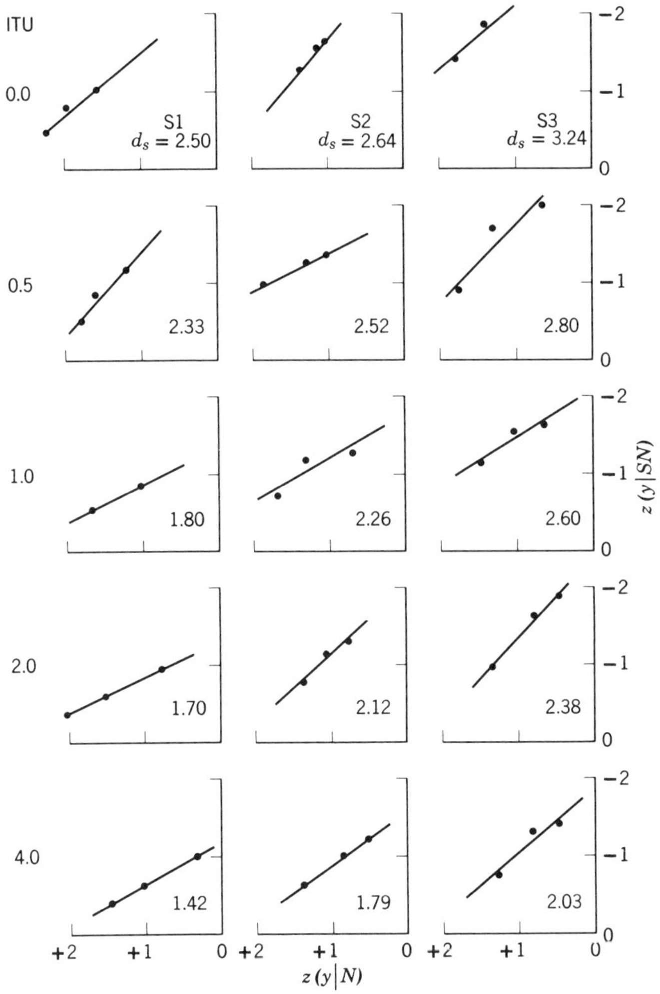

FIG. 8. Operating characteristics for three of the eight listeners who participated in the principal experiment. The five operating characteristics in a single column are based on one listener, and ITU increases from the top to the bottom of the panel. The value of E/N_0 was 20.0.

results in a decrement in performance. There are, of course, many possible interpretations of this decrement. The more reasonable of these will be examined.

In the three experiments thus far presented, the response interval HI of Fig. 3 remained constant even though ITU was varied. It might be argued, therefore, that as ITU became longer and longer, the listener

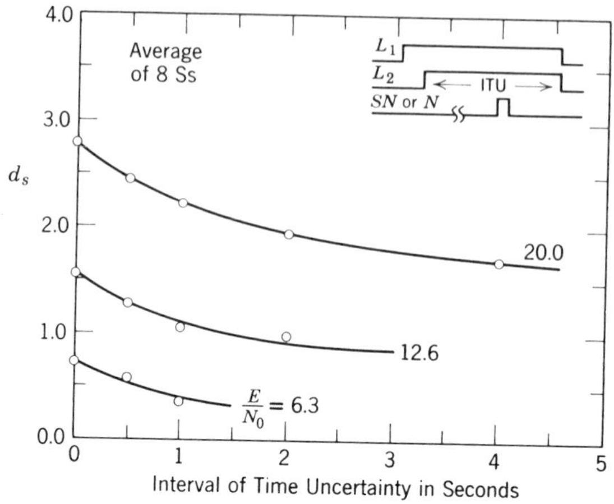

FIG. 9. The detectability index d_s as a function of the interval of time uncertainty with E/N_0 as the parameter. Each point is based on the mean of eight values of d_s, one for each listener.

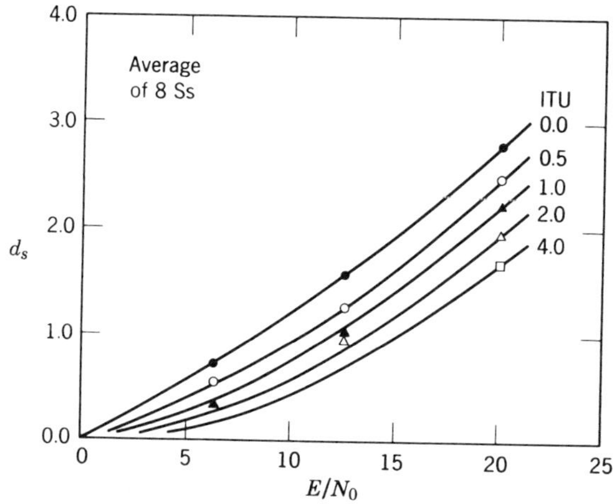

FIG. 10. The detectability index d_s as a function of E/N_0 with the interval of time uncertainty as the parameter. The curves were fitted by eye.

"fatigued" more and more rapidly over a period of trials; with the response interval held constant, the listener might not be able to recover as well at long ITU's as at short ones. This hypothesis is rather difficult to test, and only one control experiment was conducted. The interval of time uncertainty was held constant at 2.0 sec, and two response intervals were chosen, those of 4.0 and 8.0 sec. The number of trials for each listener, exclusive of practice, was 372 for a response interval of 4.0 sec and 400 for the 8-sec interval. The mean value of d_s for the eight listeners was 0.91 for the shorter response interval, and it was 1.05 for the longer interval. This difference of 0.14, although not statistically reliable, is in the direction that favors the hypothesis. Unfortunately, the effect of an increase in the response interval was tested at only one value of ITU, and it is possible that the values of d_s for other ITU's would also increase slightly with a longer response interval.

An alternative interpretation of the results is that, as the ITU becomes longer and longer, the listener's attention flags during the course of a given observation interval. This decrease in attention could result in poorer performance. As a preliminary test of this hypothesis, all data for ITU = 2.0 sec were analyzed in the following manner. Observation intervals of the *SN* type were sorted into two classes, depending upon whether the signal occurred in the first or second half of the interval. A value of d_s was then obtained for each half of the observation interval. Both values turned out to be 0.97. Evidently, the listener listens with nearly equal facility throughout the observation interval.

To us, the most reasonable interpretation of the results is that, as ITU increases, more "samples" of noise are likely to resemble and, hence, be confused with an actual signal. In other words, it would be maintained that performance declines as the time of onset of the signal becomes more and more uncertain, not because the task primarily affects the efficiency of the listener, but because the detectability of the signal itself has declined.

SUMMARY

Three experiments were conducted to measure the decrement in performance that results from uncertainty in the time of onset of a signal presented against a continuous background of noise. The fixed-interval observation experiment was employed. A light defined an observation interval for the listener during which the signal, a tone of 1000 cps, either was or was not presented [$p(SN) = 0.5$]. The signal, when presented, started at an instant randomly selected within the observation interval. Thus, the listener was uncertain as to (1) whether or not the signal would occur in the observation interval, and (2) the onset time of the signal, if in fact the signal occurred. The interval of time uncertainty (ITU) during which the tone might start was systematically varied from one series of trials to the next, and the listener knew the duration of ITU in each series. After each observation interval, the listener indicated his confidence that a tone was presented by using a rating scale. Operating characteristics $[p(y|SN)$ against $p(y|N)]$ were plotted on normal-normal coordinates, and measures of detectability were computed. The functional relation between the detectability index d_s and the interval of time uncertainty is presented for each experiment.

APPENDIX I

Experiment I was conducted in the early stages of our research in which operating characteristics were determined in the study of detection. At that time, it was felt desirable to make sure that long-term changes in performance due to practice did not markedly influence the results of our experiments on time uncertainty. We now know, after several hundred trials, that changes in d_s resulting from further practice are so small that their effects may be easily counterbalanced over experimental conditions.

Before and after Experiment I, both observers (GG and AS) were tested with ITU = 0.0 and with the signal occurrence coincident with L_2 (see upper panel of Fig. 3). Each observer was tested at E/N_0's of 7.9, 20.0, and 31.6; the signal was 0.5 sec in duration. Three "calibration sessions," one for each of the three E/N_0's, were conducted for each observer both prior to and following Experiment I. Each session consisted of 480 trials. Obtained values of d_s are shown in Table I, and these values reveal a tendency toward slightly better performance in the sessions that followed Experiment I. Figure 11 shows the mean of the first and second values of d_s in Table I plotted against E/N_0.

TABLE I. Measures of Detectability d_s Made before and after Experiment I of the Text. Although There Is Evidence That These Two Observers Improved with Long-Term Practice, the Mean Difference in d_s Is Only 0.15.

E/N_0		d_s Before	After	Difference
	AS	2.77	3.01	0.24
31.6	GG	2.14	2.53	0.39
	AS	1.68	1.80	0.12
20.0	GG	1.79	1.60	−0.19
	AS	0.57	0.70	0.13
7.9	GG	0.50	0.69	0.19

For E/N_0 = 20.0 and ITU = 0.0, a condition closely similar to one of those in Experiment I, both observers performed somewhat better in

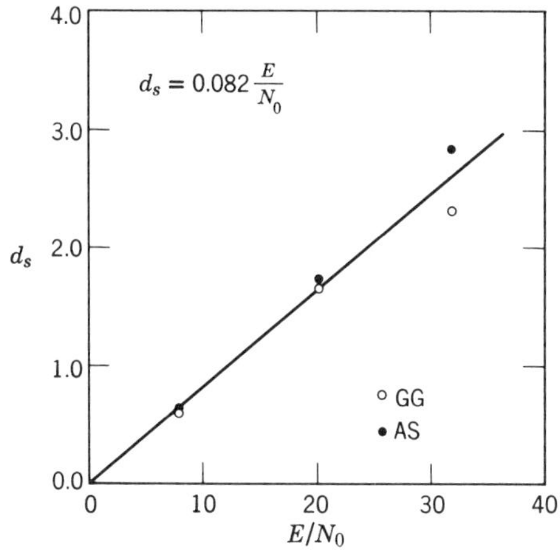

FIG. 11. The detectability index d_s as a function of E/N_0. These data are based upon Table I.

the two calibrating sessions than in Experiment I. We believe that this result is due to the fact that in Experiment I, L_2 and the signal were not coincident for ITU = 0.0. Values of d_s obtained for Observer AS in the calibrating sessions are compared in Fig. 12 with previously published data for this observer (Egan, Schulman, and Greenberg, 1959) collected under the same conditions. The slope of the straight line is relatively low because the efficiency of the human observer is not maximal for a signal whose duration is as long as 0.5 sec (Green, Birdsall, and Tanner, 1957).

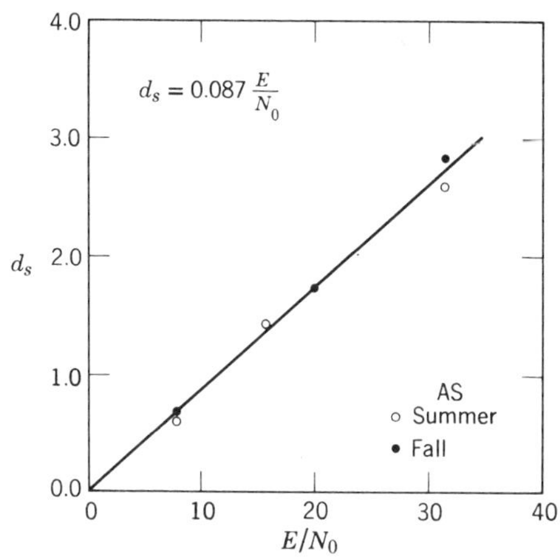

FIG. 12. The detectability index d_s as a function of E/N_0.

APPENDIX II

Eight listeners participated for a period of 11 weeks (summer, 1959) in a series of experiments related directly or indirectly to Experiment III of the text. (One listener, S8, resigned after seven weeks.) For ease of exposition, the sequence of experiments is here listed.

(*a*) General practice with fixed-interval observation experiment using four-point rating scale, five sessions.

(*b*) Practice for Experiment III with ITU's of various values, two sessions.

(*c*) Experiment III, 10 sessions.

(*d*) Control experiment for Experiment III, response interval varied, two sessions.

(*e*) Control experiment for Experiment III, long-term practice effects, two sessions.

(*f*) Experiment on memory for waveform, non-ITU (see following chapter), eight sessions.

(*g*) Experiment using the method of free response, non-ITU (see Chapter 15), 13 sessions.

(*h*) Control experiment for Experiment III, long-term practice effects, one session.

(*i*) Experiment using the method of free response, non-ITU (see Chapter 15), 11 sessions.

In all of these situations, both in practice and in actual tests, the listeners were trying to detect a sinusoid (1000 cps, 0.25 sec) in the presence of white noise.

It was felt desirable to replicate a specific experimental condition at various stages of the 11-week period in order to make sure that serious changes in performance did not occur as the result of practice or boredom. Two conditions were chosen for these "control tests." They were: ITU $= 0.0$ and 2.0 sec, with $E/N_0 = 12.6$ for both conditions. All details of the experimental conditions for these control tests were the same as those described in the text for Experiment III.

Figure 13 shows the mean performance (seven listeners) for an ITU of zero. The abscissa must be carefully interpreted. The "number of trials" refers only to those trials for which the conditions were those labeled on the graph; experience with other listening conditions also took place during the period of time over which the data for Fig. 13 were secured. For each listener, the number of trials for each point is slightly smaller than the difference between successive abscissas, because the practice trials were omitted in the computations of d_s.

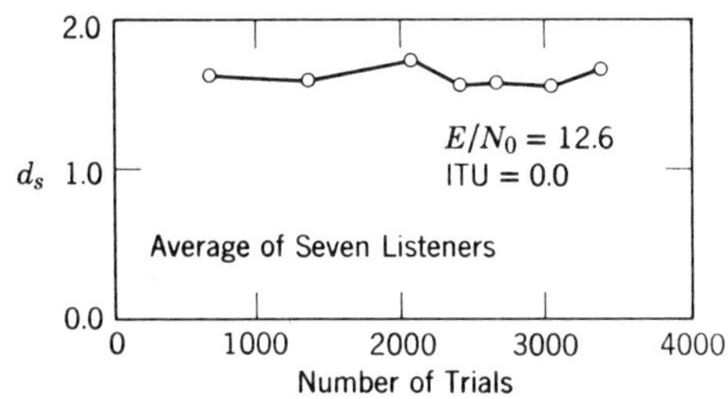

FIG. 13. Curve showing the long-term stability in the detectability index d_s. The data span a period of nine weeks.

During the first five sessions (item *a*), the listeners were given practice in the fixed-interval experiment. All details of the experiment were the same as for Experiment III. The ITU was zero, but various values of E/N_0 were employed; for about 60 per cent of the trials the value of E/N_0 was 12.6. The first three points of Fig. 13 are based on these practice trials.

The two sessions of practice with various ITU's (item *b*) did not include the experimental condition used to obtain the data for Fig. 13.

The fourth and fifth points of Fig. 13 are data taken directly from Experiment III (item *c*). The mean of these two points is 1.56, as compared with 1.65 for the first three points.

It was considered desirable to introduce a bonus for "good performance" after the control experiment in which the response interval was varied (item *d*). Listening to white noise for a signal that is near or below "threshold" is a boring task for most people, and it was hoped that the effort of the group could be maintained. The listeners were told that they could augment their base pay if they maintained a high level of performance. They were also told that the amount of the bonus would be based upon group performance. Actually, a rather standard bonus was given, and, at the beginning of each session, they were informed of the amount earned on the previous session. The bonus system was used for all remaining sessions.

The sixth point of Fig. 13 was obtained on the first two days (item *e*) after the bonus was introduced. The trials for the last point (item *h*) were run between two experiments on the method of free response (items *g* and *i*) (Egan, Greenberg, and Schulman, 1959*a*).

The second condition for which long-term practice data were available was the combination of an ITU of 2.0 sec and an E/N_0 of 12.6. Successive mean values of d_s for the seven listeners were: 0.62, 1.02, 1.04, 0.87, 0.93, and 1.08. Each of these values was based, respectively, upon the following approximate number of trials: 65, 65, 230, 355, 355, and 330.

Of course, very little effect due to practice is shown by the data presented, because the learning effect occurs in the first few hundred trials (Gundy, 1960). Furthermore, it is obvious from the data presented that the average performance level of the listeners, as measured by d_s, was maintained at a quite constant level over a period of 9 weeks of nearly daily practice in the attempt to detect the presence of a sinusoid in noise.

ACKNOWLEDGMENTS

This research was conducted in the Hearing and Communication Laboratory of Indiana University with support from the Operational Applications Laboratory of the U. S. Air Force. This article appeared as Tech. Rept. No. AFCCDD-TR-60-32, and in J. acoust. Soc. Am., *1961,* **33,** *771–778.*

References

- Clarke, F. R., Birdsall, T. G., and Tanner, W. P., Jr. Two types of ROC curves and definitions of parameters. *J. acoust. Soc. Am.,* 1959, **31,** 629–630.
- Egan, J. P. Recognition memory and the operating characteristic. Indiana University: Hearing and Communication Laboratory, 1958, Technical Note AFCRC-TN-58-51.
- Egan, J. P., Greenberg, G. Z., and Schulman, A. I. Operating characteristics, signal detectability, and the methods of free response. Indiana University: Hearing and Communication Laboratory, 1959*a,* Technical Note AFCRC-TR-59-58. [See 15]
- Egan, J. P., Greenberg, G. Z., and Schulman, A. I. Detection of signals presented at random times. *J. acoust. Soc. Am.,* 1959*b,* **31,** 1579. (Abstract)
- Egan, J. P., Schulman, A. I., and Greenberg, G. Z. Operating characteristics determined by binary decisions and by ratings. *J. acoust. Soc. Am.,* 1959, **31,** 768–773. [7]
- Green, D. M. Psychoacoustics and detection theory. *J. acoust. Soc. Am.,* 1960, **32,** 1189–1203. [2]
- Green, D. M., Birdsall, T. G., and Tanner, W. P., Jr. Signal detection as a function of signal intensity and duration. *J. acoust. Soc. Am.,* 1957, **29,** 523–531. [11]
- Gundy, R. F. Detection of an unspecified signal: A study in auditory discrimination learning. Ph.D. thesis. Indiana University: Hearing and Communication Laboratory, 1960. [See 8]
- Pollack, I. On indices of signal and response discriminability. *J. acoust. Soc. Am.,* 1959, **31,** 1031.
- Swets, J. A. Indices of signal detectability obtained with various psychophysical procedures. *J. acoust. Soc. Am.,* 1959, **31,** 511–513. [6]

- Tanner, W. P., Jr. What is masking? *J. acoust. Soc. Am.,* 1958, **30,** 919–921. [24]
- Tanner, W. P., Jr. The theory of signal detectability as an interpretive tool for psychophysical data. University of Michigan: Electronic Defense Group, 1960, Technical Memo No. 78.
- Tanner, W. P. Jr., and Birdsall, T. G. Definitions of d' and η as psychophysical measures. *J. acoust. Soc. Am.,* 1958, **30,** 922–928. [5]
- Tanner, W. P., Jr., Swets, J. A., and Green, D. M. Some general properties of the hearing mechanism. University of Michigan: Electronic Defense Group, 1956, Technical Report No. 30.
- Veniar, F. A. Signal detection as a function of frequency ensemble, I. *J. acoust. Soc. Am.,* 1958*a,* **30,** 1020–1024; II. *J. acoust. Soc. Am.,* 1958*b,* **30,** 1075–1078.

14

Memory for Waveform and Time Uncertainty in Auditory Detection

James P. Egan, Arthur I. Schulman, and Gordon Z. Greenberg

The experiment to be reported was done in the context of the fixed-interval observation experiment in which a listener decides after each observation interval whether or not the interval contained a signal (Egan, Schulman, and Greenberg, 1959). The data so obtained may be represented by an *operating characteristic*. A measure of detectability, called d_s, is derived from the operating characteristic, and the functional relation between d_s and some experimentally manipulated variable constitutes the primary result in such psychophysical experiments.

When a signal is presented in a fixed-interval experiment, it is usually coincident with the light that defines the observation interval; also, trials occur at regular intervals. In the present type of experiment, the observation interval is not coincident with the light, but it precedes the light by a fixed amount of time. When the flash of light occurs, the listener must decide whether or not a signal was presented in the observation interval which preceded the light. The time between the onset of the observation interval and the flash of light is called memory time, T_m. The top panel of Fig. 1 will help to describe the events that constitute a trial. The break in each of the lines indicates a random temporal interval between trials. The middle line shows a trial in which a signal is presented. The top line shows that the light follows the signal by a fixed temporal interval T_m which was constant and known to the listener for a given experimental condition. This fact necessitated the random spacing of trials; otherwise, the listener could use the light to estimate the onset

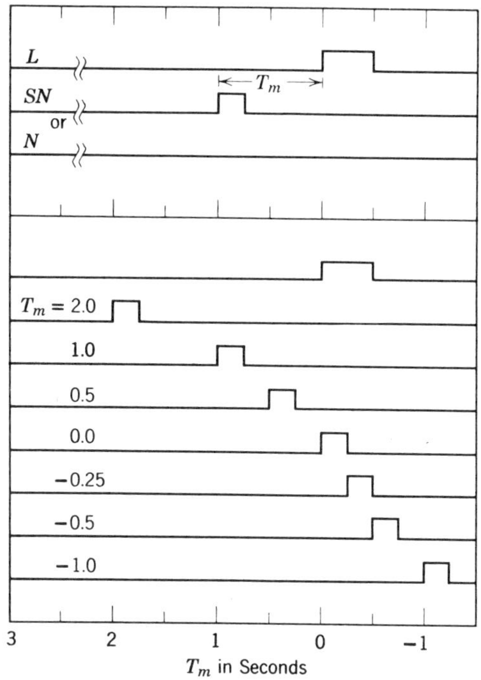

FIG. 1. Schema of the events occurring in a single trial. The top panel shows one of the seven experimental conditions. The break in each of the lines indicates the random temporal interval between trials. For this illustration, the value of T_m is 1.0 sec, which means that the onset of the signal preceded the onset of the light by 1.0 sec. On half the trials, the signal was not presented. For a given series of trials, the value of T_m was fixed and known to the listener. The lower panel illustrates each of the seven experimental conditions. For any one series of trials, only one of the conditions was used and the listener knew the value of T_m. Only trials on which a signal is presented are illustrated.

time of the subsequent observation interval. The present study investigated the effects of various amounts of memory time, as defined, on the detectability of a sinusoid presented in a background of noise.

PROCEDURE

Seven values of T_m were chosen. These were 2.0, 1.0, 0.5, 0.0, −0.25, −0.5, and −1.0 sec. These values refer to the onset time of the signal, if presented, relative to the onset time of the alerting light, as indicated in the bottom panel of Fig. 1. For example, a value for T_m of 2.0 means that the onset of the signal preceded the onset of the light by 2.0 sec.

The variable T_m is given positive values when the signal preceded the light because the emphasis here is on "memory time." The duration of the light was 0.5 sec. Therefore, when T_m was -0.5, the observation interval began with the termination of the light.

The temporal interval between successive observation intervals was determined at random by sampling from a rectangular distribution which extended from 6.0 to 13.0 sec in steps of 0.5 sec. Whether or not a signal would be presented on a given trial was also determined randomly, and the a priori probability of the occurrence of a signal was 0.5.

The signal was a sinusoid of 1000 cps, 0.25 sec in duration, and it was gated at random with respect to phase. The value of E/N_0 for all conditions was 12.6.

Testing was conducted in eight 2-hr daily sessions, the first of which was devoted to practice. A session consisted of 9 or 10 listening *periods*, each period requiring about 9 min. Because the listener had to attend nearly continuously to the input, these periods were broken up into four listening *units* of about 2 min each. Successive units were separated by a 15-sec rest interval. These units were defined for the listener by a light (not the trial light) which was turned off during the three 15-sec rest intervals. These short rests were introduced because the task required that the listener concentrate throughout nearly all of the 2-min unit. About 48 trials were presented in each 9-min period. For each listener, the total number of trials for each of the seven values of T_m ranged from 336 to 480. Two or three values of T_m were used in each session. During each session, before the first period devoted to a given value of T_m, the sequence of the signal and the light was demonstrated to the listeners with the noise turned off.

Prior to the present experiment, the eight listeners had extensive practice in the use of the rating method in the context of the fixed-interval experiment. They were used in Experiment III of the investigation of the effects of an *interval of time uncertainty* on detection (Egan, Greenberg, and Schulman, 1961 [13]). In Appendix II of Chapter 13 the experiments that the eight listeners participated in are listed; the present experiment is *item f*. All details of procedure not mentioned here were identical to those described for Experiment III of Chapter 13.

RESULTS AND DISCUSSION

Measures of detectability d_s were derived from operating characteristics which were plotted separately for each listener. For a given value of T_m, the eight values of d_s were averaged, and the results are shown in

Fig. 2. When the observation interval preceded the light (positive values of T_m), the detectability of the signal was less than when the observation interval was either coincident with the light or followed the onset of the light. Furthermore, performance was significantly better when the signal occurred during the second half of the light ($T_m = -0.25$) than when the signal and the light started simultaneously ($T_m = 0.0$). When the listener knows that the onset of the signal will be either coincident with or subsequent to the onset of the warning light, he no longer needs to listen carefully to the input during the long random intervals between the lights. When the signal starts with the light, however, the listener may be "caught unawares" and he may "miss" the first part of the signal.

The condition for which $T_m = -0.25$ is very similar to one of the conditions (ITU = 0.0) tested in Experiment III of Chapter 13. The mean value of d_s for $T_m = -0.25$ was 1.68; for ITU = 0.0, d_s was 1.56.

The present study has shown that the performance of a human listener declines when the observation interval and the alerting light are not coincident. For an ideal observer with perfect memory for the input waveform and with an unerring time sense, the situation described is no more difficult than the fixed-interval experiment in which the signal and

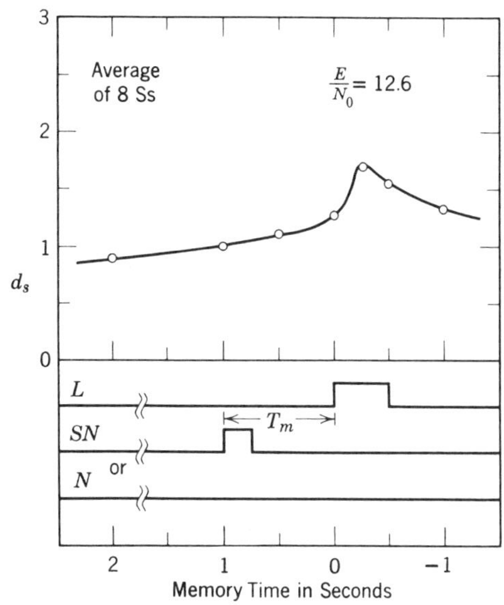

FIG. 2. The detectability index d_s plotted against memory time in seconds. Positive values of memory time T_m signify that the observation interval preceded the alerting light. Each point is the mean of eight values of d_s, one for each of eight listeners.

the trial light coincide. Such an ideal observer can record the input, note the time of the alerting light, and then measure back to the beginning of the observation interval; for him, detectability is independent of T_m. The human listener, on the other hand, has neither a perfect memory nor an unerring time sense. These imperfections are two sources of uncertainty that may be contrasted as follows: (1) The listener could have a faulty memory for the input during the observation interval, even though he might know exactly the time of onset of the interval; (2) The listener could have a faulty estimate of the time of onset of the observation interval, even though he might have a perfect memory of the input. The relative importance of these two sources of uncertainty cannot be clearly assessed from the present experiment. However, the following argument may be of value in the design of further studies on the effects of time uncertainty upon detection. Assume that the listener's error in his estimate of T_m introduces, in effect, an interval of time uncertainty (ITU) similar to that described by Egan, Greenberg, and Schulman in the previous chapter. Then, with $T_m = 1.0$ sec, assume that the listener's errors in his successive estimates of T_m are uniformly distributed over an interval extending from 0.75 to 1.25 sec. This dispersion in his estimates of T_m is equivalent to an ITU of 0.5 sec. The value of d_s for an ITU of 0.5 sec is 81 per cent of that for an ITU of 0.0 sec. Reference to Fig. 2 of the present paper shows that the value of d_s for $T_m = 1.0$ sec is only 59 per cent of the value of d_s for $T_m = -0.25$ sec. The decrement in d_s for $T_m = 1.0$ seems too large to be accounted for by an ITU of 0.5 sec.

The data for negative values of T_m provide more cogent evidence that poor memory for waveform accounts for part of the decrement in performance shown along the positive branch of the curve in Fig. 2. When the alerting light precedes the signal, the decrement would seem to be due entirely to the listener's faulty estimate of the time of onset of the observation interval. It is not unreasonable to assume that the amount of time uncertainty is about the same for $T_m = -1.0$ and $T_m = 0.5$. From Fig. 2 it may be determined that the value of d_s for $T_m = -1.0$ is 79 per cent of the highest value of d_s, whereas, for $T_m = 0.5$, the corresponding percentage is only 65. It therefore seems likely that the listener's faulty memory for waveform is responsible for a fair portion of the observed decrement in his performance.

SUMMARY

An experiment was conducted to determine how well listeners could judge whether or not a signal was presented in a noisy observation interval which had already occurred. The cardinal feature of the experiment is that the observation interval is not marked off for the listeners until some fixed time after its occurrence. The listening situation is described as follows. With a probability of 0.5, the signal (1000 cps, 0.25 sec) is presented at a randomly selected instant. A fixed time thereafter, the listener is informed (by a flash of light) of the real time at which the sinusoid may have occurred, and he responds with a rating of confidence. As compared with the typical fixed-interval experiment in auditory detection, two sources of uncertainty are emphasized in this situation: (1) The listener has a faulty memory of his transformation of the input waveform, and (2) he has a faulty estimation of the time of onset of the signal. From the results of previous experiments on the role of time uncertainty in detection, it appears that a fair portion of the decrement in performance results from poor memory for the input waveform.

ACKNOWLEDGMENTS

This research was conducted in the Hearing and Communication Laboratory of Indiana University with support from the Operational Applications Laboratory of the U. S. Air Force. This article appeared as Tech. Rept. No. AFCCDD-TN-61-1, and in J. acoust. Soc. Am., *1961,* **33,** *779–781.*

References

- Egan, J. P., Schulman, A. I., and Greenberg, G. Z. Operating characteristics determined by binary decisions and by ratings. *J. acoust. Soc. Am.*, 1959, **31,** 768–773. [7]
- Egan, J. P., Greenberg, G. Z., and Schulman, A. I. Interval of time uncertainty in auditory detection. *J. acoust. Soc. Am.*, 1961, **33,** 771–778. [13]

15

Operating Characteristics, Signal Detectability, and the Method of Free Response

James P. Egan, Gordon Z. Greenberg, and Arthur I. Schulman

This paper is concerned with an experimental analysis of the following problem in the study of the detection of signals in noise (Egan, Greenberg, and Schulman, 1959). A weak tone of brief duration is presented a number of times in a long observation interval. The temporal intervals between the presentations of the tones are randomly selected, and the listener is not given any information regarding the distribution of these random intervals. As a consequence, the listener does not know when a tone will occur, and he does not know how many tones will be presented to him for detection during the long observation interval. Only one response-key is provided for the listener, and he is instructed to press this "yes-key" just once each time he "hears a tone." In order to give further structure to this "free-responding situation," the listener is also instructed to adopt an arbitrary, but fixed, criterion according to which he can decide whether or not a tone has been presented. As here described, this entire procedure will be termed the *method of free response*.

Now, the listening situation described by the method of free response is particularly difficult to analyze simply because a trial is not defined. The data available for analysis consist solely of the time of occurrence of each signal and of each response. Many of the yes responses will surely be "detections," but some of them will be "false reports," or "false alarms." The problem consists in the determination of a procedure that allows the total number of yes responses to be partitioned meaningfully between "hits" and "false alarms." As will be seen from the present study, a wholly satisfying technique has not yet been devised for the analysis of the listener's behavior in this situation. Nevertheless, continued efforts should be devoted to an analysis of the method of free response, not because of its intrinsic value per se, but because a similar situation occurs so frequently in everyday perception.

Because the details of the analysis to be developed in the next section are rather involved, a précis follows.

Suppose that a large number of signals have been presented under the conditions prescribed by the method of free response. For the present argument, let just two intervals of equal duration be associated with each signal presentation. The first interval d_1 is taken immediately after the occurrence of each signal. The second interval d_2 is taken long after the occurrence of each signal, but always before the next signal comes along. In effect, time is reset to zero whenever a signal occurs. The number of responses in each of the two intervals is determined for a number of signal presentations.

Under a "strict" criterion, there will be a few responses in d_1, and there will be still fewer in d_2. If the listener now adopts a less strict criterion for "hearing a tone," the number of responses will increase in each of the two intervals, d_1 and d_2. Let the number of responses in d_1 be D (detections), and let the corresponding number in d_2 be O (operant level). Then, although the criterion itself cannot be directly evaluated, the use of a wide range of criteria will establish a relation between D and O.

In the present approach, an interpretation of the relation between D and O is made possible by a model that considers the task for the listener to be basically the same as that in a fixed-interval observation experiment (Egan, Schulman, and Greenberg, 1959). A trial in the fixed-interval experiment consists of a single observation interval that is well defined for the listener, who makes a response (say, *yes* or *no*) after each interval. The intervals consist of two types: (1) intervals during which the signal (SN) is in fact presented, and (2) intervals during which the signal is omitted (noise-alone intervals, N). In this context, an operating characteristic is the relation between the probability of an affirmation given a signal, $p(y|SN)$, and the probability of an affirmation given noise alone, $p(y|N)$.

In the model to be developed presently, the value of D is directly related to $p(y|SN)$, and the value of O is directly related to $p(y|N)$.

From these relations, it is possible to estimate the detectability of the signal by an index, d_s, which, unlike $p(y)$ or $p(y|SN)$, is relatively independent of the criterion adopted by the listener (Clarke, Birdsall and Tanner, 1959; Egan, 1958; Green, 1960; Pollack, 1959; Swets, 1959; Tanner and Birdsall, 1958; Tanner and Swets, 1954).[1]

THE MODEL

It is assumed that, when the listener is confronted with the task defined by the method of free response, he divides time into a succession of subjective intervals, each of duration T_σ. It will be considered that each of these subjective intervals implicitly defines a trial for the listener, and that he makes a decision after each such interval.

The duration T_σ of each subjective interval will be considered constant. Furthermore, it will be assumed that the signal always occurs wholly within one of the subjective intervals. The assumptions of the "constancy of T_σ" and of the "inclusion of the signal within T_σ" are, of course, unnecessarily restrictive, but in this presentation of the model a first approximation must suffice. Small fluctuations in the size of T_σ and the occasional overlap of a signal onto two intervals of T_σ should not seriously affect the analysis.

With a trial implicitly defined, it becomes reasonable to assume that the criterion adopted by the listener is associated with a particular point on a particular operating characteristic. The problem now consists in deriving appropriate measures of response which are related to the assumed criterial probabilities, $p(y|SN)$ and $p(y|N)$.

The rate at which the listener responds can be measured in the method of free response, and this rate, $n(y)/\text{sec}$, is related to the criterial probabilities as follows. If the listener makes a decision after each subjective interval, and if his decision is based upon some fixed criterion $[C_1: p_1(y|N), p_1(y|SN)]$, then for subjective intervals that contain the signal,

$$n_1(y|SN)/\text{sec} = p_1(y|SN)/T_\sigma \tag{1}$$

Similarly, for subjective intervals that contain noise alone,

$$n_1(y|N)/\text{sec} = p_1(y|N)/T_\sigma \tag{2}$$

[1] It is likely that some of the contradictory results obtained in experiments on vigilance are due to the failure of the experimenter to take into account changes in the "false-alarm rate" as the "watch" progresses. For example, see Bakan (1955). Actually, Bakan recorded "errors of commission," but he does not relate them to his "threshold" measures. Although his data show that the false-alarm rate decreased during the session, Bakan still concludes that the threshold increased over time.

If the listener then adopts a different criterion, $[C_2: p_2(y|N), p_2(y|SN)]$, two new equations result.

For the subsequent argument the critical assumption is made that a change in the criterion adopted by the listener does *not* affect the size of T_σ.

If ratios are taken between the appropriate equations, there result

$$\frac{n_1(y|SN)/\text{sec}}{n_2(y|SN)/\text{sec}} = \frac{p_1(y|SN)}{p_2(y|SN)} \tag{3}$$

and

$$\frac{n_1(y|N)/\text{sec}}{n_2(y|N)/\text{sec}} = \frac{p_1(y|N)}{p_2(y|N)} \tag{4}$$

where the subscripts 1 and 2 refer to the two criteria C_1 and C_2.

These equations show that, with all the assumptions made above, the ratio of the ordinates of two points on an operating characteristic and the ratio of their corresponding abscissas may be empirically determined without knowing the value of the subjective temporal interval T_σ. Unfortunately, the ratios of the respective coordinates of two (unknown) points of a function are not sufficient to determine the function. An additional assumption is necessary in order to estimate which operating characteristic is determining the behavior of the listener. The "power-law assumption" will now be considered.

Operating characteristics that describe the behavior of the real listener are typically asymmetric with respect to the negative diagonal of the square plot whose coordinate system is $[p(y|N), p(y|SN)]$. On a normal-normal plot, these asymmetric functions usually are linear with a slope less than one. Such operating characteristics are reasonably well described by a power function of the form:

$$p(y|SN) = [p(y|N)]^k, \quad 0 < k \leqslant 1. \tag{5}$$

Figure 1 shows a family of operating characteristics with k in Eq. (5) as the parameter. Figure 2 shows the relation between k and d_s.

The power function has the following unique property. Let any two points be selected on one of the curves of Fig. 1. Let the ratio of the smaller abscissa to the larger abscissa of these two points define a derived abscissa, and let the ratio of the corresponding ordinates define a derived ordinate. The derived point whose coordinates are given by these ratios will fall on the curve from which the original two points were selected.

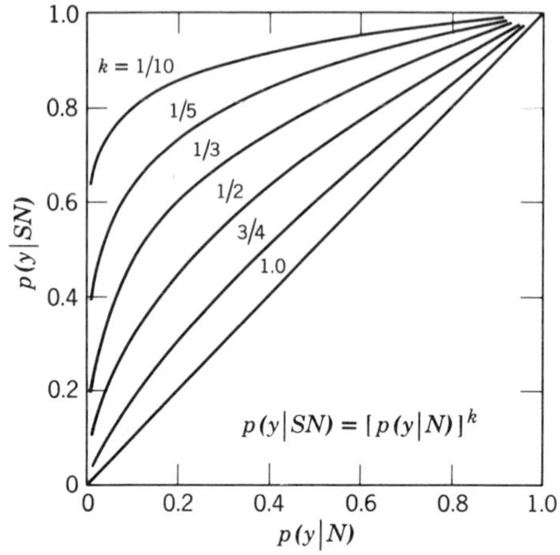

FIG. 1. Each operating characteristic of the family shown in the figure is described by a power function. The parameter k thus uniquely specifies each curve. The data obtained with the human listener are typically skewed so that the above operating characteristics may be considered fair approximations to the data.

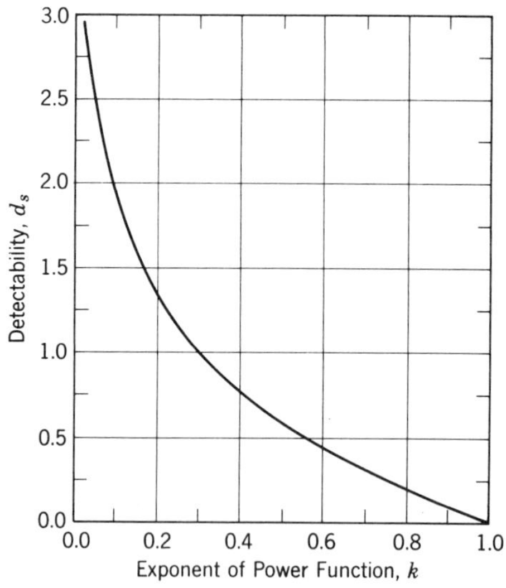

FIG. 2. As Fig. 1 shows, a complete family of operating characteristics may be generated by varying the parameter k from *one* to *zero*. The index of detectability d_s is here shown as a function of k.

If Eqs. (1) and (2) are substituted in Eq. (5) and if logarithms are then taken, the following equation results:

$$\log\,[n(y|SN)/\text{sec}] = k \log\,[n(y|N)/\text{sec}] + (k\text{-}1) \log T_\sigma \qquad (6)$$

That is to say, there should be a linear relation between the logarithm of the "rate of response ascribed to detections" and the logarithm of the "rate of response ascribed to false alarms."

Preliminary investigations made it clear that $n(y|N)/\text{sec}$ may be readily estimated by a measurement of the rate of response several seconds after the presentation of a signal. It is not at all obvious, however, how the measurement of $n(y|SN)/\text{sec}$ may be accomplished. In the development of this model, nothing was said about the reaction time of the listener in making his responses. This reaction time will vary from response to response, and its value will not be known in any particular instance. To make matters worse, the duration and the onset time of each subjective temporal interval, T_σ, are unknown. All of this means, of course, that it is not possible to associate the response of the listener with the subjective interval to which it refers.

Again, the power-law assumption makes it possible to side-step a direct measurement. Let $D = c_1 n(y|SN)/\text{sec}$, and let $O = c_2 n(y|N)/\text{sec}$, where c_1 and c_2 are constants of proportionality. Although c_1 may differ from c_2, it is assumed that, when the listener changes his criterion so that both $n(y|SN)/\text{sec}$ and $n(y|N)/\text{sec}$ change, c_1 and c_2 remain fixed at their original values.

Equation (6) may now be rewritten as follows:

$$\log D = k \log O + \log\,[c_1(T_\sigma)^{(k-1)}/c_2{}^k],$$

or

$$\log D = k \log O + c. \qquad (7)$$

Thus, the parameter k, or the related quantity d_s, may be estimated by measurements of two quantities, D and O, which are proportional, respectively, to $n(y|SN)/\text{sec}$ and $n(y|N)/\text{sec}$. If the momentary rate of response is plotted as a function of the time after the onset of the signal, then the rate should show an increase immediately after a signal. The rate should then decline to the operant level, $n(y|N)/\text{sec}$. If the listener's reaction time were constant, the rate of response immediately after a signal would show a sharp "peak" relative to the operant level, and the ordinate of this peak could be taken as proportional to $n(y|SN)/\text{sec}$. However, with a dispersion of reaction times, the value of D will be almost proportional to the area under the peak rather than proportional to the ordinate. This area will be slightly too large, because it will include responses made to a few noise-alone subjective intervals. Therefore, the analysis must involve an additional assumption, and this assumption may be rather directly verified by experimental test. It is assumed that the dispersion of reaction times is small, so that the ordinate of the peak is large relative to the width of its base. The data presented in the following pages show that this assumption is not unreasonable.

In order to test the model just given, the curve relating $n(y)/\text{sec}$ to the time after the signal is determined. A family of curves is secured by requiring the listener to change his criterion from one series of "long observation intervals" to the next. Then, according to Eq. (7), there should be a linear relation between $\log D$ and $\log O$, and the slope of this straight-line relation should identify the particular operating characteristic which is limiting the listener's performance.

In the development of the model, especially as it is represented by Eq. (7), there are four primary assumptions. These assumptions are now listed together for the sake of clarity.

(1) The listener divides time into a succession of temporal intervals T_σ, and he makes a "yes-no" decision after each of these subjective intervals.

(2) The value of T_σ is invariant with a change in the criterion adopted by the listener.

(3) There is a small dispersion of reaction times in the response. The mean of the reaction times for a given listener is irrelevant.

(4) The operating characteristic of the listener is described by a power function.

Two experiments were conducted in order to obtain preliminary tests of the model developed above. The results of Experiment I are in fair agreement with the model, in that $\log D$ turns out to be a fairly linear function of $\log O$. The results of Experiment II provide excellent support for the model, in that the relation between d_s and E/N_0 is consistent with previously established relations in a situation for which a trial is explicitly defined for the listener.

Experiment I

EXPERIMENTAL PROCEDURE. Against a continuous background of band-limited white noise, signals were presented at randomly selected points in time. The distribution of time intervals between signals was essentially rectangular, ranging in 2-sec steps from 3.5 to 7.5 sec and from 11.5 to 15.5 sec, and in steps of 0.5 sec from 7.5 to 11.5 sec. Thus, the mean time between signal onsets was 9.5 sec, but a signal could follow another by as little as 3.5 or as much as 15.5 sec. The distribution was not disclosed to the listeners, who were told merely that signals would be presented at random times, sometimes following close upon each other and sometimes spread relatively far apart.

Data were obtained daily in approximately 2-hr sessions from seven paid listeners, each of whom had listened for signals in noise for nearly six weeks prior to the start of these experiments.[2] The listeners were tested in two groups with S1, S2, S3, and S4 in one group, and S5, S6, and S7 in the other. Each listener sat in an isolated booth, and he had before him a single yes-key, which he was instructed to press just once each time he "heard a tone."

In an attempt to maintain high motivation, a bonus system was established, in which the listener could augment his regular salary. Each group of listeners was told that the size of the bonus would be determined by the performance of the group.

Each daily session consisted of 9 listening periods separated by 8 short rest intervals. Each period was subdivided into 4 listening units of approximately 2 min each. Successive 2-min units were separated by a 15-sec "time out," during which no signals were presented, although the noise was still present in the earphones. Signal lights informed the listener of (*a*) the start of a 2-min listening unit, (*b*) the beginning of a time out (end of a unit), and (*c*) the end of a period. Listeners were permitted to remove their headsets only during the rest intervals between periods. All listeners were given two sessions of practice in the method of free response before data were collected.

During the practice sessions, each listener showed that he could respond at widely divergent rates. These different rates were taken to represent different criteria for response, and each listener was asked in Experiment I to adopt four distinct criteria, designated as strict, medium, medium lax, and lax.

Eleven test sessions followed the two practice sessions. On 4 of these the listener was advised to be strict, on 3 to be medium, on 2 to be medium lax, and on 2 to be lax. The criterion for the first and last of these 11 sessions was lax, and the entire series was counterbalanced. The first of the 9 daily listening periods always served as a warm-up period so that the data to follow are based on responses made during the last 8 periods of each session.

---

[2] See Appendix II of Egan, Greenberg, and Schulman (1961) [13].

An attempt was made to confine each listener to a relatively small range of response rates for each instructional criterion. This was accomplished by advising the listener to be more or less strict, as the case might be, when in the previous period his number of responses fell outside the desired range. Most listeners, however, did respond within a narrow range of response rates for each assigned criterion, and after the initial instructions at the beginning of a session, no further instructions were usually necessary.

As will be explained later, each signal and the 7.2-sec interval that followed it were treated as the unit for analysis, and signals followed by intervals of either 3.5 or 5.5 sec were not included in the principal analysis of the data. It is for this reason that the mean number of signals per period used in the analysis of the data of Experiment I was only 39, with extremes at 28 and 48.

The signal and the noise were mixed electrically and then presented over binaural headsets with the two earphones wired in parallel and in phase. Four headsets were wired in parallel, and therefore the instantaneous, as well as the average, signal-to-noise ratio was correlated across a group of listeners. The signal was a "pure tone" of 1000 cps and was 0.25 sec in duration. The signal voltage was turned on without regard to phase and without the use of special devices, so that the (negligible) transients were determined by the response of the earphone (Permoflux Corporation, PDR-10). The white noise was generated by a 6D4 tube (noise generator, model 455-B, Grason-Stadler Company). The overall sound-pressure level of the noise (50 to 7000 cps) was about 65 db *re* 0.0002 microbar, and it was held constant for all sessions at this comfortable level for listening.

The relation between the signal and the noise will be specified by E/N_0, where E is the signal energy, and N_0 is the noise power per unit bandwidth. In Experiment I, E/N_0 was held constant at 12.6, or 11 db.

MEASUREMENT OF RATE OF RESPONSE. In order to estimate the instantaneous rate of response $n(y)$/sec the data were analyzed in the following manner. Each signal and each response was recorded upon an event recorder, and each response could be easily located in time with $d = (1/7.5)$ sec as the unit. At the onset of each signal, time was quantized into contiguous temporal intervals, each with a duration d. The successive intervals are denoted by the index i. Thus, the time in seconds of an event measured from the onset of a signal would be approximately id.

The duration of a response, as shown on the record, was variable, but for all practical purposes, the length of time that the listener held the key down for a single response was several times the duration of d. Consequently, only one response could have its onset in any particular d_i associated with a certain signal. When it is said that a response occurred "in" a particular interval d_i, it should be understood that the response had its *onset* in the interval d_i.

Figure 3 will help clarify how the records were analyzed. This figure arranges the random intervals between signals with the shortest interval at the top and the longest interval at the bottom of the schematic. On the basis of preliminary results, only the first 54 d_i's, each of length 1/7.5 sec, were analyzed. Thus, only responses occurring within 54 (1/7.5) = 7.2 sec after the onset of each signal were tabulated. The data from those signals that were followed by an interval of either 3.5 or 5.5 sec before the next signal occurred were not included in the analysis.

An example will illustrate the method of analysis. Table I displays the data obtained from the listener S4 for the first 2 seconds after the onset of the signal. (These data are from Experiment I and they are based on the 16 periods classified as "medium lax.") There were $N(S) = 634$ signals used in the analysis of these data. These 634 signals provided 634 intervals extending from 0.0 to 1/7.5 sec after the signal, 634 intervals extending from 1/7.5 to 2/7.5 sec after the signal,

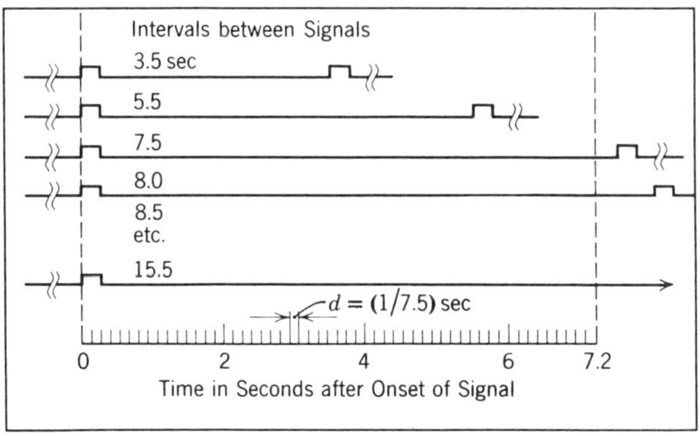

FIG. 3. Schema of data analysis. A time interval of 7.2 sec was defined for each signal (except signals followed by an interval of either 3.5 or 5.5 sec before the next signal occurred). This "long" interval began at the onset of each signal. Each long interval (associated with each signal) was then divided into 54 d_i's. The duration of each d_i was (1/7.5) sec. Of course, only one response could occur in any one interval, d_i, associated with a particular signal. The rate of response is estimated from the determination of the number of intervals, all with the same index i in d_i, in which a response occurred.

TABLE I. THE COMPUTATIONS OF THE VARIOUS MEASURES USED IN THE ANALYSIS OF THE METHOD OF FREE RESPONSE

1	2	3	4	5	6
i	id	$N(y)_i$	$\frac{N(y)_i}{N(S)}$	$\frac{n(y)}{\text{sec}}$	$\sum \frac{N(y)_i}{N(S)}$
1	1/7.5	6	0.009	0.071	0.009
2	2/7.5	10	0.016	0.118	0.025
3	3/7.5	7	0.011	0.083	0.036
4	4/7.5	38	0.060	0.450	0.096
5	5/7.5	76	0.120	0.899	0.216
6	6/7.5	81	0.128	0.958	0.344
7	7/7.5	87	0.137	1.030	0.481
8	8/7.5	31	0.049	0.367	0.530
9	9/7.5	15	0.024	0.177	0.554
10	10/7.5	13	0.020	0.154	0.574
11	11/7.5	14	0.022	0.166	0.596
12	12/7.5	7	0.011	0.083	0.607
13	13/7.5	14	0.022	0.166	0.629
14	14/7.5	3	0.005	0.035	0.634
15	15/7.5	7	0.011	0.083	0.645

and, in general, 634 intervals each having the same index i in d_i. In Table I, column 1 lists the ordinal number of the successive intervals, each of length 1/7.5 sec. Column 2 gives the time in seconds up to the end of the ith interval. Column 3 shows the raw data $N(y)_i$. For purposes of explanation of the remaining columns, consider the row for which $i = 7$. Thus, one response "occurred" in each of 87 of the 634 intervals identified as d_7. For the entry in column 4 the value of $N(y)_i$ was divided by $N(S)$, and the result in this case is 0.137. The value of $n(y)/\text{sec}$ is obtained for column 5 by dividing the value in column 4 by the size of the interval, 1/7.5 sec. The result is 1.030 responses per second. Column 6 is simply the running sum of column 4, and therefore it shows the number of responses per signal expected by the time that id seconds have elapsed after the onset of the signal.

Figure 4 summarizes the results of the computations made in Table I. In the complete analysis, the computations were extended to $id =$ 7.2 sec, and these results are also shown in Fig. 4.

The upper panel of Fig. 4 displays $n(y)/\text{sec}$ as a function of the time after the onset of the signal, and the lower panel shows the number of responses made up to the time id after the onset of the signal.[3]

[3] "Rate of response" is being used here in a special sense. The quantity $n(y)/\text{sec}$ is the momentary rate, and this rate is always referred to some particular time after the

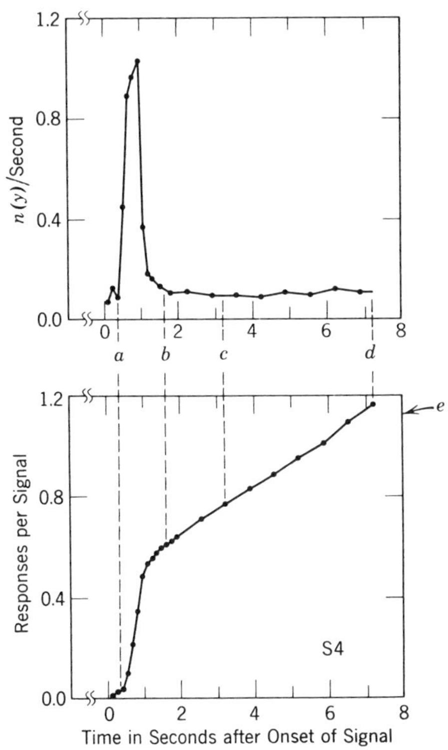

FIG. 4. Illustration of data analysis. The upper panel shows the number of responses per second as a function of the time after the signal. The lower panel shows the same data plotted in integral form. Table I illustrates the computations. In terms of the upper panel, D is taken as the area under the curve over the interval from a *to* b, and O is taken as the average value of $n(y)$/sec over the interval c to d, which extends from 3.2 to 7.2 sec. In terms of the lower panel, D is the difference between the ordinates of the two points that lie at the lower and upper portion of the sharp rise in the function, and O is the average slope of the curve over the interval from c to d.

The computations of D and of O will be illustrated with the aid of the data shown in Fig. 4. The measure D will first be considered. Now, according to the development of Eq. (7), it is sufficient to select some measure that is proportional to $n(y|SN)$/sec. Because the signals were

onset of the signal. Thus, the peak of the function shown in the upper panel of Fig. 4 does *not* mean that the listener showed a burst of responses immediately after a signal. A relatively large peak does mean that (1) he responded soon after nearly every signal and (2) he had a relatively small dispersion of "reaction times." For a fixed level of detectability of the signal, the ordinate of the peak is inversely related to the variance of the listener's reaction times. Consequently, D is taken as the area under the peak.

presented at random times, it is evident that the area under the peak of the curve that relates $n(y)$/sec to the time after onset of the signal is such a measure. The upper panel of Fig. 4 shows such a curve, and the value of D was taken as the area under this curve extending from a to b, as marked under the baseline of the figure. Of course, the interval extending from the point a to the point b varies from one criterion to another as well as from one listener to another. These two points at which the sides of the peak leave the baseline, or operant level, must be determined separately for each such curve. In most instances there is little uncertainty in the determination of the points a and b. Moreover, it should be emphasized that the determination of the measure D by this process does not involve an arbitrary definition of a "detection," such as "any response that occurs within three seconds after the occurrence of the signal."

The measure O is straightforward. An inspection of all of the data indicated that 3 sec after the onset of the signal, the listener was responding at a fairly constant average rate. Because of this fact, the measure O was always taken to be the average of $n(y)$/sec over the interval extending from 3.2 to 7.2 sec after the onset of the signal. This interval is indicated by c and d in Fig. 4.

Although the records obtained with the event recorder were read with a unit of 1/7.5 sec (Figs. 3 and 4, Table I), the data were grouped over larger units of time, either 2/7.5 or 5/7.5 sec, for the graphic presentation of the results.

CRITERIAL MEASURE AND CRITERIAL LEVEL. It is desirable to group the data obtained from several periods so that greater reliability may be obtained. Of course, the listeners were instructed to adopt some fixed criterion for a period of about 40 signals, and all periods that were run under a fixed instructional criterion could have been grouped. However, the instructions are interpreted in different ways by different listeners and the same listener may change his interpretation of a criterion from one period to the next. For this reason, it is necessary to measure the criterion adopted by the listener in terms of his performance, and a "criterial" measure was computed for each period.

The *criterial measure* of a period is defined as the number of responses per signal made in the 7.2-sec interval that begins with the onset of the signal. Figure 5 shows a grouped frequency distribution for the 88 periods for listener S3. The values along the horizontal scale represent the criterial measure of the period. The vertical scale indicates the number of periods having the same criterial measure. For purposes of analysis, the periods were grouped into four categories by the three

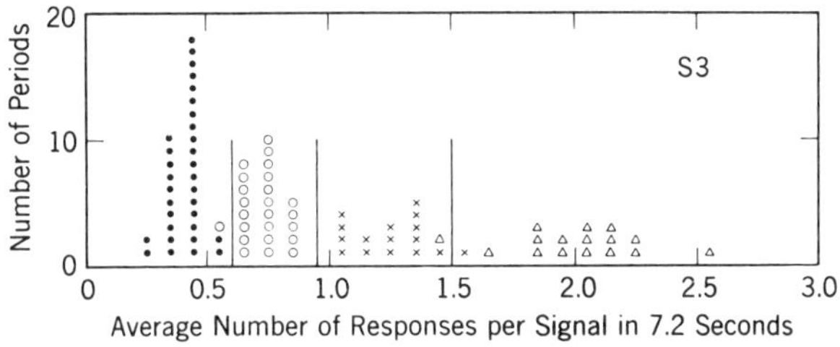

FIG. 5. Each point is based on one period (about 8 min of listening with about 40 usable signals). The values along the horizontal scale represent the number of responses per signal made during an interval that extends from the onset of the signal to 7.2 sec after the onset. This value is called the criterial measure of a period. The four different symbols represent the four instructional criteria: filled circles represent strict; open circles represent medium; x's represent medium lax; and triangles represent lax. The three vertical lines show how the periods were divided for purposes of averaging the data over a set of periods. These dividing points on the scale termed the criterial measure are called "criterial cuts."

vertical lines. A period was included within a criterial category according to the criterial measure of that period, and not according to the instructional criterion under which the period was obtained. It can be seen that there is little discrepancy between these objective cuts and the instructional category. These three cuts are termed *criterial cuts.* The set of periods between two criterial cuts is called the *criterial category.* The data for the other six listeners are similar to those shown in Fig. 5.

As will be seen below, it is convenient to have a single measure of the criterion for the set of periods that are grouped into a single criterial category. This measure, the *criterial level,* is simply the mean value of the criterial measures of those periods that belong to a single criterial category. Reference to the lower panel of Fig. 4 will clarify the meaning of the criterial level. The curve shown relates the number of responses per signal to the time after onset of the signal. Therefore, the ordinate of the point plotted at 7.2 sec after the signal (indicated by e) is the criterial level of the set of periods that were grouped in order to construct Fig. 4.

For the various functional relations to be presented, the data were first grouped into criterial categories as defined by the criterial cuts of Fig. 5 for Experiment I, and of Fig. 11 for Experiment II.

The measure O could also have been used to classify objectively each listener's 88 periods into the criterial categories. However, the criterial measure used has O as one of its components and, for a given listener, the Pearsonian correlation coefficient r between the criterial measure as defined and the values of O is about 0.97.

RESULTS. Figure 6 shows for listener S3 the rate of response as a function of time after the onset of the signal. The four panels correspond, respectively, to the four criteria of strict, medium, medium lax, and lax. The four curves, from strict to lax, are based upon 33, 23, 16, and 16 periods, respectively (see Fig. 5). The area under the peak of the curve is defined as the measure D, and, as the criterion is relaxed, the value of D increases. However, the value of the baseline, or operant level O, also increases. From these four curves, four points whose coordinates are log O, log D are obtained for the determination of a single measure of detectability, k or d_s. These four points are plotted for S3 in Fig. 9.

An important feature of Fig. 6 should be pointed out. The curve obtained under a lax criterion shows a depression in the rate of response

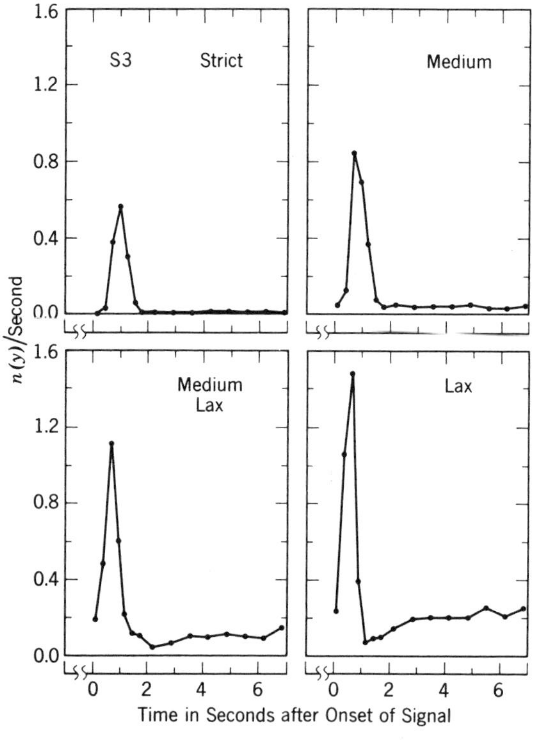

FIG. 6. Curves showing the rate of response as a function of the time after the onset of the signal. These curves were computed in the manner illustrated in Table I. The four curves correspond to the four criterial categories of strict, medium, medium lax, and lax (see Fig. 5). As predicted by the power-law assumption, the operant level O increases by a larger factor than the area under the peak D as the criterion is relaxed.

immediately after the peak. This depression in the rate also occurs, but to a smaller degree, for S3 under the criterion of medium lax. It is for this reason that the operant level O was defined as the rate of response over the interval extending from 3.2 to 7.2 sec after the onset of the signal.

The curves presented in Fig. 6 show the rate of response as a function of time after the signal. In such a form, the measures D and O are readily identifiable.

For certain purposes it is more convenient to consider the number of responses per signal as a function of the time after the signal. The method of computation is illustrated in Table I. Figure 7 shows the curves for S3, and these functions are based on the same data as are shown in Fig. 6. Thus, an ordinate of the curve labeled S in Fig. 7 taken at a given time after the signal is the area under the corresponding curve of Fig. 6 computed from zero time up to the given time. Figure 8 presents the data for the other six listeners of Experiment I.

It will be recalled from the model that Eq. (7) predicts that log D will be a linear function of log O. Furthermore, the measure of detecta-

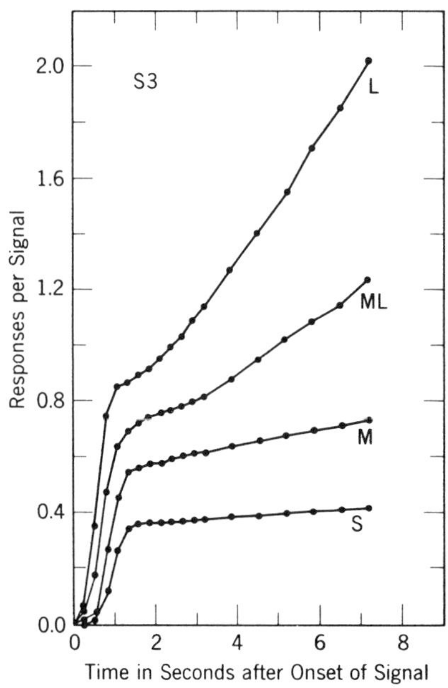

FIG. 7. Curves showing the number of responses per signal as a function of the time after the signal. The four curves correspond to those shown in Fig. 6. The measure D is the difference between the ordinates of the two points that lie at the lower and the upper portion of the sharp rise in the function. The measure O is the average slope of the curve over the interval from 3.2 to 7.2 sec.

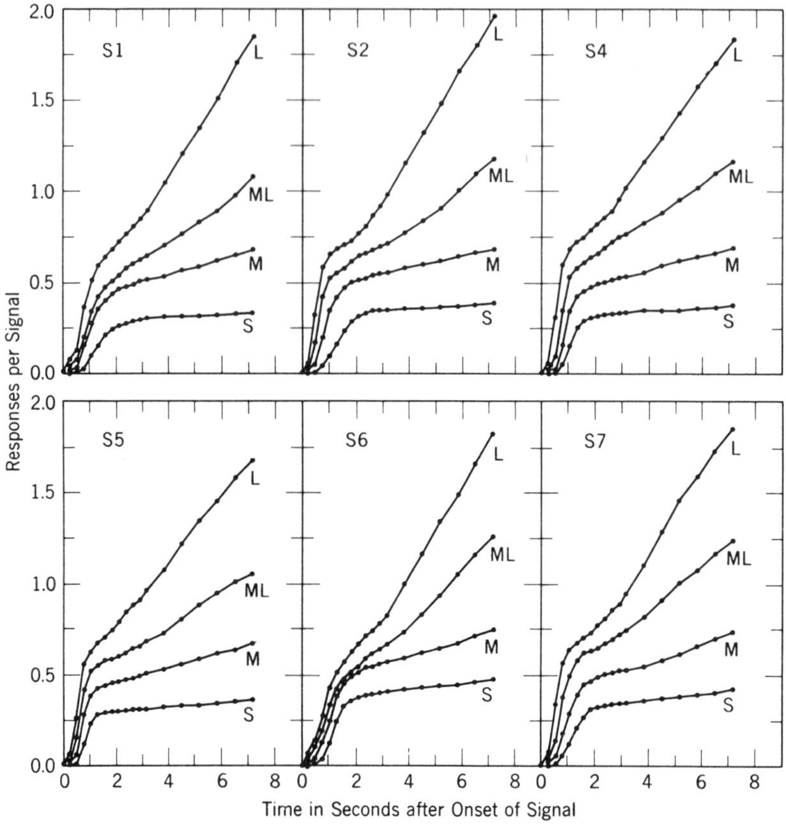

FIG. 8. The same relations as those of Fig. 7 shown for the other six listeners.

bility k will be the slope of this straight-line relation. Figure 9 shows for each of the seven listeners of Experiment I the values of (log D) and of (log O), as derived from Figs. 7 and 8.

Table II shows, for each listener, the slope k of the corresponding straight line in Fig. 9. These values of k were transformed to values of d_s by means of Fig. 2, and the mean value of d_s, based on the data for the seven listeners of Experiment I, is 1.29. When the same signal is used with the same value of E/N_0 in a fixed-interval observation experiment, the mean value of d_s for the same seven listeners is 1.55.

The "goodness of fit" of the straight lines in Fig. 9 requires further comment. In all instances the point corresponding to the condition of lax lies below the straight line. It will be recalled that the relation between the rate of response and the time after the signal for high rates of responding shows a depression in the rate immediately after

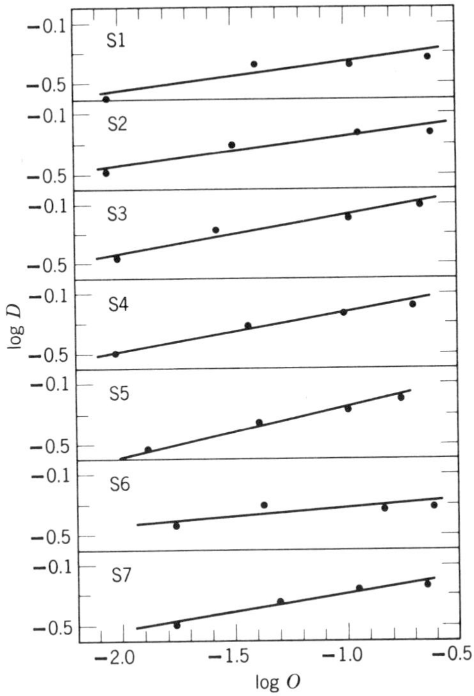

FIG. 9. Each panel shows the data for one of the seven listeners of Experiment I. The value of D is proportional to the area under the peak of a curve that relates $n(y)$/sec to the time after the onset of the signal. The value of O is the average value of $n(y)$/sec over the 4-sec interval that extends from 3.2 to 7.2 sec after the onset of the signal. In each panel, a straight line has been passed through the points by eye. The slope of this line gives the value of k for the power function.

TABLE II. THE SLOPE k OF EACH OF THE STRAIGHT LINES FITTED BY EYE TO THE DATA OF FIG. 9 IS SHOWN SEPARATELY FOR EACH LISTENER. VALUES OF k WERE TRANSFORMED TO VALUES OF d BY MEANS OF FIG. 2.

S	k	d_s
1	0.19	1.42
2	0.19	1.42
3	0.27	1.12
4	0.26	1.15
5	0.33	0.95
6	0.12	1.78
7	0.25	1.18
Mean		1.29

the peak of such a curve. This depression must mean that the listener is relatively refractory for a brief interval immediately after he makes a response. As a consequence, if the listener makes a response immediately before the presentation of a signal, he is more likely to miss the signal than if he has not made the previous response. Now, as the listener relaxes his criterion, the probability increases that a response will occur just prior to the presentation of the signal. As a consequence, the "hit rate" will not increase as rapidly as is predicted by the model. It must be said, then, that the model fails at high rates of responding, because the strong assumption is made that the process consists of a sequence of Bernoulli trials. It may be added, however, that the results of Experiment II are in excellent agreement with the model, probably because in that experiment high rates of responding were avoided.

A careful examination of the relations between the rate of response and the time after the signal (Fig. 6) indicates that the peak of the function occurs slightly earlier in time after the signal as the listener relaxes his criterion. A measure of the "reaction time" or "latency" was secured as follows. The time after the onset of the signal for each response that contributed to the area under the peak of the curve was tabulated and the mean of these times was computed. Of course, these responses may also be identified as those that make up the value of D. The mean time so computed is termed T_L, and Fig. 10 shows T_L plotted against the criterial level of those periods that were grouped into a single criterial category. As might be expected, the value of T_L decreases as the listener relaxes his criterion for "hearing a tone."

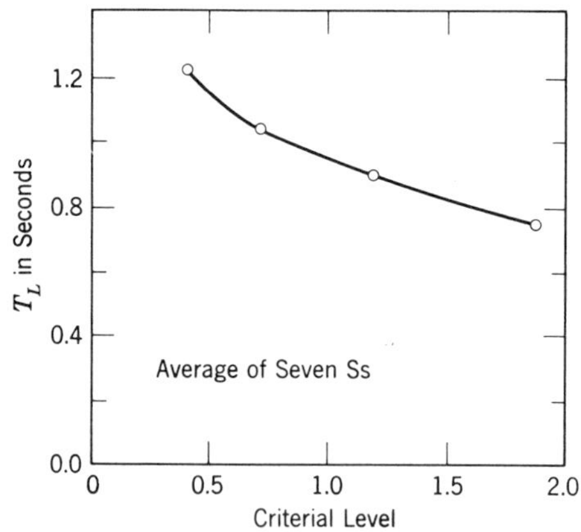

FIG. 10. Showing the decrease in "reaction time" as the listener relaxes his criterion. The value of T_L is the mean of the times of occurrence of the responses that contribute to the measure D.

Experiment II

A second experiment was conducted to test further the predictions of the model developed to analyze the data obtained by the method of free response. If the assumptions made are reasonably representative of the processes involved, then the relation between d_s and E/N_0 for weak signals should be similar to that obtained in a fixed-interval observation experiment. Experiment II was designed to determine this relationship.

EXPERIMENTAL PROCEDURE. This second experiment was conducted in much the same way as the first. All the mechanics of presenting the stimuli and of recording the responses were the same as for Experiment I. The records obtained with the event recorder were analyzed in the same manner as that already described.

There were three principal differences between the two experiments. In Experiment II: (*a*) three values of E/N_0 were used, (*b*) only three criteria were required and high rates of responding were avoided, and (*c*) data were obtained under all three criteria during each session.

Four of the listeners of Experiment I (S3, S5, S6, and S7) again served as a group of listeners. As before, they earned a bonus in addition to their regular pay. Eleven sessions of nine periods each were run, and all data were collected at one E/N_0 before moving on to the next. Again, the signal was a sinusoid of 1000 cps with a duration of 0.25 sec. The listeners were tested first with an E/N_0 of 12.6 (11 db), then with 7.9 (9 db), and finally with 20.0 (13 db). Because the listeners had not previously been exposed in a free-responding situation to the latter two values of E/N_0, a number of practice periods were given when these new E/N_0's were introduced. As in Experiment I, the first period in every session was devoted to practice.

In each session the listener was required to adopt three different criteria, designated as strict, medium, and lax. These criteria correspond to the criteria of strict, medium, and medium lax of Experiment I. In all, 78 test periods were conducted, and the number of periods run under each condition may be determined from Fig. 11. The mean number of signals used in the analysis was 40 per period.

The data obtained from several periods were grouped into a single category for purposes of analysis. Figure 11 shows the criterial measure for each of the periods (about 40 signals per period). The two vertical lines drawn in each panel mark the dividing points between adjacent criterial categories. As in Experiment I, a period was included within a criterial category according to the criterial measure of that period, and

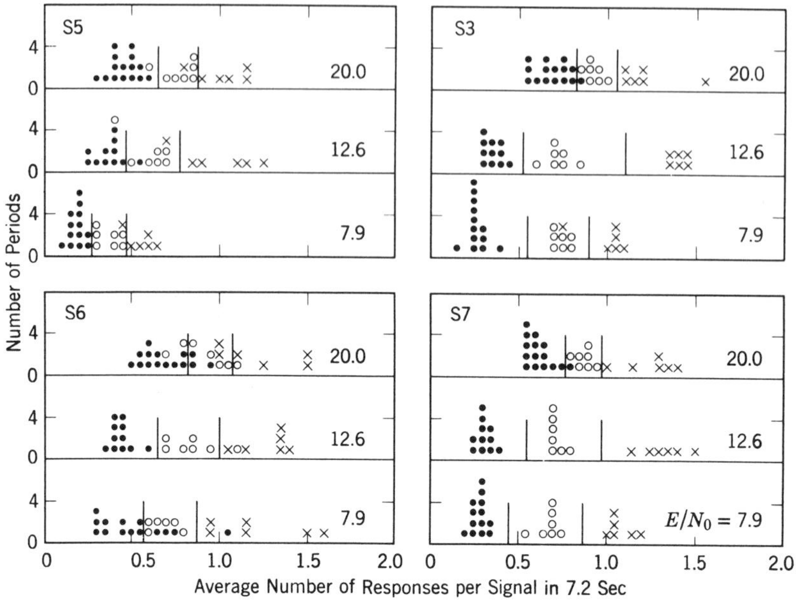

FIG. 11. Each point is based upon one period (about 8 min of listening with about 40 usable signals). The values along the horizontal scale represent the number of responses per signal made during an interval that extends from the onset of the signal to 7.2 sec after the onset. This value is called the criterial measure of a period. The three different symbols represent the three instructional criteria: filled circles represent strict; open circles, medium; and x's, lax. The two vertical lines show how the periods were divided for purposes of averaging the data over a set of periods.

not according to the instructional criterion under which the period was obtained.

The *criterial level* was defined as in Experiment I; it is the mean value of the criterial measures of those periods that belong to a single criterial category.

RESULTS. Figure 12 shows for one listener, S7, the rate of response as a function of the time after the onset of the signal. A comparison among the various curves of Fig. 12 gives support to the notion that the detectability of a signal in the free-responding situation might be specified by the utilization of one, rather than two or more, functions of the type shown. Thus, the value of D for the curve obtained with a strict criterion and with an E/N_0 of 20.0 is nearly the same as the value of D for the curve obtained with a lax criterion and with an E/N_0 of 12.6. However, it is clear that the "strict curve" in question was obtained with a higher E/N_0 than the "lax curve" because the operant

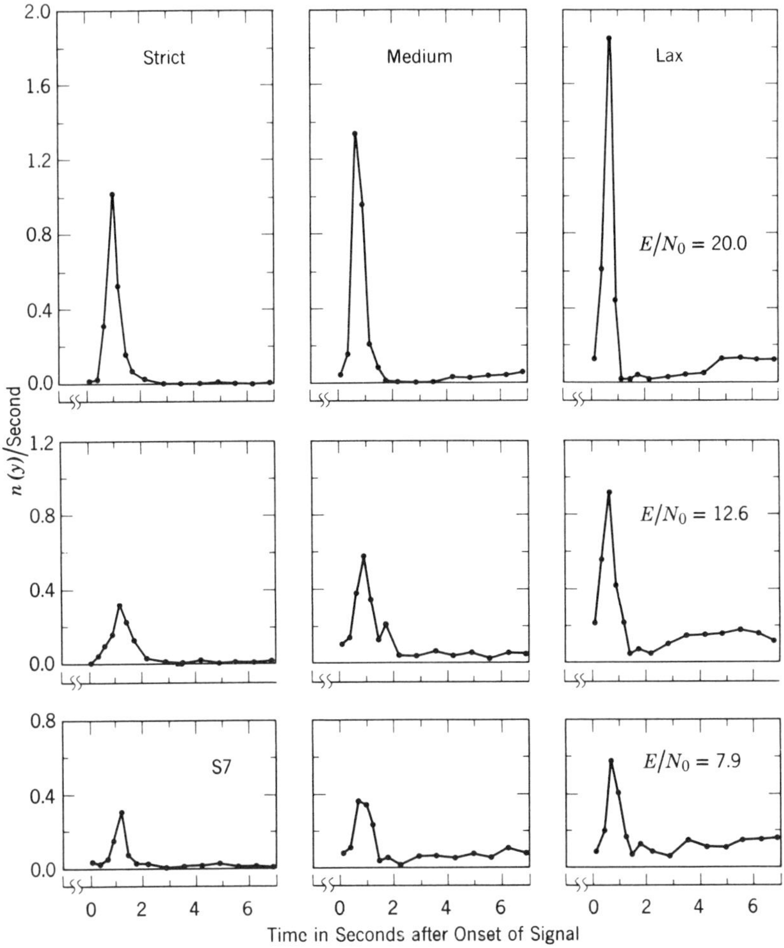

FIG. 12. Curves showing the rate of response as a function of the time after the onset of the signal. These curves were computed in the way illustrated in Table I. The three panels along the bottom of the figure show the data for the weakest signal, and the three panels along the top show the data for the strongest signal. For each E/N_0 both D and O increase as the criterion of the listener is relaxed.

levels of these two curves are so different. As yet, a model that relies upon an estimate of the parameters from only one such function has not been devised.

The number of responses per signal as a function of time after the onset of the signal is shown separately for each of the four listeners in Fig. 13. Each function represents the area under the corresponding

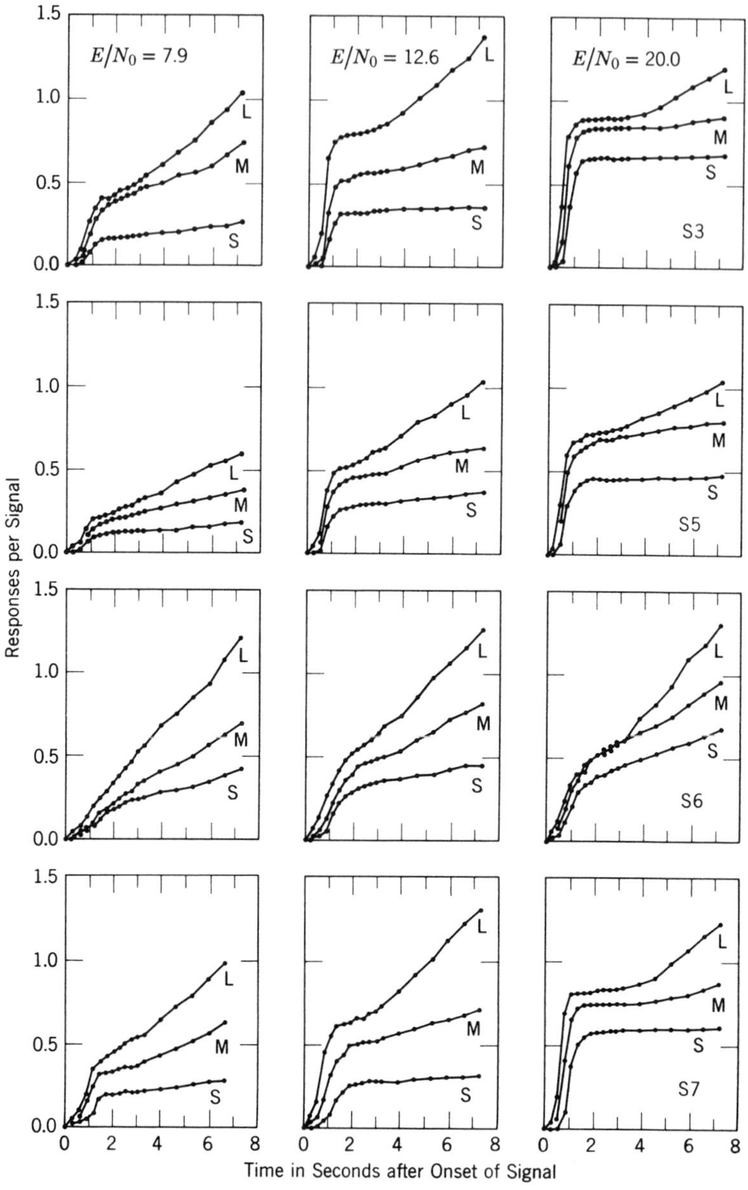

FIG. 13. Each of these curves shows the number of responses per signal as a function of the time after the signal. The three curves of each graph correspond, respectively, to the three criterial levels of strict, medium, and lax. The data in a given row of three graphs were obtained with a single listener, who is designated in the right-hand graph. The value of E/N_0 for the four graphs of a given column is indicated in the upper graph. The data for S7 are shown in a different form in Fig. 12.

curve that shows the rate of response at various times after the onset of the signal.

Values of D and of O were computed from the data shown in Fig. 13 (see Fig. 4). The results are shown in Figs. 14 to 17 for each listener separately. The slope k of each line was determined, and these values of k were converted to the corresponding values of d_s by means of Fig. 2. Table III shows the values of k and of d_s for each listener.

TABLE III. THE SLOPE k OF EACH OF THE STRAIGHT LINES, FITTED BY EYE TO THE DATA OF FIGS. 14–17, IS SHOWN IN THIS TABLE. THE VALUES OF k WERE CONVERTED TO VALUES OF d_s BY MEANS OF FIG. 2.

	E/N_0					
	7.9		12.6		20.0	
S	k	d_s	k	d_s	k	d_s
3	0.51	0.58	0.24	1.22	0.09	2.02
5	0.39	0.81	0.27	1.12	0.16	1.57
6	0.28	1.09	0.19	1.42	0.09	2.02
7	0.41	0.76	0.35	0.90	0.10	1.92
Mean		0.81		1.17		1.88

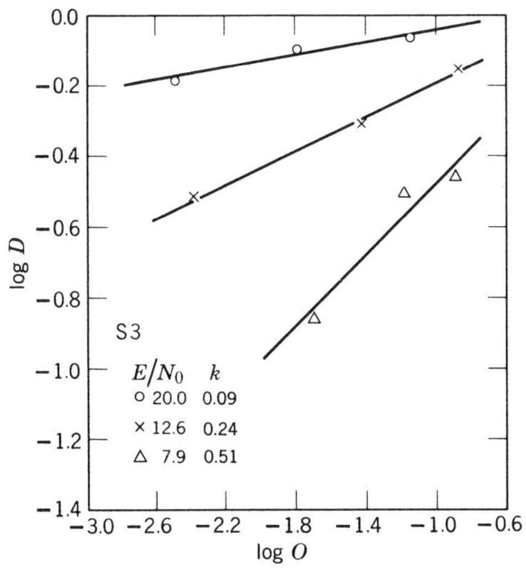

FIG. 14. According to Eq. (7), there should be a linear relation between log D and log O. This figure shows how well the data of Experiment II support the model by which Eq. (7) was derived. Each of the curves of Fig. 13 provides one value of log D and one value of log O, and these two numbers are the coordinates of one point for one of the illustrated functions.

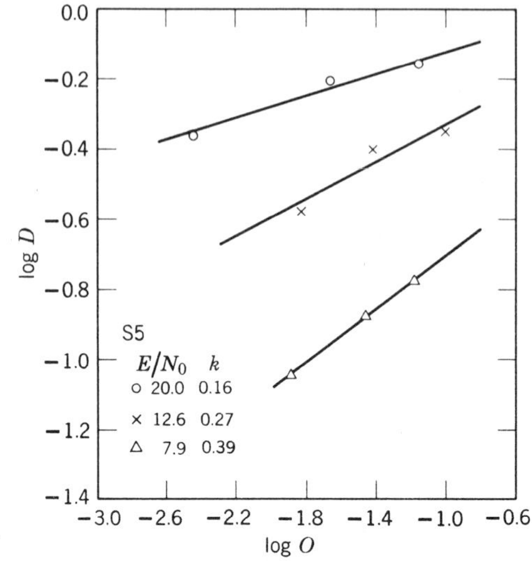

FIG. 15. These curves show the same relations as those presented in Fig. 14 for a different listener.

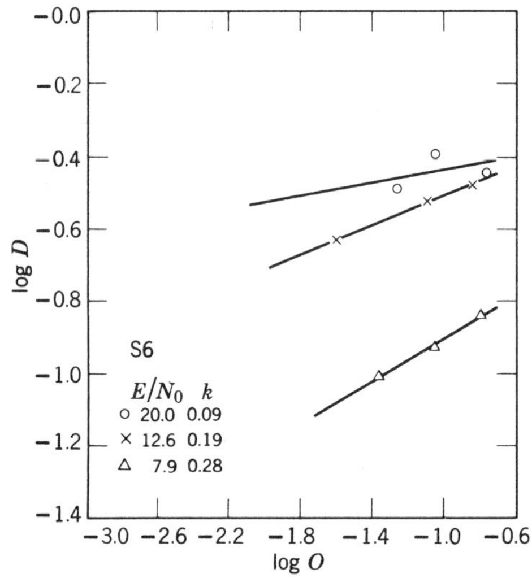

FIG. 16. These curves show the same relations as those presented in Fig. 14 for a different listener.

If the analysis which led to Eq. (7) is at all adequate, then for very weak signals the value of d_s, as determined by means of the measure k, should be an approximately linear function of E/N_0. Figure 18 shows

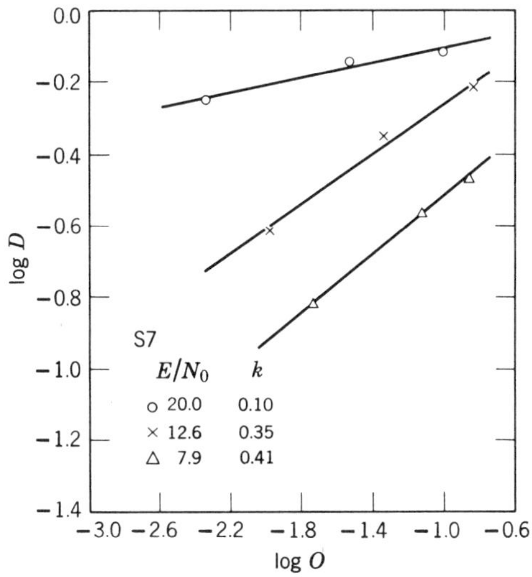

FIG. 17. These curves show the same relations as those presented in Fig. 14 for a different listener.

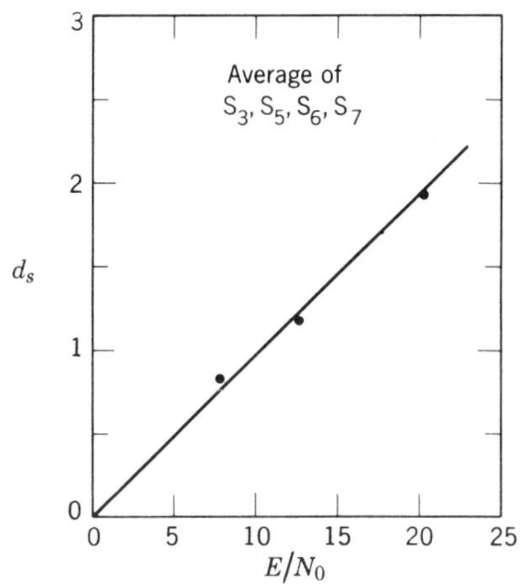

FIG. 18. Relation between d_s and E/N_0 as determined from the results of Experiment II. The points represent the mean values taken from Table III. The slope of the straight line drawn by eye through the points is 0.097.

that d_s as determined from the results of Experiment II is in fact a nearly linear function of E/N_0. This result provides support for the contention that the model, developed for the analysis of the method of free response, permits a specification of the detectability of a signal in terms of d_s.

The slope of the straight line of Fig. 18 is 0.097. For comparative purposes, Fig. 19 shows the relation between d_s and E/N_0 as secured in a fixed-interval observation experiment. The details of the procedure were similar to those described for the rating method in Egan, Schulman, and Greenberg (1959). The slope of the function in Fig. 19 is 0.137. The fact that the slope of the curve of Fig. 19 is greater than that shown in Fig. 18 provides additional empirical support for the model.

The duration of T_σ apparently corresponds to the interval of time uncertainty (ITU) as described in Egan, Greenberg, and Schulman (1961). Consequently, the functional relation between d_s and E/N_0 shown in Fig. 18 makes it possible to estimate the size of T_σ. Comparison of Fig. 18 of the present article with Fig. 10 of the article on ITU indicates that T_σ is about two seconds.

The value of $E/N_0 = 12.6$ used in Experiment I was one of the three values used in Experiment II, and four of the seven listeners of Experiment I also participated in Experiment II. Table IV shows the values of k and of d_s as determined from these two experiments. The data for Experiment I were taken from Table II, and the data for Experiment II were taken from Table III.

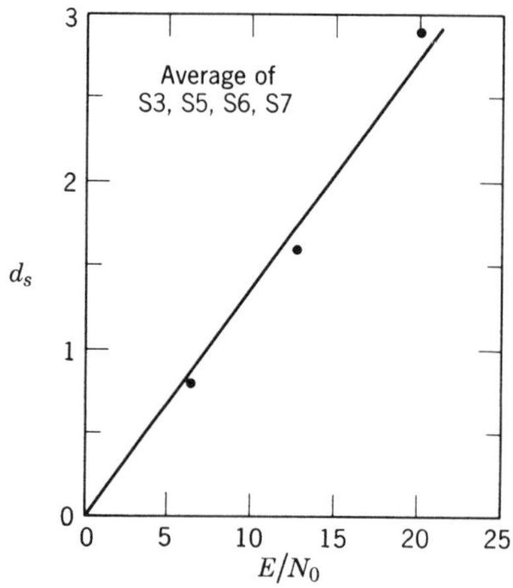

FIG. 19. Relation between d_s as determined in a fixed-interval observation experiment. The slope of the straight line drawn by eye through the points is 0.137. As expected, the performance of the listeners is considerably better in the fixed-interval situation than in the free-responding situation, but the form of the function is approximately linear in both cases.

TABLE IV. DATA WERE AVAILABLE FOR $E/N_0 = 12.6$ FROM BOTH EXPERIMENTS I AND II. THE FOUR LISTENERS OF EXPERIMENT II ALSO PARTICIPATED IN EXPERIMENT I. THE TABLE SHOWS VALUES OF k AND OF d_s AS DETERMINED IN THE TWO EXPERIMENTS.

	Experiment I		Experiment II	
S	k	d_s	k	d_s
3	0.27	1.12	0.24	1.22
5	0.33	0.95	0.27	1.12
6	0.12	1.78	0.19	1.42
7	0.25	1.18	0.35	0.90
Mean		1.26		1.17

Figure 20 shows the value of T_L as a function of the criterial level. It may be recalled from Experiment I that the value of T_L is computed from the times of occurrence (relative to the signal) of those responses that contribute to the measure D. Although T_L decreases as the listener relaxes his criterion, there appears to be no clear relationship between T_L and E/N_0.

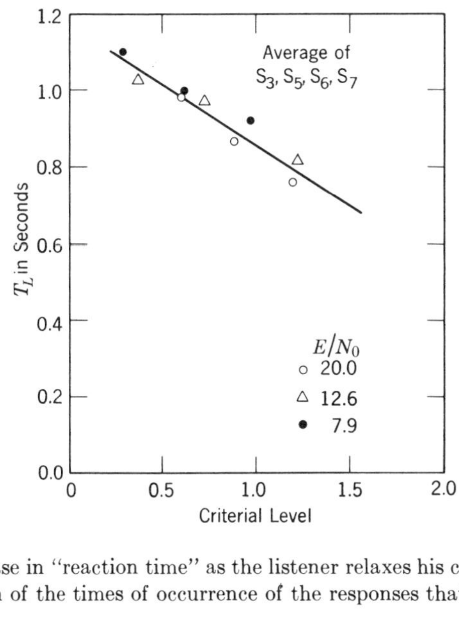

FIG. 20. Decrease in "reaction time" as the listener relaxes his criterion. The value of T_L is the mean of the times of occurrence of the responses that contribute to the measure D.

Effect of high rate of responding

It was pointed out in the discussion of the results of Experiment I that high rates of responding might result in spuriously high values of d_s. In that discussion, it was mentioned that, as the listener relaxes his criterion, the probability increases that he will make a response just prior to the presentation of a signal. If the listener is relatively refractory for a brief interval immediately after a response, then he is more likely to miss the signal than if he had not made the previous response.

After the original analysis of the data was completed, the graphic records of Experiment II were re-examined so that those signals which were immediately preceded by a response could be excluded in a second analysis. After an inspection of the available functions which showed the rate of response as a function of the time after the signal, it was decided to exclude a signal if a response had occurred in a 2-sec interval preceding that signal. For the strict criterial category, about 6 per cent of the signals had a response just prior to their onset, whereas for the lax criterial category this value increased to about 23 per cent.

It was found that the exclusion of signals which were immediately preceded by a response resulted in slightly lower values of d_s. It will be recalled that, when d_s was plotted against E/N_0 in Fig. 18, the slope of the straight line which was passed through the points was 0.097. When the mean values (0.61, 1.12, and 1.68) for the reanalysis are plotted against E/N_0, the slope of the line is 0.085. It appears reasonable, therefore, to conclude that, if very high rates of response are avoided,then the value of d_s will be only slightly overestimated.

HYPOTHESIS OF MULTIPLE RESPONSES

The present model maintains that the measure D increases as the criterial level increases because the listener responds to a greater proportion of the signals. Alternative interpretations are possible, of course, and the purpose of this section is to provide evidence against an interpretation in terms of "multiple responses to the signal."

It might be maintained that on a given presentation the signal is either above or below the "threshold." Under a strict criterion, the listener responds whenever the tone is above the threshold, and the operant level represents guesses on the part of the listener. Then, when the listener is required to relax his criterion, it might be supposed that he does two things: (1) He increases the guessing level and O increases; and (2) he gives several responses in quick succession each time he "hears a tone." The second factor is required in such a model, because, when the criterion is relaxed, the number of responses by which D increases is too large to be accounted for by an increase in the guessing level.

In order to test this hypothesis, the data for S3 of Experiment I and for all four listeners of Experiment II were analyzed as follows. Examination of Figs. 7, 8, and 13 establishes that responses that contribute to D occur almost entirely within two seconds after the onset of the signal. Therefore, the following proportions were determined from the data: (1) the proportion of signals for which no response occurred within two seconds after the onset of the signal, (2) the proportion of signals for which exactly one response occurred in two seconds, and (3) the proportion of signals for which two or more responses occurred in two seconds. This analysis showed that, averaged over all criteria, the estimated probability of two or more responses within two seconds after the onset of the signal was only 0.006. Evidently, as the listener's criterion is relaxed, the measure D increases because the listener responds to more signals, not because he responds more than once to "threshold signals." The results thus support the saying that "the listener can hear well into noise."

COMMENT

There are two matters that should be brought out, and both concern certain limitations upon the method of analysis presented in this article.

(1) It has already been mentioned that the values of d_s obtained in Experiments I and II are probably too high, because high rates of response appear to interfere with the detection process. This deficiency in the model is best realized by a comparison between the method of free response and the fixed-interval experiment. In the fixed-interval experiment, a decrease in the performance level as the criterion is relaxed will show up as a decrease in d_s. On the other hand, in the present analysis of the method of free response, a decrease in performance as the criterion of the listener is relaxed results in a decrease in the slope k of the line relating log D to log O, thereby raising the value of d_s. Fortunately, a model that makes it possible to derive d_s from a single function showing $n(y)$/sec against time should not experience this difficulty.

(2) In the preceding experiments, values of k were obtained. Granted the assumption that the power function adequately describes the operating characteristic in the free-responding situation, then a particular value of k specifies a particular operating characteristic. However, the method of analysis as presented in this study does not make it possible to specify the particular point on the operating characteristic that cor-

responds to any one of the criteria adopted by the listener. Again, a comparison with the results obtained in a fixed-interval experiment emphasizes the limitations of the model presented.

SUMMARY

The method of free response refers to the following listening situation. Against a background of noise, a weak signal is presented several times in a long (2-min) observation interval. The temporal intervals between the presentations of the tones are randomly distributed; consequently, the listener does not know when a tone will occur, and he does not know how many tones will be presented. From one series of observation intervals to the next, the listener is instructed to adopt various criteria and to press the single response-key each time he "hears a tone." The problem consists in the determination of a procedure that allows the total number of yes responses to be partitioned meaningfully between "hits" and "false alarms." A model is developed in which the measurable quantity, rate of response, is related to the "hit rate" and to the "false-alarm rate." Although the criterion adopted by the listener cannot be directly evaluated, the use of a wide range of criteria makes it possible to estimate the detectability d_s of the signal. Two experiments are described, and the results support the model.

ACKNOWLEDGMENTS

This research was conducted in the Hearing and Communication Laboratory of Indiana University with support from the Operational Applications Laboratory of the U.S. Air Force. This article is a condensed version of Tech. Rept. No. AFCRC-TR-59-58, and appeared in J. acoust. Soc. Am. *1961,* **33,** *993–1007.*

References

- Bakan, P. Discrimination decrement as a function of time in a prolonged vigil. *J. exp. Psychol.,* 1955, **50,** 387–390.
- Clarke, F. R., Birdsall, T. G., and Tanner, W. P., Jr. Two types of ROC curves and definitions of parameters. *J. acoust. Soc. Am.,* 1959, **31,** 629–630.
- Egan, J. P. Recognition memory and the operating characteristic. Indiana University: Hearing and Communication Laboratory, 1958, Technical Note AFCRC-TN-58-51.
- Egan, J. P., Greenberg, G. Z., and Schulman, A. I. Detection of signals presented at random times. *J. acoust. Soc. Am.,* 1959, **31,** 1579. (Abstract)
- Egan, J. P., Greenberg, G. Z., and Schulman, A. I. Interval of time uncertainty in auditory detection. *J. acoust Soc. Am.,* 1961, **33,** 771–778. [13]

- Egan, J. P., Schulman, A. I., and Greenberg, G. Z. Operating characteristics determined by binary decisions and by ratings. *J. acoust. Soc. Am.*, 1959, **31,** 768–773. [7]
- Green, D. M. Psychoacoustics and detection theory. *J. acoust. Soc. Am.*, 1960, **32,** 1189–1203. [2]
- Pollack, I. On indices of signal and response discriminability. *J. acoust. Soc. Am.*, 1959, **31,** 1031.
- Swets, J. A. Indices of signal detectability obtained with various psychophysical procedures. *J. acoust. Soc. Am.*, 1959, **31,** 511–513. [6]
- Tanner, W. P., Jr., and Birdsall, T. G. Definitions of d' and η as psychophysical measures. *J. acoust. Soc. Am.*, 1958, **30,** 922–928. [5]
- Tanner, W. P., Jr., and Swets, J. A. A decision-making theory of visual detection. *Psychol. Rev.*, 1954, **61,** 401–409.

section four

PHYSIOLOGICAL APPLICATIONS

Application of the general theory of signal detectability to human observers suggests certain coordinations between process descriptions in the theory and hypothetical behavioral processes. Possible correspondences between elements of the theory and physiological structures are also evident. Thus, implications of detection theory and data for physiological theory may be drawn. Moreover, the methods and measures specified by detection theory can be applied directly in physiological experiments.

In this section Tanner considers "Physiological Implications of Psychophysical Data" [16], with an emphasis on memory. FitzHugh, in "The Statistical Detection of Threshold Signals in the Retina" [17], determines several properties of the sensitivity index d′ *as measured from the responses of single nerve cells. The article by Eijkman and Vendrik ("Detection Theory Applied to the Absolute Sensitivity of Sensory Systems" [18]) is primarily concerned with physiological noise; it also presents the only experimental application of detection theory to the skin senses.*

16

Physiological Implications of Psychophysical Data

Wilson P. Tanner, Jr.

In this paper I am presenting an approach to the study of psychophysics that includes the use of mathematical models. While the individual experiments can each be interpreted as a contribution to an area in psychophysics, the program can be interpreted as an experiment testing the possibility of a profitable use of a particular scientific philosophy in the study of an area of psychology.

This philosophy involves the use of mathematical models in a manner similar to that of the physicist. It employs, first, the use of simple models describing the relations of only a few observable variables. The measures describing the relations among these variables may be measures of variables that exist only as force and gravity in physics and that can be measured only by observing their consequences. As measurement techniques become more nearly precise, or as the conditions of the experiment are extended to include a wider range, it will likely become apparent that the model had been adequate only because it was tested with coarse measurement over a restricted range of conditions. At this point it will be necessary to expand or modify the model to include the new data.

The expanded or modified model should still include the original model as applied to the limited conditions. Figure 1 is intended to illustrate this point. The large space is one that includes all possible data that might be relevant to a particular area of science. Many of the points in this space will never appear as data for they are contradictory to the "truth," whatever that may be. The shaded area in the center represents the data at hand. A model describing these data could be expanded in any of a number of directions. The large areas *A*, *B*, and *C* represent models, each of which includes the original model. If the next datum collected turns out to be at point 1, model *C* can be eliminated from consideration. If it is collected at point 2, *A* and *C* can be eliminated. Either point, however, requires an expansion of the original model.

We have tried to work with a general model that includes all of the points in the space. It is the general model of testing statistical hypotheses. The model can be expanded to specify the data that must appear if a sensory threshold exists, if Luce's (1959) axiom 1 is valid, or if the observer is intelligent. The general theory can be made specific in a number of ways; it is an experimental question that determines precisely how it should be made specific.

I shall trace one phase of the history of this program, showing how we introduced the concept of memory to modify the model to incorporate a wider range of conditions. At times I shall try to point out some of the physiological implications. However, one must not forget that I am talking about concepts that are unobservable, and the physiologist may find himself faced with similar problems to those of the physicist chasing electrons: he may have to devise physiological cloud chambers so that his electrons will create an observable phenomenon. The nerve impulse may not be sufficient.

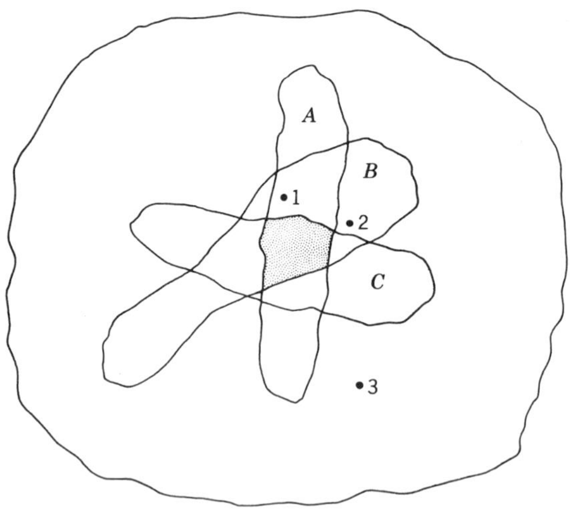

FIG. 1. Theory space.

WHAT IS A PSYCHOPHYSICAL EXPERIMENT?

Psychophysics is the study of the relations of psychological quantities to physical quantities. A block diagram of a typical experiment is shown in Fig. 2. The experimenter designates an observation interval in time, during which one of the signals from the ensemble is transmitted over the channel. At the end of the observation interval, the observer is asked to choose one of a set of responses. The joint event of the signal transmitted and the signal received (as indicated by the response) is recorded.

WHAT ARE THE MEASURES?

In the simplest type of psychophysical experiment, in which a particular signal or nothing is transmitted during the observation interval, the data may be summarized as illustrated in Fig. 3. In this figure, the rows represent the transmitted events as modified by the channel. If the signal is transmitted, the observer's input is the signal as randomly perturbed by the channel. Here we are calling this input "signal plus noise." If nothing is transmitted, the observer's input is labeled "noise."

The columns are the observer's responses. "Yes" means that he considers the input to have arisen from signal plus noise, while "No" means that he considers the input to have arisen from noise alone. The data can be summarized as percentages that, in analysis, are assumed to be estimates of probabilities. Two conditional probabilities are estimated: the probability that if the signal is transmitted the observer's input will lead to a "yes" response, $P_{SN}(A)$; and the probability that if nothing is presented, the observer's input will lead to a "yes" response, $P_N(A)$. $P_{SN}(A)$ is the detection probability and $P_N(A)$ is the false-alarm probability.

In Fig. 3,

$$P_{SN}(A) \approx \frac{n_1}{n_1 + n_2}$$

and

$$P_N(A) \approx \frac{n_3}{n_3 + n_4}$$

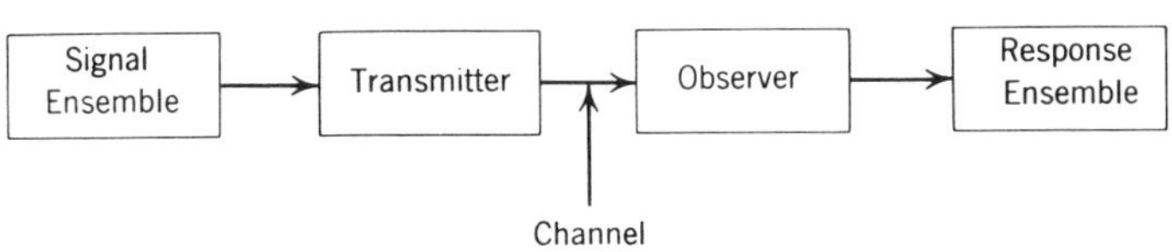

FIG. 2. Block diagram of a typical psychophysical experiment.

	Yes	No	
Signal Plus Noise	n_1	n_2	$P_{SN}(A) \approx \frac{n_1}{n_1 + n_2}$
Noise	n_3	n_4	$P_N(A) \approx \frac{n_3}{n_3 + n_4}$

FIG. 3. Data summary of a typical psychophysical experiment.

where the n's represent a counting of the various joint events occurring during the experiment.

The fact that we summarize the data as estimates of probabilities implies that the tasks the observer is asked to perform in psychophysical experiments are tasks in which there is a probability of error; consequently they satisfy Middleton's criterion (personal communication) as tasks that can be handled within the framework of decision theory. According to this criterion, whenever one is confronted with a probability of error he is confronted with a decision-theory problem.

DECISION-THEORY MODEL

Decision theory serves as a foundation for the theory of signal detectability, a theory that deals with exactly the problem with which the observer is confronted in a psychophysical experiment. An examination of the general theory of signal detectability may help us understand the observer's problem.

The problem handled in this theory is that in which an observer is asked to state which of two conditions led to a particular input, x, during a fixed observation interval, 0 to T. Any input x is considered to be a function of time, $x(t)$, since time is the dimension of the observation interval. With each $x(t)$ two numbers are associated: the likelihood of that particular $x(t)$ if the signal was transmitted, $f_{SN}[x(t)]$; and the likelihood of that particular $x(t)$ if nothing was transmitted, $f_N[x(t)]$. The decision-theory problem is to select a criterion space, A, which includes all of those $x(t)$'s that should lead to the response "yes" and excludes all of those $x(t)$'s that should lead to the response "no."

This can be stated as the problem of choosing the criterion space A such that

$$P_{SN}(A) - WP_N(A) = \text{a max}$$

where W is a number or weighting function.

The following proof, derived by Fox (1953), demonstrates that the likelihood ratio describes the information contained in the input, $x(t)$, relevant to the choice the observer must make. The equation just given can be written as

$$\int_A f_{SN}[x(t)]\, dx(t) - W \int_A f_N[x(t)]\, dx(t) = \text{a max}$$

Since both variables are over the same space, this becomes

$$\int_A f_{SN}[x(t)]\, d - W f_N[x(t)]\, dx(t) = \text{a max}$$

In this form it becomes obvious that the integral is a maximum if all positive values are included and no negative values are included. Thus the space, A, should include all of those values of $x(t)$, and only those, which satisfy the following inequality:

$$f_{SN}[x(t)] - W f_N[x(t)] \geq 0$$

or

$$l[x(t)] = \frac{f_{SN}[x(t)]}{f_N[x(t)]} \geq W$$

where $l[x(t)]$ is defined as the likelihood ratio.

WHAT IS AN IDEAL OBSERVER?

Given Fox's proof, we are now in a position to define an ideal observer, illustrated in its general form in Fig. 4. It is an observer who computes the likelihood ratio associated with the input, $x(t)$, and then matches this value to a point in the criterion space. If the point is contained in A, then it says "yes," the signal was transmitted. If it is not in A, then it is in the complement of A, CA; and the observer says "no," the signal was not transmitted. The computation of $l[x(t)]$ and the matching are performed without error.

If we were to attempt to designate in detail the construction of an ideal observer, it would be necessary to know the signals that might be transmitted, the properties of the perturbing noise, the way in which the signal and noise are combined, and the function, W, to be maximized. All of these parameters are required to specify the specific components (such as filters and integrators), and the particular criterion spaces, A and CA. Any change in the values of parameters can lead to a change in the detailed designation of the ideal observer. Thus if we want to consider the ideal observer as applied to specific situations, then there is an ideal observer for each specific case. They are all alike in that they

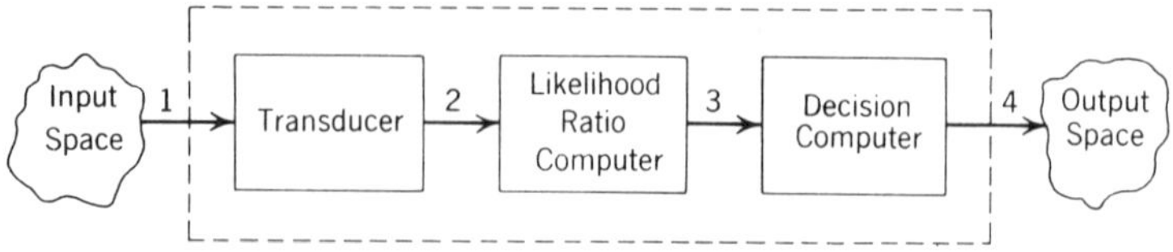

FIG. 4. Ideal observer.

compute likelihood ratios and say "yes" if the likelihood is greater than W. Whether any specific $x(t)$ leads to a "yes" or a "no" response depends on the signal and noise conditions from which it might have arisen and on the particular function, W, used in the maximization.

The whole operation is illustrated in Fig. 5. The part of the block diagram included in the dotted lines can be considered as an ideal sensory system. Those parts outside the dotted lines are the connecting links between the sensory system and the larger system that the sensory system serves. The connecting links mold the sensory system into an ideal form for the particular task at hand. It sets the parameters of the components and specifies the criterion spaces in a way that leads to optimum performance.

THE HUMAN OBSERVER AND THE IDEAL OBSERVER

We probably all agree that, in the strict sense of the word, the human observer cannot be considered as an ideal observer. Few of us would expect perfect computations of likelihood ratios and perfect matching into the criterion spaces.

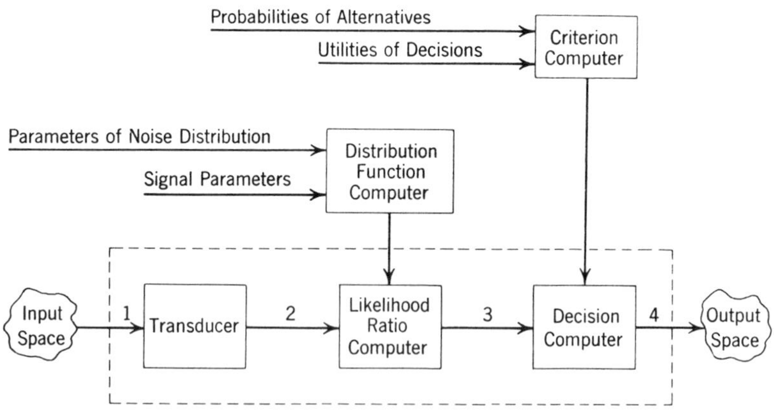

FIG. 5. The ideal observer with tie-ins to the system.

However, we might feel that the human observer's sensory system is, in a broad sense, similar to that of an ideal observer in some respects. It is, after all, a subsystem of an "intelligent" system and it seems not unlikely that the intelligent system would have some control over the form the subsystem assumes in facing any particular task. It may be molded in such a way that it exhibits a phenomenon we frequently refer to as "attention." Its performance may vary in a way that is consistent with different methods for computing W. While it may not achieve an ideal performance, it may in some ways tend toward an ideal performance.

If this is the case, then the experimenter must interpret his results in terms of the particular experimental conditions that have the potential of leading to a modification of the system. If these modifications are possible, then the physiologist is faced with a severe task in attempting to interpret data collected in experiments that eliminate the effects of the modifying agents. This line of reasoning clearly indicates physiological studies employing "consciously" behaving animals with implanted electrodes, the type of study I have heard Walter Rosenblith advocate many times.

Figure 6 shows a block diagram of an observer based on the ideal observer, but it also shows some of the places in which one might expect imperfections to exist. This diagram has as its basic structure that of the ideal observer, and the same links connecting the observer to the larger system. It has had added to it a number of memory banks that are immediately suggestive of imperfections. Let us examine the various properties an ideal memory must have in a simple detection experiment where the signal is a segment of a sine wave. This signal is specified

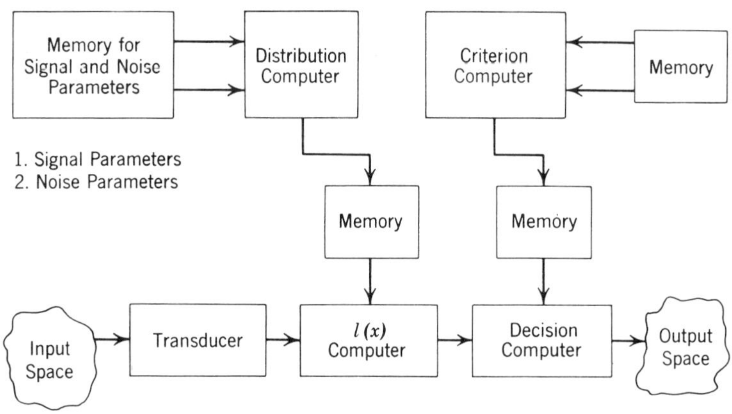

FIG. 6. The ideal observer modified to include memory.

exactly; thus when it occurs in the observation interval, 0 to T, it will occur at a precisely specified position within the interval. Its frequency, phase, and amplitude will also be specified precisely. This means that the function of time representing the signal can be positioned exactly in the observation interval. The value of this function can be precisely stated for any moment of time in the observation interval.

To be able to do this, an observer must have stored in his memory a precise representation of the function of time. He needs a clock mechanism that permits him to synchronize exactly with the observation interval, 0 to T, and to locate exactly in the interval the point at which the function of time should start, and precisely its duration. His memory must specify exactly the frequency, phase, amplitude, starting time, and duration of the segment of the sine wave. Any error in the memory will lead to a decrement in performance.

It is possible to make some inferences from psychophysical experiments regarding the role that each of these aspects of memory plays in the human observer's performance. It must be remembered, however, that these inferences are based on a model designed to describe the relation between the observables in a psychophysical experiment: the transmitted signals and the responses. The models can be looked at as mathematical equations fitting the data. As long as the data are finite, there are an infinite number of models that will fit equally well. Data collected in the future may eliminate this model, but will never confirm it. It uses words such as "memory" for the parameters because these words have intuitive appeal. The physiologist trying to correlate his observations with the parameters of the model must remember that the concept of memory arises from the model, not the data.

A PSYCHOPHYSICAL INVESTIGATION OF "MEMORY"

One of the concepts involved in using the theory of signal detectability as a tool for interpreting psychophysical data is expressed in the following "theorem":

If in two channels, one employing an ideal transmitter and an imperfect observer and the other a transmitter with statistical uncertainty and an ideal receiver, both transmitters having equal energies available, the performance as indicated by measures of the false-alarm rate and the detection rate are found to be identical, then the imperfect receiver can be said to introduce the same degree of uncertainty in its channel as the transmitter in the other channel.

The uncertainty attributed to the receiver, it was felt, would reflect the observer's memory. Consequently a series of models with specified transmitter uncertainties were studied, leading to calculations of the performance measure d' as a function of $2E/N_0$. Figure 7 shows these curves on a log-log plot, and a human observer's data superimposed. The notion was that if the human observer's data matched one of the curves, the degree of uncertainty introduced by him could be specified, and his memory characterized by a number, M, the parameter of the curves. This parameter corresponds to the number of orthogonal signals that can occur.

The concept is far too simple. The human observer's data did not fall on any one curve, but rather cut across curves. This suggested that a different model would be required for every signal level, at least in terms of the number categorizing the memory.

Careful examination of the experimental procedures under which the data were collected suggests that this is not unreasonable. Each signal level was studied in a sequence of 100 observations coming about five

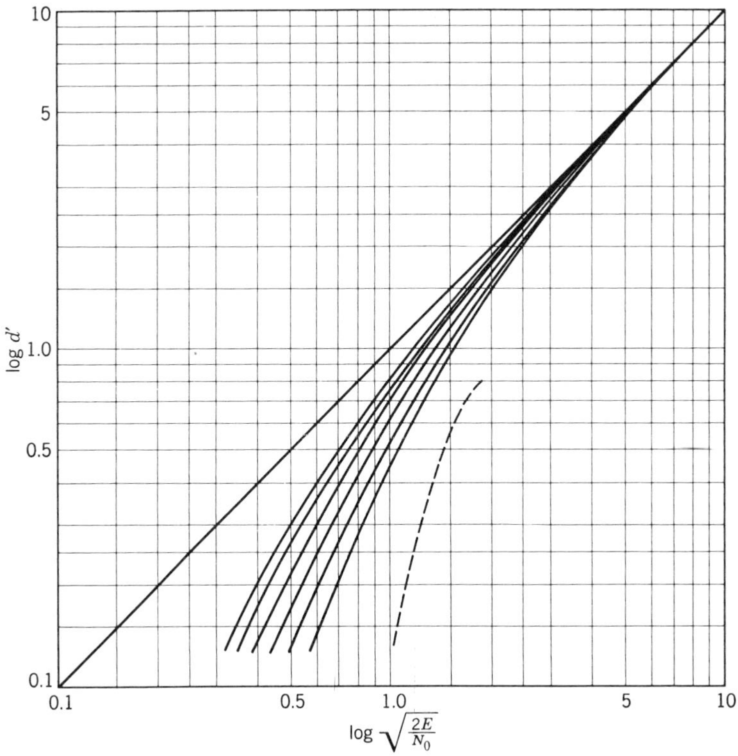

FIG. 7. Performance curves for signals specified statistically.

seconds apart. Before the sequence, the observer was permitted to listen to several samples of the signal without noise, and these noiseless samples were assumed to establish his memory.

If the signals are weak, then, as the sequence proceeds, the observer will receive few samples that are clear enough to reinforce his memory. If they are strong, he is more likely to receive some fairly good samples, and his memory on the average should be better throughout the sequence than it would be for the weak signals.

Elizabeth Shipley (personal communication) has recently performed an analysis of some data in which she considers the probability of a correct choice, given that the previous choice was correct and given that the previous choice was incorrect. She finds that a dependency exists when the signals are segments of sine waves, and does not exist when the signals are samples of noise. The dependency is in the right direction to support the hypothesis that a clear sample tends to reinforce the memory.

When Julian Bigelow saw some of the early results, he suggested a way of attacking the problem experimentally. He suggested that a sine wave of the same phase and frequency as the signal be added as a component of the noise, replacing the need for the observer's memory of frequency and phase. The signal would be superimposed on the sine wave during the observation interval. This procedure altered the slope of the psychometric function so that it agreed with one of the slopes of the computed curves of Fig. 7. However, it is positioned wrong.

There was still a need for the observer to have a memory for starting time and duration. My colleagues and I were able to extend Bigelow's suggestion in a way that could remove the need for this memory. This we have referred to as a "pulsed-carrier" experiment. In each observation interval we introduced a segment of sine wave whose amplitude was large. This segment matched the signal in frequency, phase, starting time, and duration. It was the observer's task to state whether the signal appeared on top of this pulsed carrier, or pedestal as J. C. R. Licklider calls it. In this case, the psychometric function turns out to be linear, as if there were some added noise.

This leads to an interpretation of the memories required as a function of the experimental design, as illustrated in Table I. There are three types of experiments: detection, continuous wave (CW), and pulsed carrier (PC); each with two subdivisions, "yes-no" and "two-alternative forced choice" (2AFC). The detection experiment requires a memory for frequency, phase, starting time, and duration. The CW experiment requires only starting time and duration memories, while the PC experiment requires none of these. The difference between a "yes-no" experiment and a 2AFC experiment is the need for amplitude memory in the "yes-no" experiment.

A summary of the results of the various experiments follows.

(1) In the detection experiment, the slope of the psychometric function is too great to be accounted for in terms of a fixed uncertainty. There is no difference between a "yes-no" and a 2AFC experiment, probably because the other memories are so poor that they mask the effect of amplitude memory.

(2) In the CW experiment, the slope of the psychometric function is such that it can be accounted for in terms of a fixed uncertainty. The function is misplaced, prohibiting an estimate of the degree of uncertainty. There is little, if any, difference between "yes-no" and 2AFC experiments.

(3) In the PC experiments, d' is a linear function of $(2E/N_0)^{1/2}$, a condition that can be accounted for by additive noise. Performance in 2AFC experiments is noticeably superior to that in "yes-no" experiments.

The analysis of the memory conditions shown in Table I is not precisely true for an imperfect observer, who, for example, must have some amplitude memory in the 2AFC, PC experiment; he must be able to remember the amplitude of the waveform in the first interval so that he can compare it to the amplitude of that in the second interval. In fact, the experiment can be looked at as a "yes-no" experiment in which the measure established in the first interval serves as a cutoff for

TABLE I. MEMORIES REQUIRED FOR DIFFERENT PSYCHOPHYSICAL EXPERIMENTS

Experiments		Required memories				
		Amplitude	Frequency	Phase	Starting time	Duration
Detection	"Yes-No"	+	+	+	+	+
	2AFC		+	+	+	+
Continuous wave	"Yes-No"	+			+	+
	2AFC				+	+
Pulsed carrier	"Yes-No"	+				
	2AFC					

the second. If the intervals are widely separated, this cutoff would not be precisely remembered. It might be as if noise were added to this cutoff, the amount of noise depending directly on the time between the two pulses.

Cutoff variance can be treated as additive noise, provided that all of the prior stages are linear, as illustrated in Fig. 8. There are three distributions shown: in each the abscissa is the value of the decision variable, and the ordinate is the probability density of that variable. The distribution to the left is for the second signal, given that it is the smaller of the two. The distribution to the right is for the second signal, given that it is the larger. The middle distribution is the critical value of the decision variable, x_c.

It is possible to transform to a new decision axis, $x - x_c$, where on this new axis there is a fixed cutoff at 0. There are now only two distributions, $x - x_c$ given the smaller signal, and $x - x_c$ given the larger signal. Each of these has added the variance of x_c to its original variance.

Using the form of the psychometric function for the pulsed carrier to demonstrate that the stages prior to the cutoff are linear, it should now be possible to study the variance of the cutoff as a function of the time, τ, between the observation intervals. One complication still exists, however: there must be a transducer type of operation at the input and, if τ is too small, independent observations cannot be expected. Thus the performance should drop both for very small values of τ and for very large values of τ. In between there should be a peak. In fact, the following equation should specify d':

$$(d')^2 = \eta_0(1 - e^{-e\tau}) \frac{2E_\Delta}{N_0 + k\tau}$$

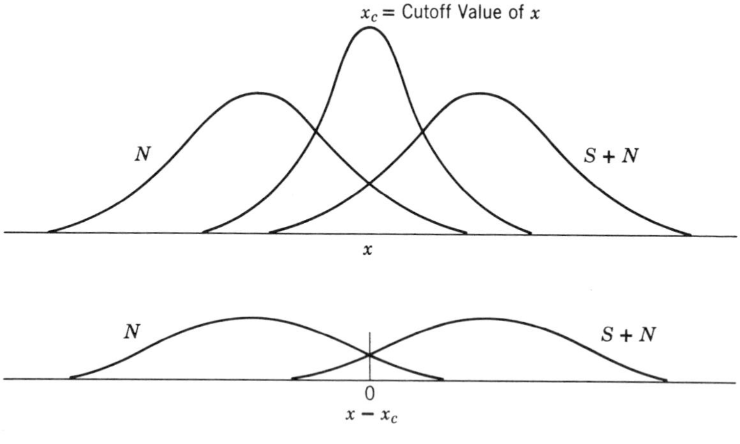

FIG. 8. Illustration of the cutoff variance as added noise.

where e is something like the time constant of the transducer, k is the noise energy per unit time added to the cutoff value, and η_0 represents the efficiency if added noise of the nervous system alone accounts for the fact that the efficiency is less than unity. A typical set of results is shown in Fig. 9.

The CW experiment, using the same observer, may be re-examined now. Suppose it is assumed that the value of $2E/N_0$ used in the experiment has been reduced to the value of $(d')^2$, as calculated by the equation with the parameters determined by the pulsed-carrier experiment. One may now plot the psychometric functions as $(d')^2$ versus the corrected value of $2E/N_0$ (Fig. 10). The misplacement of the curve is now corrected so that it is possible to estimate the degree of statistical uncertainty introduced by faulty memories of starting time and duration. The values of this parameter, M, for the four observers range from about 5 to approximately 12.

All of the experiments thus far discussed have involved acoustic signals. My colleagues and I have also made visual studies, and R. FitzHugh (1957) at the Johns Hopkins University, Baltimore, has reported some physiological data related to these studies. At first appearance there seems to be a discrepancy between FitzHugh's data and ours.

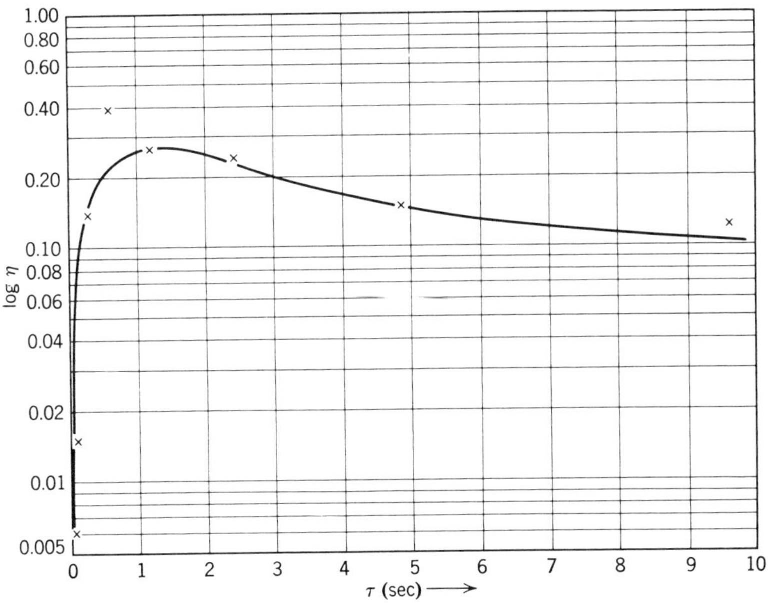

FIG. 9. Efficiency as a function of amplitude memory time.

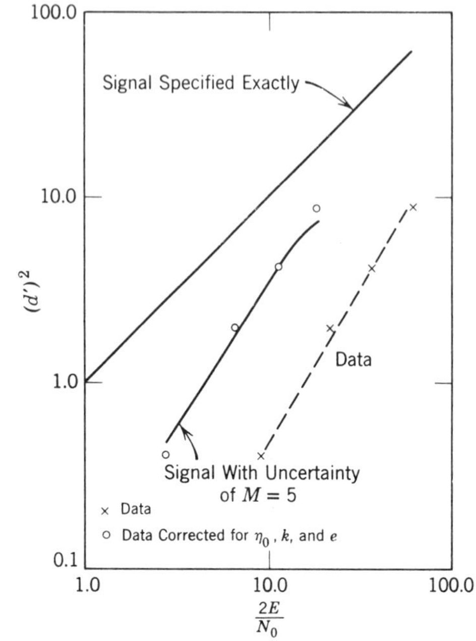

FIG. 10. Data corrected to permit an estimate of starting-time and duration uncertainty.

However, the discrepancy disappears when it is considered in terms of the memory framework.

FitzHugh studied the frequency of nerve impulses on the dark-adapted cat's eye, counted over an arbitrary time interval after a flash of light had been introduced. From his studies he was able to construct statistical distributions associated with each of a number of intensities, ΔI (including $\Delta I = 0$ or noise). He could then assign values of d' representing the separation between any one of these distributions and that for noise alone. According to FitzHugh, d' was approximately linearly related to ΔI, while in our psychophysical experiments d' varied as ΔI^p, where p was 2 or greater. An examination of our procedure indicates that there might be uncertainty both as to the time and location of the signal presentation. The slope of our curves agreed with the slope of the curves for $M = 100$. The uncertainty may be introduced at a central rather than retinal level, suggesting that one should not try to account for nonlinearities at the level of the end organ, to the exclusion of central hypotheses.

One more point on the relation between FitzHugh's results and ours. We analyzed our results on the assumption that normal distributions existed. FitzHugh's distributions started at zero, and appeared quite skewed. This is not a discrepancy, for, from the standpoint of psychophysical analysis, any distribution that can be made normal by means of a monotonic transformation of the decision variable can be analyzed in a fashion consistent with the normal assumption.

To demonstrate this point, let us consider Fox's proof, which shows that likelihood ratio is the proper decision variable. Likelihood ratio varies from 0 to infinity and, for noise alone at least, is highly skewed. However, if one considers the decision rule "say yes" if $\log_e l(x) \geq \log_e W$, every decision is the same as if it were made according to the decision rule "say yes" if $l(x) \geq W$. $\mathrm{Log}_e\, l(x)$ varies from $-\infty$ to $+\infty$, and under certain conditions is normal. Since all the decisions are the same, and since one can only observe the decisions, a normal analysis can be applied whether the decision variable is $\log_e l(x)$ or $l(x)$. The results will be the same in both cases.

ACKNOWLEDGMENTS

This article was prepared in the Cooley Electronics Laboratory of the University of Michigan with support from Wright Air Force Base of the Air Research and Development Command. It appeared in the Annals of the New York Academy of Sciences, *1961,* **89,** *752–765.*

References

- FitzHugh, R. The statistical detection of threshold signals in the retina. *J. gen. Physiol.,* 1957, **40,** 925–948. [17]
- Fox, W. C. Signal detectability: A unified description of statistical methods employing fixed and sequential observation processes. University of Michigan: Electronic Defense Group, 1953, Technical Report No. 19.
- Luce, R. D. *Individual choice behavior.* New York: Wiley, 1959.

17

The Statistical Detection of Threshold Signals in the Retina

Richard FitzHugh

The statistical variations of visual responses near threshold suggest that the sensitivity of the eye, like that of many communication systems invented by man, is limited by the presence of random energy fluctuations or "noise." This noise is a result of the unpredictable motion of the individual elementary particles of physics (atoms, ions, electrons, photons) and originates either from thermal agitation or from events to which Heisenberg's principle of indeterminacy applies. If amplified sufficiently, such noise will distort the signal being communicated. (In the remainder of this paper the word noise never refers to the purely electrical noise which arises in the recording and amplifying apparatus and obscures the action potential, but only to fluctuations of physiological processes in the retina, in particular the times of occurrence of impulses.)

For the human retina, Hecht, Shlaer, and Pirenne (1942) concluded that statistical fluctuations in response to brief flashes at the absolute threshold could be accounted for entirely by random fluctuations in the number of photons absorbed by the photoreceptors at each flash, and that "biological noise" was negligible. However, the presence of large fluctuations in the duration of intervals between successive impulses of the maintained discharge from single ganglion cells in the cat's retina

(Granit, 1947; Kuffler, 1952, 1953), both in darkness and for a wide range of light intensities, suggests that biological noise does play a part in limiting the sensitivity of the eye. A similar situation in the infrared receptors of the rattlesnake has been studied by Bullock and Diecke (1956).

This paper describes a statistical analysis of single ganglion cell discharges occurring in response to brief flashes of light of near-threshold intensity. The method of analysis used was suggested by a statistical theory of vision in man proposed by Tanner and Swets (1954). On the basis of this analysis the properties of the retina are described in terms of information theory. Finally, these deduced properties are shown to agree approximately with those observed in the experimental measurement of thresholds.

METHOD

Single ganglion-cell impulses were recorded from the eye of decerebrate cats in various stages of light and dark adaptation by methods described by Talbot and Kuffler (1952) and Kuffler (1953). Platinum-wire recording electrodes were used, except that one cell (unit E) was recorded with a KCl-filled micropipette. A flashing light stimulus having an intensity controllable with a rotating wedge filter was focussed on the retina in the form of a spot of chosen diameter (usually 0.5 to 1.0 mm) centered in the receptive field of the ganglion cell. Flashes of 5- or 10-msec duration were delivered at a repetition frequency of one per second. Photographic records were made of the discharge during ten successive flashes at a number of different stimulus intensities near threshold, and also at zero intensity.

The ganglion-cell discharge was displayed on a cathode-ray oscilloscope both in the usual way as electrical potential versus time, and also as impulse-interval duration versus time using the device of MacNichol and Jacobs (1955), in which the vertical scale of time is considerably magnified relative to the horizontal scale (Barlow, FitzHugh, and Kuffler, 1956*b*). The impulses were also audible through a loudspeaker. With the flash intensity set at a certain value, the experimenter looked at and listened to the discharge, to determine whether each flash was followed by a detectable response in the form of a momentary change in frequency or in the distribution of intervals between impulses. The experimenter chose as the threshold the lowest intensity at which he could detect a response to roughly half the flashes. It was found necessary to let at least five successive flashes occur before making up one's mind as to whether a given intensity was threshold. Although this method required some practice, the threshold values chosen by different observers agreed to within about 0.2 $\log_{10}$ unit.

Because the response was graded rather than all-or-nothing, the thresholds measured correspond to an arbitrary reference level of excitation, convenient for testing the relative light sensitivity of the photoreceptors associated with a ganglion cell. This method was adopted as being both as consistent and as sensitive as possible.

RESULTS

In this section both the experimental data and their statistical analysis will be presented. The purpose and significance of the latter will be taken up more fully in the Discussion section.

Data from five ganglion cells in different cats were analyzed statistically. The results from different units differed in detail, but for the purpose of illustration a complete analysis of one representative experiment will be given first. The experimental conditions required for a satisfactory statistical analysis will then be described and the differences between the different experiments mentioned. Finally, the results of all the experiments will be summarized in Table I.

Sample analysis

The data to be considered first were obtained from a single ganglion cell in a dark-adapted eye kept in total darkness except for 5-msec testing flashes of low intensity. The maintained discharge of this cell in the absence of light stimulation was typical; the distribution of impulse intervals fitted a gamma distribution (Pearson's type III), and the first serial correlation coefficient between successive intervals was -0.19 (Barlow, FitzHugh, and Kuffler, 1956*a*).

Figure 1 shows the discharge from this cell following five successive 5-msec flashes of intensity 1.74 times threshold, at a frequency of 1 per second. For the purpose of analysis, the period extending from 100 msec before the beginning of each flash to 400 msec after it was divided into 10-msec periods, and for every stimulus, the impulses occurring in each of these periods counted. Then for each 10-msec period the number of impulses was averaged over ten successive flashes. Figure 2 shows these averages plotted against time for five different flash intensities. The intensities are expressed as multiples of the threshold intensity, estimated by the experimenter (see Method). These curves show average

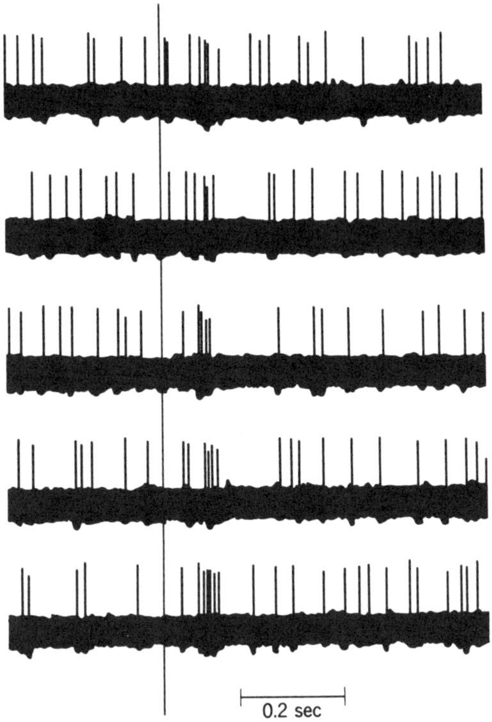

FIG. 1. Photographs of the impulses recorded from an on-center ganglion cell in response to five successive flashes at a rate of one per second. Flash duration 5 msec; flashes occur at long vertical line. Stimulus intensity 1.74 times threshold. The abscissa is time. Retouched photographs.

impulse frequency as a function of time, with the flash occurring at zero time. Counting the impulses in each 10-msec period is of course an arbitrary simplification which neglects variations in impulse time of the order of several milliseconds. The value of 10 msec was, however, small compared to the range of variation of the intervals of the maintained discharge (5 to 120 msec, mean 33.5 msec, see also Fig. 1); moreover, a shorter period than 10 msec was not necessary, because in the subsequent analysis the impulses in several of these 10-msec periods were pooled.

The following is a list of mathematical symbols used in this paper; they will be defined in more detail as used.

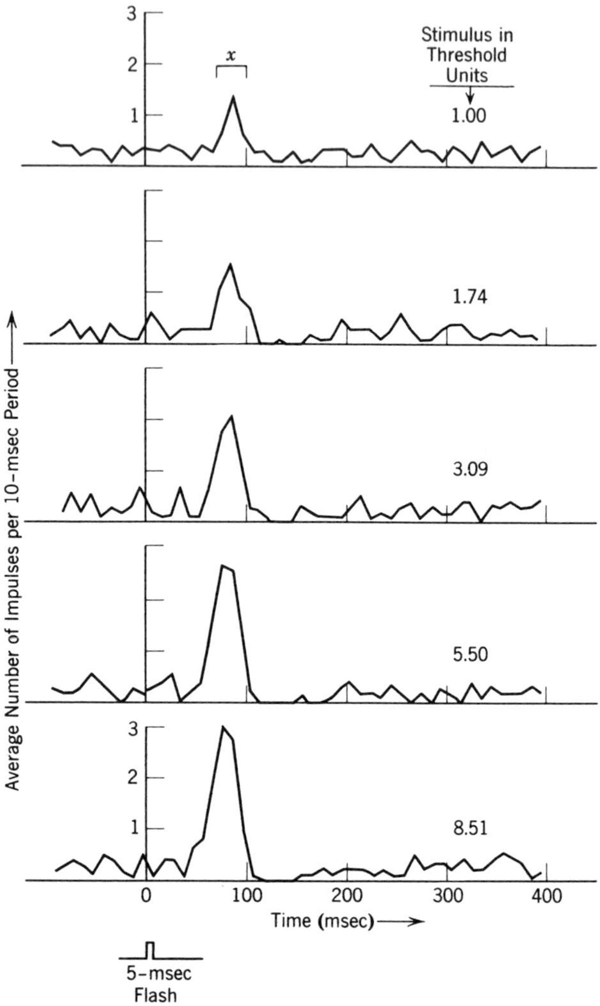

FIG. 2. Transient changes of average frequency following 5-msec flashes, plotted from data such as those of Fig. 1. On the vertical axis is plotted the mean number of impulses in each 10-msec period obtained by averaging over ten successive flashes. The relative stimulus intensity for each curve is as shown, with threshold taken as 1.00. The number of impulses (x) occurring in each discharge during the critical period marked at the top of the figure was used as an index of the response.

Symbols for ganglion cell discharge

d $= \bar{x} - \bar{x}^0$
d_N $= \bar{x}_N - \bar{x}_N^0$
I = fixed flash intensity
I_θ = threshold intensity for N cells
k, K = constants
p = slope of line obtained by plotting log d against log I
R_1 = rate of information transfer for randomized flash intensities
R_n = rate of information transfer for randomized blocks of n identical flashes
w = variable flash intensity, equal to either zero or I
x = index of response
$\bar{x}$ = mean of x over 10 flashes
$\bar{x}^0$ $= \bar{x}$ for $I = 0$
x_N = sum of x's from N cells
$\bar{x}_N$ = mean of x_N
$\bar{x}_N^0$ $= \bar{x}_N$ for $I = 0$
x' = a control index
$\bar{x}'$ = mean of x'
σ = standard deviation of x
σ_N = standard deviation of x_N

Symbols for model of Tanner and Swets

C = minimum value of X for a positive response
D $= \bar{X} - \bar{X}^0$
$f_0(X)$ = statistical distribution of X for zero intensity
$f_I(X)$ = statistical distribution of X for intensity I
P = probability of seeing flash
X = index of neural activity, corresponding to x
$\bar{X}$ = mean of X
$\bar{X}^0$ $= \bar{X}$ for $I = 0$

Figure 2 shows that following a flash of threshold intensity there occurred, on the average, first a latent period lasting 70 msec and then a burst of impulses lasting 30 msec. Since the duration and maximum frequency of the burst were the most obvious indices of the response, the index first chosen for analyzing the data of Fig. 2 was the number of impulses (x) occurring in the "critical period" from 70 to 100 msec after the beginning of each flash. For the brighter flashes, the beginning of the burst occurred sooner (shorter latency), and there was also a pronounced decrease of impulse frequency ("pause") following the burst, between 100 and 200 msec after the flash. Therefore, for flashes much above threshold, the index x neglects these parts of the response. Even at threshold it neglects the detailed course of rise and fall of average frequency within the critical period. However, in the discussion section it will be shown that the use of x provides at least as efficient a way of analyzing the response as the experimental method described above.

The histograms in Fig. 3 represent the statistical distribution of x for 10 successive records at each of 6 different stimulus intensities (I) from zero to 8.5 times threshold. As a control at zero intensity, x was taken as the number of impulses within ten 30-msec periods spaced 1 sec apart in

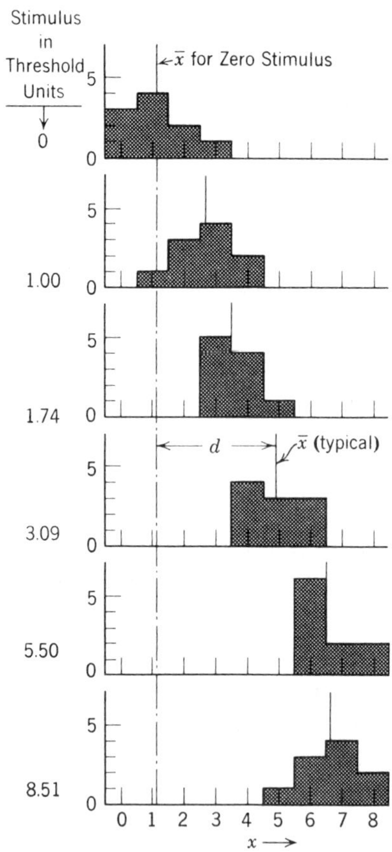

FIG. 3. Experimental distributions of the index x (see Fig. 2), obtained from records like those of Fig. 1, for six stimulus intensities.

a record of the maintained discharge. The vertical line through each histogram indicates the mean, $\bar{x}$.

The index x will be compared in what follows with the index X of Tanner and Swets (see Discussion), which has a standard deviation that is constant for all values of I. The values of the standard deviation σ of x corresponding to different values of I did not vary significantly from each other and showed no significant trend with increasing I. Details of the statistical tests used to establish this will be given in the section on Comparison of Experiments.

Let d be defined as the difference $(\bar{x} - \bar{x}_0)$, in which $\bar{x}_0$ is the mean value for x for zero stimulus (Fig. 3). In Fig. 4, d is plotted against I with logarithmic scales on both axes (filled circles). A straight line with a slope of 0.73 fits the first four of the points, but not the last one. The slope of such a line will be referred to hereafter simply as the "slope," for brevity. At the highest stimulus intensity the system may be saturating somewhere; perhaps the cell body is firing near its maximum frequency.

Sampling errors of d were not estimated directly, since the slope varied rather widely with the choice of controls and of the critical period. Two types of distributions of x were used as zero-intensity controls; they will be called "control I" and "control II." Control I is that described above, in which a distribution of x was obtained from the maintained discharge; the mean value $\bar{x}_0$ taken from this distribution was used to calculate d for all values of I. The points shown as open circles in Fig. 4 were obtained by using control II, in which a control index x' was taken

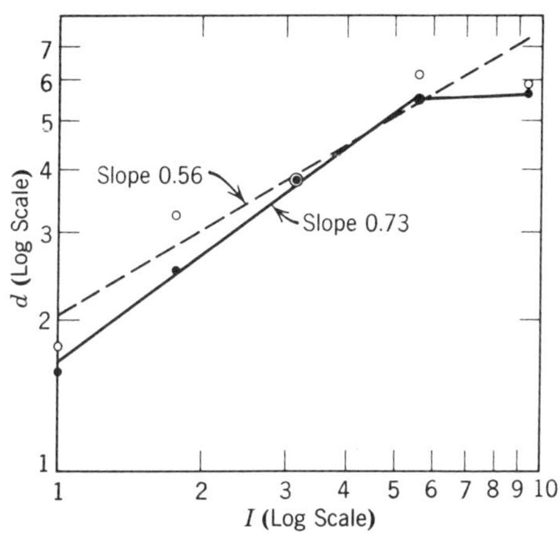

FIG. 4. The variation d of the mean value of x (see Fig. 3) as a function of stimulus intensity.

equal to the number of impulses within the period from −30 msec to 0 msec. This control period is just 100 msec earlier than the critical period used to find x, and has the same duration, but since it ends just before the flash, x' can be used as a control index for comparison with x. The mean value $\bar{x}'$ of x' was calculated; d was then taken as $(\bar{x} - \bar{x}')$ and plotted in Fig. 4 as open circles. The line drawn through these points (broken line) has the slope 0.56.

As already mentioned, the choice of the critical period from 70 to 100 msec after the beginning of the flash is arbitrary and was intended to reflect most efficiently the changes in response just at threshold. For the purpose of comparison, a second critical period from 40 to 100 msec after the flash was used. The corresponding index would be expected to be more efficient for the higher values of I, and less so for the lower ones. For this index, the slopes, corresponding to 0.73 and 0.56 in Fig. 4, were found to be 0.98 and 0.64. These figures were rounded to the nearest tenth of a unit, and the slope for each experiment was expressed as a range of values, in this case from 0.6 to 1.0 (see Table I).

The sensory system consisting of a ganglion cell, the photoreceptors of its receptive field, and the intermediate bipolar cells, forms a communication channel to which we can apply the theory of information which has been developed by Shannon and others working in communication engineering (Shannon and Weaver, 1949; Goldman, 1953; Woodward, 1953). In this theory "information" is defined numerically and its unit of measurement is the "bit"—that amount of information contained in a message which specifies one of two alternatives, both of which were equally probable before the message was received (equal a priori probabilities). This concept of information has also been extended to more complicated cases in which the number of alternatives is greater than two, their a priori probabilities are not equal, or the message is made up of many successive independent choices instead of just one. Information theory is useful in describing and comparing the properties of "noisy" communication channels; i.e., devices which distort the messages they transmit in an unpredictable, statistical manner. In the present experiments, the message to be transmitted concerns whether a flash or a blank was presented to the retina at a given moment. Our data will be analyzed assuming the statistical conditions of visual experiment done on human subjects by Tanner and Swets, the "yes-no choice" (described more fully in the Discussion section). In this experiment, a flash and a blank have equal a priori probabilities (½) and the information in each presentation is therefore one bit per flash (the term "bit per flash" will be used even when the "flash" may possibly be of zero intensity). The stimulus message is transformed or coded by the sensory system into a neural message consisting of a sequence of nerve impulses going to the brain. In the process of coding, the statistical fluctuations in the durations of the impulse intervals represent noise in engineering terminology. This noise destroys information by introducing ambiguity; one cannot always tell with certainty by analyzing a neural message whether it was caused by a flash or a blank, if the flash intensity I is too low.

Information theory provides a way to describe the statistical properties of this sensory system. We can summarize these properties in a diagram in which the average rate of transmission of information R_1 through the system in bits per flash is plotted as a function of I (Fig. 5, upper curve). This curve was calculated for the yes-no choice experiment in which flashes of intensity zero and I are randomly presented and equally frequent, and the average amount of information originally contained in each presentation is therefore 1 bit. The values of R_1 shown as filled

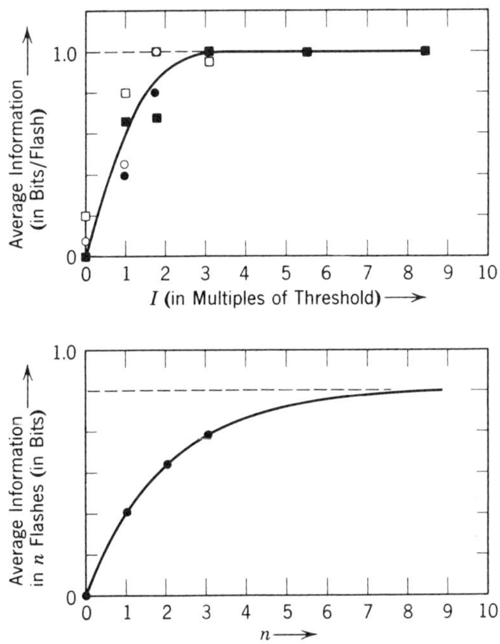

FIG. 5. Upper curve, the average information in a single flash with intensity known to be either zero or I with equal a priori probabilities, plotted as a function of I. Values of information computed from distributions of Fig. 3. Symbols are explained in the text. Lower curve, the average information in a sequence of n flashes known to be of the same intensity (either zero or I, equal a priori probabilities), plotted as a function of n.

circles were computed from the distributions of Fig. 3 by formula (1) of the Mathematical Appendix. R_1 increases with increasing I to the limit 1, showing that the higher the stimulus intensity, the less information is lost, as would be expected, since with increasing I the bursts and pauses become more accentuated and are easier to distinguish from random variations in impulse grouping.

The values of R_1 shown by the filled circles in Fig. 5 were calculated using the uppermost distribution in Fig. 3 as a "control," corresponding to zero stimulus intensity (control I). As with the slopes, the reliability of the values of R_1 was also checked by recalculating them using the zero-intensity control distributions provided by control II. These values are shown as open circles in Fig. 5. Values of R_1 were also calculated for the critical period 40 to 100 msec after the flash, with both types of controls, and these are shown as filled and open squares in Fig. 5. In Fig. 5 a smooth curve drawn through the points represents average information transfer in the yes-no choice experiment as a function of flash intensity I. (It does not necessarily follow that the uppermost value of R_1 at any I corresponds to the most efficient method of analysis; sampling errors can make R_1 either too large or too small.) The value of information corresponding to $I = 1$, or threshold intensity as estimated experimentally, is 0.4 to 0.8 bit/flash. That is, some information was being lost at this stimulus intensity, owing to noise. The experimenter was, however, able to make up for this loss of information by examining the discharges for several flashes in succession, i.e., by introducing redundancy into the message being transmitted. This will be made clearer by the following calculations.

Consider the case in which n successive flashes or blanks are presented in a block. The subject knows that all the stimuli in a given block are of the *same* intensity w, but does not know whether w is zero or a fixed value I. These two values of w have equal a priori probability (½), and therefore one bit of information is contained in this block. Let R_n indicate the average amount of information in the n nerve messages resulting from such a block of flashes, for the yes-no choice experiment. R_n is expressed in bits/block. The lower diagram of Fig. 5 shows R_n as calculated from Eq. (5) of the Appendix for $I = 1$ (threshold intensity) and for $n = 1, 2, 3$, using the histograms of Fig. 3. (For $n = 1$, R_n is R_1, the rate for one flash considered earlier.) Values of R_n for values of n greater than 3 were not calculated because the labor of computation increases rapidly with n, but the curve of R_n versus n was extrapolated with an exponential curve which closely fitted to the first three points and approached the value of 1 as n approached infinity.

Calculations of R_n were not done for all the four combinations of control distributions and critical periods that were used to get the points of Fig. 5 (upper), but if this had been done, curves of similar form would have resulted. Since the method of calculation that was used gave the lowest of the values of R_1 for $I = 1$ in Fig. 5 (upper, filled circles), curves of R_n calculated in the other three ways would all lie above that shown in Fig. 5 (lower).

The increase of information with the number of identical flashes or blanks in a block agrees with the finding of Blackwell (1953) that visual thresholds in man are lower when the stimuli are presented in blocks of twenty flashes of the same intensity, than when the intensity is varied from flash to flash.

Comparison of experiments

The five experiments will be denoted by the letters A to E. Experiment A has been analyzed in detail previously.

Because all the experiments analyzed differed somewhat, it seems advisable to mention the conditions considered necessary for statistical analysis, and how the results were affected when these conditions were not completely satisfied. This occurred either when the properties of the unit were not constant during the experiment, or when the unit was lost before all the necessary data had been gathered. The conditions are as follows.

1. The ganglion cell must have a constant frequency of maintained discharge. The frequency was monitored during the later experiments by periodically counting the impulses in a 10-sec period with an electronic counter, as described by Barlow et al. (1956*a*). No units were used which showed unusually large changes of maintained frequency. Moreover, as a control, two or three photographic records of the discharge, without stimulus and lasting for 10 sec, were made at the beginning, the end, and sometimes in the middle of the experiment. For unit A only one such control run was obtained, but its frequency remained quite constant in the other records, except for the response during 250 msec following each flash (Fig. 2).

2. The retina must be in a constant state of adaptation, with a constant threshold. This was tested by making two or three records (at beginning, end, and sometimes the middle of the experiment), using the value of the stimulus initially chosen as the threshold. Records at different stimulus intensities were made about 1 min apart, to allow any adaptation to disappear. Any change in threshold would affect the values

of $\bar{x}$ and therefore also of the slope. Again, unit A had only one such record, but had typical values for the slope. The others showed a nearly constant response to the original threshold stimulus, except for unit C. For this unit, each value of d was corrected by the amount of drift of the threshold value of $\bar{x}$, which was assumed to be changing linearly throughout the experiment. This correction changed the slope only from 0.82 to 0.75, and was unimportant compared to the other inaccuracies involved.

3. The response to one flash must be over before the next flash occurs, for the data to be applicable to the yes-no choice experiment, in which each response is used by the observer to infer the intensity of the single preceding flash only. The stimulation rate of 1 flash per second was usually slow enough to permit the original maintained frequency to be resumed after every flash. However, errors from this source were checked by using two sets of control distributions for x, as described earlier (controls I and II). Only in experiment D did requirement 3 fail, and only for the highest stimulus intensities, and the values of slope and information were not changed appreciably.

4. The temporal pattern of the frequency changes must be simple enough so that merely counting the impulses within a certain critical period will provide an efficient index of the response. This requirement, of course, only reflects the inadequacy of this method of analysis for the more complicated responses. Unit B had a response which consisted of a series of alternate bursts and pauses, the later ones appearing only in response to the brighter flashes (Fig. 6). Unit B was in a light-adapted retina; a similar response was noticed for one other light-adapted unit (not analyzed), but for no dark-adapted ones. These complex responses may have been the result of an interplay between mutually antagonistic sets of pathways from different parts of the receptive field (Barlow et al., 1956*b*). A systematic investigation of the effects on the frequency pattern of response of changing both the state of adaptation and the area of the stimulating spot might be informative. Unit B did not have a definite value of the slope, since a straight line could not be fitted to the points in the diagram of log d plotted against log I. This curve was concave downward with a slope varying from 0.3 to 1.6, but these limits are only slightly wider than those found for the other four units (see Table I), so that even this experiment is not in serious disagreement with the others.

Tanner and Swets assumed that the distribution of their index x was normal, with a standard deviation independent of I (see Discussion). The experimental distributions of x are not even approximately normal, since x is a discrete variable which varies by increments that are large

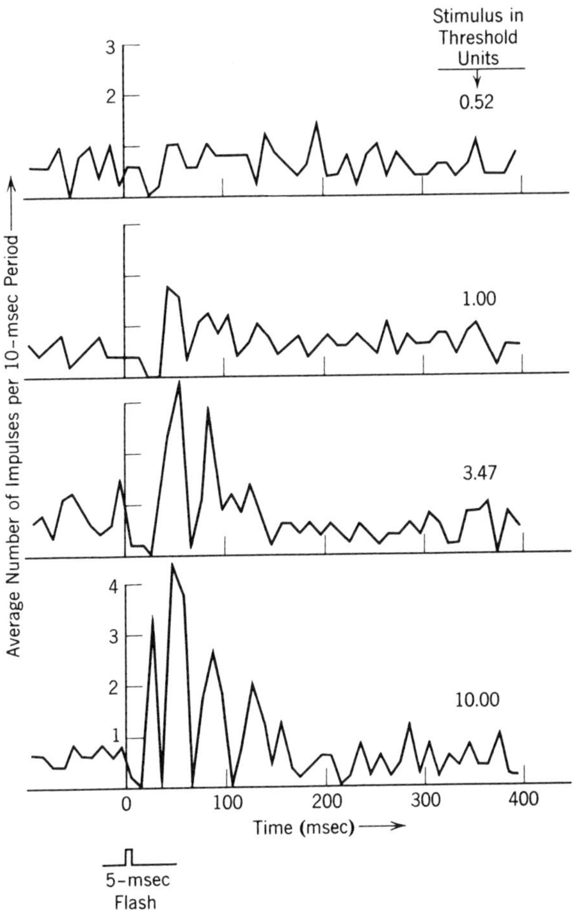

FIG. 6. Average frequency changes following a flash, plotted as in Fig. 2 for a light-adapted, off-center unit. The response to the higher intensities consists of a sequence of oscillations of impulse frequency.

compared to σ. However, the hypothesis that σ is constant was tested by Bartlett's test for uniformity of variance (Bartlett, 1937; Walker and Lev, 1953). This test is not strictly applicable to σ, since x is discrete, but from the discussion on rounding off of variables given in Eisenhart, Hastay, and Wallis (1947), this test is probably satisfactory, except when some of the values of σ are zero. Since approximating a continuous variable by a discrete one tends to increase the spread of sampled values of variance, this test will still be valid whenever its result indicates non-significance. Bartlett's test, when applied to Experiments A, B, and C showed that σ was constant to within the 10 per cent level of significance. In Experiments D and E, zero values of σ caused Bartlett's statistic to become infinite, and the test was assumed not applicable. Cochran's test for uniformity of variance, based on the maximum value of variance, was therefore applied to all experiments (Cochran, 1941; Eisenhart et al., 1947). Cochran's test showed that the maximum values of σ were not significantly large (5 per cent level) for Experiments A to D, but Experiment E showed significance at the 1 per cent level. Finally, in order to discover whether the value of σ was correlated with I, rank correlation coefficients were calculated. Again Experiments A to D showed no significant correlation at the 10 per cent level, while Experiment E did show a significant correlation (0.94) at the 3 per cent level. Thus four out of five experiments are in agreement with the assumption that σ is constant.

An interesting example of efficiency of the statistical method of analysis in preserving information was given by unit E. This unit had an unusually low maintained frequency, between 3 and 5 per second. The experimental criterion of response used was a change in impulse *frequency*, so that the response considered as "threshold" consisted of a *pair* of impulses close together. Analysis of the records showed, however, that even for a stimulus only 0.55 times the experimental threshold, a *single* impulse always occurred between 20 and 40 msec after the flash. Since the number of impulses during a random 20-msec period of the maintained discharge was nearly always zero, the calculated information was close to one even for this subthreshold intensity. Thus information was being wasted by the experimenter, and if he had used the appearance of a single impulse closely following the flash as his criterion, instead of a frequency change, he would have obtained a lower threshold.

Summary of results

In Table I, columns 4 and 5 give the limits of variation and mean values obtained by plotting log d against log I for four experiments (Experiment B did not give a straight line; see preceding section). In the Discussion, these figures will be compared with the corresponding values found for human vision by Tanner and Swets (1954).

In columns 6 and 7 are given the values for limits and mean of the rate R_1 of information transfer at the experimentally estimated threshold intensity (see Methods). In all but unit E, which was discussed as a special case in the last section, the mean value of R_1 was less than 1, which agrees with the fact that the responses to a number of successive flashes were observed before deciding on the threshold intensity setting.

TABLE I. STATISTICAL PROPERTIES OF GANGLION CELL RESPONSES NEAR THRESHOLD

Unit	Type	Retinal illumination	Slope		Information at threshold (bits/flash)	
			Limits	Mean	Limits	Mean
		foot-candles				
A	On-center	0.0	0.6–1.0	0.7	0.4–0.8	0.6
B	Off-center	4.0			0.6–0.7	0.7
C	On-center	0.0	0.5–0.8	0.6	0.9–1.0	1.0
D	Off-center	0.3	1.1–1.5	1.2	0.5–0.8	0.6
E	On-center	0.3	0.6–0.7	0.6	0.5–1.0	0.8
Overall limits			0.5–1.5		0.4–1.0	
Overall mean				0.8		0.7

The data in Table I were obtained by using the two control methods I and II, already described. Two different critical periods were used for units A and E, and one for the others.

DISCUSSION

The problem of the analysis of a nerve-fiber message by the brain is similar to the engineering problem of detection of a signal in a noisy communication channel. A theory of signal detectability in such channels, based on the principles of statistical inference (Peterson, Birdsall, and Fox, 1954), has been used by Tanner and Swets (1954) to interpret experiments on human subjects. Tanner and Swets postulate a neural mechanism in which statistical fluctuations play an essential part. The statistical properties of this mechanism can be compared with those of the retinal ganglion cell studied here. The simplest type of experiment done by Tanner and Swets was the yes-no choice, in which at each trial the observer must report whether or not a flash occurred at a known instant. For this type of experiment, Fig. 7 illustrates their assumptions, which are as follows: (1) At each stimulus, a certain quantity of neural activity (X, in the notation of the present paper) is the signal which the brain analyzes to determine whether a flash has occurred or not. (2) This signal contains noise; that is, for a given stimulus intensity, X varies randomly from flash to flash. X is distributed according to a normal

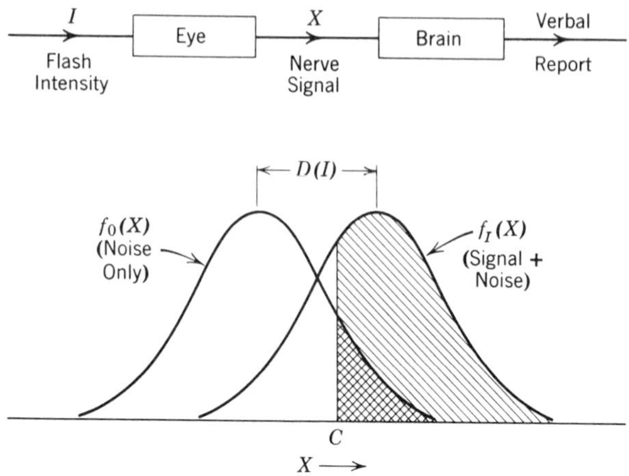

FIG. 7. Diagram illustrating the stochastic model of the visual apparatus near threshold, modified from Tanner and Swets (1954). The distribution of X is a normal probability distribution having a constant standard deviation and a mean which increases with increasing stimulus intensity I. $D(I)$ corresponds to d of Figs. 3 and 4. Whenever the value of x resulting from a flash exceeds the criterion value C, the brain reports a flash seen. The singly and doubly cross-hatched areas represent the probabilities that this will occur for flash intensities of I and zero, respectively.

probability curve, which has a standard deviation independent of the flash intensity and is equal to one, and a mean value $\bar{X}$ which increases with intensity. (3) Whenever X exceeds a certain threshold or criterion value C, the subject reports a flash seen. (4) The criterion C varies according to the observer's knowledge of the a priori probability of occurrence of a flash, and also according to his degree of motivation (the subject was paid or fined according to the correctness of his reports), and his brain adjusts C so as to maximize his average net profit. In Fig. 7, $f_0(X)$ is the probability distribution of X following a "blank" (flash of zero intensity; curve labeled "noise only"), and $f_I(X)$ is the distribution of X following a flash of intensity I ("signal plus noise"). Both curves are assumed to be normal probability curves of standard deviation (unity), but their mean values are separated by a distance D which is an increasing function of I. Once the criterion C is chosen by the brain, a flash is reported as seen whenever X exceeds C. For the yes-no choice experiment, the intensity of the flash and the relative frequency of flashes and blanks were controlled by the experimenter. According to their hypothesis, the index X can exceed C when the flash is either present or absent, with probabilities which are equal to the areas under the corresponding distribution curves to the right of C (cross-hatched in

Fig. 7). This probability is greater when a flash is present than when it is absent. If C is set very low, many blanks will be reported as flashes, whereas if C is high, many flashes will be reported as blanks.

By varying the conditions which determine C and by analyzing the resulting data according to their theory, Tanner and Swets obtained D indirectly. When they plotted log D versus log I, they obtained straight lines with slopes of from 2.1 to 3.1, which is consistently higher than the values given in Table I (0.5 to 1.5). This difference in slopes does not necessarily indicate a conflict between the present results and those of Tanner and Swets, since the slope might be different if x were defined in a different way. In general, one would expect that the more efficient x was in preserving information, the greater the slope would be, since then the mean value $\bar{x}$ of x would increase more rapidly with I, and since the rate of information transfer increases according to the decrease in overlap of the distributions to be distinguished. A second possible reason for the difference in slopes will be mentioned later, when the messages in many optic nerve fibers are considered.

It should be mentioned here that an analysis of the present data could have been done using the method of inference of Tanner and Swets, based on a criterion test, but the point of view of information theory was chosen as not requiring the choice of a particular test.

A sample of ganglion-cell discharge can be completely described by listing the times of occurrence of each impulse in it. Because of random variation in impulse intervals, many of these data represent visually useless information, or noise, and the first step in the analysis of such data was to try to choose an index or measure of neural activity x to correspond to the index X of Tanner and Swets. This index should be both reasonably simple to calculate and efficient in the sense that little significant information is lost in passing from the original message to the quantity x. This step may be roughly compared with the practice in electrical engineering of passing a signal through a filter to emphasize those bandwidths in which the signal-to-noise ratio is greatest. Some analogous process of selective analysis presumably occurs in the brain as it analyzes the optic-nerve messages.

In a previous paper (Barlow et al., 1956*a*) on the maintained discharge, the data analyzed consisted simply of the values of the successive intervals listed in order. For the present paper, however, the times of occurrence of the impulses were listed with reference to time after the flash, since the characteristic features of the response seemed to be more closely related to time than to ordinal number of the impulses. As described in the Results section, the index x was taken to be the number of impulses occurring during a certain critical period of time following the flash, and the amount of information per flash was calculated from the frequency distributions of x, by the formulas given in the Appendix.

When the a priori probabilities of a flash or a blank (i.e. flash intensities of zero and I) are each one-half, the average amount of information in each presentation is 1 bit. The average amount of information transmitted to the ganglion cell in each flash (R_1) is 1 bit/flash only when the intensity of the flash is so high that the response in the ganglion cell is never confused with the chance fluctuations in impulse grouping which can result from biological or quantal noise. For smaller intensities, near "threshold," there are certain values of x which can result from either a flash or a blank, and the corresponding rate of transmission of information is less than 1 bit/flash, since some of the information in the original signal is lost through ambiguities introduced by noise. At the intensity which was judged by the experimenter to be threshold for ganglion cell A, R_1 was 0.4 to 0.8 bit/flash (Fig. 5, upper). The average information (R_6) in six successive flashes which were known to be identical, and of intensity either zero or threshold, was estimated from Fig. 5 (lower) as 0.95 bit or higher, which may be considered as near certainty. In this way some of the information lost because of noise has been restored by the redundancy in the repeated flash. Thus the statistical method of analysis is at least as sensitive as the subjective method of the experimenters, who did not make up their minds on the threshold setting until they had considered five to ten flashes at one intensity.

Even though there is agreement between two quite different methods of analyzing optic nerve messages—the experimental (see Method) and the statistical (using a numerical index of neural activity)—this does not prove that either of them preserves as much of the information in the message as does a normal cat's brain. Both the experimental and statistical methods are limited in efficiency, although for different reasons. It is of course hard to compare the relative efficiencies of the cat's brain, as it analyzes a message in an optic nerve fiber entering its synapses, and of an experimenter's brain, which receives the same message, recoded, through his optic and auditory nerves. The experimenter is concentrating all his attention on the message in one fiber, while the cat is analyzing those in many fibers. The experimenter is using a highly unnatural method, aided by his experimental apparatus, while the cat is performing a task to which evolution has specifically adapted him. The mathematical method of calculating information is based on a knowledge of the statistical distributions of certain variables in the message, but this knowledge is limited by the sizes of the samples obtained from the data.

The information transfer might be calculated very accurately if one knew the distribution of each impulse interval following a flash. This distribution function would not be constant in time during the response, but would contain either time or ordinal number of the impulse after a flash as a parameter. The amount of data and computation required to get these distributions with sufficient accuracy would be very great. Such a method would catch more of the information in the message, but much of this would certainly be useless or noise information rather than useful stimulus information.

It is assumed here that the experimenter's actual knowledge that the flash was of intensity greater than zero did not influence his setting of the threshold. A more accurate method for measuring threshold could be used by two experimenters, if one of them were to choose flash intensities at random, either zero or I, and the other guessed the value of each intensity by observing the discharge during a block of five to ten identical flashes or blanks. To insure statistical significance, however, this process would have to be repeated so many times at each intensity as to be very time-consuming.

In addition to suggesting a method of analyzing nerve impulse data, the hypothesis of Tanner and Swets provides a link between such data and the results of experiments on human vision. These results are often expressed as frequency-of-seeing curves, with the relative frequency of seeing a flash plotted against flash intensity. If a value of the criterion C is chosen, then for each intensity I the probability of obtaining a value of X greater than C is found directly from the theoretical distribution of X. Let P be the frequency of seeing a flash of that intensity. Then P increases with increasing I, giving a frequency-of-seeing curve of the usual sigmoid form. Moreover, P increases with decreasing C, and if C is not larger than the maximum value of X obtained when I is equal to zero, then the frequency of "seeing" will be greater than zero even in the absence of a flash, as has been found experimentally (Blackwell, 1953).

For simplicity, the present analysis has been applied only to an extremely simple case of information transfer across the retina, the yes-no choice with equal a priori probabilities and only a single ganglion cell considered. The maximum rate of information transfer considered, 1 bit per second, is much less than that of which a single neuron is capable. MacKay and McCulloch (1955) estimate that under certain simple assumptions the limiting capacity of a neuron with an average frequency of 50/sec is about 450 bits/sec. This is total information and includes useless information, in the form of noise, but the useful information, due to visual signals, is probably still an appreciable fraction of this. The cases of most interest to the physiologist, however, are much more complex, and the following generalizations are possible: (1) unequal a priori probabilities of flash intensities; (2) more than two intensities to be distinguished, especially discrimination in a continuum of intensities; (3) detection of a flash when its time of occurrence is unknown to the observer; (4) detection of temporal patterns other than short flashes, generally the continuous inference of intensity from the nerve message; (5) the detection of spatial patterns by analysis of messages from many ganglion cells. These generalizations would introduce many theoretical and experimental complications, some of which have been considered by Tanner and Swets (1954), Tanner and Norman (1954), and Peterson, Birdsall, and Fox (1954). Only one of them will be touched on here.

Since in normal vision the neural activity which transmits visual activity to the brain occurs in a large number of optic nerve fibers, while the present data represent messages in a single fiber, conclusions from the latter cannot be compared directly with those of Tanner and Swets. In fact, increasing the number of independent noisy channels which all carry the same stimulus message will increase the information transfer at a given intensity, or decrease the threshold intensity, as can be shown by a rough calculation. A new index x_N is defined as the sum of the x's belonging to a number N of independently firing ganglion cells. If $d = \bar{x} - \bar{x}_0$ and σ is the standard deviation of x, if d_N and σ_N are the corresponding parameters for x_N, and if

$$d = kI^p \tag{1}$$

in which p is a positive constant (equal to the slope), then

$$\begin{aligned} d_N &= Nd = NkI^p \\ \sigma_N &= N^{1/2}\sigma \\ \frac{d_N}{\sigma_N} &= \frac{N^{1/2}kI^p}{\sigma} \end{aligned} \tag{2}$$

Assume that a certain value of average information transfer R_1 represents threshold vision and corresponds to a fixed value of d_N/σ_N. Let us keep R_1 and therefore d_N/σ_N fixed, and consider I_θ, the threshold intensity, as a function of N:

$$I_\theta = KN^{-1/2p} \tag{3}$$

in which

$$K = \left(\frac{\sigma}{k}\cdot\frac{d_N}{\sigma_N}\right)^{1/2p} = \text{a constant}$$

If the average value of $p = 0.8$ from Table I is substituted in Eq. (3), then

$$I_\theta = KN^{-0.62}$$

From this formula we can calculate, for example, that the threshold intensity for 100 ganglion cells would be 1.24 $\log_{10}$ units less than (or 0.058 times) that for one ganglion cell.

According to Eq. (2), x_N has the same value of slope as does x. Of course it may be that Eq. (1) does not hold over such a wide range of intensities. Perhaps as I increases, the response begins to saturate and p decreases, which might account for the fact that the value of the slope found here is lower than that found by Tanner and Swets. If their maximum value for p of 3.11 is substituted into Eq. (3), then the threshold value for 100 ganglion cells is only 0.32 $\log_{10}$ unit less than (or 0.48 times) that for a single cell. From these rough calculations it can be seen that the effectiveness of summation among many ganglion cells at threshold depends rather sensitively on the value of p, indicating that the value of this parameter plays an important part in determining the properties of the theoretical model of the retina.

SUMMARY

1. Photographic records of impulses from single ganglion cells in the cat's retina were made while the retina was stimulated by flashes occurring once a second. Ten flashes at each of several intensities near threshold were used.

2. For the purpose of statistical analysis, the number of impulses (x) falling within a critical period following each flash was used as an index of the response. Histograms of x were plotted and used to calculate rates of transfer of information by the ganglion cell for the case of an ideal experiment, the yes-no choice, in which flashes of intensity I and blanks are to be distinguished.

3. The information rate increased (1) with increasing stimulus intensity and (2) with the number of identical flashes or blanks presented successively in a block. The intensity chosen as threshold by the experimenter, who observed the impulses visually and aurally, corresponded to an average information rate for single flashes of 0.7 bit/flash, compared to the maximum possible rate of 1 bit/flash. A threshold intensity giving 0.4 or more bit/flash, if presented in blocks of six identical flashes, corresponded to 0.95 or more bit/block, or near certainty. Thus the calculation of information rates using the index x provides an estimate of threshold at least as sensitive as those obtained during an experiment, which were

made only after observing the responses to five to ten flashes of the same intensity.

4. The index x has statistical properties similar to those of the "index of neural activity" used by Tanner and Swets (1954) in their statistical model of human vision, and represents a possible physical interpretation of their index. However, x gave values (0.5 to 1.5) of the parameter called the slope which were consistently smaller than their values (2.1 to 3.1).

MATHEMATICAL APPENDIX

Symbols used only in Appendix

$f_w(x)$ = conditional probability of x, given w
$H(w)$, $H(x)$ = entropies of distributions of w and x
$H(w, x)$ = entropy of joint distribution of w and x
$p(w)$ = probability of w
$q(x)$ = probability of x

The formulas used to calculate the average rate of transmission of information in the optic-nerve-fiber message will be derived here. In the ideal experiment (yes-no choice) discussed in this paper, a flash intensity (I) is chosen, and a sequence of flashes and blanks is presented to the retina. w denotes the flash intensity for a particular presentation; for a flash, $w = I$, and for a blank, $w = 0$. The probabilities of a flash or a blank at a given presentation are both equal to ½. The variable x denotes the index of neural activity chosen for analysis of the data, namely, the number of impulses occurring within a certain critical period of time following the flash. The rates of information to be calculated are therefore applicable to an observer who receives only the value of x, but not the entire message.

Let $f_w(x)$ be the conditional probability that the index will have the value x, given that the flash intensity was w. Then

$$\sum_x f_w(x) = 1$$

in which x has the range of values 0, 1, 2, 3, ... The joint probability of occurrence of a given pair of values of w and x at a given presentation is $\frac{1}{2}f_w(x)$. The probabilities $p(w)$ and $q(x)$ of w and x are, respectively:

$$p(w) = \sum_x \tfrac{1}{2}f_w(x) = \tfrac{1}{2}$$

$$q(x) = \sum_w \tfrac{1}{2}f_w(x) = \tfrac{1}{2}\sum_w f_w(x)$$

From these probabilities are calculated three entropies: $H(w)$, the entropy of w; $H(x)$, that of x; and $H(w, x)$, the joint entropy of w and x. (All logarithms are to the base 2.)

$$H(w) = -\sum_{w} p(w) \log p(w) = 1$$

$$H(x) = -\sum_{x} q(x) \log q(x)$$

$$H(w, x) = -\sum_{w} \sum_{x} [\tfrac{1}{2} f_w(x)] \log [\tfrac{1}{2} f_w(x)]$$

$$= 1 - \tfrac{1}{2} \sum_{w} \sum_{x} f_w(x) \log f_w(x)$$

Let R_1 (I) be the average rate of transmission of information in bits/flash for the ideal experiment; it is a function of I. Then, according to Shannon and Weaver (1949):

$$R_1(I) = H(w) + H(x) - H(w, x) \tag{4}$$

The ideal experiment can be modified so that, instead of one flash, n successive flashes are presented in a block, known by the observer to be all of the same intensity w, either zero or I, with equal probability.

Let $x_1, x_2, \ldots, x_n$ be the values of the index obtained from the n messages. The joint probability of $w, x_1, x_2, \ldots, x_n$ is

$$\tfrac{1}{2} f_w(x_1) f_w(x_2) \ldots f_w(x_n)$$

The probability $p(w)$ of w is $\frac{1}{2}$, and the joint probability of $x_1, x_2, \ldots,$ and x_n is

$$q(x_1, x_2, \ldots, x_n) = \tfrac{1}{2} \sum_{w} f_w(x_1) f_w(x_2) \ldots f_w(x_n)$$

The corresponding entropies are

$$H(w) = 1$$

$$H(x_1, \ldots, x_n) = -\sum_{x_1} \ldots \sum_{xn} [\tfrac{1}{2} \sum_{w} f_w(x_1) \ldots f_w(x_n)]$$
$$\log [\tfrac{1}{2} \sum_{w} f_w(x_1) \ldots f_w(x_n)]$$

$$= 1 - \tfrac{1}{2} \sum_{x_1} \ldots \sum_{xn} [\sum_{w} f_w(x_1) \ldots f_w(x_n)]$$
$$\log [\sum_{w} f_w(x_1) \ldots f_w(x_n)]$$

$$H(w, x_1, \ldots, x_n) = -\sum_{w} \sum_{x_1} \ldots \sum_{xn} [\tfrac{1}{2} f_w(x_1) \ldots f_w(x_n)]$$
$$\log [\tfrac{1}{2} f_w(x_1) \ldots f_w(x_n)]$$

$$= 1 - [\sum_{w} n \sum_{x} \tfrac{1}{2} f_w(x) \log f_w(x)]$$

$$= 1 + n[H(w, x) - 1]$$

$R_n(I)$, the average information rate in bits/block, is

$$R_n(I) = H(w) + H(x_1, \ldots, x_n) - H(w, x_1, \ldots, x_n) \qquad (5)$$

In calculating $R_1(I)$ and $R_n(I)$ from the experimental data, $f_w(x)$ was assumed equal to the experimental distributions of x, as given, for example, in Fig. 3.

ACKNOWLEDGMENTS

This research was conducted at the Wilmer Institute, Johns Hopkins Hospital and University. I wish to thank Dr. S. W. Kuffler, in whose laboratory this work was done, for suggesting the problem considered in this paper. The experiments were done with Dr. H. B. Barlow, Dr. K. T. Brown, and Dr. T. N. Wiesel. Preliminary discussions of the problem with Dr. Barlow were very valuable. This work was supported by a grant from the National Institutes of Health, United States Public Health Service. This article appeared in J. gen. Physiol., *1957,* **40,** *925–948.*

References

- Barlow, H. B., FitzHugh, R., and Kuffler, S. W. Maintained activity in the light and dark-adapted cat's retina. 1956*a*, (in preparation). [Editor's note: see Kuffler, E. W., FitzHugh, R., and Barlow, H. B. Maintained activity in the cat's retina in light and darkness. *J. gen. Physiol.*, 1957, **40,** 683–702.]
- Barlow, H. B., FitzHugh, R., and Kuffler, S. W. Absolute threshold, colour sensitivity and receptive field organization in the retina. 1956*b* (in preparation). [Editor's note: see Barlow, H. B., FitzHugh, R., and Kuffler, S. W. Change of organization in the receptive fields of the cat's retina during dark adaptation. *J. Physiol.*, 1957, **137,** 338–354; and Barlow, H. B., FitzHugh, R., and Kuffler, S. W. Dark adaptation, absolute threshold and Purkinje shift in single units of the cat's retina. *J. Physiol.*, 1957, **137,** 327–337.]
- Bartlett, M. S. Properties of sufficiency and statistical tests. *Proc. Roy. Soc. London*, 1937, *Series A*, **160,** 268–282.
- Blackwell, H. R. Psychophysical thresholds: Experimental studies of methods of measurement. University of Michigan: Engineering Research Institute, 1953, Bulletin No. 36.
- Bullock, T. H., and Diecke, F. Properties of an infrared receptor. *J. Physiol.*, 1956, **134,** 47–87.
- Cochran, W. G. The distribution of the largest of a set of estimated variances as a fraction of their total. *Ann. Eugenics*, 1941, **11,** 47–52.
- Eisenhart, C., Hastay, M. W., and Wallis, W. A. *Selected techniques of statistical analysis.* New York: McGraw-Hill, 1947, Chapters 4 and 15.
- Goldman, S. *Information theory.* New York: Prentice-Hall, 1953.
- Granit, R. *Sensory mechanisms of the retina.* London: Oxford University Press, 1947.

- Hecht, S., Shlaer, S., and Pirenne, M. H. Energy, quanta, and vision. *J. gen. Physiol.*, 1942, **25,** 819–840.
- Kuffler, S. W. Neurons in the retina: Organization, inhibition and excitation problems. *Cold Spring Harbor Symp. Quant. Biol.*, 1952, **17**, 281–292.
- Kuffler, S. W. Discharge patterns and functional organization of mammalian retina. *J. Neurophysiol.*, 1953, **16,** 37–68.
- MacKay, D. A., and McCulloch, W. S. The limiting information capacity of a neuronal link. *Bull. math. Biophysics,* 1955, **14,** 127–135.
- MacNichol, E. F., Jr., and Jacobs, J. A. H. Electronic device for measuring reciprocal time intervals. *Rev. scient. Instr.*, 1955, **26,** 1176–1180.
- Peterson, W. W., Birdsall, T. G., and Fox, W. C. The theory of signal detectability. *Trans. IRE Professional Group on Information Theory,* 1954, **PGIT-4,** 171–212.
- Shannon, C. E., and Weaver, W. *The mathematical theory of communication.* Urbana, Ill.: University of Illinois Press, 1949.
- Talbot, S. A., and Kuffler, S. W. A multibeam ophthalmoscope for the study of retinal physiology. *J. opt. Soc. Am.*, 1952, **42,** 931–936.
- Tanner, W. P., Jr., and Norman, R. Z. The human use of information: II. Signal detection for the case of an unknown signal parameter. *Trans. IRE Professional Group on Information Theory,* 1954, **PGIT-4,** 222–227.
- Tanner, W. P., Jr., and Swets, J. A. The human use of information: I. Signal detection for the case of the signal known exactly. *Trans. IRE Professional Group on Information Theory,* 1954, **PGIT-4,** 213–221.
- Walker, H. M., and Lev, J. *Statistical inference.* New York: Henry Holt, 1953.
- Woodward, P. M. *Probability and information theory, with applications to radar.* London: Pergamon Press, 1953.

18

Detection Theory Applied to the Absolute Sensitivity of Sensory Systems

Egbertus Eijkman and A. J. H. Vendrik

The modern theory of signal detectability (Peterson, Birdsall, and Fox, 1954; Van Meter and Middleton, 1954) has been successfully applied to the sensory detection of signals (Green, 1960*b*; Tanner, 1960). This theory describes certain aspects of sensory perception much better than the conventional threshold theory (Tanner and Swets, 1954; Swets and Birdsall, 1956; Swets, Tanner and Birdsall, 1961).

According to threshold theory, the threshold is a fixed level of signal strength or of the corresponding neural activity, below which no detection of the signal can occur, while above this level the signal is detected with certainty. In order to explain the shape of the frequency of detection curve plotted as a function of signal strength, it is assumed that either the signal varies statistically (e.g. numbers of quanta in a light flash for the visual perception), or that the threshold level varies, or both. Possibly existing internal noise of an additive nature, which is a neural activity in the sensory channel unrelated to the presence of a signal, is not considered in threshold theory.

In the theory of signal detectability, which is based on statistical-decision theory, it is assumed that additive noise exists and that every level of noise or signal plus noise, however small, can be detected. In the so-called yes-no experiments the observer makes a decision about presence or absence of a signal by adopting a decision level or criterion which is adjustable. By adjusting this level the observer can strive for an optimum detection, which is a well-defined concept in decision theory.

This theory has been used principally to describe the observation of signals in the presence of purposely added noise. Especially the detection of sound, sine wave or noise, in band-limited Gaussian noise has been investigated in the light of detection theory (Swets and Birdsall, 1956; Green, 1960*a*; Green, 1961; Swets, Shipley, McKey, and Green, 1959; Green, Birdsall, and Tanner, 1957).

One of the main advantages of the decision model as compared with the threshold model appears to be that in the former a parameter for the signal detectability can be defined which can be experimentally determined and which is independent of the psychophysical procedure used. The shift of the decision level of an observer striving for optimal detection caused by a change in the detection situation is predicted by the detection theory. In contrast, the variation in the threshold value with the psychophysical procedure is unaccounted for in the threshold model.

The occurrence of a positive response, when no signal is presented during an observation interval, a so-called false positive response, is expected in the detection model. The threshold model can interpret these false positives only as mere guesses, i.e. a response which is not based on any information obtained from the presence or absence of a signal.

The application of detection theory to the experimental determination of the absolute sensitivity of a sense organ requires the assumption that internal noise of an additive nature exists. This internal noise is a neural activity in the sensory channel not caused by the stimulus. It adds to the neural activity caused by the stimulus. This assumption is strongly supported by electrophysiological data. But the properties of this internal noise are almost entirely unknown.

As the decision model has distinct advantages over the threshold model, it seems worthwhile to try to obtain more knowledge about the internal noise. The noise can be expressed in terms of equivalent input signals and since the input signal is the only quantity in psychophysical experiments which can be physically measured and which can be compared with the internal noise, it will often be necessary to use this measure. But as will be shown here, it is useful to think of internal noise as a neural activity, and it is possible to derive valuable information about its distribution.

The model used here is undoubtedly too simple for an ultimate description of the detectability of small signals by human observers. But at this stage of knowledge it is a fruitful way to attack the problem. It is assumed that a physical signal gives rise to a neural activity in the sensory channel and that internal noise also exists. Detection takes place on the basis of the total magnitude of the neural activity, which is characterized by a single quantity during the observation interval. The relation between the magnitude of the signal and the neural activity caused thereby is monotonic but need not be linear. Variation of this relation which is a kind of multiplicative noise is considered only when the experimental results contradict the detection model.

The psychophysical experiments which will be mentioned are of three types. In the first type one of five stimuli of different amplitudes is presented to the observer in a given time interval. The stimuli are given in random sequence. One of the stimuli has zero amplitude. The response of the observer can be either yes or no, indicating whether or not in his opinion a stimulus has been given. No costs or values are announced to the subject for a correct response, a false alarm, or a missed signal. The fact that the stimuli are given at random results in the subject's adopting a criterion, which on the average is the same for all stimuli. The aim of these experiments was to investigate the probability distribution of the noise, including the fluctuation of the criterion, by analysis based upon the decision model.

In the second type of experiment, the observer has to choose one of four possibilities. In an observation interval one of four stimuli with different amplitudes is presented to the observer, and the observer responds by stating which of the four stimuli he thinks was given. The observer is trained to the set of stimuli before the proper measurements start. The magnitudes of the stimuli are chosen in such a way that a probability of detection between 0.05 and 0.95 for each stimulus is obtained. As will be explained, this kind of experiment allows conclusions about the linearity or nonlinearity of the relation between stimulus strength and neural activity.

Finally, the third type of experiment is of the forced-choice type. In one of four observation intervals a stimulus of known magnitude is presented and the observer is asked to indicate in which interval he thinks the stimulus has been given. The observer must also make a second choice different from the first one. With the results of these measurements the important question can be answered whether the false-positive responses (saying yes when no stimulus is offered) are observations of noise indistinguishable from the signal or mere guessing. This is the crucial question for a decision between the threshold model and the decision model.

The occurrence of a stimulus interval is signaled to the observer by sound or a light flash. It is ensured that stimuli of different amplitudes differ only in amplitude, everything else being the same. Constancy of time course of the stimuli is important because of the dynamic properties of the sensitivity of the skin senses (Eijkman and Vendrik, 1960*a*; 1960*b*; 1961). All observers had thorough training before the final experiments were carried out.

The main experiments were carried out on the skin senses of touch and warmth. The stimuli were deformation, electrical current, and increase of temperature. The site of stimulation was the inner side of the forearm. A few experiments were performed on the auditory and visual sense organs. For the experiments described in this paper only the relative values of the signal strengths need be known. The relevant measure of the signal strength is considered to be the deformation for the stimulation of the touch, the electrical current strength for the electrical stimulation, the voltage across the earphone for the auditory experiments, and the light energy for the visual experiments. The adequate stimulus of the warmth sense is best expressed in terms of temperature increase of the skin (Vendrik and Vos, 1958).

The touch stimuli were linearly increasing deformations with a duration of 0.16 sec or pulse-shaped with a duration of 70 msec. The electrical stimuli were pulse-shaped with a duration of 2 msec. The warmth stimuli were given by irradiation with infrared of constant intensity resulting in a linearly increasing temperature of the skin surface during the exposure time of 0.38 sec and 1.2 sec. In order to prevent too much increase in temperature of the skin, the time between stimuli was made more than 15 sec. The experiments on hearing were done in an anechoic room. Sine-wave stimuli of 1000 cps with a duration of 0.2 sec were applied monaurally.

The observer determined the starting time of a trial by pressing a button. For a part of the experiments an electronic spinning disc was used which produced a random choice of four possibilities.

THEORY AND RESULTS OF THE EXPERIMENTS

Distribution of internal noise

In Fig. 1 the probability density of the neural activity x is plotted when both noise alone and signal plus noise are present. The magnitude of the neural activity determines whether a positive or negative response is given. If the neural activity during an observation

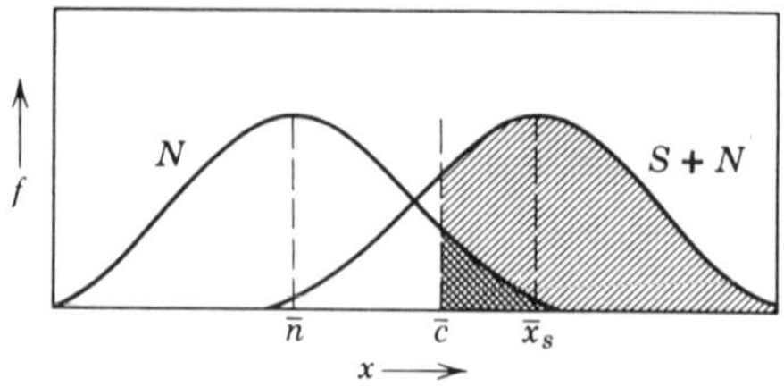

FIG. 1. Probability density of the neural activity x, for noise alone and for signal plus noise; $\bar{c}$ is the criterion.

interval is larger than a criterion c a positive response is given; if it is smaller, a negative response occurs. One of the underlying assumptions of the decision model used is that the signal itself is not noisy. The two distributions differ only in the average value.

The criterion c may not be constant. But the fluctuations of the criterion can be included in the fluctuation of the noise. It can be shown that a Gaussian noise with mean $\bar{n}$ and variance σ_n^2 and a criterion also with a Gaussian distribution with mean $\bar{c}$ and variance σ_c^2 is mathematically equivalent to a Gaussian noise with mean $\bar{n}$ and variance $\sigma^2 = \sigma_n^2 + \sigma_c^2$ and a constant criterion $\bar{c}$.

Another equivalent model is a constant noise with value $\bar{n}$ and a fluctuating criterion with mean $\bar{c}$ and variance $\sigma^2 = \sigma_n^2 + \sigma_c^2$. The variable quantity in this second model is the criterion c (Fig. 2). This c is equal to $-x + \bar{c} + \bar{x}$ in the first model, where $\bar{x} = \bar{n}$ or $\bar{x}_s$. The equivalence of the two models can easily be seen by comparing Figs. 1 and 2 and can be proved by simple mathematics. We will now use the second model. This mode of description is somewhat easier to handle when various signals with different strengths are randomly applied. The probability density of the criterion includes the variability due to the fluctuations of the noise.

If we assume that signal strength s and x are linearly related, the probability density function will have the same shape when it is plot-

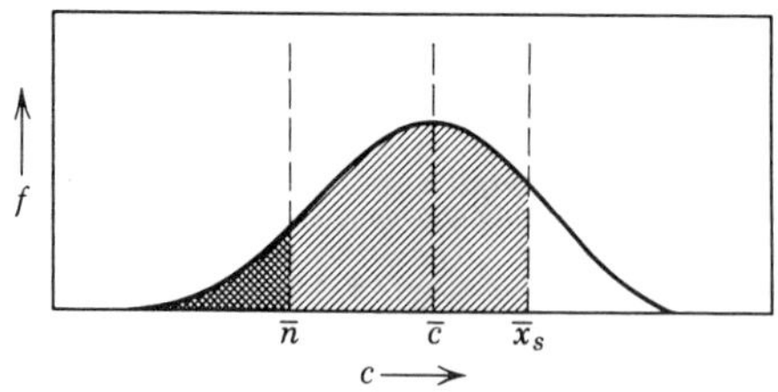

FIG. 2. Model equivalent to the model shown in Fig. 1.

ted versus s as versus x or c. The experiments of the first type are used for the measurement of this distribution function. Five signals including a signal of zero amplitude are presented at random to the observer. The observer responds with yes or no, indicating whether he thinks a signal has been given or not. The five signals are equally probable.

These experiments have been carried out on the senses of warmth, touch, and hearing, and with electrical stimulation of the skin. Some of the results are shown in Figs. 3, 4, and 5. The probability is plotted on the ordinate which has a Gaussian probability scale.

It will be seen that in first approximation the experimental points of the senses of warmth and touch lie on a straight line, which means that the distribution of the probability density is Gaussian. The standard deviation σ of this distribution is the best measure of the sensitivity of the sensory system. In our experiments the value of σ of the warmth sense was about 0.04°C, the σ of the touch sense about 60μ. But it must be emphasized that these figures are dependent on such parameters as size and shape of the stimulus, place of stimulation, and also on the time course of the stimulus (Eijkman and Vendrik, 1960*a*; 1960*b*; 1961).

Taking into account all the measurements on various subjects, it appears that for the warmth sense no significant deviation from the Gaussian distribution is found. However, the results of the experiments on the senses of hearing and touch and with electrical stimulation show a

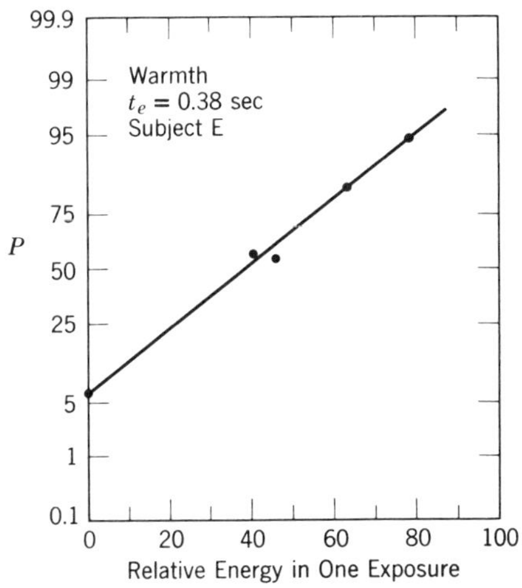

FIG. 3. Relative frequency of positive response versus signal strength, plotted on probability paper, for warmth sense.

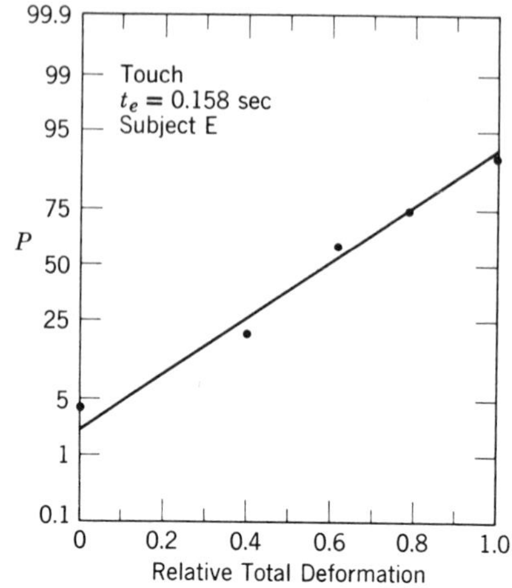

FIG. 4. Same as Fig. 3, for touch.

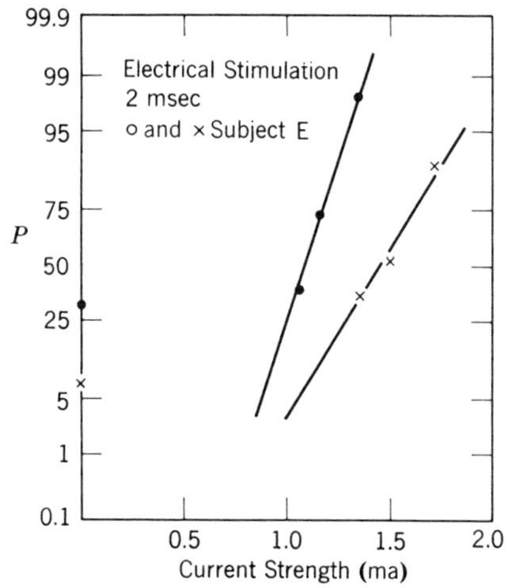

FIG. 5. Same as Fig. 3, for electrical stimulation.

deviation, which is very marked in the electrical stimulation experiments. The probability of response on the smallest signal, which is in this case a signal of zero amplitude, is too high. This deviation may be due to the following causes. First the transfer function $g(s)$ which transforms the signal s into the neural activity x, $x = g(s)$, may be fluctuating. This would be a kind of multiplicative noise, whereas the noise mentioned so far is of an additive nature. The influence of this fluctuation would, however, very likely increase with signal strength. This would cause an increase of the standard deviation of the probability density function with signal strength. The experimentally found deviation of the normal distribution, however, is entirely otherwise. Therefore this influence cannot explain the experimental results. Secondly the relation between signal strength and neural activity x may be nonlinear; or thirdly, this relation being linear, the distribution plotted versus x may be skewed (Fig. 6).

Skewness of distribution or nonlinearity

In the design of an experiment that offers the opportunity to distinguish between a skewed distribution and nonlinearity of the relation between signal strength and neural activity, the following consideration is relevant. In experiments of the first type the distribution of the criterion is determined by measuring the probability of correct responses to signals of various strengths. If one could shift the distribution of the criterion in respect to the strength of the signals and again could determine this distribution by the same measurement, a distinction between skewness and nonlinearity could be made. This is done in the following way.

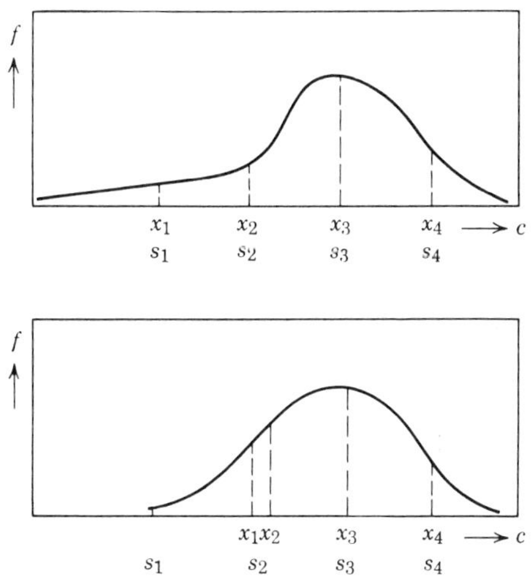

FIG. 6. Above: Probability density curve is skewed (criterion c and signal strength s linearly related). Below: Symmetrical probability density curve (relation between c and s nonlinear).

In an observation interval one of four signals S_1, S_2, S_3, S_4 with different strengths, $s_1 < s_2 < s_3 < s_4$ is presented to the subject. The subject must respond by saying which signal of the four he thinks is given. The subject needs for this response three criteria c_1, c_2, and c_3. If one of the four signals, say S_i, is presented, a neural activity x_i is caused. The subject responds by saying "four" (R_4 occurs) if $x_i > c_3$; and he responds by saying "three" (R_3 occurs) if $c_2 < x_i < c_3$. Thus R_2 occurs if $c_1 < x_i < c_2$ and R_1 if $x_i < c_1$.

The responses R_4 on the various signal strengths provide the distribution of c_3 as a function of signal strength. The responses $R_4 + R_3$ which occur if $x_i < c_2$ give in the same way the distribution of c_2, and $R_4 + R_3 + R_2$ yield the distribution of c_1. The obvious assumption is made that always $c_1 < c_2 < c_3$.

In Figs. 7 and 8 the consequences of the two possibilities, skewness and nonlinearity, for the relationship between the so-measured distributions

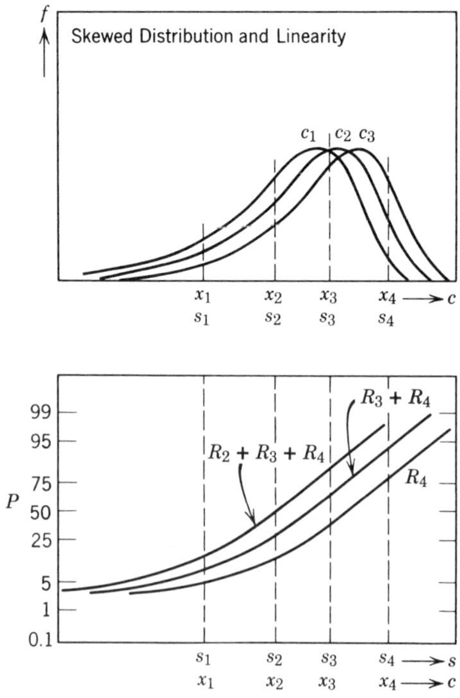

FIG. 7. Four observation categories. Skewness causes the s curves of probability versus signal strength to shift in a horizontal direction.

of c_1, c_2, and c_3 are shown. If the distribution is skewed the three curves plotted on probability paper are only shifted in the horizontal direction. This is obvious as the three distribution curves, c_1, c_2 and c_3, in the upper part of Fig. 7 are equal except for a horizontal shift. If nonlinearity exists, however, the curves are to a first approximation all shifted in the vertical direction. This is illustrated in Fig. 8. As the distribution curves c_1, c_2, and c_3 are now assumed to be symmetric Gaussian curves, the cumulative distribution curves plotted on probability paper as a function of c are straight lines. These lines are drawn in the bottom part of Fig. 8 partly solid, partly broken. However, plotted as a function of signal strength, the solid curved lines are obtained if nonlinearity between neural activity and signal strength exists as assumed in Fig. 8. In Figs. 6, 7, and 8 it is assumed for the sake of simplicity of the explanation that the signal strengths are equally spaced along the strength axis.

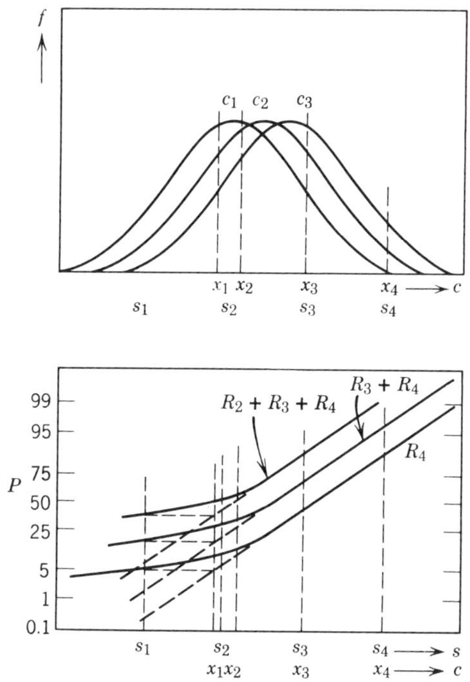

FIG. 8. Four observation categories. Symmetrical probability density curve and nonlinear relation between criterion c and signal strength s causes a shift in the vertical direction.

These experiments have been performed with the sense of touch and with electrical stimulation. Some of the results are shown in Figs. 9 and 10. Of the two possibilities considered the hypothesis of nonlinearity explains the experimental results, and skewness of the distribution is clearly excluded.

Second forced choice

If noise exists in the neural channel which is indistinguishable from the activity caused by a signal, the subject will also make false-positive responses. However, the existence of false positives does not prove the existence of this kind of noise. It could be that these false positives were mere guesses. Guesses are positive responses which are made without using any information gained from the fact that in the observation interval a signal was or was not presented.

If the threshold model were valid, false positives would only be guesses. The experiments described and other similar experiments indicate, however, that false positives should be explained on the basis of the decision model and should not be considered as guesses.

Additional evidence on this point can be obtained by the following experiment, which has been carried out by Swets with visual signals (Tanner and Swets, 1954; Swets, Tanner, and Birdsall, 1961). In a four-alternative forced-choice experiment the subject is asked not only to

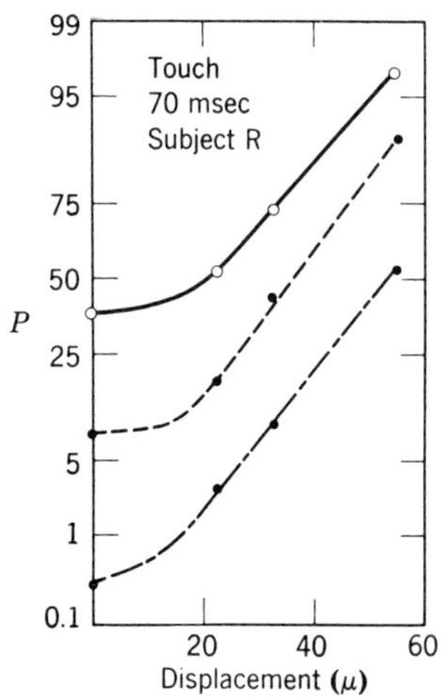

FIG. 9. Experiment on touch with four categories. Curves are shifted in the vertical direction.

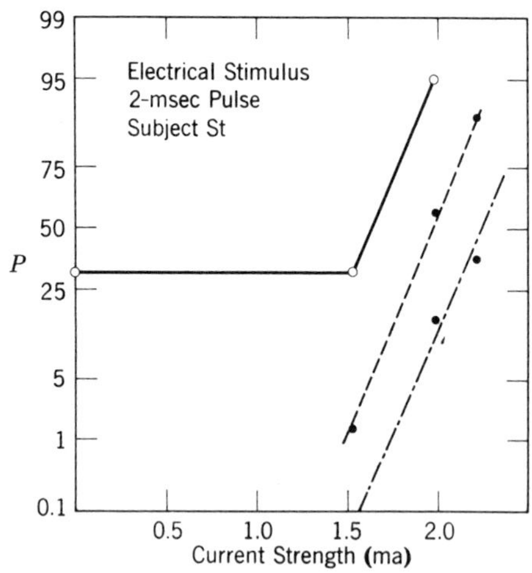

FIG. 10. The same as Fig. 9, for electrical stimulation.

state in which of the four intervals the signal is given but also to give a second choice. Assuming that the decision model holds, a correct first-choice response will occur if the neural activity due to signal plus noise is larger than the neural noise in the three other intervals. A correct second-choice response will occur if the neural activity due to signal plus noise in one interval is smaller than the neural noise in another interval and larger than the neural noise in the remaining two intervals.

If the threshold model is valid, the second-choice response can only be a guess. When the first choice is incorrect the probability of a correct second choice will then be 0.33, independent of signal strength.

The probability of the correct first choice and second choice in the four-alternative experiments will be called P_4 and P_3', respectively. The probability of the correct first choice in an experiment, which differs only from the former one in using three observation intervals, in one of which the signal is given, will be called P_3. It can be shown that very generally the relation holds $P_3' = 3(P_3 - P_4)$.

As mentioned, the threshold model predicts that $P_3' = 1/3(1 - P_4)$. If the probability of a correct response in a yes-no experiment with the same signal is called P then $P_3 = 2/3\ P + 1/3$ and $P_4 = 3/4\ \mathrm{P} + 1/4$. It follows from these three relations that $P_3' = 3(P_3 - P_4)$.

Applying detection theory and calling the probability density of the noise as a function of neural activity f_N, that of neural activity due to signal plus noise f_{SN} (Fig. 1), and the corresponding cumulative distributions P_N and P_{SN}, respectively, one obtains

$$P_4 = \int_{-\infty}^{+\infty} f_{SN} P^3{}_N \, dx, \quad P_3 = \int_{-\infty}^{+\infty} f_{SN} P^2{}_N \, dx, \quad \text{and}$$

$$P_3' = 3 \int_{-\infty}^{+\infty} f_{SN}(1 - P_N) P^2{}_N \, dx$$

Again it appears that $P_3' = 3(P_3 - P_4)$ independent of the shape of f_N and f_{SN}.

Values of P_4 as a function of the quantity d' when P_N and P_{SN} have a Gaussian distribution have been published by Green, Birdsall, and Tanner (1957). They assumed that the signal-plus-noise probability-density function has the same standard deviation, i.e. that the signal itself is not noisy. Under the same assumptions we calculated P_3. The symbol d', introduced by Tanner and Birdsall (1958), is the ratio of the strength of the signal and the standard deviation of the noise probability-density function.

Values of P_3' and P_4 have been determined by experiments using respectively touch stimuli, electrical stimuli, and warmth stimuli applied to the inner side of the forearm. Moreover, some preliminary experiments have been carried out on vision using small short light flashes with durations of 20 msec and a magnitude of 3′ stimulating the dark-adapted eye 10° nasal. The results of these experiments are partially shown in the Figs. 11 and 12. The drawn straight line gives the relation between P_3' and P_4 that holds under the threshold model. The broken line gives the relation under the decision model using the equation $P_3' = 3(P_3 - P_4)$ and the previously mentioned calculated values of P_3 and P_4. It will be seen that the experimental data differ distinctly from the drawn line. The percentage indicated in the figures beside the subject gives the level of significance of the deviation from the straight line. The experiments with the warmth stimuli fit the broken line rather well. The experimental points with touch and electrical stimuli are on the average lower.

The preliminary experiments with light stimuli also show a significant deviation of the experimental points from the straight line for one subject, but two other subjects did not.

These experiments show, therefore, that the threshold model is not adequate. The probability of a correct second choice when the first choice is wrong is significantly higher than the threshold model predicts. This is a strong argument for not considering false positives as mere guesses and accepting the significance of additive noise in the detection of small signals.

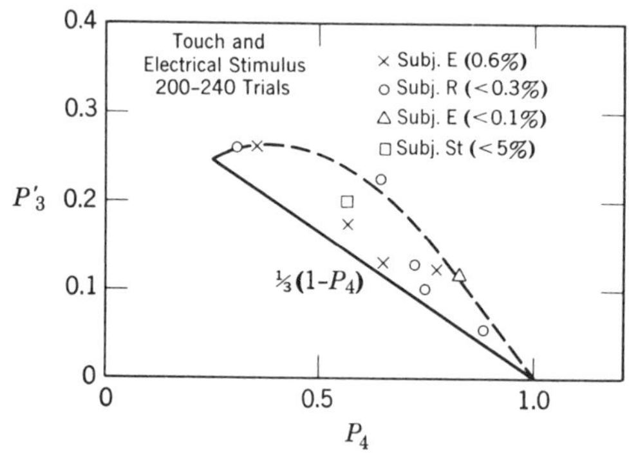

FIG. 11. Probability of correct second forced choice versus probability of correct first choice. Four alternatives. Solid line: second choice merely guesses. Broken line: theoretical line based on decision model. The x and open circle are for touch, the square and triangle for electrical stimulation.

DISCUSSION

The especially pronounced occurrence of false-positive responses in experiments on the skin senses suggests that internal neural noise exists which is indistinguishable from the neural activity caused by a stimulus. Threshold theory considers these false positives as guesses. It is shown that under the threshold theory the threshold value is dependent on the probability of false-positive responses (Swets, Tanner, and Birdsall, 1961), which is inconsistent with the underlying assumptions of this theory.

The second forced-choice experiments show clearly that the second choice contains a significant amount of information on the occurrence of a signal. This is a strong argument for accepting this internal noise. Also on the grounds of electrophysiological data it has been suggested that internal noise plays a part in limiting the sensitivity of sense organs. FitzHugh (1957, 1958) gave a statistical analysis of discharges of single ganglion cells in the retina of the cat and attempted to relate these data to the results of psychophysical measurements of visual sensitivity.

The experimental results with the warmth and touch sense can be explained to a first approximation by an internal noise (including the fluctuation of the criterion) which has a Gaussian distribution when expressed in terms of input signal. If one assumes that the internal neural activity is also normally distributed then it follows that the neural activity is proportional to signal strength.

If we accept the decision model the measure for the sensitivity of a sensory system is the standard deviation of this Gaussian distribution. If the detectability of small signals by a human observer is well described by the decision model this measure is independent of the criterion of the subject and of the psychophysical procedure.

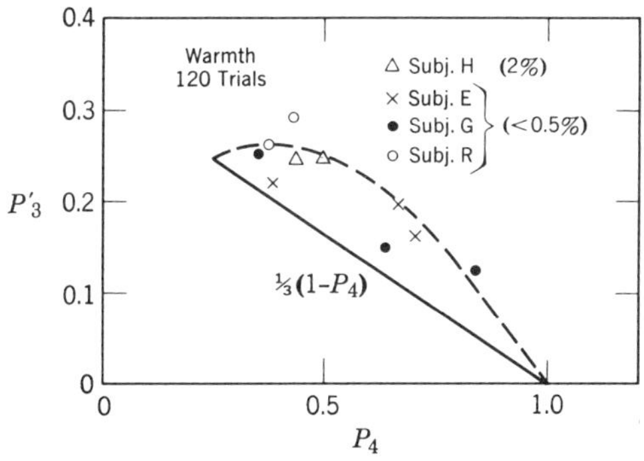

FIG. 12. The same as Fig. 11, but for warmth.

We found a small deviation from the Gaussian distribution for very small signals with the touch sense and with electrical stimulation. The experiments with four categories of magnitude of observation show that this deviation is explained by assuming that the internal neural activity is normally distributed and that the relation between signal strength and the neural activity caused thereby is nonlinear. This is shown schematically in Fig. 13. If the curve has the course of the dotted line one could speak about a threshold s_t being a value of the stimulus below which no neural activity is generated by the stimulus.

With the touch sense this nonlinearity is found using mechanical deformation and is even more pronounced with electrical stimulation, but it is not found with the warmth sense. It may be possible that this has something to do with the existence of a constant non-zero rate of action potentials of the warmth fibers when temperature is constant (Hensel and Zotterman; 1951), whereas the touch fibers show complete adaptation. Change in interval duration between action potentials may be a continuous process, whereas for the generation of action potentials in the touch fibers the stimulus has to exceed a certain threshold value.

We think it better, however, not to use the word "threshold" for the course of the curve of Fig. 13, but the broader term "nonlinearity." First, the possibility of a distinction between the solid and the dotted lines in Fig. 13 depends on the accuracy of the experiments and, in turn, on the number of observations. This is obviously very limited in psychophysical experiments. Furthermore the term "threshold" in psychophysical threshold theory has a different meaning because it refers to a cutoff in the continuum of observation.

It can be seen in Fig. 11 that on the average the probability of the correct second-forced-choice responses for the touch sense and with

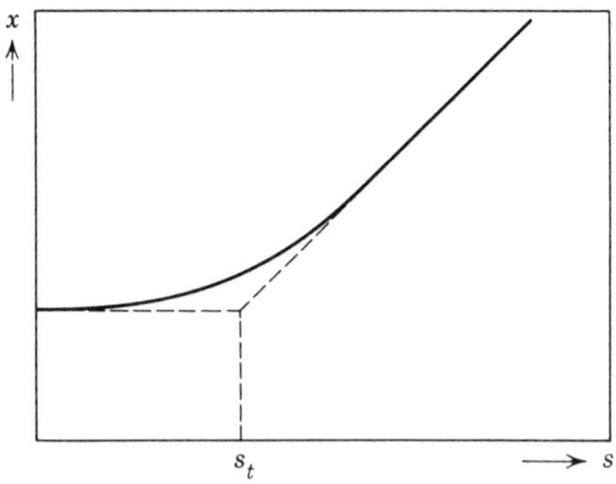

FIG. 13. Solid line: Nonlinear relation between neural activity x and signal strength, s. Broken line: Course with a stimulus threshold s_t.

electrical stimulation is lower than predicted by the decision model. We did not perform further experiments to clarify this point. We can only suggest a possible explanation. One of the observers remarked that in a part of the trials he did not get any sensation and that he thought that the responses on these trials were mere guesses. This would indeed explain the deviation but the decision model does not account for such an additional temporary high cutoff level. Future experiments should elucidate this point further.

An important question is whether, besides the internal neural noise of an additive nature, a multiplicative noise must also be assumed. This multiplicative noise would be a fluctuation which is a monotonic increasing function of signal strength, and zero when signal strength is zero. Such a noise could be due to fluctuations in the output of the signal generator but also to fluctuations in the transfer function which connects the signal with the neural activity. A multiplicative noise would cause an increase in the variance of the signal-plus-noise density function with signal strength.

As has been mentioned, the experiments on the touch and warmth senses do not justify the assumption of multiplicative noise. But it is very likely that this kind of noise is very pronounced in experiments on the absolute sensitivity of the visual sense organ because the fluctuation in the number of quanta is considerable. The second-forced-choice experiments have been also carried out in our department on the dark-adapted eye with small light flashes. Only one of the three observers showed a significantly high score of correct second responses. It is entirely possible that internal noise plays a role in one subject while in another this noise is much smaller than the fluctuations in the neural activity due to the statistics of the quanta in the light flash. We have not succeeded as yet in giving a reasonable description of the visual absolute-sensitivity measurement.

One can expect that multiplicative noise is important in the measurement of difference limens. Swets et al. (Tanner and Swets, 1954; Swets, Tanner, and Birdsall, 1961) performed second-forced-choice experiments on the detectability of light flashes against a background. The results show again that the second response conveys a significant amount of information about the signal. The data points are fitted well by a theoretical curve that is derived from the decision model on the assumption that the variance of the signal-plus-noise density function increases proportionally with signal strength. This is a kind of multiplicative noise.

Tanner (1961) applied the theory of signal detectability to auditory amplitude discrimination. He assumed, besides a noise introduced by the experimenter, a noise generated by the equipment, and a kind of multiplicative noise caused by the amplitude variation in the oscillator that is proportional to the power of the lower of two signals to be discriminated. Tanner (1961) suggests that the law of Weber should be explained on the basis of this generator inconstancy. This seems, however, not very likely.

In our opinion the most plausible explanation of the law of Weber is given by the assumption that the transfer function between the input signal and the magnitude of sensation fluctuates. The fluctuation in the sensation caused thereby is usually not perceived. The just noticeable change in stimulus has to give rise to a change in sensation which is proportional to the fluctuation in the sensation. A similar assumption is widely accepted in vision. If, furthermore, according to the investigations of Stevens (1958), the validity of the law of Plateau is accepted, which states that the sensation magnitude is a power function of the stimulus strength, the law of Weber can be easily derived. This derivation and some important consequences will be the object of a separate paper.

SUMMARY

The skin senses of touch and warmth have been investigated. It is shown that the decision model describes the experimental data better than the threshold model. The experiments lead to the assumption that an internal noise exists, which is a neural activity that is indistinguishable from the neural activity caused by small stimuli and which adds to the neural activity caused by the stimulus. The probability distribution of this internal noise can be considered to be Gaussian. The relation between stimulus and neural activity is nonlinear for the touch sense. The question of whether noise of a multiplicative nature must be assumed is discussed.

ACKNOWLEDGMENTS

This research was conducted in the Department of Medical Physics, University of Nijmegen, Nijmegen, The Netherlands. This article appeared in Biophys. J., *1963,* **3,** *65–78.*

References

- Eijkman, E., and Vendrik, A. J. H. Time constant of touch fibres in the cat. *Acta physiol. pharmacol. neerlandica,* 1960*a,* **9,** 461–472.
- Eijkman, E., and Vendrik, A. J. H. Dynamics of the vibration sense at low frequency. *J. acoust. Soc. Am.,* 1960*b,* **32,** 1134–1139.

- Eijkman, E., and Vendrik, A. J. H. Dynamic behavior of the warmth sense organ. *J. exp. Psychol.*, 1961, **62,** 403–408.
- FitzHugh, R. The statistical detection of threshold signals in the retina. *J. gen. Physiol.*, 1957, **40,** 925–948. [17]
- FitzHugh, R. A statistical analyzer for optic nerve messages. *J. gen. Physiol.*, 1958, **41,** 675–692.
- Green, D. M. Auditory detection of a noise signal. *J. acoust. Soc. Am.*, 1960*a,* **32,** 121–131. [27]
- Green, D. M. Psychoacoustics and detection theory. *J. acoust. Soc. Am.*, 1960*b,* **32,** 1189–1202. [2]
- Green, D. M. Detection of auditory sinusoids of uncertain frequency. *J. acoust. Soc. Am.*, 1961, **33,** 897–903. [28]
- Green, D. M., Birdsall, T. G., and Tanner, W. P. Jr. Signal detection as a function of signal intensity and duration. *J. acoust. Soc. Am.*, 1957, **29,** 523–531. [11]
- Hensel, H., and Zotterman, Y. The response of the cold receptors to constant cooling. *Acta physiol. Scand.*, 1951, **22,** 96–105.
- Peterson, W. W., Birdsall, T. G., and Fox, W. C. The theory of signal detectability. *Trans. IRE Professional Group on Information Theory,* 1954, **PGIT-4,** 171–212.
- Stevens, S. S. Measurement and man. *Science,* 1958, **127,** 383–389.
- Swets, J. A., and Birdsall, T. G. The human use of information: III. Decision-making in signal detection and recognition situations involving multiple alternatives. *Trans. IRE Professional Group on Information Theory,* 1956, **IT-2,** 138–165.
- Swets, J. A., Shipley, E. F., McKey, M. J., and Green, D. M. Multiple observations of signals in noise. *J. acoust. Soc. Am.*, 1959, **31,** 514–521. [9]
- Swets, J. A., Tanner, W. P., Jr., and Birdsall, T. G. Decision processes in perception. *Psychol. Rev.*, 1961, **68,** 301–340. [1]
- Tanner, W. P., Jr. Theory of signal detectability as an interpretive tool for psychophysical data. *J. acoust. Soc. Am.*, 1960, **32,** 1140–1147.
- Tanner, W. P., Jr. Application of the theory of signal detectability to amplitude discrimination. *J. acoust. Soc. Am.*, 1961, **33,** 1233–1244.
- Tanner, W. P., Jr., and Birdsall, T. G. Definitions of d' and η as psychophysical measures. *J. acoust. Soc. Am.*, 1958, **30,** 922–928. [5]
- Tanner, W. P., Jr., and Swets, J. A. The human use of information: I. Signal detection for the case of the signal known exactly. *Trans. IRE Professional Group on Information Theory,* 1954, **PGIT-4,** 213–221.
- Van Meter, D., and Middleton, D. Modern statistical approaches to reception in communication theory. *Trans. IRE Professional Group on Information Theory,* 1954, **PGIT-4,** 119–145.
- Vendrik, A. J. H., and Vos, J. J. Comparison of the stimulation of the warmth sense organ by microwave and infrared. *J. appl. Physiol.*, 1958, **13,** 435–444.

section five

RECOGNITION

The theory and methods developed for detection tasks can be applied to recognition problems in various ways. Tanner, in "Theory of Recognition" [19], shows that recognizing which of two signals occurred is formally the same as determining whether a single signal was present or absent. He describes a method for predicting recognition data from detection data and a method for determining the degree of correlation between the observations of different signals. One appendix to this chapter is devoted to the measurement of observer efficiency; a second appendix compares and contrasts detection theory to the earlier work of Thurstone. Swets and Sewall examine the substantive problem of "Stimulus Versus Response Uncertainty in Recognition" [20]; in their experiments, information about the stimulus alternatives given before the observation facilitates recognition, and information given after the observation but before the response has little, if any, effect. Pollack, in "Identification of Elementary Auditory Displays and the Method of Recognition Memory" [21], shows how the analysis procedures of detection theory provide a measure of recognition memory that is independent of the response criterion. Sorkin supplies an "Extension of the Theory of Signal Detectability to Matching Procedures in Psychoacoustics" [22], to some matching tasks of the sort frequently used to infer the attributes underlying complex choice behavior, for example, in the recognition of colors, or of synthetic speech sounds. Other applications of the theory and methods to recognition problems can be found in Section 7.

19

Theory of Recognition

Wilson P. Tanner, Jr.

Since the experiments to be described will be analyzed in terms of a variable, d', rather than thresholds, the definition of d' is first reviewed (Tanner and Swets, 1954; Tanner, 1955; Birdsall, 1955; Peterson, Birdsall, and Fox, 1954). For a signal known exactly, the ratio $2E/N_0$, is a detection index where E is the signal energy and N_0 is the noise power per unit bandwidth. Given the index, it is possible to calculate mathematically the performance one would expect of a perfect device, depending on the question asked of the device. If the device is asked to detect signals, then it is possible to state a rate of signal detection as a function of false alarm rate for a given $2E/N_0$. If the device is asked to detect in which of four intervals of time a signal appeared, then the probability of a correct decision can be calculated.

The quantity $(2E/N_0)^{1/2}$ is related to two normal probability distributions along a decision axis, one representing the conditional probability that if noise alone is present, the measure X results, the other the conditional probability distribution that if signal plus noise exists, the measure X results. The difference between the means of these distributions divided by the standard deviation of the noise distribution is $(2E/N_0)^{1/2}$.

Now, if one knows the question asked, and the performance of the device, then one can state the value of the quantity $(2E/N_0)^{1/2}$ necessary to lead to the same level of performance if the device were perfect. The assumption so far employed in the application of the theory is that the observer behaves as a mathematically perfect device. That is to say, if one could measure the input to his decision device, and determine $(2E/N_0)^{1/2}$ at that input, one could then state by means of the theory of signal detection the observer's performance. At the same time, if one knows the observer's performance, then one can state what the input to the device must be. The experimental data furnish an estimate of the observer's performance, and d' is the value of $(2E/N_0)^{1/2}$ required at the input of the decision device to lead to the estimated performance. The fact that, for given physical conditions, a d' estimated from one experimental condition specifies within sampling error expectation the prediction of an observer's performance under all of the experimental conditions so far studied, justifies the use of d' as the measure of performance in psychophysical experiments.

Recognition is, by definition, the process of classifying a signal as a member of a subset of a set. The subset may have one or more members. For example, it is possible to recognize a human being as being a member of the Chinese race, or as being an old friend John Roe with whom one attended college. In the first case the subset has many members, while in the second case the subset has one member, the particular John Roe.

The particular problem treated in this paper is the case of recognition where there are two subsets, ω_1 or ω_2, each containing one member, and each is a signal of specified frequency. Through the experimental design, the a priori probabilities of the two signals $P(S_1N) + P(S_2N) = 1.00$ and $P(S_1N \text{ and } S_2N) = 0$. The observation x,y is now associated with two probability density distributions, $f_{S_1N}(x,y)$ and $f_{S_2N}(x,y)$. The decision is based on likelihood ratio, as is shown in Eq. (1).

$$l(x,y) = \frac{f_{S_1N}(x,y)}{f_{S_2N}(x,y)} \tag{1}$$

If the decision function can be defined along an axis, the problem is similar to the detection problem with one of the probability distribution functions $f_{S_1N}(x,y)$ or $f_{S_2N}(x,y)$ substituted for $f_N(x)$ of the detection problem.

DECISION AXIS FOR TWO SIGNALS

The problem is illustrated in Fig. 1. The axis OX represents the decision axis for the detection case where the signal is known to be at ω_1. The axis OY represents the decision axis for the detection case where the frequency is known to be at ω_2.

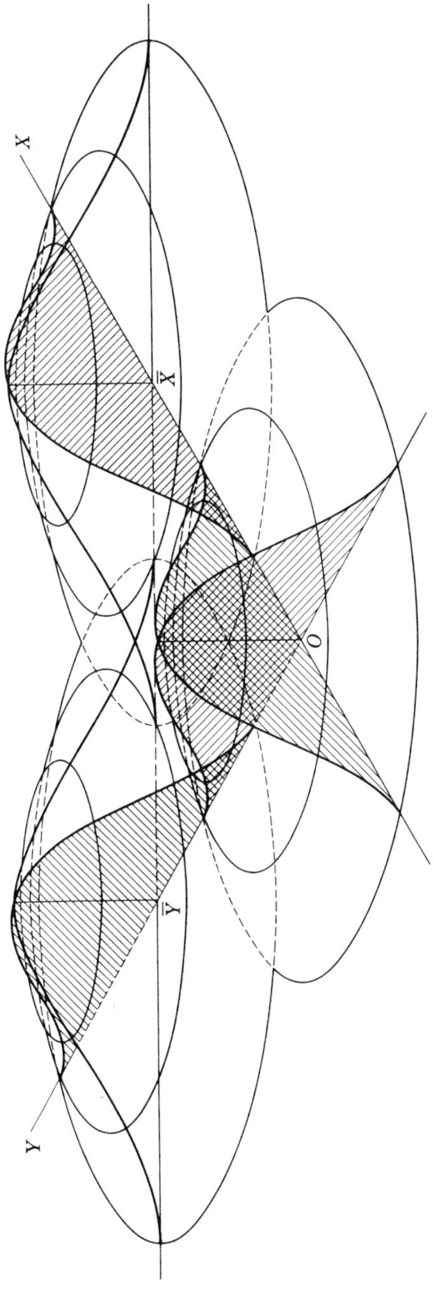

FIG. 1. The recognition space for a signal known to be one of two frequencies.

The distance OX divided by the standard deviation of the noise distribution $f_N(x)$ is called d_1', the d' for detection of frequency ω_1. The distance OY divided by the standard deviation of $f_N(y)$ is d_2' the d' for detection frequency ω_2. The d' for recognition of frequency when the signal is known to be either ω_1 or ω_2, is designated $d_{1,2}'$. The distributions $f_N(x)$, $f_N(y)$, $f_{S_1N}(x)$, and $f_{S_2N}(y)$ are all assumed to have equal variance.

First the case is discussed where the observations x and y are independent. In order to define independence, consider that the observer is essentially a narrow-band receiver at an instant in time. Illustrated in Fig. 2 is a frequency axis upon which are placed three points: ω_1, ω_2, and ω_3. At each point there are distributions shown which represent hypothetically the response curves of the observer's attention mechanism when the attention is centered at that point. The ordinate of the curve at any point represents the extent to which energy at the frequency represented by that point enters the observation. Since ω_1 and ω_2 are close together on the frequency axis there are many points at which the energy enters the observations at each frequency. Thus, observations at ω_1 and ω_2 have common variance, and consequently are correlated. The correlation arises from common variance over the shaded area in the figure. Observations at ω_1 and ω_3, which are widely separated in frequency, have very little common variance, and consequently can be said to be independent.

The problem considered is the fixed-observation-interval problem. An observation x, y, a function of time for T seconds, is the datum upon which the decision is based. The signal is known to be either ω_1 or ω_2, but not both. Thus, $f_{S_1N}(x,y)$ is the joint probability density function $f_{S_1N}(x)$ and $f_N(y)$, while $f_{S_2N}(x,y)$ is the joint probability density function $f_{S_2N}(y)$ and $f_N(x)$, assuming x and y are independent.

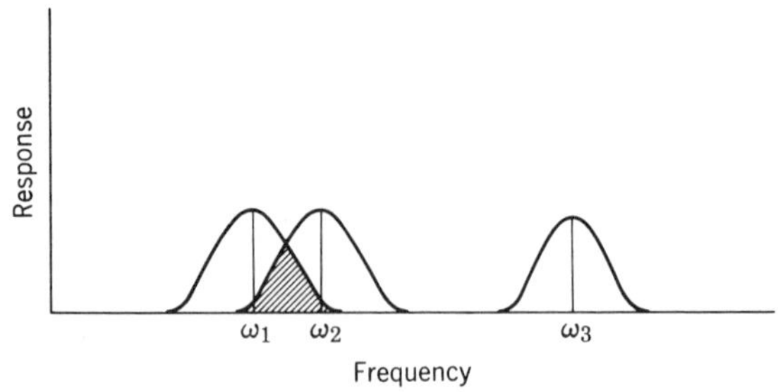

FIG. 2. Observer's response curves for three frequencies.

If

$$f_{S_1N}(x,y) = \frac{1}{2\pi} \exp\left[\frac{-(x - d_1')^2}{2}\right] \exp\left(\frac{-y^2}{2}\right) \tag{2}$$

and

$$f_{S_2N}(x,y) = \frac{1}{2\pi} \exp\left[\frac{-(y - d_2')^2}{2}\right] \exp\left(\frac{-x^2}{2}\right) \tag{3}$$

then, from Eq. (1),

$$\begin{aligned} \log_e l(x,y) &= \frac{x^2}{2} + xd_1' \\ &\quad - \frac{(d_1')^2}{2} - \frac{y^2}{2} + \frac{y^2}{2} - yd_2' + \frac{(d_2')^2}{2} - \frac{x^2}{2} \\ &= xd_1' - \frac{(d_1')^2}{2} - yd_2' + \frac{(d_2')^2}{2} \end{aligned} \tag{4}$$

If $d_1' = d_2'$ and $d' \neq 0$, then

$$y = x - \frac{\log_e l(x,y)}{d'} \tag{5}$$

Thus, if $l(x,y)$ is held constant, this is the equation for a straight line with slope 1.00, and intercept $\log_e l(x,y)/d'$. This line passes through the origin when $l(x,y) = 1.00$.

By Eq. (5), each value of $l(x,y)$ is represented by a line of slope 1 which intersects the line connecting $d_1' = \bar{x}$ and $d_2' = \bar{y}$ at right angles. From this, it follows that the decision axis for the recognition problem can be mapped on the line, with S_1 normally distributed $(\bar{x},1)$, and S_2 normally distributed $(\bar{y},1)$.

Part of Fig. 1 has been reproduced as Fig. 3*a* to illustrate this point more simply. The dotted lines on this figure are lines of constant likeli-

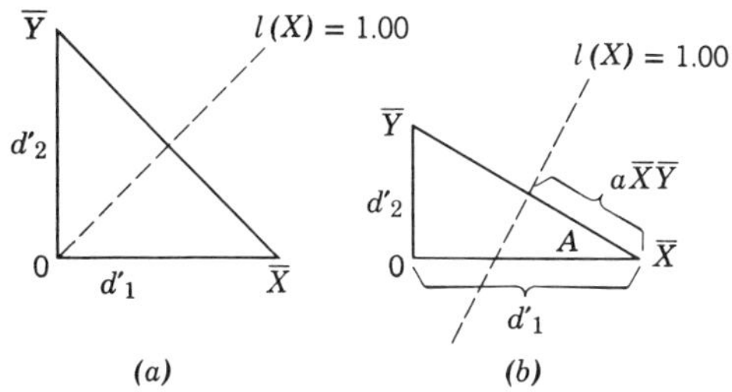

FIG. 3. Simplified diagrams for the orthogonal cases.

hood ratio. The slope of the line $\bar{x}$, $\bar{y}$ is -1 while the slope of the lines of constant likelihood ratio are $+1$ [by Eq. (5)]. Therefore, these lines intersect at right angles. If the value of y is held constant, say at $y = 0$, then the values of x are normally distributed along the x axis, indicating the normality of the mapping along the $\bar{x}$, $\bar{y}$ axis.

The assumption of independence implies that the angle $\theta(XOY) = 90°$. Therefore,

$$(d_{1,2}')^2 = (d_1')^2 + (d_2')^2 \tag{6}$$

If $d_1' \neq d_2'$, then Eq. (5) becomes

$$y = x\frac{d_1'}{d_2'} - \frac{\log_e l(x,y) + (d_1')^2 - (d_2')^2}{d_2'} \tag{7}$$

and it can be shown that $l(x,y)$ constant is represented by a line which intersects the line $\bar{x}$, $\bar{y}$ at right angles, the line $l(x) = 1.00$ intersecting at the midpoint. Thus, Eq. (6) also applies to this case.

Again, part of Fig. 1 has been reproduced as Fig. 3*b*. The line connecting $\bar{x}$, $\bar{y}$ is a slope $-\, d_2'/d_1'$, while the lines of constant likelihood ratio are at slope $+\, d_1'/d_2'$, and again the two lines intersect at right angles. In the figure, the distance $\bar{x}$, $\bar{y} = (d_1')^2 + (d_2')^2$. Solving for the intersection of the line $l(x,y) = 1.00$ and the line $\bar{x},\bar{y}$:

$$\cos A = \frac{d_1'}{\bar{x},\bar{y}}$$

$$\cos A = \frac{a(\bar{x},\bar{y})}{(d_1') - \dfrac{(d_1')^2 - (d_2')^2}{2d_1'}} = \frac{2ad_1'(\bar{x},\bar{y})}{(d_1')^2 + (d_2')^2}$$

Equating:

$$\frac{d_1'}{\bar{x},\bar{y}} = \frac{2ad_1'(\bar{x},\bar{y})}{(d_1')^2 + (d_2')^2}$$

$$1 = \frac{2a(\bar{x},\bar{y})^2}{(d_1')^2 + (d_2')^2}$$

Since $(x,y)^2 = (d_1')^2 + (d_2')^2$, $a = \frac{1}{2}$ and thus, if $l(x,y) = 1.00$, the line $\bar{x}$, $\bar{y}$ is intersected at the midpoint.

If the two signals are not independent, or in other words, if there is a common factor in the observations x and y, then the signal spaces x and y are correlated. The degree of correlation is defined by the cosine of the angle θ. For this case,

$$(d_{1,2}')^2 = (d_1')^2 + (d_2')^2 - 2\cos\theta d_1'd_2' \tag{8}$$

Equation (8) is the general form. For the orthogonal or independent case, $\cos\theta = 0$ and Eq. (8) is identical with Eq. (6). For the perfectly correlated case, such as two signals of the same frequency differing only in d' as a result of different intensity, $\cos\theta = 1.00$ and

$$d_{1,2}' = |d_1' - d_2'| \tag{9}$$

Thus, in each case, the decision function has been defined along a single axis, showing that each recognition case is essentially the same as the detection case.

This discussion furnishes the basis for the development of the theory. So far, it is based on the assumption that the process of observing one frequency does not interfere with the process of observing at other frequencies.

MODIFICATION TO ALLOW FOR OBSERVATION AT BOTH FREQUENCIES

Some experiments previously reported suggest that for a signal 0.1 sec in duration, at a frequency of either 900 cps or 1000 cps, the detection rate is as if both frequencies can be observed simultaneously. When the frequencies are separated by more than 100 cps, the detection performance is lower until the separation reaches 300 cps ($\omega_1 = 700$ and $\omega_2 = 1000$), at which point the performance is such that only one frequency can be observed during the duration of the signal. The results first reported by Tanner and Norman (1954) are illustrated in Fig. 4, because

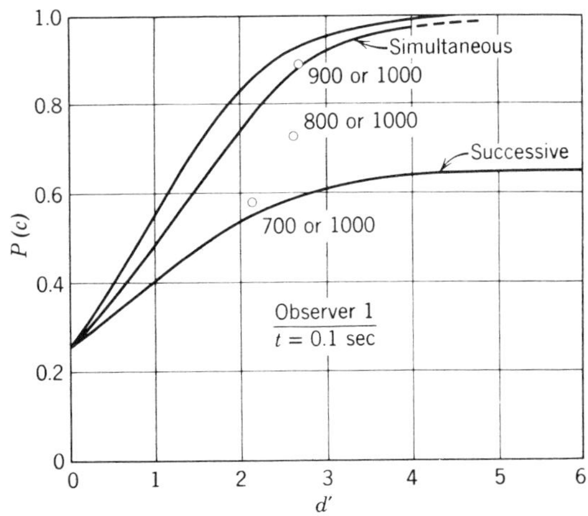

FIG. 4. Illustrative results of the "unknown frequency" experiment, Observer 1, $t = 1$ sec.

they relate closely to the data to be reported below. The top curve is the forced-choice curve for a signal of known frequency. The middle curve is for a signal known to be at one of two frequencies when it is possible to observe at both frequencies simultaneously. The lower curve is for a signal known to be at one of two frequencies when it is possible to observe at only one frequency. Thus, if the observer happens to be observing at the wrong frequency, he is forced to make his choice without relevant information.

The data are placed on the graph as follows. First, the d' is determined for the signals when the frequency is known exactly, and then the percentage correct for the experiment in which the signal is known to be at one of two frequencies is entered for that d'. Two durations were reported with the results virtually the same. It should be noted that it is likely that both of the durations are within the range for matching of observation to duration and the results for the durations should not be markedly different.

Thus, for a signal 0.1 sec in duration, the signal space is expected to show the angle of correlation, θ, increasing until the frequencies are separated by 100 cps (900 to 1000 cps) at which point a maximum of $\theta = 90°$ is expected. For frequencies further separated, the calculations are expected to yield a decrease in θ until at a separation of 300 cps, θ should appear to be 60°. An apparent 60° can be achieved if the observer attends to one frequency, effectively performing a yes-no experiment. If he accepts a signal at that frequency, he states so. If he does not, then he indicates that the signal was at the other frequency. After the maximum is reached the decrease in θ does not represent correlation, but rather a loss due to the observer's inability to observe both x and y. If the signal is sufficiently long in duration, the observer should be able to observe both x and y regardless of the separation, so that once θ reaches 90° it should stay there for frequencies of wider separation.

EXPERIMENTAL DESIGN

The experimental design involves first a two-alternative, forced-choice experiment at each of the frequencies, until approximately equal d's are determined. Then a signal known to be at either one of the two frequencies is presented at a specified time, the observer's task being to state whether the signal is ω_1 or ω_2. The two-alternative, forced-choice experiment is actually the choice of one of two signals orthogonal in time. The d_1' and d_2' are determined as follows. The percentage correct is used as an estimate of the probability of a correct response. This figure is used to enter normal tables, and the corresponding x/σ is determined. This value is multiplied by $\sqrt{2}$ giving the equivalent yes-no d'. For the recognition experiment, the same procedure is used, except in this case the value of x/σ is multiplied by 2.

From a rearrangement of Eq. (8) the d's are then used to find θ.

$$\cos\theta = \frac{(d_1')^2 + (d_2')^2 - (d_{1,2}')^2}{2d_1'd_2'} \tag{10}$$

Thus, θ is shown as a function of frequency separation.

EXPERIMENTS

Four durations, 0.05, 0.1, 0.5, and 1.0 sec were studied for frequency separations of 25, 50, 100, 200, 300, 400, 500, and 600 cps. Two observers served for the entire set of experiments. Approximately 200 observations are contained in each determination of d'. The results are tabulated in Table I, and are presented graphically in Fig. 5*a-h*. No effort has been made to fit curves to data, so that the reader can have an unbiased look at the data.

Occasionally the results show θ's greater than 90°. In all except one case there is the impression that the deviation is within the range of sampling error. The one case of serious deviation can be accounted for largely on the basis of a single run of 100 in which one observer dropped appreciably in the detection experiment from the other run of 100 at that frequency. The result is an indeterminate θ, explaining the absence of a data point for a frequency separation of 400 cps in Fig. 5*h*. Aside from this, the data conform roughly to predictions.

GENERALITY OF THE THEORY

In the introduction, it is suggested that while the study is in audition, the application extends generally to human information-collecting systems. In order to illustrate the anticipated generality, the following discussion is presented on the problem of color vision in terms of experimental design and data interpretation. Suppose that instead of presenting two frequencies, two monochromatic light signals are studied in an experiment. Exactly the same procedure is to be followed, ending with a determination of $\cos\theta$.

For each of the two monochromatic light signals, the detection d' is obtained experimentally. The recognition d' is also determined. These values can now be used to determine θ by Eq. (10). If the angle θ turns

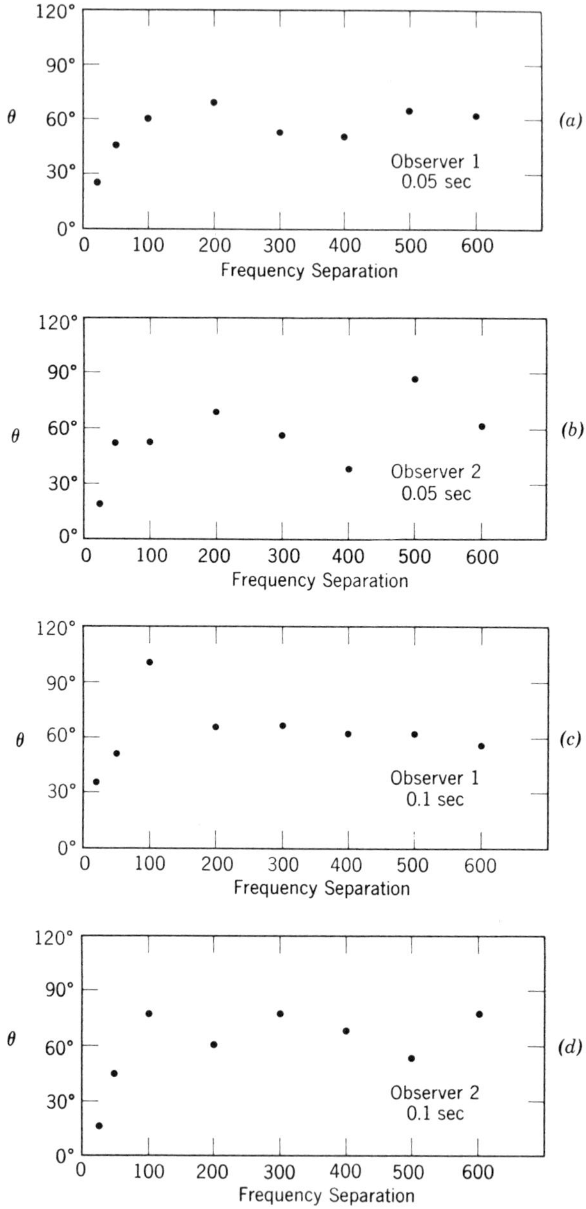

FIG. 5. Recognition of one of two frequencies near 1000 cps by two observers at four durations.

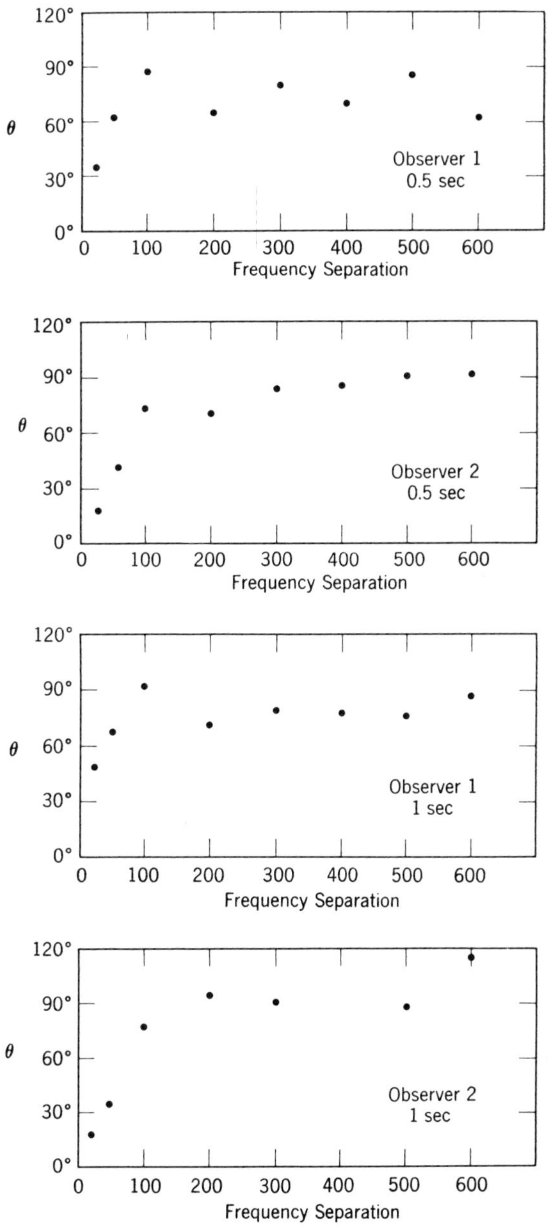
θ
120°
90°
60°
30°
0°
0 100 200 300 400 500 600
Frequency Separation
Observer 1
0.5 sec
Observer 2
0.5 sec
Observer 1
1 sec
Observer 2
1 sec

(e)

(f)

(g)

(h)

TABLE I. RESULTS OF THE EXPERIMENTS.[a] N_0 = 52.3 db *re* 10^{-16} watt/cm^2

Frequency separation	f_1	f_2	$\left(\frac{2E_1}{N_0}\right)^{1/2}$	$\left(\frac{2E_2}{N_0}\right)^{1/2}$	No. of trials N_1	N_2	$N_{1,2}$	Observer 1 d_1'	d_2'	$d_{1,2}'$	θ	Observer 2 d_1'	d_2'	$d_{1,2}'$	θ
						Duration 0.05 sec									
25 cps	975 cps	1000 cps	3.16	3.16	198	198	198	1.85	1.85	1.13	35	1.15	1.15	.50	25
50	950	1000	3.16	3.16	198	198	197	1.77	1.85	1.53	50	1.00	1.15	.89	51
100	900	1000	3.10	3.16	197	198	198	1.69	1.85	1.84	62	.85	1.15	.91	51
200	800	1000	3.05	3.16	198	198	198	1.97	1.85	2.18	69	1.12	1.15	1.27	67
300	700	1000	3.02	3.16	198	198	198	2.14	1.85	1.81	53	1.33	1.15	1.03	49
400	700	1100	3.02	3.25	198	198	198	2.14	1.80	1.37	40	1.33	1.23	.61	28
500	700	1200	3.02	3.42	198	198	197	2.14	1.80	2.12	64	1.33	.95	1.63	89
600	700	1300	3.02	3.42	198	198	198	2.14	1.80	2.05	62	1.33	1.35	1.41	63
						Duration 0.10 sec									
25	975	1000	3.44	3.44	197	196	196	2.19	2.19	1.31	35	1.80	1.80	.51	16
50	950	1000	3.44	3.44	197	196	197	2.19	2.19	1.78	48	1.80	1.80	1.37	45
100	900	1000	3.43	3.44	191	196	292	2.06	2.19	3.27	102	1.32	1.80	1.95	76
200	800	1000	3.36	3.44	197	196	198	2.91	2.19	2.80	63	1.46	1.80	1.68	60
300	700	1000	3.23	3.44	197	196	194	2.46	2.19	2.52	72	1.73	1.80	2.20	78
400	700	1100	3.23	3.60	197	198	198	2.46	2.40	2.61	65	1.73	1.69	1.89	69
500	700	1200	3.23	3.67	197	194	196	2.46	2.17	2.38	62	1.73	1.14	1.39	53
600	700	1300	3.23	3.67	197	195	195	2.46	2.55	2.28	54	1.73	1.54	2.08	79

							Duration 0.5 sec								
25	975	1000	5.37	5.37	197	198	197	2.62	2.62	1.49	33	2.38	2.38	.69	17
50	950	1000	5.37	5.37	197	198	197	2.75	2.62	1.56	61	2.10	2.38	1.56	40
100	900	1000	5.14	5.37	197	198	296	2.91	2.62	3.76	86	1.84	2.38	2.51	74
200	800	1000	4.93	5.37	197	198	197	2.79	2.62	2.80	62	1.68	2.38	2.38	69
300	700	1000	4.60	5.37	197	198	197	2.67	2.62	3.38	80	1.76	2.38	2.78	83
400	700	1100	4.60	5.37	197	197	297	2.67	2.66	3.04	70	1.76	1.73	2.39	87
500	700	1200	4.60	5.90	197	196	197	2.67	2.42	3.74	94	1.76	1.65	2.42	91
600	700	1300	4.60	5.90	197	197	197	2.67	2.91	2.86	61	1.76	2.13	2.86	93
							Duration 1.0 sec								
25	975	1000	5.81	5.85	198	198	198	2.65	2.56	2.15	48	1.52	1.73	.48	16
50	950	1000	5.76	5.85	197	198	198	2.25	2.56	2.74	68	1.73	1.73	1.03	35
100	900	1000	5.63	5.85	197	198	198	2.19	2.56	3.49	93	1.23	1.73	1.86	76
200	800	1000	5.06	5.85	198	198	198	2.61	2.56	3.02	71	1.55	1.73	2.44	93
300	700	1000	4.93	5.85	198	198	196	2.25	2.56	3.38	80	1.40	1.73	2.22	90
400	700	1100	4.93	5.99	198	196	197	2.25	2.25	2.86	79	1.40	1.28	2.72	*
500	700	1200	4.93	6.38	198	198	198	2.25	2.40	2.80	76	1.40	1.73	2.15	86
600	700	1300	4.93	6.38	198	197	198	2.25	2.47	3.28	88	1.40	1.55	2.49	115

[a] See Appendix I for explanation.

out to be 90°, then the implication is, according to the theory, that the two signals lead to transmission over uncorrelated sensory pathways. Different receptors and different pathways are involved. The theoretical framework offers a method of psychological determination of the number of independent systems involved in color vision, or the number of different types of color receptors. There are many other problems to which such an approach may be useful.

SUMMARY

The theory of statistical decision is expanded to include the problem of recognition. A method of predicting recognition data from detection data is described, and experimental data are reported. The experimental data are not inconsistent with the theory.

Since the method of approach to the recognition problem is considered by the author to be generally applicable regardless of the sensory process involved, an experimental design is described, suggesting how the author feels the method of study might be applied in an experimental approach to color vision.

APPENDIX I

OBSERVER EFFICIENCY. Table I is self-explanatory except for columns headed by $(2E/N_0)^{1/2}$. This column indicates a mathematical upper bound for expected performance. A perfect detector operating on the output would be expected to achieve this level of performance. Any detector which achieves this level of performance is using all of the available information. This quantity represents a standard which can be used for purposes of evaluation of either an operator, a receiver, or a combination of an operator and a receiver. The significance of these columns is thus worth some discussion. Consider

$$d_0' = \sqrt{d} = \left(\frac{2E}{N_0}\right)^{1/2} = \left(\frac{2V^2T}{N_0}\right)^{1/2} \tag{A.1}$$

in which d_0' is the optimum d', d is the detectability index, E is the signal energy, N_0 is the noise power per unit bandwidth, V is the signal voltage, and T is the pulse duration. The right-hand member of the equation is that used for the calculation of the column head $(2E/N_0)^{1/2}$, with the subscript of E referring to the signal.

The columns headed d' indicate the value of $(2E/N_0)^{1/2}$ which would be required to lead to the same level of performance as that achieved if a perfect device were placed on the output of the system. The observed

d' is thus always equal to, or less than, the calculated value of $(2E/N_0)^{1/2}$. The ratio of the inferred value to the calculated value can be used as an index of the efficiency of the operating device.

The calculations of $(2E/N_0)^{1/2}$ are based on measurements made of the output of the earphones used in the experiments. It has thus been possible to calculate efficiency ratings for the observers' performance for the different durations and the different frequencies studied in the experiments. These are listed in Table II. These tables are not intended to

TABLE II. Observer Efficiency as a Function of Pulse Duration and Center Frequency

Pulse duration in sec / Center frequency	Observer 2				Observer 1			
	0.05	0.10	0.50	1.00	0.05	0.10	0.50	1.00
700	0.503	0.536	0.383	0.284	0.596	0.762	0.762	0.456
800	0.367	0.435	0.341	0.306	0.646	0.866	0.566	0.516
900	0.274	0.385	0.358	0.218	0.545	0.601	0.566	0.389
1000	0.364	0.523	0.443	0.296	0.585	0.637	0.488	0.438
1100	0.378	0.469	0.322	0.213	0.554	0.667	0.495	0.376
1200	0.234	0.310	0.280	0.271	0.526	0.591	0.410	0.376
1300	0.376	0.420	0.361	0.243	0.526	0.695	0.493	0.387

represent a complete study. They are suggestive of a method of study to approach most nearly the optimum use of signal energy in a system involving the human observer. Of the durations studied, the observers are most efficient at a duration of 0.1 sec, and tend to be more efficient at the lower frequencies. These studies involve one particular noise level, and the interpretation of the table should be made with this in mind.

The discussion in this appendix is presented as a contribution to methodology rather than as a contribution of content.

APPENDIX II

THURSTONE'S LAW OF COMPARATIVE JUDGMENT. In two papers, Thurstone (1927*a*,*b*) presents and develops the law of comparative judgment. Similarities between Thurstone's subject matter and that of this paper, and in particular, between the form of Thurstone's equations and those of this paper, justify a discussion of the content of this paper in terms of Thurstone's earlier work.

By the expression "comparative judgment," Thurstone describes the experimental design with which he is concerned. It is an experiment of the type in which the observer is presented first with a signal of frequency f_1 and then with a signal of frequency f_2. He is then asked to state whether f_2 is higher or lower than f_1. Another variation of this experiment is where the observer is presented first with a signal of energy E_1 and then with an energy E_2. He is then asked to state whether $E_2 > E_1$ or $E_2 < E_1$. For the case where either E_1 or E_2 is zero (or noise alone), this is the two-choice, forced-choice experiment employed in determining the detection d' used in this paper.

The definition of d' is $(M_{SN} - M_N)/\sigma$, where M_{SN}, in Thurstone's language, is the *modal discriminal process* for signal plus noise, M_N is the *modal discriminal process* for noise alone, and σ is a measure of the discriminal dispersions, σ_N and $\sigma_{SN}(\sigma_N = \sigma_{SN})$. The observations x are assumed in the paper to be a continuous variable corresponding to Thurstone's discriminal processes.

The analysis of forced-choice experiments presented in earlier papers (Tanner and Swets, 1954; Tanner and Norman, 1954) can be expressed in terms of comparative judgments. Suppose that a signal of energy $E > 0$ is presented in one of four intervals in time, while in the other three intervals signals of energy $E = 0$ are presented, and that the observer is asked to state which interval contained the signal $E > 0$. Observations x are made in each of the four intervals. Three comparative judgments are required. First, a comparative judgment involving the first and second intervals is made. Whichever is judged greater is compared to the third interval, and the greater of this comparison is then compared to the fourth interval. The greater of the last comparison is then judged to be the signal $E > 0$. This is equivalent to the analysis presented in the previous papers.

The main interest in the theory developed in this series of papers is not in comparative judgments, however. It is in detection and recognition. These are subjects not discussed by Thurstone, although had he recognized the existence of a noise distribution such as the one postulated in the theories of detection and recognition, it seems likely that he would have developed essentially the same theory as that developed in the current set of papers, only Thurstone would have been thirty years earlier. It is essentially the noise assumption, along with the denial of the fixed threshold, which has led to this development.

The detection and recognition theories developed in these papers involve experiments in which the observer has a single observation, x, and is asked to state which of a set of alternatives existed to lead to the observation x. It is not a comparative judgment in the Thurstone or forced-choice sense. Analysis of this type of experiment led to the interest in a priori probabilities and risk functions, variables which are not immediately obvious in Thurstone's discussion of the law of comparative judgments. Thurstone has assumed that, of two stimuli (S_1 and S_2), the a priori probabilities [$P(S_1 > S_2)$ and $P(S_2 > S_1)$] are equal, and that type I and type II errors are equally costly. Due reflections and experimentation should show that these variables (a priori probabilities and risk functions) also play a part in comparative judgments. The criterion for judgments $S_1 > S_2$ may not contain all values $S_1 - S_2 > 0$ or only values $S_1 - S_2 > 0$, but rather all values $S_1 - S_2 > \alpha$ where α is some function of β as defined in the section entitled "Decision Axis for Two Signals."

One further point requires discussion. Thurstone considers a correlation factor which he considers safe to assume equal to zero. The assumption, in view of the noise assumption, is satisfactory for comparative judgments. If signals of two frequencies are presented successively in time, the correlation is likely to be zero because of the autocorrelation function of the noise. However, if a single observation is made, and the choice is between two frequencies close together, the presence of a signal at one frequency influences the observation of the components of the other frequency. In these experiments it is necessary to take into account the correlation factor. It is, in fact, this correlation factor which determines the "distance" Thurstone discusses. Equation (8) is a general equation for Thurstone's "distance," given the distance of the signals from the noise, and given the correlation between the detection axes. It is not the same as Thurstone's general equation, which looks very much like Eq. (8).

ACKNOWLEDGMENTS

This research was conducted in the laboratories of the Electronic Defense Group of the University of Michigan with support of the U. S. Army Signal Corps. This article appeared as Tech. Rept. No. 50 of the Electronic Defense Group, and in J. acoust. Soc. Am., *1956,* **28,** *882–888.*

References

- Birdsall, T. G. The theory of signal detectability. In H. Quastler (Ed.), *Information theory in psychology.* Glencoe, Ill.: Free Press, 1955.
- Peterson, W. W., Birdsall, T. G., and Fox, W. C. The theory of signal detectability. *Trans. IRE Professional Group on Information Theory,* 1954, **PGIT-4,** 171–212.

- Tanner, W. P., Jr. On the design of psychophysical experiments. In H. Quastler (Ed.), *Information theory in psychology*. Glencoe, Ill.: Free Press, 1955.
- Tanner, W. P., Jr., and Norman, R. Z. The human use of information: II. Signal detection for the case of an unknown signal parameter. *Trans. IRE Professional Group on Information Theory,* 1954, **PGIT-4,** 222–227.
- Tanner, W. P., Jr., and Swets, J. A. A decision-making theory of visual detection. *Psychol. Rev.,* 1954, **61,** 401–409.
- Thurstone, L. L. Psychophysical analysis. *Am. J. Psychol.,* 1927*a,* **38,** 368–389.
- Thurstone, L. L. A law of comparative judgment. *Psychol. Rev.,* 1927*b,* **34,** 273–286.

20

Stimulus versus Response Uncertainty in Recognition

John A. Swets and Susan T. Sewall

Several experiments in recent years have shown that the detectability of a tonal signal suffers when the observer is uncertain about its frequency (Tanner, Swets, and Green, 1956; Tanner, 1956; Veniar, 1958; Swets, Shipley, McKey, and Green, 1959; Creelman, 1960). In the typical experiment a trial consists of two temporal intervals, one of which contains the signal. In one series of trials the signal has a fixed frequency throughout the series. In another series of trials a different frequency is used, but again the same frequency is presented on each trial of the series. Under the condition of principal interest the signal on a given trial is equally likely to be either of these two frequencies. In any case, the observer indicates only the interval in which he believes the signal occurred; he is not required to indicate which frequency was presented. The measure of performance is simply the proportion of correct responses, denoted $P(c)$.

The consistent result is that the $P(c)$ obtained when uncertainty exists is lower than that obtained when the signal frequency is known. Moreover, the size of the decrement that results from uncertainty depends upon the difference between the two frequencies. When the frequency separation is increased from one group of trials to another, $P(c)$ drops steadily until it reaches a minimum that depends on the duration and the general frequency range of the signal.

These experiments were undertaken within the framework of the general theory of signal detectability, specifically, within the context of two models of the auditory process that were appended to the general detection theory in its psychophysical application. The first of them was conducted to test a *single-band* model of the auditory process (Tanner, Swets, and Green, 1956). This model is reminiscent of the searchlight analogy to the process of attention. The observer attempting to detect a weak tonal signal is viewed as sensitive at any instant to only a narrow band of frequencies—as if he has at his disposition a single filter of fixed bandwidth, but adjustable frequency location. In order to change the band of sensitivity, the observer must sweep the filter through the intervening frequencies. Effecting a change of any consequence requires a measurable amount of time that increases with the extent of the change.

Given the values of $P(c)$ obtained when no uncertainty exists, the single-band model predicts the minimal $P(c)$ that will result from uncertainty. This minimum is obtained, presumably, when the two frequencies are sufficiently separated that the observer cannot listen for both during the duration of the signal; in this case the observer will not be listening at the frequency presented on half of the trials. The results of the first experiment were regarded as supporting this model. They showed $P(c)$ to decrease with increasing frequency separation until it approximated the predicted minimal level.

Subsequently, Green (1958) developed a *multiband* model for predicting the detectability of a signal compounded of several frequencies. According to this model, the observer is capable of listening at once to any number of frequency bands. He selects the number and frequency location of the bands to which he listens, and he bases his decision upon a linear combination of the outputs of the filters he has selected. When the multiband model is applied to the task of concern here, it predicts a smaller decrement from uncertainty than does the single-band model.

At this point, with a competing model on the scene, the force of the data was less obvious; the results of some observers were better fitted by one model, some by the other, and the results of the remaining observers lay between the two predictions. The later studies cited were carried out in an attempt to distinguish more clearly between the two models, but they failed to produce conclusive evidence for either, and a standoff was declared.[1]

Interest in the problem of frequency uncertainty was then revived by

---

[1] See Section 6 for further discussion of these models.

Luce's (1959) development of a theory of individual choice behavior, and particularly by Shipley's (1960) adaptation of the choice theory to the task under discussion. Shipley showed that the choice theory leads to two predictions, one exactly coincident with the prediction of the single-band model, and the other practically coincident with the prediction of the multiband model. The predictions from the detection and choice theories are displayed in Fig. 1.

The great similarity between these two sets of predictions is surprising for, whereas the models associated with detection theory base their predictions on a concept of perceptual filtering, the choice theory achieves its predictions by a manipulation of response probabilities. The choice theory asserts explicitly that uncertainty concerning signal frequency affects a response mechanism rather than a perceptual mechanism. For the task in question, the choice theory leads to the prediction that there will be no decrement as a result of uncertainty about frequency if the observer is informed *after* the observation, but before his response, which of the two frequencies was presented (Shipley, 1960). The single-band model, of course, predicts that frequency information given after the observation will have no effect whatsoever. Similarly, the multiband model, which assumes an irrevocable combination of the outputs of the

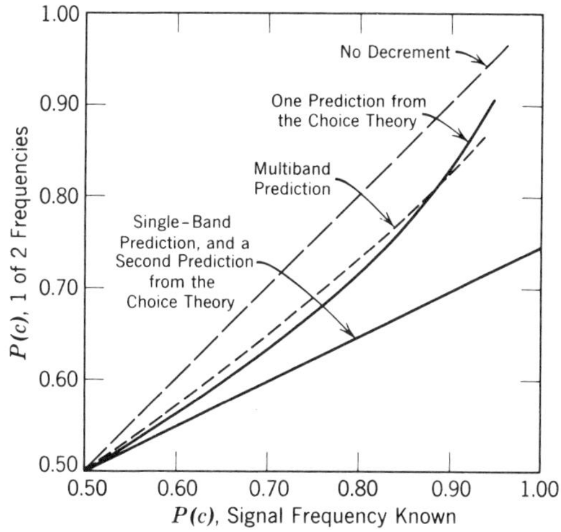

FIG. 1. The various predictions, for $P(c)$ when the signal is either one of two frequencies, are shown as a function of the average value of $P(c)$ obtained when no uncertainty exists. In the latter case only one of the frequencies, known to the observer, is presented on a series of trials. The figure shows the predictions from the single-band and multiband models associated with detection theory and the two predictions derived from choice theory.

relevant filters, predicts that this information will not remove any of the decrement.

We report in the following some experiments conducted to test these divergent predictions of the detection and choice theories. The experiments compare the relative effects of frequency "cueing" provided before and after the observation. They are of particular interest because very few—in fact, only two—instances have been uncovered to date for which the grossly different assumptions of the two theories lead to noticeably different results. Over a wide range of experimental situations to which both detection theory and choice theory apply, they make almost identical numerical predictions. After reporting the results of the cueing experiments, we describe briefly the outcome of the other experiment for which the difference in predictions is large enough to make a test reasonable. It, too, is concerned with the distinction between perceptual and response mechanisms in what was first regarded to be a perceptual process.

THE CUEING EXPERIMENTS

In Experiment I, the $P(c)$ obtained when the observation is followed by information about the frequency that was presented, is compared with the $P(c)$ obtained when no frequency information is given. The frequency cueing is supplied by two lights, with the simple code that the left light corresponds to the lower of the two frequencies and the right light to the higher. Experiment II examines the effects of cueing after the observation when the cueing is provided by the tones themselves; the frequency that was presented on a given trial is re-presented, this time clearly audible, before the response is made. Experiments III and IV serve as controls; they examine the effects of frequency cueing provided before the observation, by lights and by tones, respectively.

In describing the results, we are not concerned with distinguishing between the single-band and multiband models or, correspondingly, between the two predictions from choice theory. The present data, like previous data, are inadequate for this purpose; on the whole, the results fall between the two predictions. We confine our attention now to determining whether the results implicate a perceptual mechanism or a response mechanism as underlying the effects of uncertainty. A quantitative account of the decrement caused by uncertainty, in terms of either a perceptual or a response model, will be postponed.

In all four experiments the signal was a tone burst of 0.1-sec duration, of either 500 or 1100 cps. It was presented in a continuous background of white noise of approximately 50 db *re* 0.0002 d/cm^2. The same three practiced observers served in all of the experiments, two hours a day, five days a week. A two-interval, forced-choice task was used throughout.

Experiment I. Cueing by lights after the observation

METHOD. Eight groups of trials, of 100 trials each, were presented in a two-hour experimental session. In every session four experimental conditions were employed in a counterbalanced order: In the first and eighth groups of trials only the 500-cps signal was presented; in the second and seventh groups only the 1100-cps signal was presented; in groups 3 and 6 the two frequencies were equally likely to appear on a given trial with no frequency cueing provided; in groups 4 and 5 either of the two frequencies was presented, and frequency cueing was given.

Preliminary sessions established the signal levels required to yield values of $P(c)$ of approximately 0.75, 0.85, and 0.95 for each frequency. These signal levels were 9.5, 10.5, and 11.5 db, respectively, for the 500-cps signal, and 10.5, 11.5, and 12.5 db for the 1100-cps signal. These signal levels are expressed in terms of 10 log E/N_0; E is the signal energy or time integral of power, and N_0 is the noise power in a one-cycle band.

Five tests were conducted at these signal levels, in the order 0.75, 0.75, 0.85, 0.95, and 0.75. Each test occupied two experimental sessions, so each value of $P(c)$—for the 500-cps signal, for the 1100-cps signal, for either without cueing, and for either with cueing—is based on 400 trials.

The sequence of events on each trial and their durations were: warning light, 0.5 sec; space, 0.5 sec; observation interval, 0.1 sec; space, 0.5 sec; observation interval, 0.1 sec; space, 0.5 sec; an interval which (depending on the condition in force) was either empty or filled by a cue light to indicate the frequency presented, 1.5 sec; response period, 1.5 sec; an interval in which another pair of cue lights indicated the correct response, 0.5 sec. The total duration of a trial was 5.7 sec.

RESULTS. The results for the three observers are shown in Figs. 2 to 4. The crosses mark the values of $P(c)$ obtained on the trials without frequency cues; the dots represent the trials in which frequency cues were supplied.

It is apparent that frequency information given by cue lights after the observation removes little, if any, of the decrement in performance that results from uncertainty prior to the observation. The average discrepancies between values of $P(c)$ obtained with and without information, for the three observers, are +0.02, 0.00, and +0.04. On the whole,

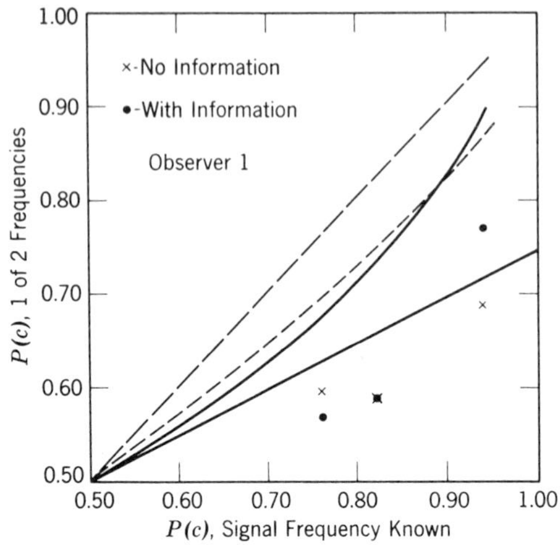

FIG. 2. The results, for Observer 1, of cueing by lights after the observation. This observer was absent during the first two of the five tests conducted.

the deviations associated with frequency information are positive, but they are not significant.[2]

Experiment II. Cueing by tones after the observation

It seemed reasonable at the conclusion of the first experiment to suspect that the coded lights might not provide adequate frequency cueing. A shorter experiment was therefore conducted in which the tones themselves were used as the cues to frequency.

METHOD. The cue tone occurred after the observation, with the same intensity it possessed during the observation, while the masking noise was attenuated 10 db. For comparability, tones were also presented after the observation in the control conditions of the experiment, although in these conditions they did not supply additional information about the frequency that was presented. On those sets of trials in which only the 500-cps signal occurred, the 500-cps tone was re-presented while the

---

[2] Tests of significance, t tests, were applied to the data. The estimates of variances used in these calculations were obtained directly from the data. Binomial statistics were not used because they tend to underestimate the variance, especially when groups of trials comprising an experimental condition are distributed over time. Of 13 t tests one yielded a (one-tailed) $p = 0.01$; the others yielded values of $p > 0.10$. A combination of all the values of p according to the chi-square model (Jones and Fiske, 1953) led to $0.20 > p > 0.10$.

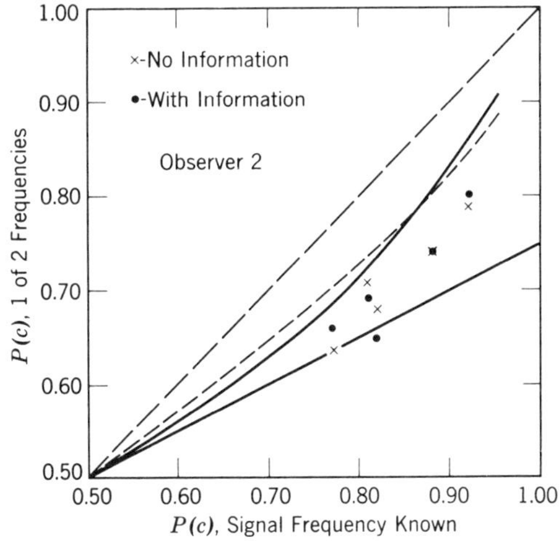

FIG. 3. The results, for Observer 2, of cueing by lights after the observation.

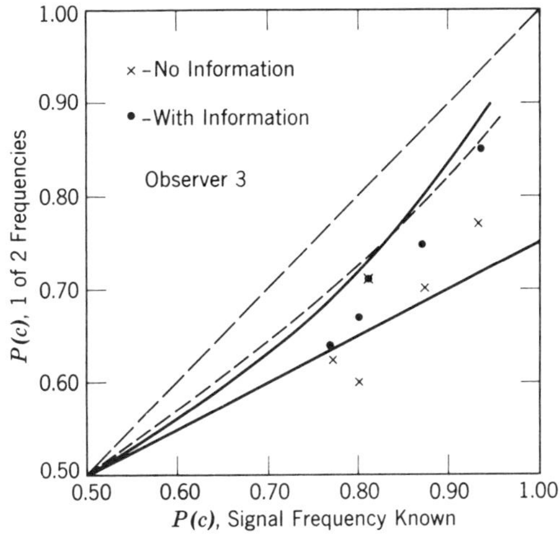

FIG. 4. The results, for Observer 3, of cueing by lights after the observation.

noise was attenuated; similarly, on those sets of trials containing only the 1100-cps signal, the 1100-cps tone was re-presented; on the sets of trials in which the signal could assume either frequency but no cueing was to be provided, *both* tones were presented after the observation on every trial. The sequence of events on each trial and their durations were: warning light, 0.5 sec: observation interval, 0.1 sec: space, 0.5 sec: observation interval, 0.1 sec; space, 0.5 sec; cue tone, 0.1 sec; space,

0.5 sec; a second cue tone or not depending on the condition, 0.1 sec; space, 0.5 sec; response period, 2.0 sec; cue light indicating correct response, 0.5 sec. The total duration of a trial was 5.4 sec. The period during which the noise was attenuated extended from immediately after the second observation interval until the beginning of the response period.

Only one signal level was used for each frequency, that corresponding to a $P(c)$ of 0.85 in the preliminary test. The experiment consisted of 10 groups of 100 trials and was completed in a single two-hour session. Only the 500-cps signal was presented in groups 1 and 10; only the 1100-cps signal was presented in groups 2 and 9; in groups 3, 5, and 7 either frequency could appear on any trial with no frequency cueing provided; in groups 4, 6, and 8 either of the frequencies could occur, and frequency cueing was given. Thus the values of $P(c)$ for the 500-cps signal alone and for the 1100-cps signal alone are based on 200 trials; the values of $P(c)$ for the two conditions with uncertainty before the observation are based on 300 trials.

RESULTS. The results for two observers (observer 3 was not present for this experiment) are shown in Fig. 5. We observe there a result like that obtained in the first experiment. Frequency cueing given after the observation interval by the tones themselves removes little, if any, of the decrement associated with uncertainty prior to the observation. The discrepancy between the values of $P(c)$ for cueing and no cueing is −0.04

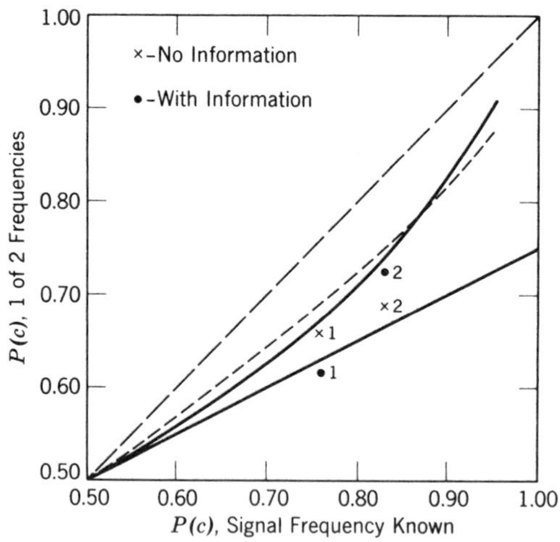

FIG. 5. The results, for two observers, of cueing by tones after the observation. The numerals on the data points refer to the observers as numbered in previous figures.

for observer 1 and +0.04 for observer 2. Apparently the cueing provided by tones is no more effective than the cueing provided by coded lights.[3]

Experiments III and IV. Cueing before the observation by lights and by tones

This section reports the results of two control experiments in which frequency cueing was given before the observation, in one by lights and in the other by tones.

METHOD. Except for the fact that the cueing was given before the observation, the procedures used in Experiments III and IV were like those used in Experiment II. The only other difference of note is that the signal levels used in Experiment III corresponded to a value of $P(c)$ of 0.95 in the preliminary test.

RESULTS. Figure 6 shows that cueing by lights before the observation aids performance substantially more than cueing after the observation. The average differences between the values of $P(c)$ with and without

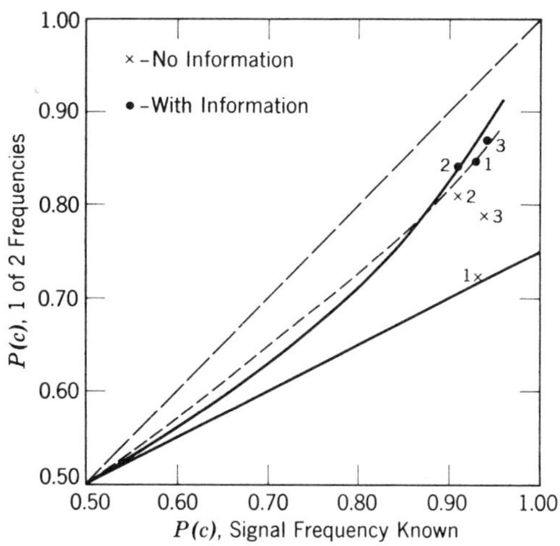

FIG. 6. The results, for three observers, of cueing by lights before the observation.

[3] A t test applied to the data obtained with cueing by tones yields $p = 0.50$. A combination of the results for cueing by lights and by tones after the observation led to $0.20 > p > 0.10$.

cueing for the three observers are +0.13, +0.04, and +0.80. Figure 7 shows a similar result for prior cueing by tones; the relevant differences in $P(c)$ are +0.02, +0.07, and +0.07.[4]

Partial summary and comment

An experimental procedure in which the stimulus presented is specified before the observation, and a procedure in which the stimulus is specified after the observation, were compared with a procedure in which no trial-by-trial specification is made. In each case, two different ways of specifying the stimulus were used. It was found that a reduction in uncertainty before the observation facilitated performance, and that reduction in uncertainty after the observation led to little if any effect. This result indicates that the effects of stimulus uncertainty in this task are mediated by a perceptual mechanism rather than by a response mechanism. The result is consistent with detection theory, and it is inconsistent with choice theory.

The fact that the data points representing prior cueing fall consistently below the 45° line in Figs. 6 and 7 is worthy of comment. It indicates that the observer performs less well when two frequencies are

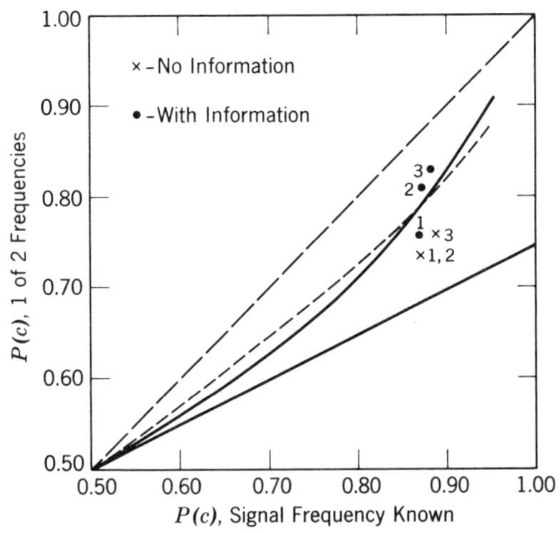

FIG. 7. The results, for three observers, of cueing by tones before the observation.

[4] The differences connected with cueing by lights have associated a $p \approx 0.001$. Cueing by tones yielded $0.05 > p > 0.02$. Considering both types of cueing given before the observation, $p < 0.001$.

presented in random order over a group of trials, even when he is informed before each trial which frequency will be presented on that trial, than he performs when the same frequency is used throughout a group of trials. This result suggests that the observer sacrifices precision in adjusting his set if he must do so on a moment's notice. In this respect it is in agreement with certain other results we have obtained.

In an experiment such as the ones described here, but without frequency cueing (Swets, Shipley, McKey, and Green, 1959), a contingency analysis was made to determine the probability of a correct response on a given trial for each of the four conditions that could have held on the previous trial: (*a*) same frequency, correct response, (*b*) same frequency, incorrect response, (*c*) different frequency, correct response, and (*d*) different frequency, incorrect response. It was found that if the same frequency was presented on two successive trials, the observer was more likely to be correct on the second if he had been correct on the first; if different frequencies were presented on two successive trials, the observer was more likely to be correct on the second if he had been incorrect on the first. This analysis indicates that the observer is differentially sensitive to the two frequencies at a given point in time, in particular, that he perseveres to some extent in listening to a given frequency band.

In another experiment, this one using only a single frequency, Shipley (1959) tested the hypothesis that the effective signal intensity on one trial influences the probability of a correct response on the next. Relatively strong and weak signals were presented at random, and a higher $P(c)$ was observed on those trials following a correct response to the strong signal than on those trials following a correct response to the weak signal. This result was interpreted to mean that stronger signals provide better cues to the nature of the signal than weaker signals, and that the observer's perceptual set, following a strong signal, is correspondingly better. Swets describes other experimental results which indicate that the set for detecting a weak tone is quite labile: even when the same signal is used throughout a series of trials, performance can be significantly improved by continually providing the observer with additional cues to the signal's frequency, starting time, duration, and amplitude (Swets, 1961).

The fact that the observer performs less well when the frequency, though known, is changed randomly from trial to trial is not predicted by either of the theories we have considered. As a matter of fact, it had been assumed in connection with both theories, in deriving the original quantitative predictions for the effects of uncertainty without cueing, that the 45° line is an adequate baseline. We have not been concerned here with distinguishing between the single-band and multiband predictions or, alternatively, between the two predictions from choice theory. We note, however, that if data collected with the present technique are to be used in an attempt to distinguish between the two models associated with each theory, it will be necessary to make a correction in deriving their predictions; in particular, it will be necessary to use an empirically determined baseline to represent the case of no uncertainty with trial-to-trial changes in frequency.

ANOTHER EXPERIMENT RELATED TO THE DETECTION AND CHOICE THEORIES

An experiment was conducted to investigate the other known instance for which the detection and choice theories make divergent predictions. In this case, the problem for theory is to predict the function that relates $P(c)$ to the number of observation intervals in a forced-choice test. Again the prediction from detection theory is based upon a consideration of the mechanism of observation, and a different prediction is derived from choice theory on the basis of a response mechanism.[5]

METHOD. Since some analyses of the data of this experiment have been reported previously (Swets, 1959), the experimental procedure is not described in detail here. In general, it is like the procedure used in the experiments reported previously. Only one frequency was used (1000 cps), but other aspects of the procedure such as the signal and noise levels, the signal duration, the counterbalancing of experimental conditions, and the previous training of the observers were similar. The essential facts are that values of $P(c)$ were obtained from three observers in a number of forced-choice tests having 2, 3, 4, 6, or 8 observation intervals; these values of $P(c)$ were based, respectively, on 300, 500, 600, 900, and 1200 trials.

RESULTS. The results are shown in Fig. 8. They may be compared with the two families of curves shown in the figure, the dashed-line curves representing choice theory and the solid curves representing detection theory. It can be seen that the shallow curves from detection theory approximate the data more nearly than the steeper curves from choice theory.

---

[5] The derivation of the prediction from detection theory has been reported in Elliott (1959); the prediction from choice theory follows from Luce's (1959) discussion. W. S. Torgerson suggested to us that this experiment would provide a contrast of the two theories.

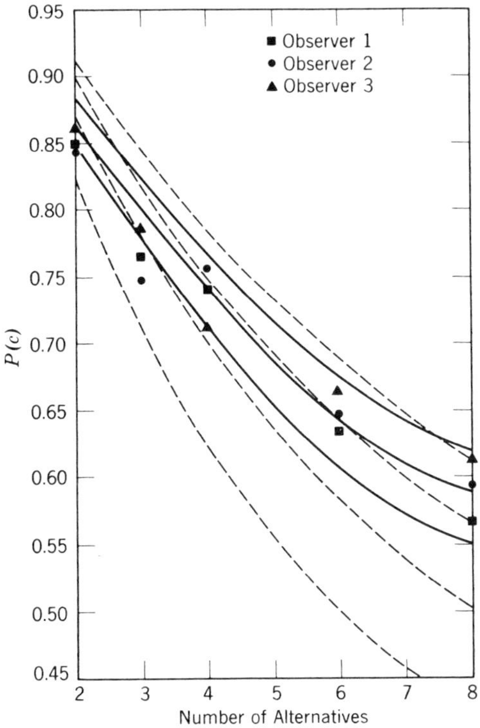

FIG. 8. The results of forced-choice tests with various numbers of observation intervals compared with the predictions from detection theory and choice theory. The solid curves represent detection theory; these curves correspond to values of d' of 1.5, 1.6, and 1.7. The dashed curves represent choice theory and correspond to values of α of 5.0, 7.0, 9.0, and 11.0. The parameters of d' and α are the indices of detectability in the respective theories.

DISCUSSION

It has been known for a long time, of course, that the recognition of a brief stimulus is facilitated when the observer is told in advance that it will be one of a restricted set of alternatives. Külpe (1904) and many others since (e.g. Chapman, 1932) have suggested that the facilitative effect depends upon a perceptual mechanism, upon a perceptual tuning. For almost as long a time, the interpretation in terms of a perceptual mechanism has been questioned. The procedure used in the present study, that of comparing the effects of restrictive instructions presented before and after the observation, has been used several times to determine whether a response process might instead be responsible (Lawrence and Coles, 1954; Pollack, 1959). This procedure has also been used in an attempt to determine whether or not a memory mechanism, some modification of the memory trace, underlies the facilitative effect (Chapman, 1932; Lawrence and Coles, 1954).

We should mention that we have not been concerned here with the memory hypothesis because we believe the before-after procedure to be insensitive to it. A consideration of the possible results of the procedure leads us to the conclusion that, whereas it permits a perceptual mechanism or a response mechanism to be ruled out altogether, it leaves the memory hypothesis invulnerable. As this hypothesis has been stated, memory could be, with any result, the only process involved. Neither of the other hypotheses can be supported at its expense, and it cannot be supported at the expense of both of the others.

The other principal difference between the present approach and the approach taken in the earlier studies is the level of generality implied. We have not asked, "What is the mechanism for the facilitative effect of restrictive instructions?" for we believe that the answer depends on the task chosen for study. Although the contradiction between certain of the earlier results (Chapman, 1932; Lawrence and Coles, 1954) may not have forced this conclusion, it seems unavoidable given the recent reports of Long, Reid, and Henneman (1960), Long, Henneman, and Garvey (1960) and Reid, Henneman, and Long (1960). These investigators performed a number of experiments in which they used different numbers of alternatives and a variety of stimulus materials. In about half of their tasks instructions given before the observation were found superior to instructions given after the observation; in the other half, the two were equally effective. Thus, we would restrict our conclusions concerning the mechanism to the task that we employed. We see the general problem as requiring a large amount of parametric exploration, to which we have added a single case.[6] This case is of particular interest because the stimuli are much simpler than any used in previous studies. It also led to a result not encountered before, namely, that information given after the observation had very little, if any, effect.

[6] Unfortunately, not all of the results that have been reported can be accepted at face value; Long, Henneman, and Garvey (1960) obtained a result for words presented aurally that stands in flat contradiction to that obtained by Pollack (1959).

SUMMARY

We raise again, in the framework of a very simple recognition task, the question of the relative efficacy of specifying the stimulus alternatives before and after the stimulus is presented. Our experiments show information given before the observation to facilitate recognition and information given after the observation to have little, if any, effect. We conclude that the facilitative effect of restricting alternatives, in the task studied, depends on a perceptual mechanism rather than on a response mechanism. These experiments are discussed in connection with two current psychological theories: the theory of signal detectability, which is essentially a perceptual theory, and the theory of individual choice behavior, which is essentially a response theory. The results of another experiment, the only other experiment discovered to date for which these two theories make different predictions, are also reported. In this experiment, too, the results are in agreement with the detection theory.

ACKNOWLEDGMENTS

This work was conducted in the Research Laboratory of Electronics, Massachusetts Institute of Technology, with support from the U. S. Army Signal Corps, the Air Force (Operational Applications Laboratory and the Office of Scientific Research), and the Office of Naval Research. This article appeared as Tech. Rept. No. AFCCDD-TR-60-44, and in J. acoust. Soc. Am., *1961*, **33,** *1586–1592. We gratefully acknowledge the assistance of Elizabeth F. Shipley in the design of this research.*

References

- Chapman, D. W. Relative effects of determinate and indeterminate aufgaben. *Am. J. Psychol.,* 1932, **44,** 163–174.
- Creelman, C. D. Detection of signals of uncertain frequency. *J. acoust. Soc. Am.,* 1960, **32,** 805–810.
- Elliott, P. B. Tables of *d'*. University of Michigan: Electronic Defense Group, 1959, Technical Report No. 97. [34]
- Green, D. M. Detection of multiple component signals in noise. *J. acoust. Soc. Am.,* 1958, **30,** 904–911. [25]
- Jones, L. V., and Fiske, D. W. Models for testing the significance of combined results. *Psychol. Bull.,* 1953, **50,** 375–383.
- Külpe, D. Versüche über Abstraktion. *Ber. Kongr. Psychol.,* 1904, 56–68.
- Lawrence, D. H., and Coles, G. R. Accuracy of recognition with alternatives before and after the stimulus. *J. exp. Psychol.,* 1954, **47,** 208–214.

- Long, E. R., Reid, L. S., and Henneman, R. H. An experimental analysis of set: Variables influencing the identification of ambiguous, visual stimulus-objects. *Am. J. Psychol.,* 1960, **73,** 553–562.
- Long, E. R., Henneman, R. H., and Garvey, W. D. An experimental analysis of set: The role of sense-modality. *Am J. Psychol.,* 1960, **73,** 563–567.
- Luce, R. D. *Individual choice behavior.* New York: Wiley, 1959.
- Pollack, I. Message uncertainty and message reception. *J. acoust. Soc. Am.,* 1959, **31,** 1500–1508.
- Reid, L. S., Henneman, R. H., and Long, E. R. An experimental analysis of set: The effect of categorical restriction. *Am J. Psychol.,* 1960, **73,** 568–572.
- Shipley, E. F. Cueing as a determiner of apparent variability in sensitivity. Massachusetts Institute of Technology: Research Laboratory of Electronics, 1959, Quarterly Progress Report No. 53.
- Shipley, E. F. A model for detection and recognition with signal uncertainty. *Psychometrika,* 1960, **25,** 273–289.
- Swets, J. A. Indices of signal detectability obtained with various psychophysical procedures. *J. acoust. Soc. Am.,* 1959, **31,** 511–513. [6]
- Swets, J. A. Detection theory and psychophysics: A review. *Psychometrika,* 1961, **26,** 49–63.
- Swets, J. A., Shipley, E. F., McKey, M. J., and Green, D. M. Multiple observations of signals in noise. *J. acoust. Soc. Am.,* 1959, **31,** 514–521. [9]
- Tanner, W. P., Jr. Theory of recognition. *J. acoust. Soc. Am.,* 1956, **28,** 882–888. [19]
- Tanner, W. P., Jr., Swets, J. A., and Green, D. M. Some general properties of the hearing mechanism. University of Michigan: Electronic Defense Group, 1956, Technical Report No. 30.
- Veniar, F. A. Signal detection as a function of frequency ensemble, I. *J. acoust. Soc. Am.,* 1958*a,* **30,** 1020–1024; II. *J. acoust. Soc. Am.,* 1958*b,* **30,** 1075–1078.

21

Identification of Elementary Auditory Displays and the Method of Recognition Memory

Irwin Pollack

A stumbling block to many experimental examinations of the identification of elementary auditory displays is that the listener is forced to employ a set of arbitrary designations, e.g., numerals, in the identification of the displays. The present study presents a procedure which circumvents the assignment of arbitrary designations to the display and presents illustrative results obtained with the procedure.

METHOD

The method presented for circumventing the assignment of arbitrary designations is the "method of recognition memory." This method has long been employed in psychological studies of learning and memory. The exact form of the present application parallels the development of Egan (1958).

Members of a defined set of objects—the exposure set—are initially exposed to the observer. An equal number of members outside the exposure set—the confusion set—are randomly intermixed with the exposure set. Members of the combination of the two sets—the combined set—are then presented, one at a time, to the observer. His task is to report which items belong to the exposure set and which items do not belong to the exposure set, i.e., which items were, or were not, exposed previously.

The application of the method to the identification of elementary auditory displays is direct. The observer is exposed to a set of tones, one at a time, e.g., a set of six different sound levels. To the set of six initially exposed sound levels, an additional set of six sound levels is intermixed. The listener's task is simply to indicate whether a given tone was, or was not, presented in the initial exposure period, i.e., whether a given tone was, or was not, from the exposure set. The measure of the listener's identification performance is the extent to which he can successfully discriminate among the two classes of tones.

Egan extended the method of recognition memory to permit the determination of decision relationships. In particular, if the listener is instructed to assign a confidence rating, rather than a simple two-way discrimination, the entire receiver operating characteristic (ROC) can be obtained (Egan, 1958; Pollack and Decker, 1958). In this case, the ROC describes the discrimination between the exposure and confusion sets at several decision criteria or confidence levels.

TREATMENT OF DATA

The treatment suggested by Egan is illustrated in Fig. 1 for the results of one of the test series with a 6-point confidence rating. For each of five

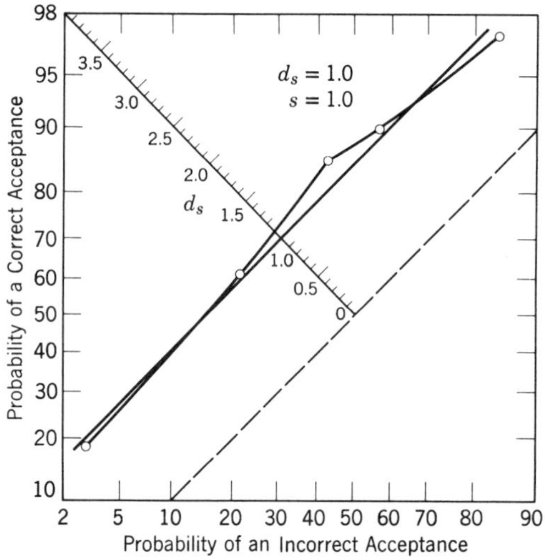

FIG. 1. A typical receiver-operating characteristic for the recognition memory of an exposure set of sound levels. The ordinate and abscissa present the percentage of correct and incorrect acceptances, respectively. Each point represents a single decision criterion. The dashed 45° reference line represents a chance level of performance. The axis, perpendicular to the reference line, is the performance axis, and is scaled in terms of the d_s index. This example illustrates the results of the top group of listeners with an exposure set of four sound levels. The empirical function is based upon 128 items—four presentations of eight sound levels to four listeners.

confidence ratings (the sixth rating is not employed because all items are accepted as members of the exposure set), two quantities are obtained. The first is the probability of a correct acceptance—the tone was selected from the exposure set and was accepted by the listener as a member of the exposure set. The second is the corresponding probability of an incorrect acceptance—the tone was selected from the confusion set and was accepted by the listener as a member of the exposure set. Only a single condition (an exposure set of four tones with the best group of listeners) is illustrated in Fig. 1. The coordinates are scaled in terms of the cumulative normal probability function. The dashed 45° reference line represents a chance level of performance. The 135° line, perpendicular to the reference line, represents the locus of points for symmetrical two-way classifications; e.g., 90 per cent correct acceptances and 10 per cent incorrect acceptances, or alternatively, 70 per cent correct acceptances and 30 per cent incorrect acceptances. This line is scaled in terms of standard deviation units and will be termed the d_s axis.[1]

The index of performance employed was obtained by projecting the individual points to the d_s, or discriminability axis, and obtaining the mean d_s score. In the particular example chosen, a smooth curve of slope s, equal to 1.0, cuts the d_s axis at about 1.0.[2]

APPARATUS AND PROCEDURE

The exposure and confusion sets were constructed from a battery of 24 sound levels of a 1000-cps tone. This battery of sound levels was obtained by a 24-position selector switch and a bank of 24 potentiometers. The sound levels ranged in 2.5-db steps from 52 to 109.5 db.

The exposure and confusion sets were constructed such that the maximum range was sampled and the distances between successive levels were identical among the stimuli in both the exposure set and the con-

---

[1] It is useful to distinguish between two indices. The first is the index of signal discriminability, d_s, which reflects the extent to which items of the information source are discriminated. The second is the index of response discriminability, d_r, which reflects the extent to which a listener can discriminate the correctness of his own responses to the information source. The method of recognition memory yields a hybrid of these indexes. While the steps in the treatment of the data of the method of recognition memory are identical with the steps leading to d_r, the method reflects the discrimination of the information source, d_s, rather than among the listener's responses.

[2] In a recent Letter to the Editor, Clarke, Birdsall, and Tanner also recommend the description of the receiver operating characteristic in terms of the slope, s, and in terms of the intercept with the d_s axis, which they define as $d_e^{\frac{1}{2}}$ (Clarke, Birdsall, and Tanner (1959).

fusion set. In terms of the battery of 24 levels, for example, one of the exposure sets with 3 sound levels consisted of levels 8, 16, and 24 and its confusion set consisted of levels 4, 12, and 20. Different versions of the exposure sets were presented to different listeners; e.g., a second exposure set with 3 sound levels consisted of levels 1, 9, and 17 and its confusion set consisted of levels 5, 13, and 21.

TABLE I. RECOGNITION MEMORY FOR SOUND LEVEL OF A TONE[a]

Exposure set	Listener group I d_s	I %	II d_s	II %	III d_s	III %
2	2.2	(87)	2.5	(90)	2.3	(88)
3	0.95	(68)	1.0	(69)	0.70	(64)
4	1.0	(69)	0.60	(62)	0.07	(51)
6	0.36	(57)	0.32	(56)	0.10	(52)

[a] Results are presented for three groups of listeners with four exposure sets of sound levels. Each entry, outside the parentheses, represents the d_s index. Each entry, within the parentheses, represents the equivalent percentage correct acceptance level in a two-way classification. Each entry is based upon $(32 \times n)$ observations, where n is the size of the exposure set.

Each exposure set was presented in ascending order and descending order to the listeners for the purpose of acquainting the listener with the set. The procedure was repeated until the listener felt that further exposure would not be helpful to him. The listeners were not informed that the tones were drawn from a set of 24 sound levels. The duration of presentation of each tone was controlled by the listener. A sharp band-pass filter (General Radio 830-R) eliminated sharp transients.

To each sound level, each listener responded with a 6-point confidence rating ranging from +3 or "I am sure this is one of the tones previously presented," to −3 or "I am sure this is not one of the tones previously presented." After a single presentation of all members of the combined set, the same exposure set was again presented. The procedure was repeated until the exposure set and the combined set were presented four times.

The order of experimental sessions was exposure sets of 1 tone, 2 tones, 3 tones, 4 tones, and 6 tones. All listening was carried out in a quiet room with binaural earphones (PDR-8).

Twelve young university students served as listeners. For purposes of analysis, the twelve listeners were subdivided into three groups on the basis of a weighted error score for the larger exposure sets.

RESULTS

Twelve empirical functions were examined: results for the three groups of listeners with exposure sets of 2, 3, 4, and 6 sound levels. Perfect discrimination was obtained with an exposure set of one sound level. Ten of the 12 empirical functions were reasonably linear: the median slope was 1.0; the 10 to 90 per cent range was 0.66 to 1.05.

The results of the experimental tests are summarized in Table I in terms of the normalized d_s index (outside the parentheses) and in terms of the equivalent percentage discrimination level with a two-way symmetrical classification (within the parentheses). For example, the d_s axis of Fig. 1 indicates that a d_s of 1.65 corresponds to an 80 per cent correct acceptance level. The results for exposure sets of 2, 3, 4, and 6 sound levels are presented for three groups of listeners.

As expected, the d_s index decreases as the size of the exposure set is increased. A low performance level was approached with even the most proficient group of listeners for an exposure set of six sound levels—a total set of twelve sound levels.

DISCUSSION

One of the questions often addressed to the results of identification studies is, "How many sounds can be identified by the listener?" Since the d_s index will vary with the size of the exposure set in the method of recognition memory, any statement about the equivalent number of identifiable tones must also include the d_s criterion required. If a 75 per cent correct two-way symmetrical classification—equivalent to a d_s of 1.32—is employed, as is often the case in psychophysical studies, we would conclude that the listeners can employ an exposure set of 2 to 3 sound levels, or a combined set of about 5 sound levels. This result matches closely with studies which required the listener to assign arbitrary designations to the sound levels (Garner, 1953). Finally, it may be noted that the method of recognition memory, itself, has not imposed the final ceiling upon performance. Nearly perfect discrimination has been obtained with this method, for example, for exposure sets of several hundred sentences.[3]

SUMMARY

The "method of recognition memory" is considered as a procedure which permits the examination of the identification of elementary audi-

[3] Roger Shepard (private communication).

tory displays without requiring the assignment of arbitrary designations to the displays. The procedure is described and illustrative results are presented.

ACKNOWLEDGMENTS

This research was conducted in the Operational Applications Laboratory of the U. S. Air Force. This article appeared as Tech. Note No. 59-7, and in J. acoust. Soc. Am., *1959,* **31,** *1126–1128.*

References

- Egan, J. P. Recognition memory and the operating characteristic. Indiana University: Hearing and Communication Laboratory, 1958, Technical Note AFCRC-TN-58-51.
- Clarke, F. R., Birdsall, T. G., and Tanner, W. P., Jr. Two types of ROC curves and definitions of parameters. *J. acoust. Soc. Am.*, 1959, **31,** 629–630.
- Garner, W. R. An informational analysis of absolute judgments of loudness. *J. exp. Psychol.*, 1953, **46,** 373–380.
- Pollack, I., and Decker, L. R. Confidence ratings, message reception, and the receiver operating characteristic. *J. acoust. Soc. Am.*, 1958, **30,** 286–292. [31]

22

Extension of the Theory of Signal Detectability to Matching Procedures in Psychoacoustics

Robert D. Sorkin

One problem in classical psychophysics is that of specifying performance across different tasks or experimental procedures. For example, one might want to predict performance in a discrimination task on the basis of observed data from absolute judgment or detection experiments. The success of the theory of signal detectability (TSD) and its wide range of application to such problems led us to investigate a related problem involving a "matching" task (Swets, Tanner, and Birdsall, 1961; Swets, 1959). The observer's job in the matching situation is to state whether, after two signal presentations, the signals were the same or different. One reason for interest in such procedures arises because recent investigators are employing the matching procedure to make inferences about the attributes underlying choice behavior and general perceptual evaluation (Coombs, in press). Success at generalizing the TSD may help clarify some of the important assumptions implicit in using "matching" data for scaling purposes.

The interest of the present study is in evaluating the TSD as an interpretive tool for describing human performance in a simplified matching situation. Specifically, the study was designed to consider the usefulness of the model of the ideal observer as applied to human matching performance, and to test application of the model's rules for generalizing matching performance from experiments involving the detection and discrimination of acoustic signals in noise.

PREVIOUS RESEARCH

A series of experiments employing the matching procedure was performed by Hefner (1958). Hefner extended Thurstone's law of comparative judgment to the matching situation. When two stimuli are presented to an observer, it is assumed each generates a point drawn from an appropriate discriminal process distribution. If the Euclidean distance between that pair of points is greater than some criterion distance, the observer says they are different; if not, he says they are the same. Hefner showed that, under the assumptions of Thurstone's Case V, the squared differences between these pairs of points are noncentral chi-square distributed, with r degrees of freedom, where r is the dimensionality of the space. The noncentrality parameter is the squared distance between the means of the two multivariate normal distributions from which these points were sampled. Hefner's stimuli consisted of tachistoscopically exposed Munsell hues presented in pairwise fashion. The resulting square data matrix consisted of the relative frequencies of a stimulus pair being judged different. (Actually only half of the matrix plus a diagonal composed each matrix, since the stimuli were presented together.) Hefner's method of analysis consisted of assuming $r = 1$, computing the interpoint distances between stimuli, then testing for satisfaction of a unidimensional fit, and if no fit, assuming $r = 2$, and continuing through this iterative process until a reasonable solution is reached. However, since for $r > 1$ tables of the noncentral chi-square distribution (with $df > 1$) are required, this method is not feasible without considerable approximation. The first step of the interpoint-distance analysis is to establish the criterion distance, and this criterion is assumed by the model to be constant for all pairs of stimuli. This is estimated from the diagonal entries of the matrix, the probability that a pair of identical stimuli is judged different. Hefner noted that these diagonal probabilities often were not consistent, indicating the violation of either the constant-criterion or the constant-variance assumption in "fallible data." After deciding on the criterion distance, one proceeds with computations directly analogous to those of the law of comparative judgment. Hefner concluded from his study that the matching procedure was probably of more use in investigating the judgmental process than as a practical method for scaling stimuli.

Although an aim of the Hefner model and similar scaling models is to obtain metric information relating particular perceptual or psychological variables to particular physical variables, this relationship is usually an empirical, a posteriori affair. The theory of signal detectability, on the other hand, allows for predictions of functional relationships between specified physical measures on both the input and output sides of the receiver under study. Hence, a major interest of the present study was to evaluate a TSD extension to such procedures in order to place matching tasks within the large framework of interrelated psychophysical methods successfully covered by the model. The larger the descriptive capability of such a theoretical framework, the closer we will come to reasonable models of the perceptual process.

The general approach that the TSD makes to the matching task is similar to Hefner's, but differs in some important ways. The signal space consists of points in a $2WT$ dimensional space, where the $2WT$ correspond to the number of independent samples specifying the observed waveform. (All relevant signals are assumed to be within the low passband 0 to W in frequency.) The relevant decision space is assumed to be composed of multivariate normal distributions, where the dimensions of the space are likelihood ratio or some monotone transformation of likelihood ratio, and the dimensionality of the space has an upper bound of M-1, where M is the number of decision alternatives available to the observer. Now the situation for the simple detection of a signal in noise can be simply visualized as in Fig. 1, where both hypothesis distributions are assumed normal with unit variance, and τ is some monotonic transformation of the likelihood ratio,

$$l(x) = \frac{f_{SN}(x)}{f_N(x)}$$

and x is the raw datum of the observation. The ideal observer sets a cutoff β according to the particular value function to be maximized in the decision situation, the costs and values of the possible outcomes, and the a priori probability of each hypothesis. When $\tau[l(x)]$ is greater than $\tau(\beta)$, the observer reports "signal plus noise"; when $\tau[l(x)] < \tau(\beta)$, he

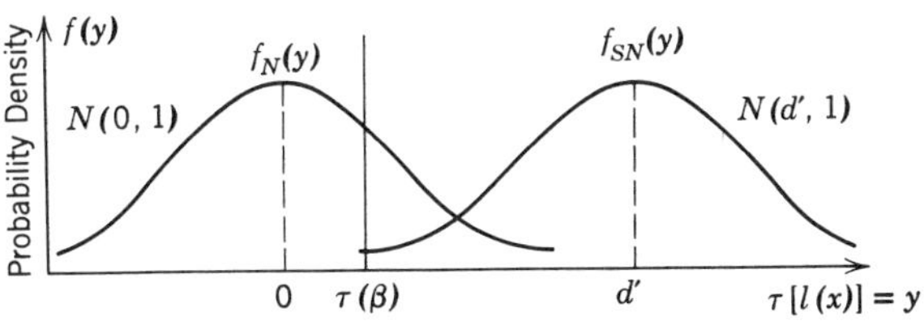

FIG. 1. Signal- and noise-hypothesis distributions in a detection task.

reports "noise alone." It can be shown that for an ideal observer detecting a sine-wave signal in Fourier-series band-limited white Gaussian noise the detectability d' is equal to $(2E/N_0)^{1/2}$, where E is the signal energy and N_0 is the average noise power. From the parameters of these distributions one can construct a receiver-operating-characteristic curve (ROC) completely describing performance at different levels of β or d'. Figure 2 shows a family of such curves for different values of d'. A more complete discussion of the theory and the crucial underlying assumptions may be found in many recent references (Tanner and Birdsall, 1958; Tanner and Swets, 1954; Tanner, Birdsall, and Clarke, 1960; Tanner, 1960; Peterson and Birdsall, 1953).

The matching task can be visualized in similar fashion. A signal from some specified set of possible signals is randomly presented in an observation interval. The observer's task is to state whether or not two such intervals contained the same signal. Figure 3 shows one way of con-

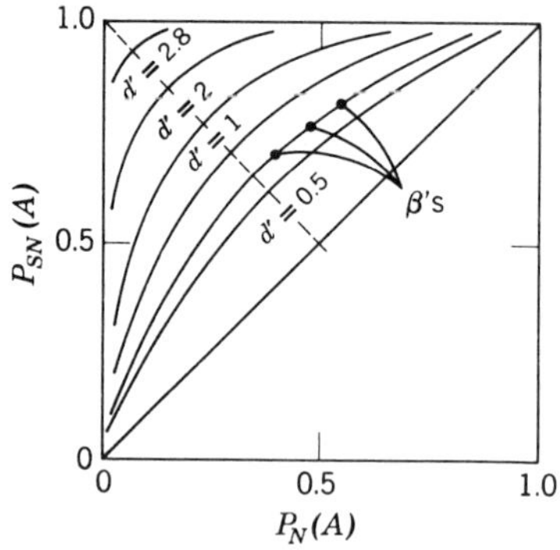

FIG. 2. Receiver-operating-characteristic curves. $P_{SN}(A)$ = probability of correctly identifying signal. $P_N(A)$ = probability of incorrectly reporting an observation as signal when it was noise.

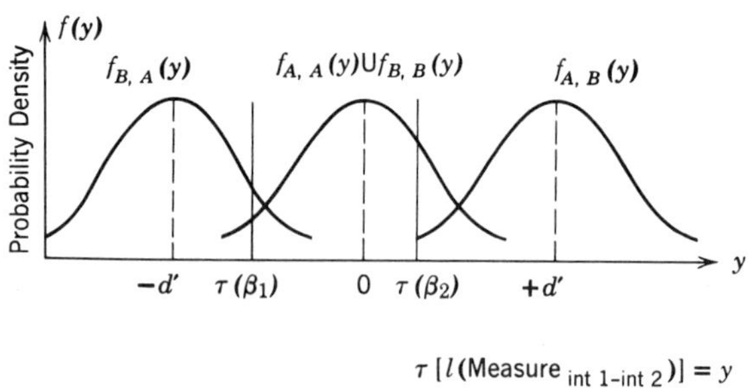

FIG. 3. Hypothesis distributions in a matching situation: $f_{i,j}(y)$ = probability of the observation y given signal i in first interval and signal j in second.

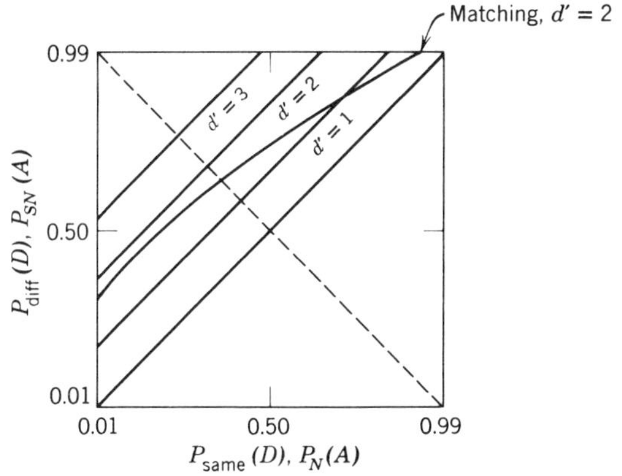

FIG. 4. ROC curve for matching compared to ROC curves for detection. $P_{\text{diff}}(D)$ = probability of saying "different," given different signals, $P_{\text{same}}(D)$ = probability of saying "same," given different signals.

ceptualizing the problem. That is, let the observer compare the input from each interval and form likelihood estimates that the difference measure was due to either the "same" or the "different" hypothesis. Whenever the relevant measure on the observation y is $>\tau(\beta_2)$ or $<\tau(\beta_1)$, the observer says "different," whenever $\tau(\beta_1) < y < \tau(\beta_2)$, he says "same." The two cutoffs $\tau(\beta_1)$ and $\tau(\beta_2)$ may not be symmetric around 0; however, if they are, that is if $|\tau(\beta_1)| = |\tau(\beta_2)| = \tau(\beta)$, it is possible to construct an ROC curve just as in the detection case. Figure 4 provides an example of such a curve, where ROC curves for detection are compared to a matching ROC curve (symmetric β's). For convenience, normal probability coordinates are used which result in linear ROC curves for the detection situation. One may then plot an unknown observer's data points directly on such a graph; for any $\tau(\beta)$, the d' line intersecting the data point defines the separation of the observer's hypothesis distributions. At this point we may simplify further discussion by dropping the τ transformation, remembering that it may be a requirement for achieving normality of the hypothesis distributions on the likelihood-ratio dimension.

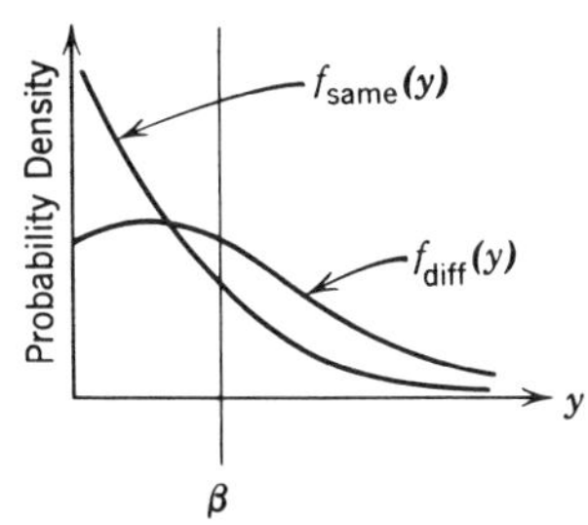

FIG. 5. Complex-hypothesis distributions in a matching task.

Figure 5 shows an alternative way of examining the problem. Let the observer look only at the absolute value of the difference measure. Whenever this measure is greater than β he says "different"; whenever it is smaller he says "same."

The hypothesis distributions $f_{\text{same}}(y)$ and $f_{\text{diff}}(y)$ may be constructed by examination of the distributions underlying them, $f_{B,A}(y)$, $f_{A,B}(y)$, etc. A comparable situation leading to the same functions is discussed by Clarke, Birdsall, and Tanner (1959). Lamphiear and Birdsall (1960) apply a noncentral chi-square analysis to related problems in detection and discrimination. For the purpose of this study, however, the double-cutoff approach was thought more appropriate. A more the precise theoretical statement of the matching problem follows in next section.

THEORY

Ideal observer

Discussion of ideal behavior in yes–no (YN) and two-alternative forced-choice (2AFC) signal-detection experiments appears in many related papers and will be briefly reviewed here in order to demonstrate application of the model to the more complex matching situation (Tanner and Birdsall, 1958; Tanner, 1960). In the yes–no experiment, a sine-wave signal of voltage ΔV may occur in an observation interval, against a background of white Gaussian noise. The hypotheses of noise alone and signal plus noise are conceptualized as in Fig. 1, where d' is then related to the actual signal, ΔV, i.e., $d' = (2E/N_0)^{1/2} = k\Delta V$. In a two-alternative forced-choice pulsed-carrier (2AFC-PC) experiment, there are two observation intervals. Two signals differing only in voltage occur in this experiment, signal V_1 and signal V_2, where $V_2 - V_1 = \Delta V$. The larger signal may occur in either the first observation interval or the second; the observer must specify which. Both intervals contain white Gaussian noise. The relevant observation then consists of observing interval one and interval two, and subtracting one measure from the other, i.e., $y = x_1 - x_2$, as shown in Fig. 6. Because of the additional noise in the added observation, the variance of the new hypothesis distributions will be twice that of the YN case. The means of the hypothesis distributions are found by finding the mean of $f_{V_i,\, V_j}(y)$ when the signal i is indeed in the first interval. For example, $(x_1 - x_2)$, given V_2 in the first interval, will clearly be distributed around a value equal to the difference between the mean of the signal distribution kV_2 minus the mean of the second signal distribution kV_1. This difference is simply equal to $k\Delta V$, or $+d'$. Similarly for the case of V_2 in the second interval, the mean of the difference distribution is a function of $-\Delta V$, specifically, $-d'$. Converting both distributions to unit variance, we have means of $+d'/\sqrt{2}$ and

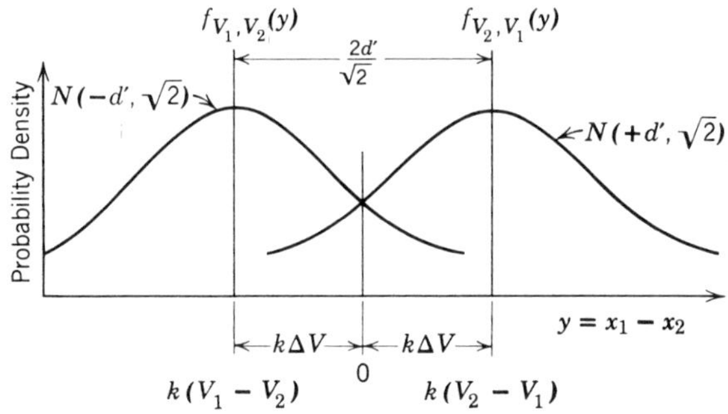

FIG. 6. Hypothesis distributions in 2AFC-PC situation.

$-d'/\sqrt{2}$; the difference is then $2d'/\sqrt{2}$. Thus in the 2AFC-PC experiment having the same ΔV as a YN experiment, ideal performance should be $\sqrt{2}$ times the performance in the YN situation.

It will be remembered that the ideal observer is assumed to possess a perfect memory, in order that the signal-specified-exactly condition be met. This assumption is important in understanding the difference between the next two tasks to be considered. The first of these will be specified as the fixed-base matching experiment (FBM). In this experiment three signals may appear: V_0, $V_0 - \Delta V$, and $V_0 + \Delta V$. There are again two observation intervals. In the first interval, V_0 always appears against the noise. In the second interval, either V_0, $V_0 - \Delta V_0$ or $V_0 + \Delta V$ may appear with noise. The observer's task is to specify whether or not the second interval contained V_0 and noise, i.e., whether or not it is the same as (matches) the signal in the first interval. The crucial point in conceptualizing this experiment is to realize that an observation of the first interval is unrelated to optimum behavior. The ideal observer already has available to him a noise-free recording of the signal (V_0) with which to compare the second interval observation; why should he use a noisy observation instead? The answer is, he should not; hence his performance is based solely on an observed measure of the second interval. Following the reasoning of the YN case, we can see that the hypotheses will be distributed as in Fig. 7. Clearly, had the observer used the first interval as a relevant measure to compare with the second, the variances involved would have doubled, with a resulting decrement in performance. We can conceptualize an alternative experiment in which such behavior would be required. Consider the random-base matching situation (RBM) where V_0 is randomly chosen from a set of possible values and ΔV is constant. That is, whenever V_0 appears in the first

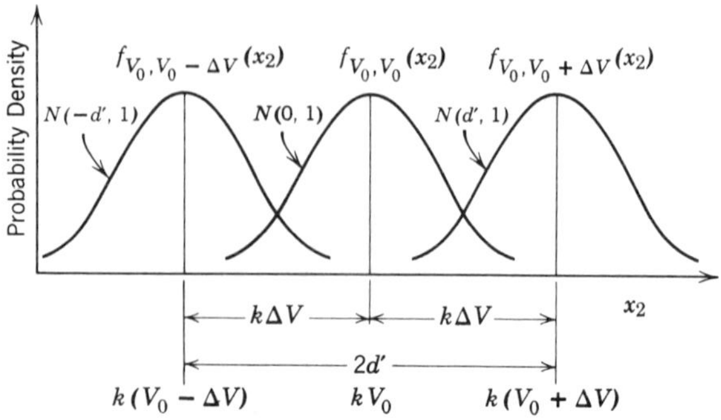

FIG. 7. Hypothesis distributions in matching, fixed-base condition.

interval, the second will contain either V_0, $V_0 + \Delta V$, or $V_0 - \Delta V$. Now the ideal observer needs to know what V_0 has occurred in a particular trial of this experiment in order to determine a same or different response in the second interval. Since there is noise in both intervals, the comparison measure on the first interval will be noisy and his performance will be degraded. As in the 2AFC-PC experiment, the relevant measure is the difference between the measures made on each interval $y = x_1 - x_2$. The new hypothesis distributions can be conceptualized as in Fig. 8. The distribution means are calculated as in the 2AFC case: $\mu_{V_0-\Delta V}(x_1 - x_2) = k\Delta V = d'$, $\mu_{V_0} \times (x_1 - x_2) = 0$, etc. It can be seen that the maximum difference between the distributions is $\sqrt{2}d'$, just as in the 2AFC case.

Human observer

In the 2AFC-PC experiment, factors which degrade human performance in comparison with ideal are the filter's time constant, short-term memory, and added noise. These factors can be conveniently pooled, for the human observer, in the relation $(d')^2 = \eta(2E/N_0)$, where η is an efficiency term incorporating these factors and E is the energy of the difference signal. If we were to construct a new experimental situation (e.g., matching), where so far as is possible the factors affecting η were held constant, we should expect that performance in the new situation would be completely specified by the η of the 2AFC-PC experiment; that is, d' should be constant across all situations, provided we have accurately described the particular situation in terms of the model's assumptions and have held those factors affecting efficiency constant.

Consider then what would result if human observers were given a matching task paralleling the fixed-base matching situation. A naive

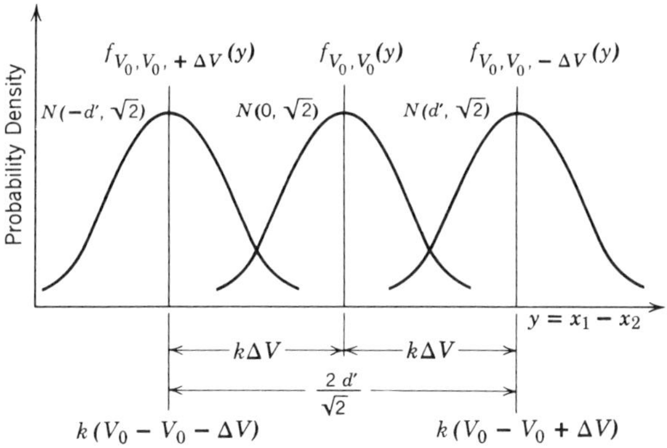

FIG. 8. Hypothesis distributions in matching, random-base condition.

expectation might be that the resulting separation between the distant hypotheses would be $\sqrt{2}$ times that of the parallel 2AFC-PC experiment. Yet the memory assumptions underlying each of these situational applications of the model are quite different. The pulsed carrier or base voltage V_0 in the 2AFC-PC experiment completely specifies the signal's frequency, starting time, phase, and duration, and hence eliminates all memory requirements for the signal parameters except amplitude. Use of the two-alternative forced-choice procedure further eliminates the long-time amplitude-memory requirement, and requires amplitude-memory specification only for the short time between the two intervals upon which the comparison observation is based. The fixed-base matching model of the ideal observer, however, assumes perfect amplitude specification in the memory prior to the matching trial. Thus, we should expect the fixed-base model's prediction of ideal performance to be at best only an upper bound on the separation of the human observer's hypotheses in this situation. Consideration of the random-base model's assumption, however, seems more reasonable. That is, assuming that the observer has some, perhaps noisy, recording of the signal's amplitude prior to a trial of the experiment, his separation should be somewhere between that predicted by the random-base model and that of the fixed-base model—since now an observation of the first interval is quite relevant. If additional uncertainty is somewhere present in the matching situation, the observed separation would be even less than that predicted by the random-base model. If in a fixed-base experiment some observers are performing at levels better than those predicted by the random-base model, an interesting test of the amplitude-memory assumption presents itself. Placing these same observers in a task which is situationally identical to the random-base case should place a new upper bound on their performance equal to that predicted by the random-base model, since they would now be forced (as was the ideal observer) to use an observation of the first interval. Indeed, if the efficiency as estimated by the 2AFC-PC experiment is correct and if this η is constant in the random-base matching experiment (as it should be by control over the factors affecting η), then the predicted separation in the random-base task should not just be an upper bound on the observed separations, but should be identical to it.

EXPERIMENTAL PROCEDURE

The experimental plan consisted of three steps. The first step was to place the observers in a two-alternative forced-choice pulsed-carrier situation to allow calculation of d' at different signal energies. The experimental procedures and laboratory equipment have been extensively described elsewhere (Green, Birdsall, and Tanner, 1957). During the second and third phases of the study, the observers were given matching tasks. During these tasks the same base voltages, time intervals, and noise level were used as in the 2AFC-PC experiments. The experimental situation present in the first of these matching tasks is identical to that of the fixed-base experiment discussed in the theory section of this report. That is, a 50-msec signal of 0.020 V at 1000 cps always occurred with noise $(2E/N_0)^{1/2} = 2.7$, for $\Delta V = 0.005$ in interval one, and either a signal of 0.020V + ΔV, 0.020V − ΔV, or 0.020V plus noise occurred in the second interval. The prior probabilities involved were $P(\text{same}) = 0.5$, $P(\text{different}) = 0.5$, and a symmetrical payoff matrix was employed. The required response was "same" or "different" via the appropriate response pushbuttons. Correct-answer information was provided to the observers following each experimental trial. The last step of the experiment was a matching task identical to the random-base situation. In this situation, the base or standard signal was chosen randomly from among 4 signals equal to 0.014, 0.017, 0.023, and 0.026 V. The signal occurring in the second interval was either the same as the one appearing in the first interval or that signal plus or minus the particular ΔV under study. Voltages of 0.005 and 0.007 were employed.

ANALYSIS OF DATA

The matching data for each observer and each condition consist of three probability measures from which it is possible to derive the three independent parameters relevant to observer performance in the matching situation: the two cutoffs β_1 and β_2, and the separation between the comparable hypotheses in the 2AFC-PC experiment. The separation between the "same" hypothesis and either of the "different" hypotheses is assumed to be half of that of the most distant hypotheses. One could write the equation for each obtained probability and solve the resultant equations simultaneously for the desired parameters:

probability of saying "different" given signal

$$V_0 - \Delta V = P_1(\mathrm{D}) = \int_{-\infty}^{\beta_1} f_1(x)dx + \int_{\beta_2}^{\infty} f_1(x)dx \tag{1}$$

probability of saying "same" given signal

$$V_0 = P_2(\mathrm{S}) = P_s(\mathrm{S}) = \int_{\beta_1}^{\beta_2} f_2(x)dx \tag{2}$$

probability of saying "different" given signal

$$V_0 + \Delta V = P_3(\mathrm{D}) = \int_{-\infty}^{\beta_1} f_3(x)dx + \int_{\beta_2}^{\infty} f_3(x)dx \tag{3}$$

where X_i is $N(\mu_i,1)$, $\mu_1 = -d'$, $\mu_2 = 0$, $\mu_3 = +d'$ under FBM assumptions, $\mu_1 = -d'/\sqrt{2}$, $\mu_2 = 0$, $\mu_3 = +d'/\sqrt{2}$ under RBM assumptions. Since such a procedure requires a pair of graphical solutions for each determination of d', an alternative approach was employed. The cutoffs were found by solving Eqs. (1) and (3) graphically using the d' obtained from the 2AFC-PC experiments performed early in the experiment (run at the same time interval between observations, base voltage, signal energy, and noise level). Specification of the cutoffs then allowed calculation of a predicted value for $P_s(\mathrm{S})$ by simple substitution of β_1, β_2, and d' in Eq. (2). This method was used to predict $P_s(\mathrm{S})$ values from $d'_{\mathrm{PC-2AFC}}$ under the assumptions of the random-base matching model (RBM). Predicted values of $P_s(\mathrm{S})$ were also calculated using a simpler, one-tailed approximation technique with the larger d''s generated by the fixed-base matching model. An approximation ignoring the tail of the distant hypothesis distribution is allowable in the latter case because of the much larger distances to the distant cutoffs. The results for the 2AFC-PC experiments are tabulated in Table I. Table II presents the observed values of $P_s(\mathrm{S})$ for the fixed-base experiment together with predicted

TABLE I. 2AFC-PC EXPERIMENTAL RESULTS

Observer	ΔV	d'
K	0.003	0.869
	0.005	1.413
	0.007	2.139
B	0.003	0.951
	0.005	1.610
	0.007	2.073
H	0.003	1.250
	0.005	1.775
	0.007	2.571

values under the assumption of the fixed- and random-base models. Table III consists of similar data for the random-base experiment. Figure 9 presents some examples of the hypothesis separations and cutoffs for the random-base condition. Approximately 1400 observations form the basis for each probability estimate.

DISCUSSION

It can be seen from Table II that the fixed-base model predictions provide an upper bound on the observed $P_s(S)$ for the first matching experiment. In the random-base matching experiment, summarized in Table III, close agreement between the random-base model predictions and the actual probabilities may be noted. Since the 2AFC-PC d''s served as a basis for calculation of these predicted values, the generality of the model across these experimental procedures is supported.

The data lend considerable support to the validity of the assumption that, for the human observer, η is constant between discrimination and

TABLE II. MATCHING RESULTS FOR FIXED-BASE CONDITION COMPARED TO PREDICTED VALUES UNDER BOTH FIXED- AND RANDOM-BASE ASSUMPTION

			$P_s(S)$	
Observer	ΔV	Observer	FBM[a]	*RBM*[a]
K	0.005	0.553	0.827	0.584
	0.007	0.591	0.958	0.697
B	0.005	0.548	0.775	0.468
	0.007	0.673	0.913	0.567
H	0.005	0.834	0.865	0.801
	0.007	0.822	0.992	0.848

[a] Predicted values.

TABLE III. MATCHING RESULTS FOR RANDOM-BASE CONDITION COMPARED TO PREDICTED VALUES UNDER RANDOM-BASE ASSUMPTION

Observer	ΔV	P_s(S) Observer	P_s(S) RBM[a]
K	0.005	0.507	0.492
B	0.005	0.488	0.487
H	0.005	0.844	0.863
B	0.007	0.478	0.502
H	0.007	0.834	0.899

[a] Predicted values.

matching experiments. Taking advantage of this result, one might employ experiments utilizing the matching procedure to replicate the results of studies in quite different areas of signal detectability theory, e.g., the determination of the degree of correlation, cos Θ, between non-independent signals in recognition or identification tasks (Tanner, 1956).

Another result can be seen in Fig. 9: the subjects' cutoffs β_1 and β_2 are clearly not symmetric around the "same" hypothesis. Thus one

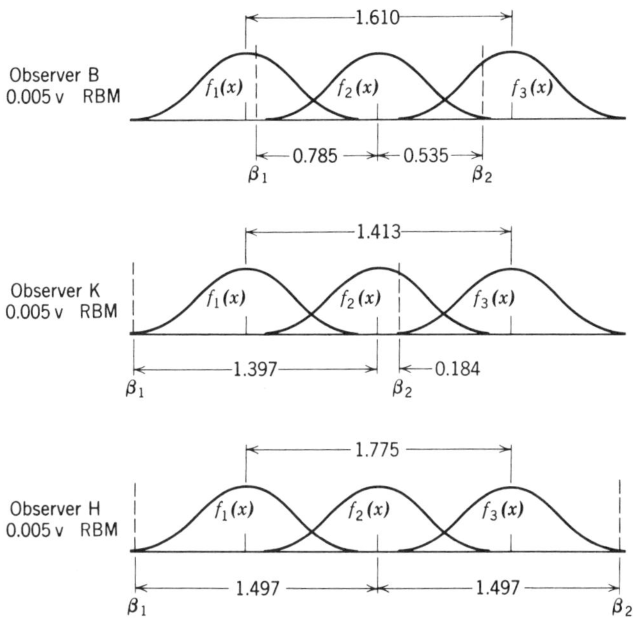

FIG. 9. Representative hypothesis distributions in random-base matching experiments.

cannot plot ROC curves based on the symmetry assumption and employ them to estimate separations from raw matching data. However, in the more complex experiment, where one of two or more signals is randomly chosen for each interval, the asymmetry of cutoff would not effect differences between $P_{A,A}(\mathrm{D})$ and $P_{B,B}(\mathrm{D})$, the characteristic of "fallible" data that Hefner had noted. A possible explanation for these differences, if they occurred in acoustic data, might be in consideration of the effect of base-voltage differences, in experiments requiring greater sampling of widely differing base signals. For example, it has been shown that an effective added noise may be introduced in the discrimination task equal to kV_0^2, where k is a constant and V_0 is the voltage of the base signal (Tanner, 1961). These differential effects, suggestive of Weber's Law, might be described by one of the distributions $[H_{B,B}(y)]$ making up $H_{\text{same}}(y)$ as having a higher variance (due to kV_0^2) than the other $[H_{A,A}(y)]$. Future experiments could test the reasonableness of this hypothesis.

Problems exist in extending the theory to more complex matching tasks, where random signals chosen for each interval come from a large set of possible ones. In such a situation, the TSD may become as unwieldy, for purposes of computing hypothesis separations, as Hefner's procedure was for scaling multidimensional stimuli. But the advantages of the TSD approach over the classical ones are obvious. The dimensionality of the relevant decision space is a function only of the number of decision alternatives; the theory allows a priori specification of the function relating the response variables to the relevant input variables; it allows generalization to and from other experimental procedures and situations; its pertinent measures do not confound criterion with sensitivity; and it provides a general theoretical framework for studying the crucial theoretical issues and incorporating new experimentally-obtained information into a broadly applicable descriptive model.

SUMMARY

The theory of signal detectability is used to analyze experiments where the observer's task is to state, after two signal presentations, whether the signals were the same or different. A model is suggested for predicting human performance in auditory "matching" tasks using data from detection and discrimination experiments. Three experiments are discussed which lend support to the model's application. The first, a two-alternative, forced-choice, pulsed-carrier experiment, serves to determine each observer's efficiency. The efficiency η is assumed constant provided certain observation-interval and signal characteristics are held fixed, as they were during the entire experimental sequence. The second was a simple matching task, where the first observation interval always contained a specified signal and the second sometimes contained a signal identical to the first. In the third experiment the signal appearing in the first interval was randomly chosen from a set of possible signals, thus removing the long-term memory requirement, and necessitating a comparison observation based on both intervals. The results are consistent with the assumption of constant efficiency across different tasks, and close agreement with the model's predictions for matching performance is demonstrated. Also discussed are some interesting side issues raised by the experimental data which are relevant to current use of the matching procedure in other areas of psychology. Consideration is made of possible further applications of the matching procedure, such as in determining the correlation among observations in recognition experiments.

ACKNOWLEDGMENTS

This research was conducted in the Cooley Electronics Laboratory of the University of Michigan with support from the Operational Applications Laboratory of the U. S. Air Force. This article appeared as Tech. Rept. No. ESD-TDR-62-210, and in J. acoust. Soc. Am., *1962,* **34,** *1745–1751.*

References

- Clarke, F. R., Birdsall, T. G., and Tanner, W. P., Jr. Two types of ROC curves and definitions of parameters. *J. acoust. Soc. Am.*, 1959, **31,** 629–630.
- Coombs, C. H. *A theory of data.* New York: John Wiley and Sons (in press), Chap. 19.
- Green, D. M., Birdsall, T. G., and Tanner, W. P., Jr. Signal detection as a function of signal intensity and duration. *J. acoust. Soc. Am.*, 1957, **29,** 523–531. [11]
- Hefner, R. A. Extensions of the law of comparative judgment to discriminable and multidimensional stimuli. University of Michigan: Doctoral dissertation, 1958.
- Lamphiear, D. E., and Birdsall, T. G. Approximations to the noncentral chi-square distributions with applications to signal detection models. University of Michigan: Electronic Defense Group, 1960, Technical Report No. 101.
- Peterson, W. W., and Birdsall, T. G. The theory of signal detectability. University of Michigan: Electronic Defense Group, 1953, Technical Report No. 13.
- Swets, J. A. Indices of signal detectability obtained with various psychophysical procedures. *J. acoust. Soc. Am.,* 1959, **31,** 511–513. [6]
- Swets, J. A., Tanner, W. P., Jr., and Birdsall, T. G. Decision processes in perception. *Psychol. Rev.,* 1961, **68,** 301–340. [1]

- Tanner, W. P., Jr. Theory of recognition. *J. acoust. Soc. Am.*, 1956, **28,** 882–888. [19]
- Tanner, W. P., Jr. Theory of signal detectability as an interpretive tool for psychophysical data. *J. acoust. Soc. Am.*, 1960, **32,** 1140–1147.
- Tanner, W. P., Jr. Application of the theory of signal detectability to amplitude discrimination. *J. acoust. Soc. Am.*, 1961, **33,** 1233–1244.
- Tanner, W. P., Jr., and Birdsall, T. G. Definitions of d' and η as psychophysical measures. *J. acoust. Soc. Am.*, 1958, **30,** 922–928. [5]
- Tanner, W. P., Jr., Birdsall, T. G., and Clarke, F. R. The concept of the ideal observer in psychophysics. University of Michigan: Electronic Defense Group, 1960, Technical Report No. 98.
- Tanner, W. P., Jr., and Swets, J. A. A decision-making theory of visual detection. *Psychol. Rev.*, 1954, **61,** 401–409.

section six

FREQUENCY ANALYSIS

Of the substantive problems studied within the framework of detection theory, auditory frequency analysis has received the most attention. Several different approaches have been used in an attempt to refine the concept of the critical band.

Swets, Green, and Tanner ("On the Width of Critical Bands" [23]) combine the classical masking experiment with new methods of analysis. They show that the estimated width of the auditory filter depends on the shape that it is assumed to have. Tanner, after noting that masking has been viewed as the opposite of analysis, asks "What is Masking?" [24]. He analyzes three different kinds of experiments in terms of the conventional definition of masking, and points out that three different processes are involved.

Green, in "Detection of Multiple Component Signals in Noise" [25], compares three mathematical models, all of them extensions of the concept of the critical band, with data on the detection of signals consisting of two sinusoids. The model favored by these data is also supported by results obtained with signals having larger numbers of components, as shown by Green, McKey, and Licklider in "Detection of a Pulsed Sinusoid in Noise as a Function of Frequency" [26], and by results obtained with signals consisting of bands of noise, as shown by Green in "Auditory Detection of a Noise Signal" [27].

In "Detection of Auditory Sinusoids of Uncertain Frequency" [28], Green reports results that cannot be accounted for by any of the existing models. Swets reviews the models and data, particularly with regard to their implications for "Central Factors in Auditory Frequency Selectivity" [29], and concludes that the number, the frequency locations, and the widths of the critical bands operative in a given task reflect substantially the strategy of listening that is adopted by the observer for that particular task.

23

On the Width of Critical Bands

John A. Swets, David M. Green, and Wilson P. Tanner, Jr.

For the better part of a century, attempts to specify the process of auditory frequency analysis were based almost exclusively on anatomical and physiological evidence. Then, in 1940, Fletcher presented psychophysical data that gave a new form to the problem. He reported an experiment showing that only noise components in a narrow region about a pure tone are effective in masking the tone. This region he termed the "critical band" (Fletcher, 1940).

The existence of a critical band of frequency has since been clearly established in a variety of psychophysical experiments, including experiments on masking by tones or noise, on loudness summation, on phase sensitivity, and on detection of multiple tones and tones of uncertain frequency. Estimates of the width of the critical band, however—even those estimates obtained from experiments of the same type—have varied widely.

The present study approached the problem of the width of the critical band by repeating Fletcher's basic experiment, but with a different method of analysis. Before discussing the results, we shall consider the setting of this study in terms of the procedures used and the results obtained in previous experiments.

A BRIEF HISTORY OF THE PROBLEM

Fletcher determined the threshold of a tone in the presence of bands of noise of various widths centered at the frequency of the tone. For bands wider than some critical value, the amplitude of the just-detectable tone was constant; as the bands were made progressively narrower than this value, the amplitude of the tone could be progressively decreased and still the tone would remain detectable. Fletcher found the critical band to be approximately 65 cps wide for a tone of 1000 cps, to remain relatively constant at lower frequencies, and to increase sharply for higher frequencies, reaching a width of 500 cps for a tone of 8000 cps.

Fletcher summarized his data in another form by stating that, at least for moderate levels of noise power, the noise in the critical band equals in acoustic power the just-detectable tone. This conclusion, perhaps better termed an assumption since it was based on very few data, suggested that the critical band could be measured indirectly in masking experiments that used only broad-band noise. Fletcher later reported measurements based on broad-band noise; the critical bands so determined showed a similar dependence upon frequency and, again, the critical band in the region of 1000 cps was estimated to be approximately 65 cps wide (Fletcher, 1953).

The estimates made by Fletcher were subsequently confirmed by other investigators in both types of experiment. Schafer et al. (1950) measured the critical band directly, with noise bands of various widths, and obtained an estimate of 65 cps at a center frequency of 800 cps. Their experiment also provided support for Fletcher's assumption about the acoustic power in the critical band. Using this assumption along with broad-band noise, Hawkins and Stevens (1950) estimated the critical band to be 63 cps at 1000 cps.

Several experiments were then performed using quite different methods. These experiments—on loudness summation, detection of multiple tones, masking of noise by tones (the inverse of Fletcher's experiment), and phase sensitivity—have been reviewed by Zwicker, Flottorp, and Stevens (1957). All these experiments show dependence of the critical bandwidth on frequency similar to previous observations. However, the critical bands reported as the average result of these four experiments were approximately 2½ times as wide as those observed previously; in particular, the critical band at 980 cps was taken to be 160 cps in width. At the same time, Hamilton (1957), using Fletcher's direct method, obtained an estimate almost as large as that reported by Zwicker et al.; he reported the critical band to be 145 cps wide at 800 cps. Hamilton had begun a trend, for recently Greenwood (1961), also by means of

Fletcher's direct method, obtained estimates essentially the same as those reported by Zwicker et al.

WHY THE DIVERSE ESTIMATES?

We should perhaps expect the measures of the critical bandwidth to vary from one kind of experiment to another. For one thing, it seems unlikely that all of these experiments are measuring *the* critical band, a fixed property of the auditory system that exists independent of experiments. It seems more reasonable to suppose that the parameters of the auditory system are not fixed, specifically, that they may vary from one sensory task to another under intelligent control (Swets, Shipley, McKey, and Green, 1959; Green, 1960). That the system is adaptable is suggested by the high degree of efficiency exhibited by human observers in very different sensory tasks. An adaptive system is also consistent with the evidence (as pointed out by Licklider, 1950) that the high degree of frequency selectivity displayed by the auditory system is contributed by the neural part of the system: Békésy's direct observations show the cochlea to have a selectivity curve that is an order of magnitude wider than the critical bands we have been considering (von Békésy and Rosenblith, 1951).

Moreover, even if the auditory system were fixed, we might expect it to manifest itself differently in different types of experiments. If, for example, the edges of the critical band are not perfectly sharp (if frequencies farther from the center are progressively more attenuated rather than passed fully up to a point and attenuated infinitely beyond that point), then the role played by these edges would vary with the stimuli used. We may note Greenwood's (1961) finding that his measures of the critical band depended on the level of the masking noise.

Nor should it be surprising that diverse estimates of bandwidth are obtained in different experiments of the same type. Hamilton (1957) has pointed out that the small variations in measurements which would result from differences in experimental method and filter characteristics can lead to large differences in critical band values. Still another source of variability is the shape of the critical band which is assumed in the analysis. As we shall see, even if a single sensory task is employed so that the parameters of the auditory system are likely to be relatively constant throughout the experiment, the single set of data that is obtained can lead to substantially different estimates of critical bandwidth which correspond to different assumptions about the shape of the critical band.

THE SHAPE OF THE CRITICAL BAND

With one exception, among the studies mentioned it has been assumed or concluded that the response characteristic of the auditory system (or the critical band) is rectangular. The assumption of a rectangular band is certainly justified as a first approximation, but it does not receive strong support from the data; a sharp discontinuity at the critical value is not evident. Schafer et al. (1950) likened the auditory response characteristic to that of a single-tuned, or universal-resonance, filter. Their results were in fair agreement with the assumption; their experiment indicated, at the least, that the assumption of some kind of filter with sloping skirts was in better agreement with the data than was the assumption of a rectangular filter.

Schafer et al. used the electronic-filter model advisedly. They stated: "This interpretation is for analytical purposes only, and is not intended to suggest the mechanism by which the selectivity is obtained. The fact that the mechanism is a complex interrelation of peripheral elements of hydrodynamical and mechanical nature, neural elements electrochemical in nature, and central neural processes discourages attempts to carry the analogy further." They go on to say, however: "Because the pure tone probably excites a restricted region of the basilar membrane in a manner somewhat resembling a simple resonance curve, the noise power effective in masking this tone should be analogous to the noise power in a simple resonant circuit having a response curve of the proper width."

We subscribe both to the disclaimer and to the spirit of the positive statement. Models are no more than "as-if" representations; even if a model is in close agreement with all available data, it does not specify exactly, and probably not even approximately, the mechanism that actually exists. In principle, a large number of models will fit any set of data equally well. By the same token, we need not restrict a consideration of filter models to the available and simple single-tuned filter. The advantages of a filter model in this instance—economy, simplicity, and accuracy in description and calculation—are provided by any filter that can be specified in mathematical terms, whether or not it can be physically realized.

EXPERIMENT

Procedure

The procedures followed in the present experiment differed in several ways from those used previously. Fletcher filtered the masking noise with a filter that was necessarily, for his purpose, a rather poor approximation to a rectangular filter; his treatment of the data requires the use of a perfectly rectangular, and thus nonexistent, filter. Schafer et al. constructed a more nearly rectangular masking stimulus, a pseudo-noise, by adding sinusoids. In the study reported here, a simple filter with gradually sloping skirts (single-tuned) was used along with white noise, and the actual characteristic of the filter was taken into account in the calculations. This study also used an index of detectability that is not dependent upon the validity of the concept of a sensory threshold (Swets, 1961).

The problem is treated mathematically as two filters in series—one representing the real, external filter, the other representing an assumed internal or auditory filter—intervening between a detector and the sources of tone and noise.

The reduction in total noise power from source to detector which is effected by a serial arrangement of any two specified filters can be calculated. Figure 1 shows, for four different pairs of filters, the reduction in noise power as a function of the ratio of the widths of the two filters. One of the filters used in each of these calculations was a single-tuned filter; this filter corresponds to the filter actually used as the external filter in the experiment to be reported. The various functions shown in the figure represent several different shapes of the second filter; these correspond to different assumptions about the shape of the internal filter. Given these relations, and given the width of the external filter, an experimental determination of the change in noise power at the

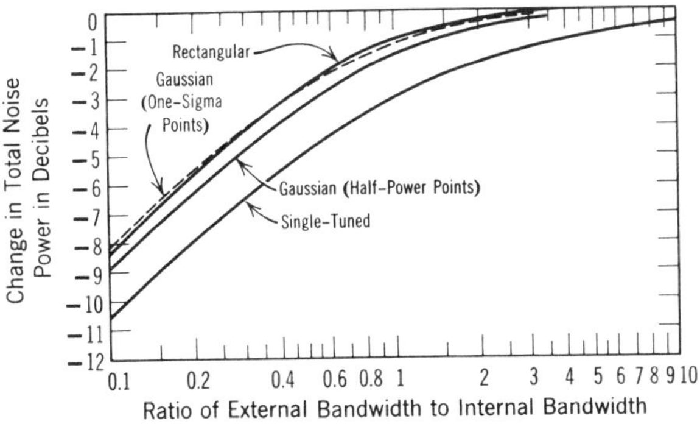

FIG. 1. The reduction in noise power from source to detector, which results from a pair of filters intervening between the source and the detector, is shown as a function of the ratio of the width of the two filters. The four curves represent the combination of a single-tuned filter with the four different types of filters indicated in the figure.

detector which results from varying the width of the external filter will enable one to estimate the width of the internal filter under any of the several assumptions about its shape.

The change in the noise power at the detector which is caused by varying the width of the external filter can be determined indirectly if it is assumed that the changes produced by varying an external filter on the noise are comparable to changes produced by simply varying the power of a broad-band noise. Then, by means of an experimentally determined function relating the detectability index to the power of broad-band noise, the changes in the detectability index which are produced by external filtering can be translated into changes in noise power at the detector.

In order to fix these ideas, let us describe the procedure in terms of the operations performed. We first determined how the detectability index increased as the width of the external filter (on a broad-band noise of constant power) was decreased from one group of trials to another, say, from a very large value (equivalent to no filtering), to 90, 80, and 70 cps, etc. We assume that the detectability increased because the total noise power at the detector was successively reduced by the filtering. Then, in a second experimental condition, we determined how the detectability index increased as a broad-band noise, first at the same level as used in the previous experimental condition with the filtering, was simply decreased in power from one group of trials to another. Now the increase in the index that is produced by an external filter of a given width can be expressed in terms of a decrease in noise power at the detector. The two values—the width of the external filter and the reduction in noise power that it effects—were then used in conjunction with the curves of Fig. 1 to estimate the width of the internal filter under a particular assumption about its shape. If, for example, an external filter 20 cps wide results in an increase in the detectability index (compared to no filter) which equals the increase in the index brought about by reducing the spectrum level of the wideband noise by 7 db, then according to Fig. 1, the ratio of external to internal bandwidth—assuming the internal filter has the shape of a single-tuned filter—is 0.25. Thus, the internal filter, under this assumption about its shape, would be estimated to be 80 cps wide.

We estimated the width of the critical band, or of the internal filter, under each of four assumptions about its shape: (1) single-tuned; (2) rectangular; (3) Gaussian, with the width taken as the distance between the plus and minus one-sigma points; (4) Gaussian, with width as determined by the half-power points. Under each assumption, for each of three observers, we obtained seven values representing the width of the critical band. These seven values correspond to the seven different values of external bandwidth employed: 10, 20, 30, 40, 50, 60, and 90 cps. We took the average of the seven values calculated on the basis of each particular assumption about the shape of the critical band as an estimate of the width of the band given that particular assumption.

Throughout the experiment, the tonal signal was presented at a frequency of 1000 cps and at a duration of 0.1 sec. The signal-to-noise ratio, before filtering and at the reference level of the noise, was $10 \log E/N_0 = 7.15$. E is the signal energy, or time integral of power, and N_0 is the noise power in a one-cycle band. The spectrum level of the noise at the reference level was approximately 50 db *re* 0.0002 d/cm². The signal was always passed through a filter 10 cps wide.

The method of stimulus presentation and response used was the four-alternative forced-choice method. On each trial, the signal was presented in exactly one of four time intervals, and the observer was required to state in which interval he believed the signal was presented. The percentage of correct responses was converted, by a simple transformation, into the detectability index d'. The definition of d' has been given elsewhere (Tanner and Birdsall, 1958). A table showing the relation of d' to the percentage of correct responses in a four-alternative test has also been reported previously (Green, Birdsall, and Tanner, 1957).

Results

In the first condition of the experiment, the broad-band noise was held constant at 50 db *re* 0.0002 d/cm², and the width of the external filter was varied from one group of 100 trials to another in a counterbalanced order. At each of the seven values of the external bandwidth already mentioned, a total of 400 trials were presented, and a value of d' was determined. The seven values of d' obtained from each observer are shown in Fig. 2. The eighth value of d' shown, at the point on the abscissa labeled "wide," was obtained from 400 trials in which the noise was not filtered at all.

The second experimental condition enables us to translate these values of d' into the reduction in the noise power at the detector. The broad-band noise was reduced from the reference level of 50 db *re* 0.0002 d/cm² by 1, 2, 3, 4, 6, or 8 db. A total of 400 trials was presented at each noise level. The values of d' obtained are shown in Fig. 3.

Using these data and the curves of Fig. 1, we have determined a value of the critical band for each value of the external filter. Table I shows,

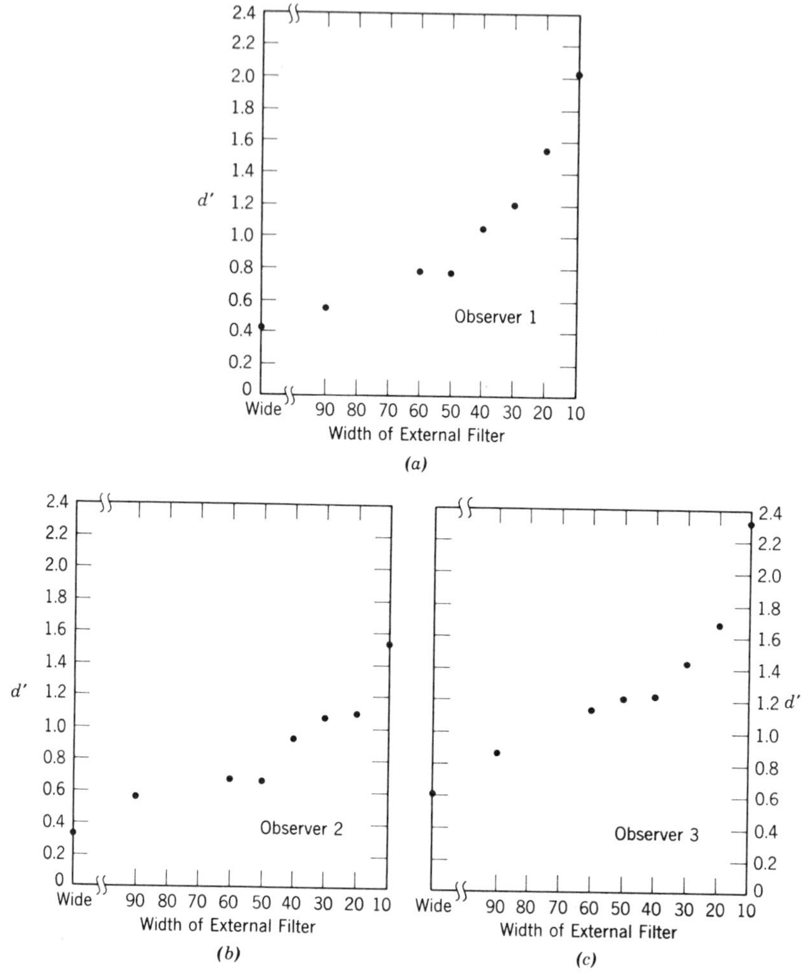

FIG. 2. The detectability index d' obtained with external filters of various widths from three observers.

for each observer, these seven values of the critical band as calculated under each assumption about its shape. The means and standard deviations of the values and the ratios of the means to the standard deviations are also given in the table.

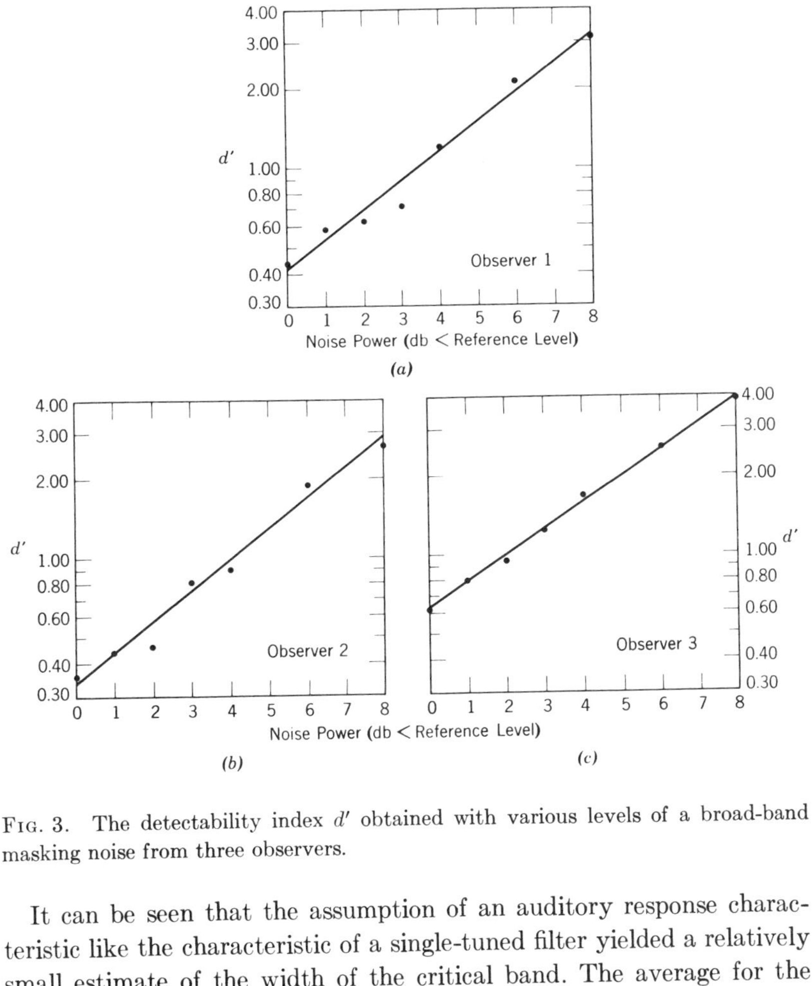

FIG. 3. The detectability index d' obtained with various levels of a broad-band masking noise from three observers.

It can be seen that the assumption of an auditory response characteristic like the characteristic of a single-tuned filter yielded a relatively small estimate of the width of the critical band. The average for the three observers is 41 cps. The average under the Gaussian (half-power) assumption is 79 cps. On the basis of the Gaussian (one-sigma) assumption, and also on the basis of the rectangular assumption, the average value is 95 cps. It can also be seen that the ratios of mean to standard deviation under the four assumptions are comparable.

TABLE I. ESTIMATES OF INTERNAL BANDWIDTH ON THE BASIS OF VARIOUS EXTERNAL BANDWIDTHS

Assumed internal bandwidth characteristic		Width of external filter[a]							Mean	Standard deviation	M/S.D.
		10	20	30	40	50	60	90			
Single-tuned	Observer 1	37	44	49	53	37	44	26	41	8.3	4.9
	Observer 2	31	35	53	58	42	50	50	46	9.2	5.0
	Observer 3	28	32	37	37	43	44	33	36	5.4	6.6
Rectangular	Observer 1	64	87	100	114	94	113	95	95	15.7	6.1
	Observer 2	58	71	107	124	102	122	138	103	26.9	3.8
	Observer 3	55	65	82	89	104	113	106	88	20.2	4.4
Gaussian (one-sigma points)	Observer 1	73	91	103	117	91	109	86	96	13.8	7.0
	Observer 2	61	74	111	124	100	120	130	103	24.3	4.2
	Observer 3	58	67	82	87	102	109	97	86	17.2	5.0
Gaussian (half-power points)	Observer 1	60	77	86	98	77	92	69	80	12.2	6.6
	Observer 2	55	61	94	105	83	100	107	86	19.5	4.4
	Observer 3	50	56	69	73	86	92	78	72	14.1	5.1

[a] The bandwidths of the external filter listed as column headings here, and along the abscissa of Fig. 2, are nominal. It was not practicable in the experiment to attempt to adjust the bandwidths to be exactly equal to any given figure. The actual values of external bandwidth employed in the experiment and in the calculations were 12, 20, 31, 41, 50, 60, and 90, respectively.

SUMMARY AND DISCUSSION

This study has demonstrated a different technique of analysis for use with Fletcher's basic experiment on the critical band. The results reverse the recent trend toward obtaining estimates of the width of the critical band which are considerably larger than those obtained in the earliest studies.

Under one assumption about the shape of the critical band, its width (in the neighborhood of 1000 cps) was determined to be approximately 40 cps. This estimate is somewhat smaller than the estimate of 65 cps obtained in the first studies by Fletcher (1940; 1953), Schafer et al. (1950) and Hawkins and Stevens (1950). Under another assumption about its shape, the critical band was measured as approximately 80 cps. Two other assumptions about its shape led to estimates of 95 cps. These values, while larger than those obtained originally, are still smaller than the estimate of 145 cps made by Hamilton (1957), and the estimate of 160 cps made by Zwicker et al. (1957) and by Greenwood (1961).

It is clear that the estimated value of critical bandwidth is highly sensitive to the shape that the band is assumed to have. It would be desirable, therefore, to have a good basis for choosing among the several similar assumptions. Unfortunately, there seems to be no independent basis for choice, and the results of this study do not provide one. However, the fact that we cannot discriminate among the various assumptions in this study does not appear to us to be the major problem. We believe that what might turn out to be the best assumption in any given study will depend upon the stimuli used and upon the task posed for the observer. We would suggest a consideration—in theory construction and in research strategy—of the possibility that the parameters of the mechanism of frequency selectivity vary from one sensory task to another under intelligent control. If they do, then, of course, we cannot speak of, or measure, *the* critical band.

ACKNOWLEDGMENTS

The authors are indebted to T. G. Birdsall, R. R. MacPherson, J. A. Lauder, and G. A. Roberts of the University of Michigan for various contributions to this research.

The experiment reported here was conducted in the laboratories of the Electronic Defense Group of the University of Michigan with support received from the U. S. Army Signal Corps. This paper was prepared in the Research Laboratory of Electronics, Massachusetts Institute of Technology, with the support of the U. S. Army Signal Corps, the Air Force (Operational Applications Laboratory and Office of Scientific Research), and the Office of Naval Research. This article appeared as Tech. Rept. No. ESD-TR-61-34, and in J. acoust. Soc. Am., *1962,* **34,** *108–113.*

References

- Fletcher, H. Auditory patterns. *Revs. mod. Phys.*, 1940, **12,** 47–65.
- Fletcher, H. *Speech and hearing in communication.* New York: D. Van Nostrand Co., 1953.
- Green, D. M. Auditory detection of a noise signal. *J. acoust. Soc. Am.*, 1960, **32,** 121–131. [27]
- Green, D. M., Birdsall, T. G., and Tanner, W. P., Jr. Signal detection as a function of signal intensity and duration. *J. acoust. Soc. Am.*, 1957, **29,** 523–531. [11]
- Greenwood, D. D. Auditory masking and the critical band. *J. acoust. Soc. Am.*, 1961, **33,** 484–502.
- Hamilton, P. M. Noise masked thresholds as a function of tonal duration and masking noise band width. *J. acoust. Soc. Am.*, 1957, **29,** 506–511.
- Hawkins, J. E., and Stevens, S. S. The masking of pure tones and of speech by white noise. *J. acoust. Soc. Am.*, 1950, **22,** 6–13.
- Licklider, J. C. R. On the mechanism of auditory frequency selectivity. *J. acoust. Soc. Am.*, 1950, **22,** 83. (Abstract)
- Schafer, T. H., Gales, R. S., Shewmaker, C. A., and Thompson, P. O. The frequency selectivity of the ear as determined by masking experiments. *J. acoust. Soc. Am.*, 1950, **22,** 490–496.
- Swets, J. A., Is there a sensory threshold? *Science,* 1961, **134,** 168–177. [4]
- Swets, J. A., Shipley, E. F., McKey, M. J., and Green, D. M. Multiple observations of signals in noise. *J. acoust. Soc. Am.*, 1959, **31,** 514–521. [9]
- Tanner, W. P., Jr., and Birdsall, T. G. Definitions of d' and η as psychophysical measures. *J. acoust. Soc. Am.*, 1958, **30,** 922–928. [5]
- von Békésy, G., and Rosenblith, W. A. The mechanical properties of the ear. In S. S. Stevens (Ed.), *Handbook of experimental psychology.* New York: Wiley, 1951.
- Zwicker, E., Flottorp, G., and Stevens, S. S. Critical band width in loudness summation. *J. acoust. Soc. Am.*, 1957, **29,** 548–557.

24

What Is Masking?

Wilson P. Tanner, Jr.

According to Licklider (1951), "Masking is thus the opposite of analysis; it represents the inability of the auditory mechanisms to separate the tonal stimulation into components and to discriminate between the presence and the absence of one of them." He continues by pointing out that the "degree to which one component of a sound is masked by another is determined by measuring two thresholds"; that of the masked tone with the masking agent present and without the masking agent present.

In view of a result first reported by Tanner and Norman (1954) it appears to be worthwhile to re-examine the masking concept. In that experiment the detectability of a tone appears to be changed when the observer is uncertain of the frequency of that tone. Is this uncertainty a masking agent in the same sense that one usually conceives of a masking agent which actually introduces physical energy into the ear at the same time that detection occurs? Certainly the result is the same.

However, if one is not willing to accept the similarity of results as an indication that the same type of phenomenon is occurring in the two cases, then one might extend his doubts to the question concerning the similarity between masking by white noise and masking by pure tones. This paper is intended to treat the differences among these three types of experiments: (1) the change in the detectability of a tone through the introduction of an additional white noise, (2) the change in detectability of a tone in the presence of an additional pure tone, and (3) the change in the detectability of a tone when the observer knows that it might have been a different tone.

The measurements employed in the experiments reported below depend on the definitions of η and d' presented by the author (Tanner and Birdsall, 1958). η is the ratio of the energy required of the ideal observer (Peterson, Birdsall, and Fox, 1954) to the energy employed in an experiment, leading to equal performances for the ideal observer and the observer in the experiment. For purposes of comparison over the three types of experiments, the masking index M is defined as

$$M = (\eta_1 - \eta_2)/\eta_1$$

where η_1 is the efficiency of performance without the masking signal, and η_2 is the efficiency of performance with the masking signal present.

THREE MASKING EXPERIMENTS

All of the experiments to be reported are of the class referred to as "temporal forced choice" (Blackwell, 1953). A signal is known to occur in one of n positions in time. It is the observer's task to state in which of the n positions in time the signal occurred. Since in all the experiments each of the positions was equally likely to be that of the signal, and each had associated an equal risk function, d' could be obtained from the percentage of correct responses and the approximations of Peterson and Birdsall (see Appendix 1) for the probability of a correct choice among one of n alternatives.

Masking by white noise

The first problem treated is that of masking by white noise. In this problem, the data of Green, Birdsall, and Tanner (1957) are employed. In the experiments reported in that paper, involving weak signals, d' is found to vary approximately linearly with signal energy for every case in which signal duration is held constant. Since d' ideally should vary linearly with the square root of signal energy, this means that η is a small number when d' is small, and increases as d' increases. Actually, η has been observed to be as large as 0.3 in some of these experiments. This result, along with the result that d' varies in nearly the same manner with the ratio $2E/N_0$ when the ratio is varied by varying the noise level rather than the signal level (Tanner, Swets, and Green, 1956), suggests that only the higher values of η should be used in computing the masking index if one is interested in signal masking as such. The reason for the low values of η appears to exist in some effect other than masking of the signal itself.

Alternate-frequency masking

Next, consider the decrement in performance which results from the fact that the signal might have been at another frequency. In this experiment the signal appears in one of n positions in time. The observer knows that the signal will be selected randomly from one of two possible frequencies. He is graded as being correct if he states the correct position in time; he need not state the frequency. The masking index, calculated from data of Tanner and Norman (1954), is zero when the two frequencies are the same, and increases as the two possible frequencies become farther separated. The effect of a 1000-cycle tone on 1000, 900, 800, and 700 cps is shown in Fig. 1. Surely, this tone which might have been the *signal* is not masking in the usual sense. It appears rather that it is serving to distract the attention of the observer from the signal. Of course, in these experiments involving two tones either signal can be considered to be the masking tone.

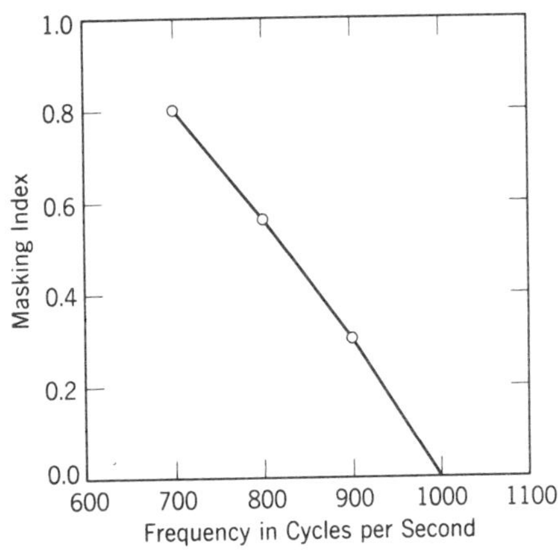

FIG. 1. Masking by a 1000-cps tone which might have been the signal.

Masking by pure tone

The third type of masking experiment is like that performed by Wegel and Lane (1924). In this experiment, a pure tone is employed as the masking signal. It is added to a noise background present to permit the calculation of η. The effect of the presence of this tone on the performance in two types of experiment, each employing the same information-carrying component, is studied. One of these experiments is a detection experiment; the other, a recognition or discrimination experiment.

The two experiments are illustrated in Fig. 2. The first experiment has presented, in two positions in time, the signals illustrated in lines 1 and 2, in a random order. The observer states whether the larger signal (line 2) came first or second. The difference signal, the one that carries the information, is shown in line 3. The second experiment presents in the same way the signals shown in lines 4 and 5. Again the observer is asked to state whether the larger came first or second. The difference signal, carrying the information, is illustrated in line 6. Note that the signals in line 6 and line 3 are the same.

Perhaps a little discussion will help the reader see that, ideally, the two experiments lead to the same results. In the second experiment,

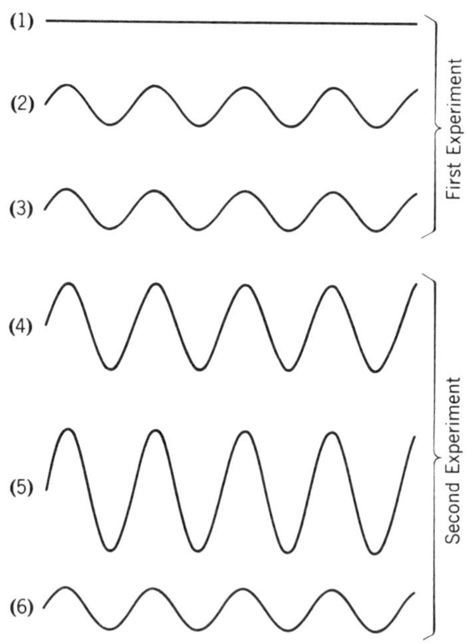

FIG. 2. Two masking experiments.

the smaller of the two signals (line 4) appears in both positions in time. In one of the time positions the information-carrying signal (line 6) is added to the smaller. The ideal observer subtracts the smaller signal from the observation in each of the two positions in time. This leaves in one position the signal in line 1, plus noise, of course, and in the other the signal of line 2 plus noise. Ideally, he now tests to determine whether the signal in line 2 is more likely to be in position 1 or position 2. This is, of course, the identical task required of the observer in the first experiment.

Experiment 1 involved two signals: zero volts and 0.05 volt. The other experiment employs signals of 0.20 volt and 0.25 volt. The difference in each case is 0.05 volt. Each experiment was performed with masking tones at 1200 cps, first with the masking tone at 0.10 volt, and then at 0.40 volt. The sound pressure level of these two tones at the output of the earphones is approximately 65 and 77 db *re* 0.0002 d/cm^2. The masking tone was continuously present in the noise, and the signals were 0.1 sec in duration. The determination of each η involved 200 observations for the unmasked condition and 200 observations for the masked condition.

DISCUSSION OF RESULTS

The results of these experiments are shown in Figs. 3 and 4. It is obvious at a glance that the "masking" tone does not appear to be affecting the signal equally in the two cases. When the weak signal is presented at the same frequency and in phase with the weaker of the two masking tones, the masking index is less than -1. In other words,

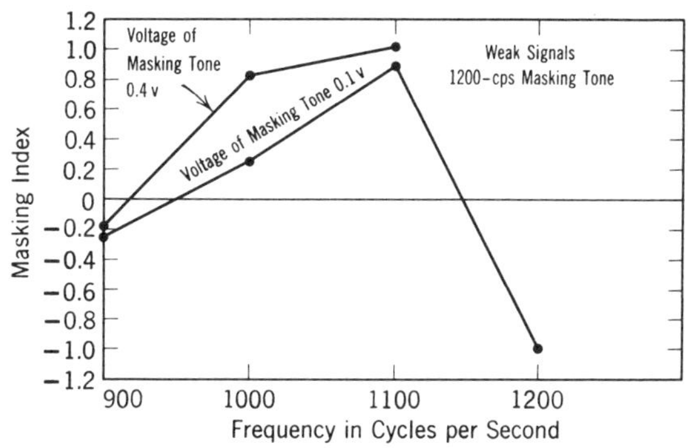

FIG. 3. Masking of weak signals by a pure tone.

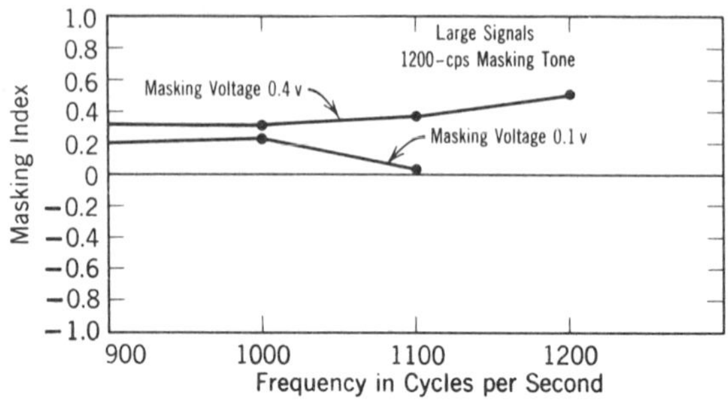

FIG. 4. Masking of large signals by a pure tone.

performance is enhanced rather than decreased. However, when the two signals are separated by 100 cps, the masking index is nearly 1.00, and with the larger masking tone is 1.00. As the separation becomes greater, the effect decreases faster for the lower masking tone than for the larger tone.

For the second experiment, the "masking" effect is much less, except for that case in which the large signals are at the same frequency and in phase with the masking tone. The sum of the two is sufficient to place the two in the range in which distortion might be expected, more than 80 db above 0.0002 d/cm². Other than this case, there appears to be relatively little effect, particularly for the smaller masking tone.

Reviewing all three types of experiments, there appear to be at least three types of effects involved. One of these is the signal masking[1] accomplished by white noise. The size of this effect probably is not much greater than one would predict on the basis of the theory of signal detectability (Peterson, Birdsall, and Fox, 1954).

The second is the distraction of the observer from the signal he is trying to detect. Some of this effect may exist when only noise is used to mask, since the noise may tend to disturb the observer's memory for the signal frequency. In the case where the signal frequency is uncertain, it seems fairly clear that this type of effect may exist. The notion is further supported in the third type of experiment. When the signal is weak, the masking tone interferes except in that case where it serves as the memory of the signal frequency. When the signal has the carrier, as in experiment 2 of the third type, the carrier is strong enough to resist the distraction.

[1] Gunnar Hok (personal communication) distinguishes between masking of the signal and other processes which interfere with the operation of the receiver.

The third effect is that illustrated when the large signals are added to the larger masking tone, a distortion effect. This leads to a spreading of energy which could cause a decrease in performance.

The masking by white noise appears to be both physical and psychological. When noise is introduced, the signal is masked even for an ideal receiver. In addition, noise seems to have a further effect on the human observer, perhaps reducing the effectiveness of his memory for signal parameters, or reducing his ability to resist distraction by undesired signals. The noise may also be so powerful that it overdrives the auditory mechanism.

SUMMARY

Masking appears to take place in all three of the experiments reported. Still, careful analysis suggests that there are three different processes involved. Should all three be accepted as masking? If so, then masking theories should take into account the fact that they must consider these processes. If not, then masking should be redefined.

It seems to the author that the difficulty lies not so much in the definition as it does in the acceptance of an operational definition based on the method of measure. Does masking occur merely because conditions are established leading to a change in performance?

ACKNOWLEDGMENTS

This research was conducted in the laboratories of the Electronic Defense Group of the University of Michigan with support from the Operational Applications Laboratory of the U. S. Air Force. This article appeared as Tech. Rept. No. AFCRC-TN-57-64, and in J. acoust. Soc. Am., *1958,* **30,** *919–921.*

References

- Blackwell, H. R. Psychophysical thresholds: experimental studies of methods of measurement. University of Michigan: Engineering Research Institute, 1953, Bulletin No. 36.
- Green, D. M., Birdsall, T. G., and Tanner, W. P., Jr. Signal detection as a function of signal intensity and duration. *J. acoust. Soc. Am.*, 1957, **29,** 523–531. [11]
- Licklider, J. C. R. Basic correlates of the auditory stimulus. In S. S. Stevens (Ed.), *Handbook of experimental psychology.* New York: Wiley, 1951.
- Peterson, W. W., Birdsall, T. G., and Fox, W. C. The theory of signal detectability. *Trans. IRE Professional Group on Information Theory,* **1954, PGIT-4, 171–212.**

- Tanner, W. P., Jr., and Birdsall, T. G. Definitions of d' and η as psychophysical measures. *J. acoust. Soc. Am.*, 1958, **30,** 922–928. [5]
- Tanner, W. P., Jr., and Norman, R. Z. The human use of information: II. Signal detection for the case of an unknown signal parameter. *Trans. IRE Professional Group on Information Theory,* 1954, **PGIT-4,** 222–227.
- Tanner, W. P., Jr., Swets, J. A., and Green, D. M. Some general properties of the hearing mechanism. University of Michigan: Electronic Defense Group, 1956, Technical Report No. 30.
- Wegel, R. L., and Lane, C. E. The auditory masking of one pure tone by another and its probable relation to the dynamics of the inner ear. *Phys. Rev.*, 1924, **23,** **226–285.**

25

Detection of Multiple Component Signals in Noise

David M. Green

While there are a great deal of data available concerning the detectability of simple auditory signals, little information is available concerning the detectability of complex signals. There are at least two reasons why the detectability of complex signals in noise is an important problem. The first reason is a practical one; almost all of the sounds one hears outside the laboratory are other than single sine-wave signals. The second reason is theoretical; the critical band concept, which provides a model for explaining the detection of single sine wave signals, is not specific in how this concept should be extended to encompass complex signals.

The complex signals investigated in this paper are generated by adding two sine-wave signals. The data obtained with these signals are compared with three mathematical models. These models reflect quite different sets of basic assumptions concerning how the ear operates. By comparing the obtained results with the predictions of these models it will, perhaps, be possible to suggest the more promising approaches which one may use to predict the detectability of complex signals.

Admittedly, a two-component signal represents only a small class of all complex auditory stimuli. Nevertheless this modest approach provides a simple condition for testing theoretical formulations which may be applicable to more general conditions.

All of the models predict the detectability of the complex signal in terms of the detectability of the single components which comprise the complex signal. Such a method of prediction allows one to make use of the considerable quantity of data already available on the detectability of sine-wave stimuli. While it is possible that some aspect of the complex signal, such as "patterning," plays a significant role in determining its detectability, it is not considered in any of the three models presented. This does not imply any particular bias of the author. Rather, it reflects the author's opinion that it is prudent to attempt the explanation with models which do not include this additional factor. If the models fail, then, by necessity, this additional factor will have to be included.

The three models can be briefly summarized as follows. The first model, the no-summation model, may be considered the null hypothesis. This model asserts that the detectability of a complex signal is no better than the detectability of the most detectable component of the complex. The second model, the multiple-independent-thresholds model, asserts that an increase in the detectability of the complex signal will result because only one threshold need be exceeded by the complex signal. The third model, the statistical-summation model, asserts that the detection of a complex signal may be predicted by assuming that the outputs of several critical bands may be linearly combined.

In order to clarify the conditions under which the models apply, the experimental procedure and the results will be presented first. Then the three models and the predictions of these models will be explained. A comparison of the obtained results and the predicted values will be used to test the models. Before presenting this material, the history of the problem will be reviewed briefly. This review will help establish the basic frame of reference for the several models.

HISTORY OF THE PROBLEM

Schafer and Gales (1949) measured the detectability of multiple component signals masked by noise. They concluded that for two tones, separated by a critical band or more, the energy of each component can be reduced by 0 to 2 db and the composite signal remains as detectable as the signals when they are presented separately. The value for 4 to 8 tones is between 0 and 3 db. If one accepts the 0-db figure in all cases, then one would conclude there is no summation, i.e., a complex tone is no more detectable than the most easily detectable component of the complex. If a power-summation model explained the data, two tones should be 3 db, 4 tones 6 db, and 8 tones 9 db easier to hear than the single components. Schafer and Gales found their data fell, on the average, somewhere between these two extremes.

Marill (1956) used four frequencies: 500, 540, 1060, and 1100 cps. If the frequency difference were small, such as with the frequency pair 500 and 540, then the results supported the power-summation model. If the frequency pairs were widely separated, such as 500 and 1100 cps, then the no-summation model appeared to predict the data. This latter finding is not consistent with the results of Schafer and Gales.

Fletcher's (1940) critical-band model may be interpreted as asserting that the auditory system may be likened to a narrow band-pass filter. When explaining the detection of a single sine-wave stimulus in noise, one can neglect all components of the interference with the exception of a narrow band of frequencies centered around the signal to be detected. This model has been tested and appears to be adequate. How this model should be applied when the signal consists of two or more sinusoids widely separated in frequency is not stated. One possible extension is to assume that the observer can listen with only a single critical band. When a composite signal is presented, the observer's behavior might then be explained by assuming that he is listening to only one narrow frequency region where the signal-to-noise ratio is most favorable for detecting the signal. Such a hypothesis is completely consistent with the results obtained by Marill's experiment.

Tanner, Swets, and Green (1956) have also reported data which support the conclusion that, for widely separated frequencies, the observer apparently listens to only one frequency region. Their experimental situation required the observer to detect one of two possible signals presented in one of four time intervals. The observer was asked only to detect the signal's presence, never to state which frequency it was. For signals of sufficiently short duration, and of sufficiently wide frequency separation, the observers behaved as though they were listening to only one or the other of the two possible frequency regions where the signal might have been presented.

The studies just discussed have provided a basis for the models considered in the later sections. It is unfortunate that all the results do not agree, because the answer to the question of multiple-tone detection is necessary if one is ever going to explain the detection of anything but the simplest of auditory signals. The research reported below is both a repeat of the previous studies, and an investigation of two more parameters of the process which may be a source of interaction. These parameters are (1) the duration of the signals, and (2) the relation of the frequencies in the complex signal.

EXPERIMENTAL PROCEDURE

The experiment was conducted at the Psychophysical Laboratory, Electronic Defense Group, University of Michigan. The basic apparatus has been described elsewhere (Green, Birdsall, and Tanner, 1957). A four-alternative forced-choice method was used to measure the detectability of a signal. Two changes were made from the procedure employed in the previous study. Each sequence of four test intervals was preceded by an interval in which the noise dropped 10 db in level and the signal was presented: This served to remind the observers of the frequency characteristics and duration of the signal. Also, the signal was simply gated for the specified duration without regard to phase.

Four frequencies were employed: 500, 1000, 1823, and 2000 cps. The complex signal was generated by adding the voltages of two of these signals. The frequencies were generated by two independent oscillators. All possible pairs were employed. For each signal duration, each frequency was used as a signal and was adjusted in amplitude so that about 75 per cent correct detections were obtained. One of the six possible pairs of frequencies, using the amplitudes previously determined, was then used as the complex signal. The percentage of correct detections for this complex signal was determined. There are therefore ten signals used in this experiment, four single-frequency signals and six complex signals. Four blocks, each of one hundred trials, were used to estimate the probability of a correct detection for each signal. Each signal received one block of trials before a second block was conducted for any other signal. The choice of conditions was determined by a random sequence. Signal durations of 50, 200, and 1000 msec were employed. Four hundred observations were completed for each signal before another duration was selected.

Measurement of amplitude has been described (Green, Birdsall, and Tanner, 1957). Measurements of frequency and duration of the signals were made with a Hewlett-Packard model 521C Frequency Meter. Frequency drift throughout an experimental session was less than about 3 cps. Permoflux PDR-8 headphones were used. The observers listened binaurally. A noise spectrum level of about 55 db *re* 0.0002 d/cm^2 was used throughout all tests.

RESULTS

The data are summarized in graphical form in Fig. 1. In Table I the entries are E/N_0; E is the signal energy, or time integral of power, and N_0 is the noise power per unit bandwidth (dimensions of energy). All

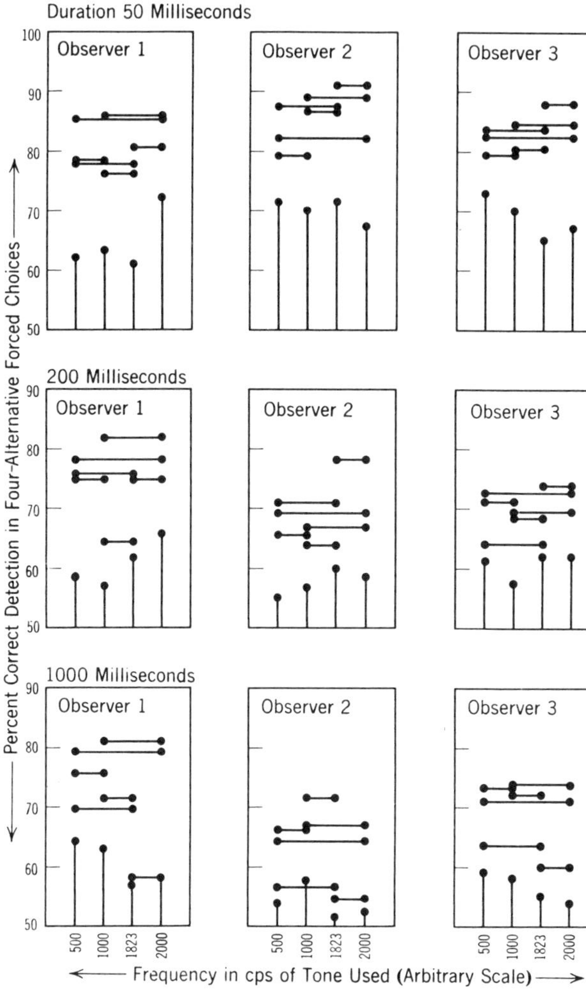

FIG. 1. The points attached to the vertical lines represent the percentage of correct detections obtained when the stimulus was a single sine wave. The frequency of this signal is given by the abscissa (arbitrary scale). The points connected by the horizontal line give the percentage of correct detections obtained for the complex stimulus. The two end points represent the frequencies of the pair of sine waves used to generate the complex stimulus.

subjects were tested under the conditions shown in the table. In the figure, each entry is based upon 400 observations. For each single-component signal, the percentage of correct detections is represented by a vertical line. For example, with the 50-msec, 500-cps signal, Observer 1 obtained 62 per cent correct detections. The percentage of

TABLE I. Experimental Conditions: Entries are E/N_0.

Frequency (cps)	Duration in milliseconds 50	200	1000
500	8.7	6.2	13.2
1000	10.7	8.8	19.8
1823	15.6	15.4	30.8
2000	15.8	15.8	33.0

correct detections for the complex signal is represented by a horizontal line connecting the two frequencies which were used to generate the complex signal. For the same conditions, and the same observer, the complex signal of 500 and 1000 cps yielded 79 per cent correct detections. The complex signal is generated by using the same physical parameters for each component of the complex as were used when an individual component was presented. Thus, if the horizontal line representing the complex is above both of the vertical lines representing the single component signal, the complex is easier to detect than either single component. These graphs show the individual data obtained from three observers at three durations. About the only point that can be made with the data in this form is that the detectability of the complex signal is somewhat better than the detectability of either single component of the complex. For a finer analysis of the data it is obvious that some procedure must be adopted to normalize the data so that the amount of increase in detectability for the complex is independent of the value of detectability for the single-component stimuli. There is no accepted method of accomplishing this result. In the next section of the paper, however, three models will be considered. These will allow a form of normalizing the data so that the detectability of the complex signals may be compared.

MODELS

Three models will be used to analyze the data. All of these models make predictions which are independent of the duration or frequency separation of the components. The predictions of two models will then be compared with the data obtained in the various conditions of the experiment; such a comparison will allow for the evaluation of the models and the determination of whether the amount of improvement is indeed independent of these other factors.

Model 1: No-summation model

This model predicts that the percentage correct obtained on the complex signal will be no greater than the percentage correct obtained on the most easily detectable component of the pair. This statement of the prediction assumes the conditions which prevailed in this experiment; that is, the level of the individual components is the same when the complex is tested as when the individual stimuli are tested. The rationale for such a prediction might be that the observer can listen with a critical band to only one frequency region at any given time. When faced with detecting a complex signal, where the frequencies involved are more than a critical band apart, he listens at that region in frequency where the signal is easiest to detect.

The data collected in the experiment indicate that this hypothesis is incorrect. Of the 54 instances tested, the detectability of the complex was greater than the detectability of the most detectable component in 53 cases. Thus, for the conditions employed in this experiment, the no-summation model is definitely rejected.

Model 2: The two-independent-thresholds model

Shafer and Gales (1949) suggested that such a model predicted fairly accurately the data collected in their experiment. This model asserts that, in order to detect a single component signal, some hypothetical variable must exceed some critical value. This value is called a threshold. Assuming that the variable rarely exceeds this critical value when no signal is presented, the probability of a correct detection, $P(C)$, in a forced-choice test employing n temporal alternatives is given by

$$P(C) = p + (1/n)(1 - p) \tag{1}$$

where p is the probability of the signal causing the threshold to be exceeded. The second term of the equation is the probability of not obtaining a supra-threshold value $(1 - p)$ times the probability of correctly guessing the correct alternative with no information $(1/n)$.

Now, consider the case where two or more signals are presented simultaneously and the hypothetical variables associated with each signal are independent. Four cases can arise: (1) the first signal can cause a supra-threshold value and the second not, or (2) the second signal can lead to a supra-threshold value and the first not, or (3) and (4) both signals can lead to either supra-threshold or sub-threshold values for the hypothetical variable.

Several combination rules could be used, but the one investigated is that a correct response will result if either or both signals lead to a supra-threshold value of the variable. The probability of either or both signals exceeding threshold is, therefore, given by Eq. (2),

$$p_m = 1 - \prod_{i=1}^{m} (1 - p_i) \tag{2}$$

where p_i is the probability that the ith signal will be supra-threshold, and m is the number of signals.

Hence, the probability of a correct choice, $P_m(C)$, among n temporal alternatives with m signals, can be written by substituting p_m of Eq. (2) for p of Eq. (1),

$$P_m(C) = 1 - \prod_{i=1}^{m} (1 - p_i) + \frac{1}{n} \prod_{i=1}^{m} (1 - p_i) \tag{3}$$

For the temporal four-alternative forced-choice method ($n = 4$) used in these studies, and for complex signals using two components ($m = 2$), this formula reduces to

$$P_2(C) = 1 - \tfrac{4}{3}[1 - P_1(C)][1 - P_2(C)]. \tag{4}$$

This model allows us to predict the percentage of correct detections obtained on the complex from the percentage correct obtained on the single-component signals.

If the hypothetical variables of this model are not independent these predictions will not be correct. If the variables are perfectly correlated, only two cases could arise. Both variables would either exceed the threshold or they would not. The predictions obtained from this model would then be identical to those obtained with the first model.

Other changes could be made in the model. We have assumed that the observer guesses only when both components fail to reach the threshold. If more than two components are used for the complex signal it is possible that the signal would be detected only when a majority of the signals cause a supra-threshold value of the variable. Such a model becomes considerably more complicated. Yet another alternative is to assume that, even without a signal, the threshold is exceeded some constant percentage of the time. Depending, then, upon the value of this constant, the model would predict quite different values for the detectability of the complex.

Model 3: A statistical-summation model

This model will be explained in some detail because it appears to predict the data obtained in this experiment better than either of the other two models. This model is a logical extension of the statistical decision theory proposed by Tanner and Swets (1954), and especially of the ideas expressed by Tanner (1956). The critical-band hypothesis is used as an interpretive device in explaining several assumptions of the model. These are, strictly considered, assumptions, and hence do not depend upon the critical-band hypothesis being correct. However, the assumptions are consistent with some sort of auditory filtering process, and the interpretations will be used so as to make the model less abstract.

Before explaining how the model is extended to encompass the problem of detecting multicomponent signals in noise, a brief review of how the model explains the detection of a single-component stimulus will be given. Presumably, the energy located in a narrow frequency region (critical band) is transformed to a single variable so that the value of this variable will be greater when a signal is present than when noise alone is present. Let this variable be denoted $X(f_1)$. As a convenience for a later part of the discussion, this notation will make obvious the dependency of X on the frequency region of f_1. Now, since noise is a random variable, $X(f_1)$ will have some distribution of values. Actually, it will have two distributions of values, one when the signal (f_1) is present in the noise and another when there is no signal. When no signal is present the condition will be termed noise alone. It is assumed that in the noise-alone condition the variable $X(f_1)$ will be normally distributed. When signal plus noise is present, $X(f_1)$ will also be normal with a greater average value but the same variance.

The parameter of importance is d', the difference in the means of the two distributions divided by the standard deviation. In order to avoid unnecessary notation, the noise-alone distribution may be normalized so that the mean is zero and the standard deviation unity. Then the parameter d' becomes simply the mean of the signal-plus-noise distribution. This parameter will be denoted d'_{f_1}.

In a temporal four-alternative forced-choice test the observer listens to four temporal intervals. In one and only one of these intervals the signal is added to the noise. The observer is instructed to choose the interval in which the signal occurred. The model assumes that in each interval the variable $X(f_1)$ is measured. It is assumed that the observer operates with a decision rule which is equivalent to choosing the interval in which the largest value of the variable $X(f_1)$ occurred. Hence, the probability that the largest value of $X(f_1)$ will occur when the signal (f_1) plus noise is present is simply the probability that a sample taken from a normal deviate with mean d' and variance unity will be larger than any of the other three samples from a normal deviate with mean zero and the same variance. A table relating the probability of a correct decision in a four-alternative forced-choice test and the parameter d' has been presented elsewhere (Green, Birdsall, and Tanner, 1957).

In extending the model to a situation involving more than a single sine-wave stimulus the problem is essentially that of determining the distribution associated with the complex signal plus noise and the distribution associated with noise alone. Particularly, the parameter which characterizes the difference divided by the standard deviation of the distributions must be determined.

The extension of the model will be discussed for two-component complex signals. This limitation will greatly simplify the mathematics, and the extension of this result to signals involving many component signals will be obvious once this derivation is complete.

If two components are widely separated in frequency the output of the critical band associated with each will be independent. This statement is simply a way of interpreting the assumption that $X(f_1)$ and $X(f_2)$ are independent. When noise alone is presented both variables are normally distributed with some mean and variance. When signal $(f_1 + f_2)$ plus noise is presented the mean values of both variables, $X(f_1)$ and $X(f_2)$, will increase, compared with the noise-alone conditions, and will have the same variance. The correlation of the variables when the complex signal plus noise is presented will still be zero.

One reasonable method of combination is simply to add each variable, weighted by a constant. It is presumed that each variable is normalized so that the noise-alone distribution has zero mean and unit variance before the summation. Actually, such normalization could be included in the constants of the addition, but it greatly simplifies the following derivation to assume such a normalization at this point in the argument. The two variables, therefore, have the following properties.

Noise alone: $X(f_1)$ is normally distributed with zero mean and unit variance; $X(f_2)$ is normally distributed with zero mean and unit variance.

Signal plus noise: $X(f_1)$ is normally distributed with mean d'_{f_1} and unit variance; $X(f_2)$ is normally distributed with mean d'_{f_2} and unit variance.

Consider the linear combination, $Z = aX(f_1) + bX(f_2)$, where a and b are constants.

With noise alone: Z is normally distributed with mean zero and unit variance: $a^2 + b^2 + 2r[X(f_1)X(f_2)]ab$, where $r[X(f_1)X(f_2)]$ is the correlation of the variables $X(f_1)$ and $X(f_2)$. Since $r[X(f_1)X(f_2)] = 0$, the variance of Z is $(a^2 + b^2)$.

With signal $(f_1 + f_2)$ plus noise: Z is normally distributed with mean $(ad'_{f_1} + bd'_{f_2})$ and variance $(a^2 + b^2)$.

Hence, in the variable Z the difference between the means of the two distributions divided by the standard deviation, or d'_Z, is given by

$$\frac{ad'_{f_1} + bd'_{f_2}}{(a^2 + b^2)^{1/2}} \tag{5}$$

The d' for the combination is now determined except for the constants a and b. In order to predict anything about the detectability of the complex from the detectability of the individual components, a and b will be chosen so as to maximize d'_Z. This is equivalent to assuming that the probability of a correct detection is maximized since d' and this probability are monotonically related.

To accomplish this maximization it is convenient to write a and b as a function of a single variable. Consider a and b as two sides of a right triangle.

$$\frac{a}{(a^2 + b^2)^{1/2}} = \sin \gamma \tag{6}$$

$$\frac{b}{(a^2 + b^2)^{1/2}} = \cos \gamma \tag{7}$$

The maximum occurs when

$$(\cos \gamma)d'_{f_1} = (\sin \gamma)d'_{f_2} \tag{8}$$

$$\frac{d'_{f_1}}{d'_{f_2}} = \tan \gamma = \frac{a}{b} \tag{9}$$

One solution is to set

$$a = d'_{f_1}, \quad b = d'_{f_2} \tag{10}$$

then,

$$d'_Z = \frac{(d'_{f_1})^2 + (d'_{f_2})^2}{[d'_{f_1})^2 + (d'_{f_2})^2]^{1/2}} = [(d'_{f_1})^2 + (d'_{f_2})^2]^{1/2} \tag{11}$$

Thus, an expression for the detectability of the complex signal has been determined in terms of the detectability of each component of the complex. The geometric interpretation of this result is very simple. Consider $X(f_1)$ and $X(f_2)$ as the coordinates of a plane. If the two values associated with each frequency region are plotted in this plane, one finds the noise-alone distribution centered about the point (0, 0). When the complex signal plus noise is present the values form a new distribution centered about the point (d'_{f_1}, d'_{f_2}). Now suppose that each observation taken by the observer yields a value for $X(f_1)$ and $X(f_2)$. The maximum d' for the combination is obtained by projecting such points in the space on a line running from the point (0, 0) to (d'_{f_1}, d'_{f_2}). The distribution functions for such projections are normal when either noise alone or signal plus noise is present. The difference in the means of these two distributions divided by the standard deviation has the value d'_Z.

If this line of argument is extended to a situation where many components are used for the signal, and assuming each component affects independent processes, then the maximum d' for the linear combination is simply the square root of the sum of the squares of d' for the individual components.

Since the frequency separations between components used in the experiments reported in this paper are wide compared with the width of a critical band, $r[X(f_1), X(f_2)]$ will be assumed to equal zero. The model may be extended to handle cases where the correlation is not zero. The following gives a brief discussion of the manner in which the model handles such cases. Presumably such cases arise when the components are located near each other in frequency so that the outputs of the critical bands associated with each component are affected by energy which is common to both bands. In other words, the filter bands overlap. One result of such a condition is to make the correlation coefficient $r[X(f_1), X(f_2)]$ greater than zero. The second result is that the signal energy associated with one frequency, say f_1, influences the variable $X(f_2)$, which is associated with the other band. Since the frequencies f_1 and f_2 are very close together it may be assumed that this influence is symmetric; that is, f_2 affects $X(f_1)$ in the same way that f_1 affects $X(f_2)$.

When the signals were widely separated in frequency, the mean of the signal-plus-noise distribution was d'_{f_1}. For the case now being considered, it will be assumed that the mean of the signal-plus-noise distribution for $X(f_1)$ will be $d'_{f_1} + kd'_{f_2}$. The positive constant k has a value somewhere between zero and unity. It reflects the amount of overlap between the critical bands. Both $r[X(f_1), X(f_2)]$ and k should be a monotonic decreasing function of the distance in frequency between the two components, f_1 and f_2. If the difference in the frequency of the two components is very small both r and k should be near unity.

In order to simplify the following derivation it will be assumed that $d'_{f_1} = d'_{f_2} = d'$. Proceeding as before one finds the difference in means divided by the standard deviation, d'_Z.

$$d'_Z = \frac{d'(a + b)(1 + k)}{(a^2 + b^2 + 2rab)^{1/2}} \tag{12}$$

Using the same method to maximize d'_Z, the maximum occurs when $a = b$, letting $a = b = 1$.

$$d'_Z = \frac{d'2(1 + k)}{(2 + 2r)^{1/2}} = \sqrt{2}d' \frac{1 + k}{(1 + r)^{1/2}} \tag{13}$$

If both signals are nearly the same in frequency, $k \approx 1$ and $r \approx 1$, then $d'_Z = 2d'$. The result agrees with Marill's finding for the frequency pair 500 and 540 cps. If the frequency pair is very far apart, $k \approx 0$, $r \approx 0$, and $d'_Z = \sqrt{2}d'$, which agrees with the previous Eq. (11).

This model, therefore, gives a plausible derivation of the detectability of a complex signal using any two frequencies. No quantitative predictions are made when the frequency pair is close together in frequency since the relation between k, r, and frequency separation is not known. This relation depends theoretically only upon the shape of the critical band.

In summary, the model makes it possible to predict the detectability of a complex signal from the detectability of each component of the complex. The application of the model to those cases where the noise affects both correlated and uncorrelated processes is explained. For components separated by several critical bands one may assume k and r are zero. Once this separation has been reached, the predictions of the model are independent of any further separation. These are the types of separations used for the complex signals discussed in the experimental section of this paper. Thus, the predictions cited in the following sections assume both k and r equal to zero, as in Eq. (11).

EVALUATION OF THE MODELS

Only the two-independent-thresholds and the statistical-decision model will be compared with the obtained data. The no-summation model in this experiment could be rejected as being inadequate in 53 out of 54 cases as discussed previously.

For each of the three observers and three durations there are six possible pairs of tones used as the complex signal. For both models the detectability for the single-component stimuli was used to generate a prediction concerning the detectability of the complex tone. The difference between the predicted per cent correct detections and those actually obtained is displayed in Fig. 2. Two points appear for each complex stimulus and condition, one for each of the models used to generate predicted values. At the extreme right of each condition the average

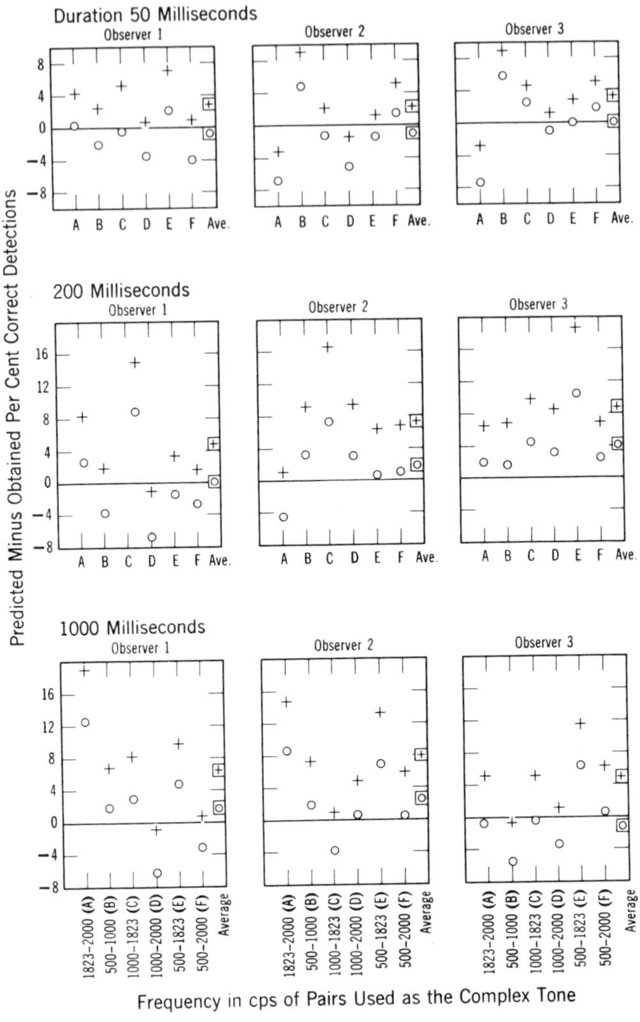

FIG. 2. The ordinate is the difference between the predicted and the obtained percentage of correct detections. Two points are plotted for each complex signal, one point when the threshold model is used, another when the statistical-decision model is used. The abscissa is the pair of frequencies used for the complex signal. Plus sign: threshold model; open circle: statistical-decision model.

error in prediction is plotted. The average error over all conditions and subjects is about 1.5 per cent for the statistical-decision model and about 5 per cent for threshold model. A t test was calculated for the entire set of data. The value of the parameter t was about 1.25 for the threshold model and about 0.25 for the statistical-decision model. The threshold model can thus only be rejected at the 20-per-cent confidence limit while the statistical-decision model can only be rejected at the 80 per cent confidence limit. In terms of the likelihood ratio, the statistical-decision model is to be preferred about 4 to 1 over the threshold model. Obviously an experiment involving more than two components will provide a stronger test of the differences between the theories. With only two components used for the complex signal, the difference between the predictions of the two theories never exceeds 10 per cent and averages much less than that.

The predictions made by both models are independent of the frequency separation and of the duration of the complex stimuli. Such a position can be checked to some extent by using the graphs of Fig. 3. The statistical-decision model is employed since it best predicts the available data and conveys essentially the same picture that one would obtain with the other model. The per cent error as plotted in the previous figures has simply been averaged across observers and plotted as the ordinate of Fig. 3. The combination signals are plotted as the abscissa in the order of their frequency differences. The scale is arbitrary. As one can observe, there is no dependence upon frequency separation or signal duration.

DISCUSSION

The statistical-decision model is tentatively accepted as the most adequate model for predicting the detectability of a complex signal in noise. This model is consistent with the detection theory previously proposed for single-component stimuli. It is also consistent with a critical-band model which asserts one can linearly combine the outputs of several critical bands. The model has the advantage of incorporating all the variables which affect the detectability of a single component, because the detectability of each signal component is used in determining the detectability of the complex. The manner of combination is theoretically linear and no interaction term is used.

Since d' is roughly proportional to signal energy, the level of two equally detectable components can be lowered by 1.5 db in a threshold experiment and the same detectability can be maintained for the complex signal. This result agrees with the average values cited by Schafer and Gales (1949) but is inconsistent with the results obtained in Marill's work (1956).

The statistical-decision model has been applied to an experiment in which the observer is asked to detect one of two possible signals. If the

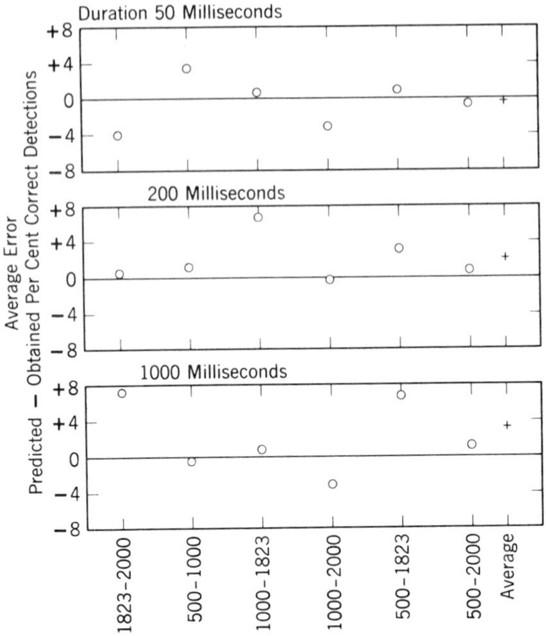

FIG. 3. The ordinate is the average over the subjects of the obtained minus the predicted percentage of correct detections. The abscissa is the pair of frequencies used to generate the complex signal. Only the predictions of the statistical-decision model are used.

two variables $X(f_1)$ and $X(f_2)$ are combined, the d' for the combination will be decreased, as compared with the d' associated with either component, because only one signal is presented on any series of trials. Thus, the observer listens to twice as much noise power when only one of the two signals is present. The predictions generated by such considerations are similar to those made when one assumes that the observer listens to only a single frequency region at any instant in time. Thus, the present model is consistent with most of the data obtained by Tanner, Swets, and Green (1956).

The use of only two components as a complex signal does not provide the best condition for attempting to choose between models. Rather, it provides a simple condition for formulating a theory which will work in the more general case. The discrepancy between the results obtained in this study and those obtained by Marill provides an interesting challenge. Assuming both results are correct, it is obvious that some factor neglected by both Marill and the author plays an important role in this situation.

SUMMARY

The detectability of a complex signal, one generated by adding two sinusoids, and partially masked by white noise, is determined. Several frequencies and three durations are used for the signal. The experimental determinations are compared with three mathematical models. These models are all interpretable as an extension of the critical-band concept. The data are best explained by a model in which it is assumed that two or more critical bands may be linearly combined. This implies that the auditory mechanism may change the appropriate parameters of the analysis process in order to match the signal to be detected.

ACKNOWLEDGMENTS

This research was conducted in the laboratories of the Electronic Defense Group of the University of Michigan with support from the U. S. Army Signal Corps and from the Operational Applications Laboratory of the U. S. Air Force. This article appeared in the J. acoust. Soc. Am., *1958,* **30,** *904–911.*

References

- Fletcher, H. Auditory patterns. *Revs. mod. Phys.*, 1940, **12,** 47–65.
- Green, D. M., Birdsall, T. G., and Tanner, W. P., Jr. Signal detection as a function of signal intensity and duration. *J. acoust. Soc. Am.*, 1957, **29,** 523–531. [11]
- Marill, T. Detection theory and psychophysics. Massachusetts Institute of Technology: Research Laboratory of Electronics, 1956, Technical Report No. 319.
- Schafer, T. H., and Gales, R. S. Auditory masking of multiple tones by random noise. *J. acoust. Soc. Am.*, 1949, **21,** 392–398.
- Tanner, W. P., Jr. Theory of recognition. *J. acoust. Soc. Am.*, 1956, **28,** 882–886. [19]
- Tanner, W. P., Jr., and Swets, J. A. A decision-making theory of visual detection. *Psychol. Rev.*, 1954, **61,** 401–409.
- Tanner, W. P., Jr., Swets, J. A., and Green, D. M. Some general properties of the hearing mechanism. University of Michigan: Electronic Defense Group, 1956, Technical Report No. 30.

26

Detection of a Pulsed Sinusoid in Noise as a Function of Frequency

David M. Green, Mary J. McKey, and J. C. R. Licklider

Hawkins and Stevens (1950) and investigators at the Bell Telephone Laboratories (French and Steinberg, 1947; Fletcher, 1953) measured the auditory detectability of a continuous sinusoid of indefinite duration in white noise as a function of the frequency of the sinusoid. The relation between signal detectability and signal frequency is important in current auditory theory because it is used as a basis for inferring how the critical bandwidths of the human auditory system vary with frequency (Hawkins and Stevens, 1950; Fletcher, 1953). In one experiment we determined how the detectability of a pulsed signal of definite duration varies as a function of signal frequency. With such measurements, we can answer an important substantive question: does the variation of the critical bandwidths with signal frequency as estimated from the data on the detection of indefinitely-continued tones agree with the variation as estimated from the data on the detection of fixed-duration tones?

In this first experiment 16 signal frequencies were used. Each signal frequency was one of the harmonics of 250 cps. The data obtained in the first experiment provide the foundation for the second. In the second experiment, measurements were made of the detectability of pulsed compound signals. The components of the compound signal were of the same frequencies as the sinusoids used in the first study. The data obtained from the measurements with compound signals prepare us to consider another question: what rule does the auditory system follow in integrating signal energy over frequency?

One of the reasons for conducting these studies with pulsed sinusoids was to obtain data in terms of signal *energy*. In order to relate human performance in signal detection to the theory of ideal detectors, it is essential to control and specify the duration of signal presentation because energy, rather than power, is the basic variable in the theory. An ideal detector can detect a sustained signal of prespecified parameters in random noise at any ratio of signal power to noise power density. Accordingly, one purpose of the experiments was to measure the detection performance of human listeners using signals of definite duration so that the performance might be described in terms of the energy ratio.

EXPERIMENT WITH SINGLE SINUSOIDS

Procedure and equipment

In the experiments, the signals were presented, and the listeners' responses were tallied, by an automatic two-interval, forced-choice audiometer. The audiometer presents the signal successively at 10 sound pressure levels in a stepwise, descending pattern. Each signal in a sequence of 10 is 1.5 db weaker than the preceding one. After the audiometer reaches the tenth and lowest level, it recycles and begins at the highest level once more.

An experimental session consisted of 40 practice trials and 250 test trials, 25 test trials at each of the 10 signal levels. The signal duration was 0.1 sec. The signal was gated without reference to the zero crossings of the sinusoid, so the phase of the signal presented to the observer in each trial can be considered random. Two or three sessions were run each day. The rest periods were approximately as long as the experimental sessions. The observers used Permoflux PDR-8 earphones in Grason-Stadler type 001 semiplastic earphone cushions and observed monaurally with their untested ears covered by dummy earphones.

In the sequence of 40 practice trials given before each series of test trials, the signal started in a range 12 to 15 db higher than the highest level employed in the test trials. After each block of 10 practice trials, the signal was attenuated 4 or 5 db so that, at the beginning of the fourth block, the level was the same as the highest level selected for the test trials. The fourth practice block then consisted of 10 trials, one for each of the 10 levels to be used in the subsequent test. Then the series of 250 test trials was begun.

In each trial of the tests, the two 0.1-sec intervals were marked off for the observer by lights. Each observer was asked to select the interval he believed to contain the signal. In each trial, the signal occurred just once, either in the first interval or in the second; the two alternatives were equally likely. The temporal pattern of the events within a trial is shown in Table I.

TABLE I. SEQUENCE OF EVENTS IN A TRIAL

Interval	Duration (in sec)
1. Warning	0.15
2. Waiting	0.25
3. Signal	0.10
4. Waiting	0.25
5. Signal	0.10
6. Response	1.75
7. "Right or wrong" feedback	0.50
8. Recycle	0.50

Measurements of signal and noise

The signal energy (E) and the noise-power density (N_0) are the basic physical parameters of the stimuli used in the experiment. Actually, it is the ratio E/N_0 that is of primary interest. Both E and N_0 were calculated from measurements of voltage across the listeners' earphones. The impedance of the earphones is not relevant, since it cancels itself out when the ratio E/N_0 is formed. Since the earphones are assumed to be linear, the ratio E/N_0 derived from the electrical measurements should be the same as the ratio derived from sound pressure measurements. Note that N_0 (power/cps) has the same dimensions as E (power·seconds). We shall work with the decibel equivalent of this ratio, namely, $\mathcal{E} - \mathfrak{N}_0 = 10 \log_{10} E - 10 \log_{10} N_0 = 10 \log_{10} E/N_0$.

A Ballantine True Root-Mean-Square Voltmeter model (320) was used in all the measurements. In order to obtain a measure proportional to the signal energy, we squared the steady-state rms voltage of the sinusoidal signal and multiplied by the signal duration, 0.1 sec. In order to obtain a measure proportional to the noise power density and having the same constant of proportionality as the signal-energy measure, we employed a single-tuned R-L-C band-pass filter, centered at the frequency of the signal. The noise was passed through the filter, and the rms voltage at the output was determined. In order to correct for the gain of the filter, the voltage was then divided by the voltage gain measured at the peak of the filter-selectivity curve. The resulting quantity was then squared and divided by the equivalent rectangular bandwidth of the filter. (The equivalent rectangular bandwidth of an *R-L-C* filter is $\pi/2$ times the 3-db bandwidth.) Measures of the noise-power density, of the type just described, were obtained at four center frequencies. They were all the same within ± 0.2 db. The noise, which was continuous throughout each experimental session, had a spectrum level of about 45 db *re* 0.0002 microbar.

Observers

In the experiments involving single pulsed sinusoids, three groups of subjects were used. Group A, three male college students, had observed in other, similar experiments prior to participation in these tests. Group A was joined, for the measurements reported in this paper, by group B, five male college students, who had no previous listening experience. The subjects in groups A and B observed at the same time. After the tests involving group A and group B were complete, three female technical assistants, group C, repeated the same series of tests and participated in the experiment involving compound signals.

A piecework remunerative system was used to motivate the listeners in groups A and B. In each 250-trial test, each listener was paid nothing for incorrect responses and nothing for his first 125 correct responses. In the equally likely two-alternative test, even if the observer does not listen, about 50 per cent of his responses will be correct. He received 2 cents for every correct response beyond 125. There was, however, a minimum salary of 1 dollar per test. The technical assistants, group C, were not given any special monetary incentive.

All the members of each group participated in 2 experimental sessions, of 250 test trials each, at each of 16 different signal frequencies. The frequencies were tested in a random order, with the restriction that each of the 16 frequencies was tested once before any frequency was tested a second time.

Results

For each listener in each experimental session, the basic experimental results were the percentages of correct responses in the 25 trials at each of the ten values of $\mathfrak{S} - \mathfrak{N}_0$. The values of $\mathfrak{S} - \mathfrak{N}_0$ were separated, as mentioned earlier, by steps of 1.5 db. The percentages were plotted

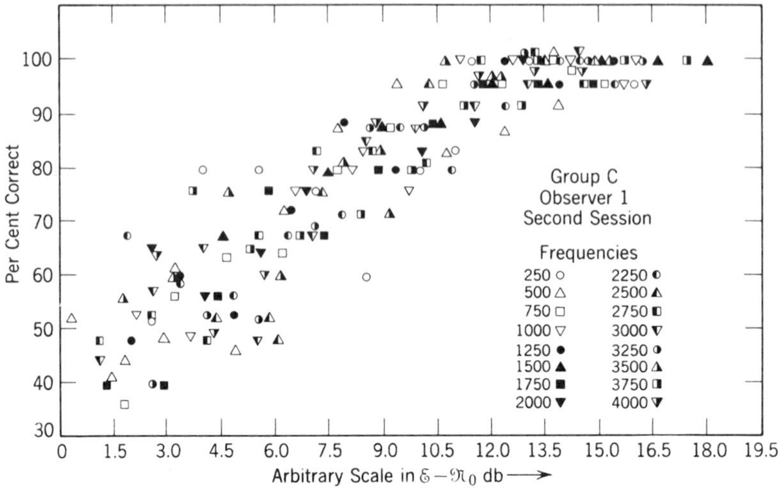

FIG. 1. The psychometric functions of a single observer at various signal frequencies. Each data point represents 25 observations. For each signal frequency the abscissa has been shifted by an arbitrary amount so that the scatter of points appears minimum.

against the values of $\mathcal{E} - \mathfrak{N}_0$ and smooth lines were fitted by eye. The fitted lines were not specified exactly; the only restriction was that they be monotonic increasing functions with asymptotic approaches to 50 and 100 per cent correct. From the fitted lines the values of $\mathcal{E} - \mathfrak{N}_0$ necessary for 65, 75, and 85 per cent correct were determined. All three were obtained for each listener in each of the two experimental sessions at each of the sixteen frequencies. Figure 1 shows one listener's psychometric functions for all 16 frequencies, second test session. The listener was subject 1 of group C.[1] If the listener's response process conforms to a binomial model, the variance about a given value of per cent correct is

$$\sigma^2 = P(c)[1 - P(c)]/25$$

and the standard deviation is therefore about 10 for $P(c) = 50$, 9 for $P(c) = 75$, and 4 for $P(c) = 95$. The scatter in the figure appears consistent with the assumption of a binomial process.

Figures 2, 3, and 4 present the data relating the value of $\mathcal{E} - \mathfrak{N}_0$ necessary for 75 per cent correct response to signal frequency. We could

[1] A listener from group C was selected in order to provide a comparison of the psychometric functions obtained with single sinusoids and the compound signal. The results obtained with this listener are typical of the other observers.

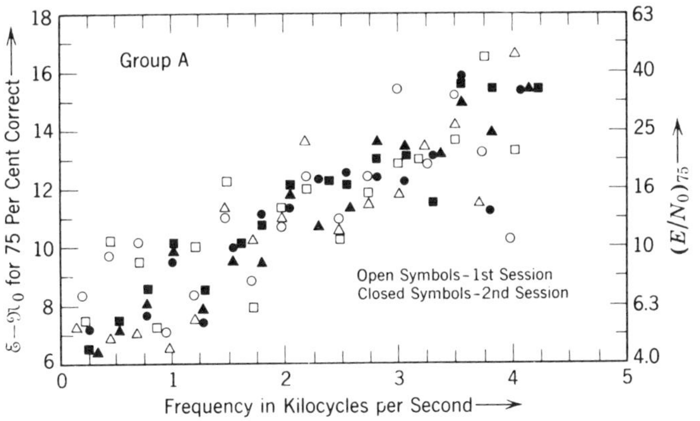

FIG. 2. For each subject of group A, the value of $\mathcal{E} - \mathcal{N}_0$ necessary for 75 per cent correct at each frequency is displayed for each experimental session. The different symbols represent different subjects. The repeatability of data for a single subject at any frequency can be judged by comparing the open and closed values for a single symbol.

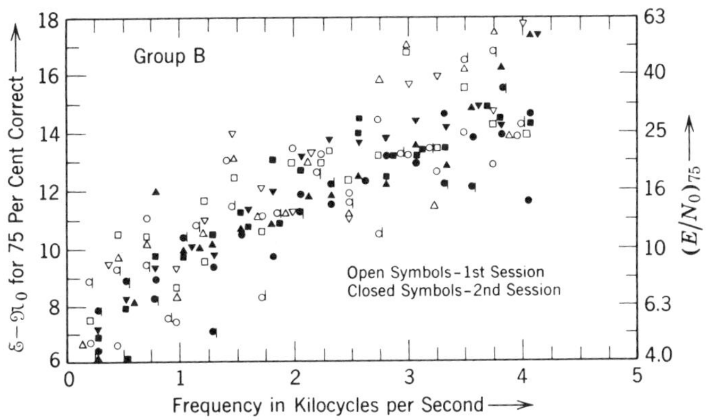

FIG. 3. For each subject of group B, the value of $\mathcal{E} - \mathcal{N}_0$ necessary for 75 per cent correct at each frequency is displayed for each experimental session. The different symbols represent different subjects. The repeatability of data for a single subject at any frequency can be judged by comparing the open and closed values for a single symbol.

plot similar graphs for 65 and 85 per cent correct response, but it is simpler and more direct to work with the main parameters of the several functions as determined by a curve-fitting technique, as we shall describe in the following.

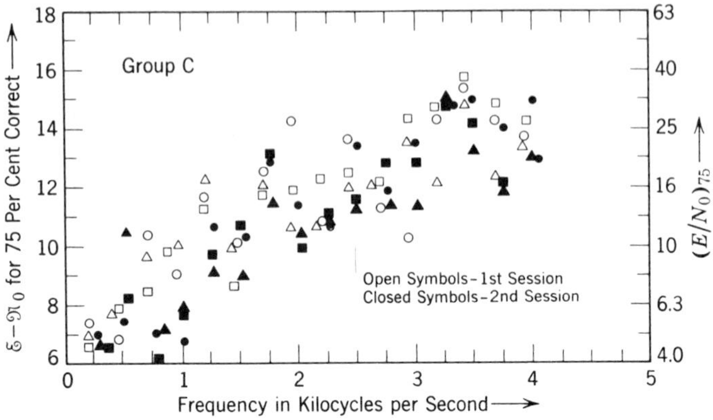

FIG. 4. For each subject of group C, the value of $\mathcal{E} - \mathfrak{N}_0$ necessary for 75 per cent correct at each frequency is displayed for each experimental session. The different symbols represent different subjects. The repeatability of data for a single subject at any frequency can be judged by comparing the open and closed values for a single symbol.

For each group, each frequency, and each session, the average value of $\mathcal{E} - \mathfrak{N}_0$ required for each of the three levels of detectability (65, 75, and 85 per cent) was found. Since there were three groups, two sessions, and three levels of detectability, these averages determine 18 functions relating $\mathcal{E} - \mathfrak{N}_0$ to signal frequency.

We used a least-squares technique to fit curves of specified form to the 18 sets of averaged data. In the absence of a theoretical rationale, we used the polynomial of arbitrary order as the function form. That is, we used

$$\mathcal{E} - \mathfrak{N}_0 = a_0 + a_1 f + a_2 f^2 + a_3 f^3 + \cdots + a_n f^n$$

Actually, we employed Fisher's (1954) orthogonal polynomials, since they allow us to consider the terms of higher order without changing the coefficients of the terms of lower order. The coefficients of the terms of successive orders of the polynomial were computed, and at each state in the process the residual variance was obtained. About 85 per cent of the variance was accounted for by the constant and the first-order term. Computation was continued to determine the coefficients associated with the terms up to sixth order. Both the magnitude of the coefficient and the reduction in residual variance indicated that terms of order above the first do not justify their inclusion in this first approximation to the form of the data.

TABLE II. $\mathcal{E} - \mathfrak{N}_0 = 10 \log_{10}(E/N_0) = a + b(f/F)$, $250 < f < 4000$, F IS 1000 cps

			a	Ave a	b	Ave b	Residual variance (per cent)
Group A $N = 3$	65%	Session 1	5.3	4.8	1.9	2.1	19
		Session 2	4.2		2.3		17
	75%	Session 1	7.2	6.9	1.8	2.0	19
		Session 2	6.5		2.2		7
	85%	Session 1	8.9	8.4	1.9	2.2	18
		Session 2	7.8		2.5		15
Group B $N = 5$	65%	Session 1	6.4	6.0	2.0	2.1	15
		Session 2	5.6		2.1		8
	75%	Session 1	8.0	7.8	1.9	2.0	17
		Session 2	7.5		2.0		6
	85%	Session 1	9.7	9.7	2.0	2.0	20
		Session 2	9.7		1.9		8
Group C $N = 3$	65%	Session 1	6.4	6.2	1.6	1.7	18
		Session 2	5.9		1.8		26
	75%	Session 1	7.8	7.6	1.8	1.8	16
		Session 2	7.4		1.8		20
	85%	Session 1	9.4	9.2	1.8	1.8	13
		Session 2	9.0		1.8		19

Average
$\mathcal{E} - \mathfrak{N}_0 = 5.6 + 2.0(f/F)$ for 65% correct response.
$\mathcal{E} - \mathfrak{N}_0 = 7.4 + 2.0(f/F)$ for 75% correct response.
$\mathcal{E} - \mathfrak{N}_0 = 9.1 + 2.0(f/F)$ for 85% correct response.

Table II presents the coefficients obtained with the technique just described. The main point to be noted is that the slope (b) does not seem to be influenced systematically by changing the level of detectability. Therefore, had figures for 65 and 85 per cent correct response been presented along with Figs. 2, 3, and 4 (75 per cent correct response), they would have appeared similar except for intercept value (a). This conclusion is consistent with the view that the psychometric function [relating $P(c)$ to $\mathcal{E} - \mathfrak{N}_0$] is the same at all frequencies except for a signal attenuation factor which is dependent on frequency and which has the effect of shifting the abscissa scale. Implicit in the manner in which Fig. 1 was constructed is the assumption that this conclusion is justified.

Comparison with other data

The two previous studies (Hawkins and Stevens, 1950; French and Steinberg, 1947) provided results showing how the audibility of a sinusoidal signal in noise changes with signal frequency. In both studies the stimulus was presented continuously and the subject adjusted the intensity of the signal until it was audible in the noise. In Hawkins and Stevens' study the "subject was instructed to report as the threshold for a given tone in the presence of noise the attenuator setting at which the tone could be recognized as having a definite pitch." The criterion used in the tests at the Bell Telephone Laboratories (BTL) was not precisely specified, but it appears that the BTL data were obtained under conditions similar to those of Hawkins and Stevens' tests.

It is impossible to compare directly the critical $\mathcal{E} - \mathfrak{N}_0$ values of tests with pulsed signals with the physical measurements employed in tests with continuous signals. When a pulsed signal is used, one can specify the signal energy. When an indefinitely continuing signal is used, the signal has no definite energy value. Values of signal power may be specified for either type of signal, pulsed or indefinitely continuing. The signal power of a pulsed signal may be considered the "signal power while the signal is being presented." It is thus operationally the same measure as that used in tests with indefinitely continuing signals.

Figure 5 compares the Harvard and BTL data with the results obtained in the present experiment. The slope of the function relating

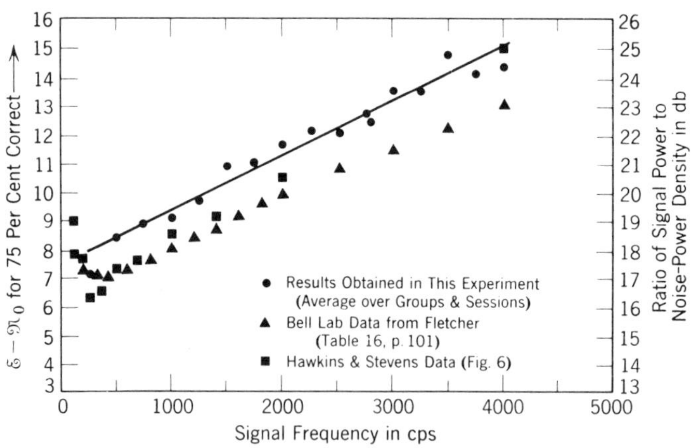

FIG. 5. A comparison of the present and previous data. The solid line is the best fitting linear function to the average data obtained in this experiment (filled dots). The key explains the source of the various data points.

detectability to signal frequency is very nearly the same in all three instances. Thus it appears that the fundamental dependence on frequency remains unchanged even when we go from an indefinitely continuing signal to a signal that is a pulsed segment of a sinusoid 0.1 sec in duration. The most important consequence of this result is to suggest that, down to 0.1 sec, the shape of the function relating critical bandwidth to center frequency is not heavily dependent upon signal duration.

Let us now consider the Harvard, BTL, and present data with reference to signal power required for detection. At the signal frequency of 1000 cps, the required value of $\mathcal{E} - \mathfrak{N}_0$ was 9.2 db in the present study. This corresponds to $\mathcal{P} - \mathfrak{N}_0 = 19.2$ db where $\mathcal{P}$ is 10 times the logarithm (base 10) of the signal power while the signal is present. Hawkins and Stevens obtained 18.5 db. The BTL value is 18.0 db. But the similarity of the first value to the second and third is accidental. Had we used another duration in the present study, our value of $\mathcal{P} - \mathfrak{N}_0$ would have been quite different. We can infer from the results of Green, Birdsall, and Tanner (1957), that had we used a 3-sec signal, for example, the value of $\mathcal{P} - \mathfrak{N}_0$ required for detection would have been about 11.7 db. That is 7.5 db lower than the value we obtained with our 0.1-sec signal.

EXPERIMENT WITH COMPOUND SINUSOIDS

About the time the single-component tests with group C were being conducted, equipment was completed which enabled us to generate compound signals consisting of the first 16 harmonics of 250 cps, i.e., the same frequencies used in the previous test. Each component of the compound could be adjusted independently of the others in amplitude and in phase.

Equipment and procedure

The equipment consisted of a signal generator which produced a train of 250 impulses per second. This pulse train was delayed in time by a selected amount and used to ring a sharply tuned electronic filter, a feedback circuit on the verge of oscillation. There were sixteen such delays and filters. Each filter was tuned to one of the harmonics of 250 cps. The delay associated with each harmonic allowed us to shift the starting point of the sinusoidal output of the filter with respect to the impulse train and hence, in effect, to adjust the phase of any component with respect to any other component. The output voltage waves of the sixteen filters were adjusted in amplitude and then superposed in a linear adder. The compound signal was recorded on tape for later playback to the observers in the test sessions.

The same procedure was used to determine the detectability of the compound signal as was used to determine the detectabilities of the single sinusoidal signals. The duration of the compound signal was 0.1 sec; the noise background was held at the same level as in the tests with single sinusoids.

Two patterns of amplitude versus frequency were employed. One pattern was produced by adjusting the amplitudes of the individual components in such a way as to make them all equally detectable when presented singly. The amplitude used for each component was determined from the data presented in the first part of this paper. The other amplitude pattern was produced simply by making all the components equal in voltage amplitude. In addition to the 16-harmonic pattern, we prepared 12-harmonic patterns by turning off the components at 2250, 2750, 3250, and 3750 cps.

Two patterns of phase versus frequency were investigated. One was an all-cosine-phase pattern. To produce it, we adjusted the phases in such a way as to make all the components have maxima at a particular instant of time. The compound wave approached the form of a pulse train with a pulse repetition frequency of 250 cps. In setting up this pattern, we observed on the screen of a cathode-ray tube the voltage across the headphones, not the output of a coupler or the sound pressure at the listeners' eardrums. The second pattern was generated by adjusting the phase of each component haphazardly. We term this second pattern a random phase pattern.

Results

Table III gives the values of $\mathfrak{S} - \mathfrak{N}_0$ necessary for 75-per-cent-correct detection of eight recorded samples of compound tones. The entries represent the values of $\mathfrak{S} - \mathfrak{N}_0$ necessary for 75-per-cent-correct response in two-interval forced-choice tests. Each row refers to a particular tape recording of a compound signal having the amplitude and phase patterns and the number of components indicated. For each of the two all-cosine patterns, two recorded samples were used. These were recorded at different times, and the generating equipment was set up independently for each recording session. The difference between the results obtained with tapes 2 and 3, and the difference between the results obtained with tapes 4 and 5, may reflect in part our inability to duplicate recording conditions exactly. Fortunately, these differences are small. The main difficulties

TABLE III. ENTRIES ARE $\mathcal{E} - \mathfrak{N}_0$ NECESSARY FOR 75 PER CENT

Record[a]	Phase	No. of components	Observer 1	Observer 2	Observer 3	(a) Average	(b) Predicted	Difference (b-a)
Equal amplitude								
1	Cosine	16	15.3	16.5	16.8	16.2	16.0	−0.2
Equal detectability								
2	Cosine	16	18.4	18.5	19.1	18.7	17.9	−0.8
3	Cosine	16	17.0	17.0	17.3	17.1	17.9	0.8
4	Cosine	12	16.5	16.6	16.5	16.5	17.0	0.5
5	Cosine	12	15.8	17.7	17.3	16.9	17.0	0.1
6	Random_1	16	15.7	16.9	17.0	16.5	17.9	1.4
7	Random_2	16	15.2	16.4	16.1	15.9	17.9	2.0
8	Random_3	12	17.0	17.6	18.5	17.7	17.0	−0.7
							Average	+0.4

[a] Three 250-trial tests were conducted with each record.

encountered were due to drifts in the center frequencies of the electronic filters. Some components changed in amplitude during the recording session. If a change of 1 db or more was noted in any component between beginning and end of a recording session, the recording made during that session was not used.

The next-to-final column of Table III is a prediction based on the summation model presented by Green (1958). In generating the predictions, it was necessary to make an assumption concerning the relation between d', a measure of signal detectability, and E/N_0. It was assumed that these two quantities are linearly related. This is approximately true (Green, Birdsall, and Tanner, 1957), and since the extrapolation was only over a 4 to 1 range of energy, the linear relation was considered to be a reasonable simplifying assumption. It was further assumed that each component of the compound tone stimulated independent auditory processes (Fisher, 1954). The equation used to generate the predictions was

$$d'_c = \Big[\sum_{i=1}^{n} (d'_i)^2 \Big]^{1/2}$$

where d'_i is a measure of the detectability of the ith component, d'_c is the corresponding measure of the compound signal, and n is the number of components used in the compound signal.

Since a d' of unity is equivalent to $P(c) \approx 75$ in two-interval forced-choice tests, if there were 16 harmonics, then d'_c, the value of d' for the compound, would be $[(16)(1)]^{1/2} = 4$. Alternatively, to produce a $d'_c = 1$, each d'_i should be $\frac{1}{4}$. In other words, for a 16-component compound, each individual component should be attenuated approximately 6 db in order to make the compound tone as detectable as the components were as individuals before they were attenuated. A model involving perfect energy summation over frequency would lead to the figure 12 db, instead of the 6 db predicted by this model.

The total energy of the compound signal is, of course, the sum of the energies of the components. Consider the compound signal when the energy is adjusted for 75 per cent correct. Each individual component of the compound has been attenuated about 6 db from the energy used to achieve 75 per cent correct when that component was used alone. Nevertheless the total energy of the compound signal may be, and in general is, greater than the energy of any component before attenuation.

The results are consistent with the assumption that variations in phase pattern, which are ignored in Green's model, do not affect the detectability of a compound signal. Obviously, however, the meager evidence does not permit us to conclude that phase is not important in detection. "All-cosine phase" is descriptive of the waveform impressed upon the earphones. The earphones and the ear, itself, undoubtedly introduce relative phase shifts. Whether or not some particular phase pattern is unusual in respect of detectability remains a difficult and unresolved experimental question.

Bearing of the data upon another model

The data obtained with the compound signal allow us to consider as unlikely one model that has been proposed to explain the detection of multicomponent signals. This model is the so-called independent-threshold model (Schafer and Gales, 1949). Briefly, the model asserts that the increase in detectability resulting from the addition of more components is due to the increase in the probability that at least one component will exceed the threshold and hence be detected. Assuming equal detectability—that the probability p that any component will exceed its threshold is the same as the probability that any other component will exceed its threshold—and that the probabilities are independent, we have

$$p_c = 1 - (1 - p)^n$$

where p_c is the probability that the compound signal will exceed the threshold and n is the number of components. The important aspect of this model is that it requires, in general, that the psychometric function (the relation of p to some physical measure) change in shape as n is varied. Obviously, the relation between p and p_c for $n = 16$ is highly nonlinear. The independent-threshold model therefore appears to dictate that the psychometric function obtained with a compound signal having $n = 16$ or $n = 12$ will be quite different from the psychometric function obtained with a single sinusoidal component. The only way to escape that dictate is to assume that the psychometric function has a very special nonlinear shape that lets the combination rule transform one segment of it into another. Such a happy accident seems unlikely, even for a fixed value of n. If variation in n is admitted, this way of escape seems even more dubious. Figure 6 shows the psychometric function obtained with observer 1, group C for the compound signal. The psychometric function obtained with the same observer for the single component signal is displayed in Fig. 1. A comparison of Figs. 1 and 6 shows that the shape of the function relating per cent correct to $\mathcal{E} - \mathfrak{N}_0$ does not change markedly.

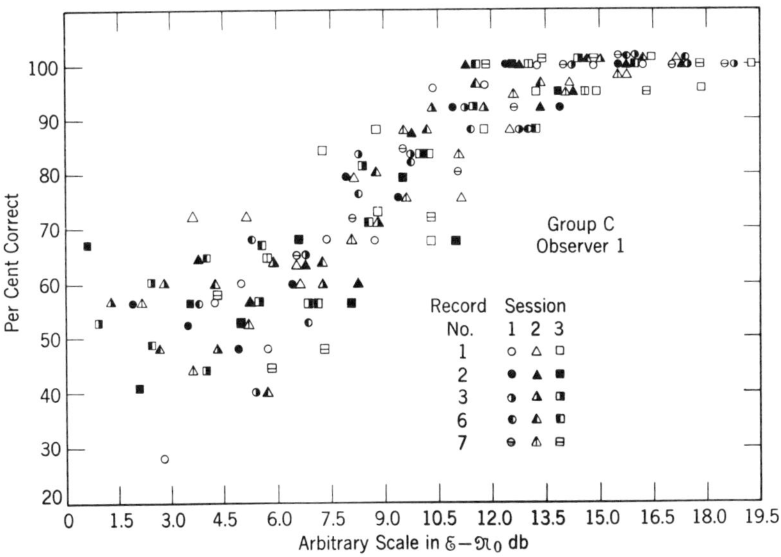

FIG. 6. The psychometric functions of a single observer for various compound signals, each containing sixteen components. Each data point represents 25 observations. The abscissa has been shifted by an arbitrary amount for each recording number and session so that scatter of points appears minimum. Table III gives the amplitude and phase pattern used for each recording number. A comparison of this figure and Fig. 1 shows that the psychometric function does not seem to depend on the number of components used for the signal.

SUMMARY

The detectability of a pulsed sinusoid (0.1 sec) in white noise was measured at sixteen frequencies ranging from 250 to 4000 cps. The measurements are compared with the results previously obtained from experiments in which continuous sinusoids of indefinite duration were used. The dependence of detectability on frequency appears to be very similar in all the experiments. We also measured the detectability of compound signals, i.e., signals with 12 and 16 sinusoidal components. A comparison of the detectability for the single and combined sinusoids allows us to determine approximately how the auditory system sums energy over frequency.

ACKNOWLEDGMENTS

This research was conducted in the Research Laboratory of Electronics, Massachusetts Institute of Technology, with support from the Operational Applications Laboratory of the U. S. Air Force. David M. Green held a fellowship from the National Science Foundation. This article appeared in J. acoust. Soc. Am., *1959,* **31,** *1446–1452.*

References

- Fisher, R. A. *Statistical methods for research workers.* 12th edition. New York: Hafner Publishing Co., 1954, 147–156.
- Fletcher, H. *Speech and hearing in communication.* New York: D. Van Nostrand Co., 1953.
- French, N. R., and Steinberg, J. C. Factors governing the intelligibility of speech sounds. *J. acoust. Soc. Am.*, 1947, **19,** 90–119.
- Green, D. M. Detection of multiple component signals in noise. *J. acoust. Soc. Am.*, 1958, **30,** 904–911. [25]
- Green, D. M., Birdsall, T. G., and Tanner, W. P., Jr. Signal detection as a function of signal intensity and duration. *J. acoust. Soc. Am.*, 1957, **29,** 523–531. [11]
- Hawkins, J. E., Jr., and Stevens, S. S. The masking of pure tones and of speech by white noise. *J. acoust. Soc. Am.*, 1950, **22,** 6–13.
- Schafer, T. H., and Gales, R. S. Auditory masking of multiple tones by random noise. *J. acoust. Soc. Am.*, 1949, **21,** 392–398.

27

Auditory Detection of a Noise Signal

David M. Green

Noise has no rival in psychoacoustic experiments as a masking agent for such stimuli as speech and sinusoids. Despite the popularity of noise as a *masking* stimulus, there are comparatively few studies using noise as a *masked* stimulus. The use of noise in both roles is an interesting situation because the bandwidths of the two stimuli establish a kind of continuum. At one extreme, where the masking and masked stimulus have identical bandwidth, one may study the noticeable increment in intensity. Where the bandwidths of the two differ, one can study the detectability of the masked stimulus, or equivalently the effectiveness of the masking stimulus. Thus either the detectability of a masked stimulus or the difference limen for intensity may be investigated in the same experimental situation simply by changing one parameter of the stimulus.

In some of the studies to be reported, noise signals with narrow bandwidths were used in a wide-band masking noise. The question of whether the center frequency of the signal band influences the detectability was investigated. In other studies both signal and background noise had identical frequency characteristics. Here the study involved determining how detection depends upon signal duration.

It is hoped that a study of how the detection of a noise signal depends upon certain parameters such as power, bandwidth, center frequency, and duration will permit conclusions to be drawn concerning the nature of the auditory system. To further this objective an optimum-detection model is introduced. As a consequence of the optimum nature of the model the resulting equations are stated in terms of the physical parameters of the detection situation without any arbitrary constants or free parameters. Thus, because of the optimum condition, it is possible to state exactly what percentage of correct responses this detection process should obtain by a measurement of only the physical parameters. This model thus serves to identify the physical parameters which are of first importance, and provides a convenient upper bound for comparison with the experimental results.

The paper is divided into three major parts. First the model is explained and the optimum equations are derived. Next the experimental procedure and the results are presented. Finally the data are compared with the equations of the model and the implications of such a comparison discussed. In this last section certain conclusions are drawn concerning the critical-band concept. In particular, the data, considered in the light of the model, suggest that these critical bands are not fixed in width but are adjustable so as to match the particular detection situation. This conclusion, based on noise signals, is an extension of the critical-band concept which has previously been investigated by studies employing single sinusoidal signals.

MODEL

Analysis of the detection problem

Before presenting the mathematical model, we shall briefly review the formal analysis of this detection problem. This introduction will provide an abstract statement of the problem and will discuss the general objectives of the mathematical derivation which follows. The rationale of the more important assumptions made in the derivation will also be presented.

To begin, we must state what the detection task involves. A sample of noise having a certain duration and bandwidth is added to a continuous background of noise in either one or the other of two nonoverlapping time intervals. The detection problem is to state which interval contained the added segment of noise. It will be convenient to call the added sample of noise the signal, and the background noise simply noise.

The problem is basically a choice between two waveforms; did the waveform in the first time interval or the one in the second time interval contain the signal? For the sake of simplicity, let us assume that both signal and noise have the same frequency characteristics. Now both waveforms are Gaussian and have zero means. The noise waveform has some average power and the signal plus noise has a greater power since the power of the signal is added to the power of the noise. Thus, it is intuitively plausible that the waveform having the larger variance or power is the waveform more likely to contain the signal. Now, owing to random fluctuation, the sample of noise alone will sometimes have a greater power than the sample of signal plus noise. A statement of the *probability* that the waveform with the larger variance is the one containing the signal is therefore the strongest statement that can be made. This probability depends, in turn, on the distribution of the variance in the waveform for each condition: (1) when the waveform is noise alone or (2) when the waveform is signal plus noise. The first part of the derivation involves determining the distribution function of waveform variance or power, assuming each hypothesis.

Mathematical derivation

During one of the two time intervals, the observer receives some single-valued function of time, $f(t)$, which may be either signal plus noise or noise alone. We wish to derive the distribution of power in the obtained waveform under both hypotheses. We shall use a discrete approximation to the continuous waveform so that each sampled waveform can be represented by a sequence of $n = 2W_sT$ numbers, where W_s is the signal bandwidth and T is the signal duration. One manner of accomplishing this result is first to filter the waveform with a filter of bandwidth W_s. We then measure the magnitude of the waveform at n discrete points along the time axis. The spacing of these sample points along the time axis could be Δt, where $\Delta t = 1/2W_s$. When the waveform is sampled in this way, the magnitude of the waveform at each sample point is statistically independent of the magnitude at any other sample point.

If noise alone is presented, let us denote X_i as the magnitude of the ith sample point in time. Since Gaussian noise is used, X_i will be normally distributed with a mean zero and variance N.[1] One should note that the quantity N refers only to that noise power which is in the signal band.

In deriving the distribution of the power in the sample waveform it will be more convenient to work with a variable P_N, which is linearly related to waveform power, rather than with power itself:

$$P_N = \sum_{i=1}^{2WT} X_i^2$$

P_N is a random variable, since it is a transformation of the random variables X_i^2. Since the summation involves a series of independent normalized Gaussian variables, i.e.,

$$\sum_{i=1}^{2WT} \left(\frac{X_i}{N^{1/2}}\right)^2$$

it is distributed as chi square with $2W_sT$ degrees of freedom. The expected value of the distribution is $2W_sT$, or,

$$E(P_N) = E \sum_{i=1}^{2WT} X_i^2 = 2W_sTN \tag{1}$$

Since the variance of a chi-squared distribution is simply twice the number of degrees of freedom,

$$E[\text{variance of } P_N] = 4W_sTN^2 \tag{2}$$

For $2W_sT$ greater than 30, a chi-squared distribution closely approximates a normal distribution; thus P_N is normally distributed.

The distribution of power when signal plus noise is presented may be determined by a derivation parallel to that just given for noise alone. If signal plus noise is presented, let the magnitude of the waveform at the ith sample point be Y_i. Since both signal and noise are Gaussian, Y_i will be normally distributed with mean zero and variance $S + N$.[2] Note that $S + N$ refers only to the power in the signal band.

---

[1] To be consistent, if N is the average power of the noise, the average total energy in the sample must be

$$E\left[\int_0^T X(t)^2 dt\right] = NT$$

where T is the duration and $X(t)$ is the voltage wave form. A Riemann sum must approximate this integral; thus

$$E[\sum_{i=1}^{n} X_i^2 \Delta t] \approx NT$$

where X_i is the discrete approximation to $X(t)$, and $n = 2WT$. Since $t = 1/2W$,

$$E[\sum_{i=1}^{n} X_i^2 \Delta t] = n(X^2)\frac{1}{2W} = T(X^2), \text{ where } (X^2) = E(X_i^2)$$

but then X^2 must equal N, which is the variance of X_i.

[2] An argument similar to that given in the first footnote leads to the result $E(Y_i^2) = S + N$.

In the case of the signal plus noise, we will again use a variable linearly related to the waveform power,

$$P_{S+N} = \sum_{i=1}^{2WT} Y_i^2$$

The summation,

$$\sum_{i=1}^{2WT} \left[\frac{Y_i}{(S+N)^{1/2}} \right]^2$$

is distributed as chi-squared with $2WT$ degrees of freedom. The expected value of this distribution is $2W_sT$, or

$$E(P_{S+N}) = E(\sum_{i=1}^{2WT} Y_i^2) = 2W_sT(S+N) \tag{3}$$

and the expected value of the variance

$$E[\text{variance of } P_{S+N}] = 4W_sT(S+N)^2 \tag{4}$$

As long as $2WT$ is greater than 30, P_{S+N} will also be normally distributed.

Figure 1 shows the results of these derivations. The distribution of power in the sampled waveform, under each hypothesis, is displayed.

The approach used in this derivation rests entirely upon the work presented by Peterson and Birdsall (1953). In their paper it is shown that a discrete approximation to the continuous waveform is an optimum procedure. This result was used in the mathematical derivation to obtain the n discrete numbers used in calculating the distribution of power. In addition, Peterson and Birdsall demonstrate that a decision rule based on the power of the waveform is optimum. In this derivation there is calculated the distribution of power since selecting the interval with the

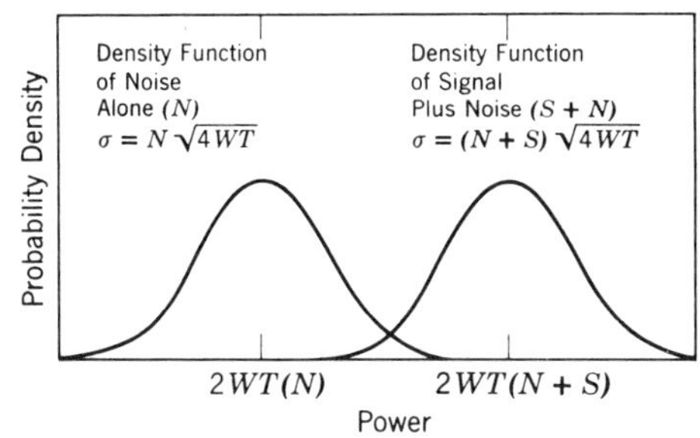

FIG. 1. The distribution of power in a sampled waveform when noise alone or signal plus noise is sampled. The bandwidths of both the signal and noise are assumed to be the same in this figure.

larger waveform power will maximize the percentage of correct decisions. These two factors are in essence what give the following approach its optimum character and hence deserve some discussion.

There are really two aspects of the optimum approach that should be distinguished. The first aspect involves the way in which the waveform is represented or analyzed by the detection device. Somehow the continuous waveform must be analyzed or represented and all the relevant properties included as a basis for detection.

The manner in which the continuous waveform is represented or summarized obviously determines in large part the quality of the resulting decision. One way of representing the waveform would be to record the initial, middle, and final value of the waveform during the interval. Such a scheme is extremely inefficient since it obviously ignores a great deal of relevant information.

It is demonstrated by Peterson and Birdsall that, if the waveform is assumed to be of the class of waveforms that can be represented by a finite series in a Fourier expansion, in short, if the waveform is Fourier-series band-limited, then a so-called "sample plan" may be employed which provides a discrete representation of the waveform. Roughly speaking, the waveform can be represented by a finite set of numbers and still preserve all of the information. While the assumption is fairly broad in character, Slepian (1958) has demonstrated that it is not trivial. Slepian has worked some very similar problems, relaxing only this series band-limited condition, and comes to very different conclusions.

The second factor involves how, or on what basis, the decision is made. Once the representation problem has been solved, there still remains the very important problem of somehow reducing all of the numbers obtained by the discrete representation to some single quantity, and using this quantity in making the final decision. In the present case it turns out that the power of the sampled waveform is the optimum quantity. One can conceive of a more realistic model of auditory detection, such as that accomplished by the human observer, which does not obtain as complete a representation of the waveform but nevertheless is optimum in the sense that it treats the obtained information in an optimum manner. One could, for example, devise optimum decision rules based on the rather incomplete information obtained from the initial, middle, and final value of the waveform. One might say in this case that the analysis or representation mechanism was not optimum but that the decision mechanism was. Such a partially optimum model would result in equations having various parameters which reflect the particular non-optimum quality of the model. The present model is optimum in both senses, and thus permits derivation of the expected percentage of correct detections based only on a knowledge of the physical parameters of the detection situation.

Finally, in the situation in which the signal noise is a band-limited signal, for example, when the signal noise is first filtered and then presented as a narrow-band noise signal in a wider band of noise, the optimum approach is to start with a filter that is matched to the signal's bandwidth. This then eliminates much of the background noise which could not contain any power due to the signal and hence could not be relevant in making a decision.

Probability of a correct choice

In the experiments reported in this paper a two-alternative forced-choice technique was used. Two time intervals were marked off for the observers, and, in one of these intervals, the signal was added to the noise. As was previously discussed, the optimum decision rule would be to say that the sample having the largest variance or power was the one that contained the signal. The probability that this decision is correct is simply the probability that a random sample from the signal-plus-noise distribution will be larger than the drawing from the distribution of noise alone.

This probability is most conveniently determined by considering the *difference* between the distributions of signal plus noise and noise alone. When the drawing of signal plus noise is greater than the drawing from noise alone, the difference sample will be greater than zero. Thus, the problem is to determine the distribution of the quantity $(P_{S+N}) - (P_N)$.

Now since both P_{S+N} and P_N have normal distributions, their difference also has a normal distribution. The probability of a correct decision is then the probability that a drawing from this normal deviate will be greater than zero. The mean of the differences is the difference of the means, and since the samples are taken at two different intervals in time, they are uncorrelated; therefore, the variance of the difference is the sum of the individual variances. It is convenient to normalize this difference distribution so that the variance is unity. The mean of this normalized distribution is then

$$M = \left(\frac{W_s T}{2}\right)^{1/2} \frac{S}{N} \frac{1}{[\frac{1}{2}(S/N)^2 + (S/N) + 1]^{1/2}} \tag{5}$$

Both the signal power (S) and the noise power (N) are measured in the same bandwidth. Therefore the noise power density, or spectrum level of the noises, may be used in Eq. (5). Letting $N_0W = N$ and $S_0W = S$, the equation may be rewritten as

$$M = \left(\frac{W_sT}{2}\right)^{1/2} \frac{S_0}{N_0} \frac{1}{[\frac{1}{2}(S_0/N_0)^2 + (S_0/N_0) + 1]^{1/2}} \tag{6}$$

This is the form that is used in analyzing the data.

Let the quantity d'_{opt} (d' optimum) be defined in the following way:

$$d'_{\text{opt}} = \sqrt{2}M \tag{7a}$$

The quantity d' has been introduced in other papers on signal detection (Tanner, Swets, and Green, 1956; Tanner and Swets, 1954; Green, Birdsall, and Tanner, 1957). Previously this quantity was used only when the distribution of signal plus noise and noise alone both had the same variance. For the types of signals considered in the present paper, this condition may not be true. However, when the ratio of signal power to noise power per unit bandwidth becomes small (i.e., $S_0/N_0 \ll 1$), the radical in Eq. (6) becomes unity. Then d'_{opt} has the following value:

$$d'_{\text{opt}} = (W_sT)^{1/2} \frac{S_0}{N_0}, \quad \frac{S_0}{N_0} \ll 1, \quad W_N > W_S \tag{7b}$$

In this case the variances of the signal-plus-noise and noise-alone distributions are nearly the same (see Fig. 1); thus the quantity d'_{opt} is consistent with the previous definitions as S_0/N_0 approaches zero.

Using either the quantity M or d'_{opt}, a table of the normal probability integral can be used to determine the expected percentage of correct detections for the ideal receiver. For example, at the value of $d'_{\text{opt}} = 1$ the expected percentage correct is 75 per cent.

This last equation best lends itself to an intuitive interpretation of the derivations. If d'_{opt} is thought of as the detectability of the signal, we see that this quantity is monotonically related to the signal-to-noise ratio. Also, for some fixed signal-to-noise ratio the detectability increases as the square root of either signal duration or bandwidth. This corresponds to the familiar statistical result that the standard deviation of the sample mean decreases as the square root of the number of samples. For an optimum detection device, more sample values can be obtained by extending the signal either in time or frequency. This result can be anticipated, since there must exist a symmetry between the time and frequency domain for an optimum receiver.

Review of assumptions

Before considering the experimental results, let us review briefly the essential operations used by an optimum detection device in order to make at least plausible the comparison of the optimum device and the human auditory system.

Basically the device for optimum detection measures the power in two waveforms and selects the larger of these two powers. As a matter of fact, the device need not even measure power. If the device measures any quantity that is strictly monotonic with power, then the decision as to which waveform has the largest power will still be the same. This is true because order relations are preserved on scales monotonic with power; thus decisions as to which waveform caused the largest power would be the same. The decisions generated by such a procedure would agree, decision by decision, with a device which measured power directly.

It seems reasonable to suppose that the auditory mechanism provides some transformation of the acoustic waveform which is monotonic with waveform power. It seems even more reasonable to assume that the human observer can rank such transformations. Subjective scales of loudness, in particular, assume the subject can do a great deal more than establish an order. Furthermore, it is *not* assumed that the optimum device samples the waveform discretely according to some "sampling plan." This is simply the way in which the *analysis* of such an operation proceeds in the development of the statistical properties of the power of a waveform.

The optimum-decision device must, of course, know the exact duration and starting time of the two waveforms, and must filter according to the signal bandwidth. The human observer, who is notified by a light flash of the signal presentations, can hardly be expected to know with any real precision the duration or the starting times of the signal. This discrepancy will probably lead to some difference between the human performance and the optimum performance. This discrepancy certainly does not vitiate the attempt to apply the optimum model. Rather, it suggests that a comparison of the optimum equation and the human's performance for different signal durations might provide some insight into this difference. The question of filtering to match signal bandwidth is entirely similar.

Though it is hardly to be expected that the human observer will perform as well as the optimum receiver, this inequality does not mean that there is no reason to compare human observers and the optimum model. It is entirely reasonable to expect that the man might perform like the ideal receiver with respect to certain physical parameters. The following experiments were conducted to investigate this possibility.

EXPERIMENTS

Two experiments were performed to test various aspects of the theory. Both experiments will be described and the data presented before any discussion of the implications of the results of the experiments is undertaken.[3] The first experiment was conducted to determine how the duration of the noise signal influences its detectability. The signal and noise had the same bandwidth; hence one could say that the study investigated how duration influences the observer's differential sensitivity to noise. The second experiment was conducted to determine how the detectability of the signal is influenced by center frequency. A narrow-band signal was presented in wide-band noise and the detectability of the signal at seven center frequencies was investigated. In addition, one test was conducted in which the noise and signal had the same wide bandwidth. By analyzing several different conditions of the two experiments, we can also determine how detectability is influenced by different bandwidths of the signal. Thus the variation of signal detectability with signal duration, center frequency, and bandwidth may be determined from these two experiments.

Experiment I

The parameter investigated in this experiment was the duration of the noise signal. Both signal and noise were passed through the same filter which had an equivalent square bandwidth of about 3800 cps. Six signal durations were employed. At each duration the signal power was set at five or six different levels so that the percentage of correct detection could be determined at each level.

The equipment used in this experiment is similar to that already reported (Green, Birdsall, and Tanner, 1957), except that, instead of an oscillator to generate the signal, a noise source was employed. The

---

[3] The experiments were not conducted in the order reported. The first experiment was conducted at the Psychophysical Laboratory of the Electronic Defense Group, University of Michigan, in the fall of 1957. The second experiment was conducted at the Bell Telephone Laboratories, Murray Hill, New Jersey, where the author was a temporary employee during the late summer of 1957.

signal and noise were filtered at the input to the power amplifier. The masking noise which was present throughout an experimental session had a spectrum level of about 50 db *re* 0.0002 d/cm^2.

MEASURED QUANTITIES. Listed here are the definitions of the various quantities used in the experiment.

S_0/N_0 = the ratio of signal power to noise power in a 1-cps band. [Both quantities were measured at the same point in the circuit (the headphones) with a true-rms meter. The equivalent square bandwidth of both noise and signal, where they differed, was taken into account. The logarithm of this quantity expressed in decibels is the spectrum level of the signal with respect to the noise.]

W_s = the equivalent square bandwidth of the signal.

W_n = the equivalent square bandwidth of the noise.

T = the duration of the signal.

RESULTS OF EXPERIMENT I. Figures 2 to 4 show how with duration held constant the percentage of correct detections depends upon signal power. The abscissa is presented in terms of d'_{opt} in order to include all the data points on a single graph. For any one signal duration, the experimental variable is the signal level. Thus the psychometric function, the variation of percentage correct and signal level, appears similar for all durations if the signal level is transformed in the manner indicated.

Three hundred observations were used to define each point presented on the graphs. Some of the observers were unable to complete all of the experimental conditions owing to illness.

A summary of these data is presented in Fig. 5. The points in this figure represent, as a function of duration, the signal-to-noise power ratio in a 1-cps band necessary to obtain 75 per cent correct detections. Miller (1947) has obtained similar data for the 1-sec duration. He found the ratio of S_0/N_0 to be 0.102 for one subject, and 0.107 for another, at this noise level.

The solid line found below the data points is the expected performance of the optimum detector, which was discussed in the previous section, and is obtained by applying Eq. (7) to the present experiment. The optimum detector appears to reflect the variation of signal level and signal duration (Fig. 5). If one selects the 75-per-cent-correct detection point for each duration, the optimum detector seems to be about 5 or 6 db better than the human observer for all but the longest duration. It may be seen that the optimum model does not appear to predict the observed variation of per-cent-correct detections as a function of signal intensity (Figs. 2 to 4). The psychometric function appears to be somewhat

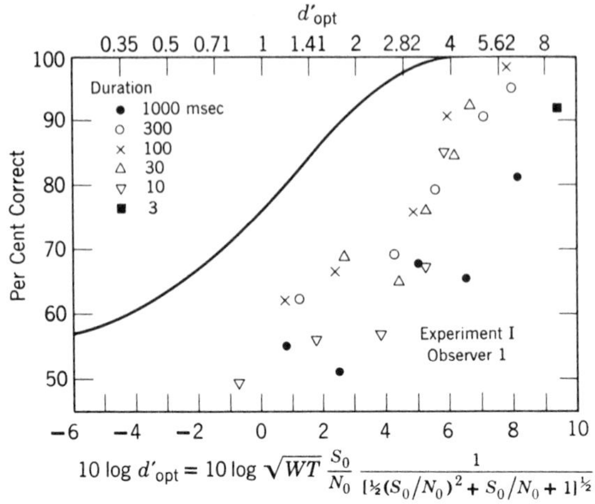

FIG. 2

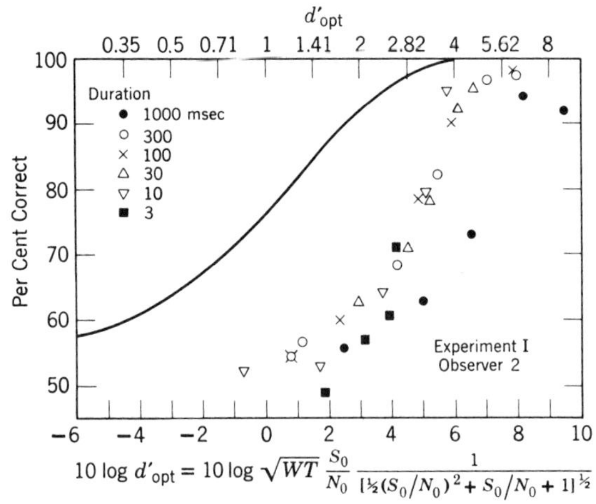

FIG. 3

steeper than that suggested by the model. The implications of these results and particular modifications of the model to account for the obtained data will be discussed after the presentation of the results of the second experiment.

Experiment II

This experiment was conducted in order to determine in what way, if any, the center frequency of a narrow-band noise signal influenced the

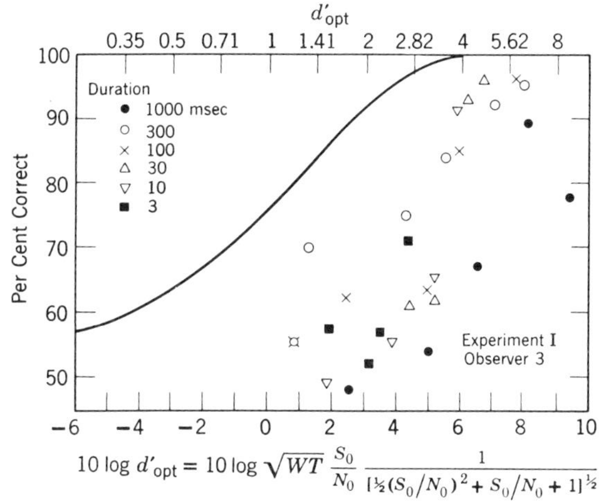

FIG. 4

FIGS. 2–4. The ordinate is the percentage of correct responses obtained in a two-alternative forced-choice test. The abscissa represents a transformation of the physical parameters used in the test. The solid curve represents the expected behavior of the ideal detector.

detectability of the signal. According to the mathematical model of the optimum detector, the center frequency of the signal is unimportant as long as the receiver first filters the incoming waveform so as to match

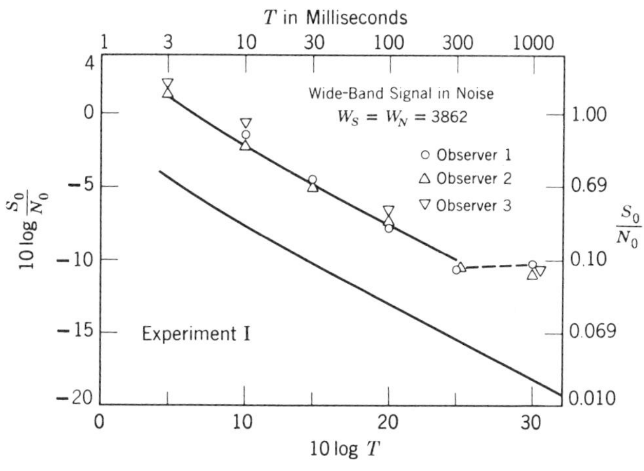

FIG. 5. The points represent the ratio of signal to noise power per unit bandwidth necessary for 75-per-cent-correct detections. The abscissa is the duration of the signal. The solid curve represents the expected behavior of the ideal detector.

the signal in bandwidth and center frequency. If one assumes that the detector accomplishes this filtering operation, then only the *bandwidth* of the signal influences detection, *not the center frequency*. When this assumption is considered in connection with the critical-band hypothesis, it is at least questionable whether the human observer will produce results at all comparable with the optimum detection scheme. The results obtained from experiments on the detection of pure tones in noise indicate that the critical bands become wider at the higher frequencies, so that, even if the observer can adjust the center frequency of the critical band, perhaps the bandwidth will not be optimally adjusted.

In order to investigate this problem, the audio circuit displayed in Fig. 6 was constructed. The noise source provided a Gaussian output with an approximately flat power spectrum up to 200 kc. This noise was passed through a fairly sharp passive filter with a center frequency at about 30 kc and a bandwidth of about 650 cps. This band of noise was then modulated and the low-frequency components were passed through a low-pass filter. If the oscillator connected to the modulator was set at a frequency X cps above 30 kc, the output of the headphones would be a band-passed noise with a center frequency at X cps and a bandwidth of 650 cps. The spectrum of this noise on a linear frequency scale would then be the same for any value of X or center frequency. Therefore the total power of the noise signal is independent of the center frequency of the band. The spectrum level of this background noise was held constant at about 40 db *re* 0.0002 d/cm^2.

After the experiment with the narrow-band signals had been completed, a wide-band signal was used in order to determine how signal bandwidth per se influenced the observer's performance. The wide-band signal, which was the same width as the background noise, had a bandwidth of about 5100 cps.

The signal duration was held constant at 0.25 sec in the experiments with both wide- and narrow-bandwidth signals.

The psychophysical procedures were similar to those used in Experiment I. In each condition of the experiment a psychometric function was obtained by varying the intensity of the signal. Each function was obtained at a single center frequency before the next center frequency was investigated. The order in which center frequencies were tested was determined by a random sequence. Two female employees of the Bell Telephone Laboratories served as subjects. They were not the same observers as were used in the first experiment.

RESULTS. The results of this experiment are presented in Figs. 7 and 8. The data for all the conditions of the experiment are presented for each

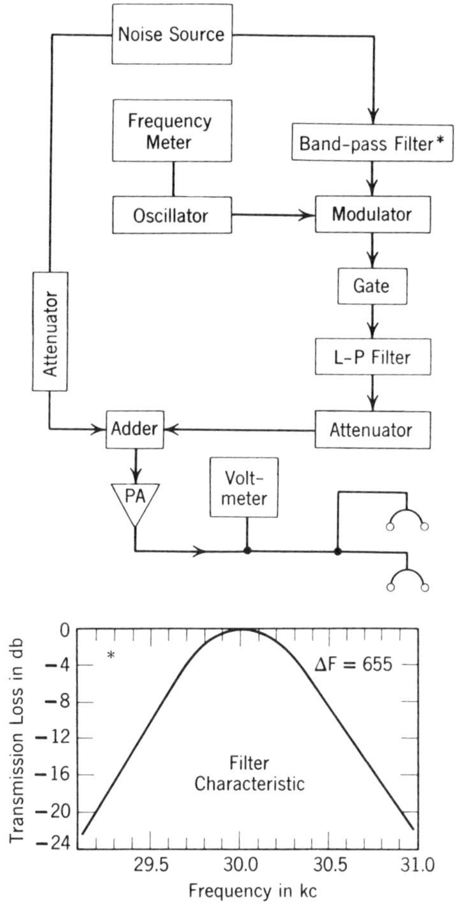

FIG. 6. Block diagram of the equipment used in the second experiment.

observer. The ordinate is the percentage of correct decisions. Three hundred observations were used to define each point. The abscissa is again the logarithm of d'_{opt}. This scale is used because it permits one to plot the results of both the narrow-band and wide-band noise signal on the same graph. Once again the psychometric function appears similar for all experimental conditions. It is also quite similar to the form of the psychometric function obtained in the previous experiment (Figs. 2 to 4).

The same inconsistency between the model and the observer's performance is evident in these psychometric functions as was observed in the first experiment. The observer does not respond to a change in signal

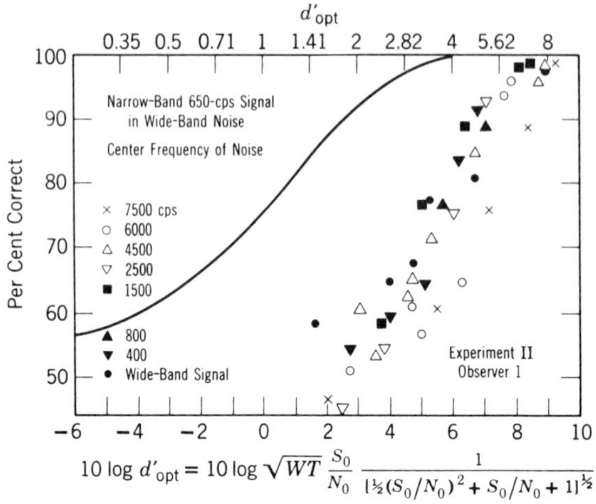

FIG. 7

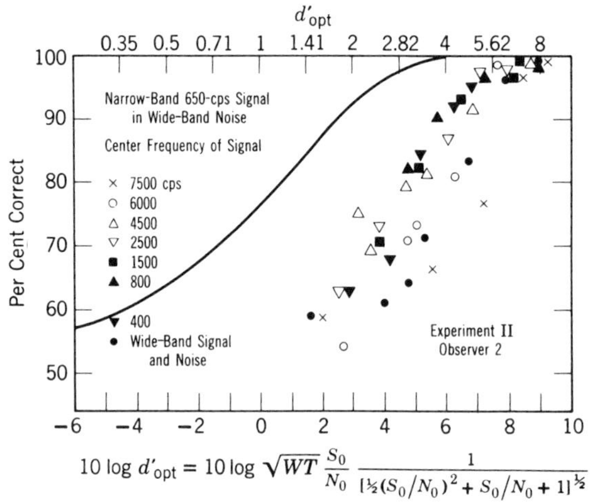

FIG. 8

FIGS. 7 AND 8. The ordinate is the percentage of correct responses obtained in a two-alternative forced-choice test. The abscissa represents a transformation of the physical parameters used in the test. The solid curve represents the expected behavior of the ideal detector.

intensity in the same way as would be expected from Eq. (7). This point will be discussed more fully in a later section.

Figure 9 is a summary of the data presented in Figs. 7 and 8. It is similar to the summary previously presented for the duration data. In

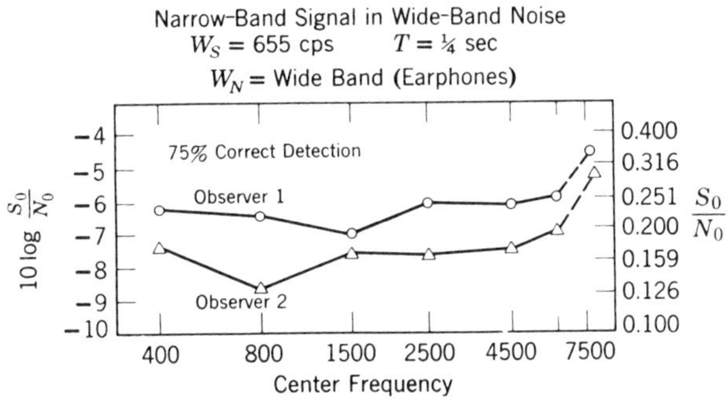

Wide-Band Signal in Wide-Band Noise
$W_S = W_N$ = 5143 cps, T = ¼ sec

Observer	10 Log S_0/N_0	S_0/N_0
1	−10.0	.100
2	−9.6	.1096

FIG. 9. The points represent the signal to noise power per unit bandwidth necessary to obtain 75-per-cent-correct detections. The abscissa is the center frequency of the band of noise used as the signal. The table is the summary of the data when a wider bandwidth is used for the signal.

Fig. 9 the ratio of signal-to-noise power in a 1-cps band necessary for 75-per-cent-correct detections is plotted against the center frequency of the narrow-band noise signal. Clearly, for a narrow-band signal, the center frequency of the signal had little to do with the signal's detectability. Only the data obtained at a center frequency of 7500 cps seem to disagree with this conclusion. Here the frequency-response characteristics of the headphones may contribute heavily to the results. Anomalous data at such frequencies have been obtained in another study (Hawkins and Stevens, 1950). No complete explanation of such a result can be suggested at this time.

The table in Fig. 9 expresses the same data for a wide-band signal. These data were obtained by passing both signal and noise through the same filter; hence these data represent the differential intensity sensitivity for a noise stimulus. S_0/N_0 is thus equivalent to the Weber function $\Delta E/E$ for sound energy. In order to avoid confusion it should be pointed out that the measure S_0/N_0 is independent of signal bandwidth. This ratio is about 0.25 for observer 1 with the 655-cps bandwidth signals, and about 0.11 for the 5134-cps bandwidth signal. In terms of the total energy of the signal (W_sS_0T), the wide-band signal has a total energy of about 3.3 times the total energy of the narrow-band signal.

Signal detectability and bandwidth

The results obtained with the two signal bandwidths in the second experiment combined with the data obtained from the first experiment allow us to present data on the question of how signal bandwidth influences detection. In Table I we have presented the spectrum level of the signal, with respect to the noise, necessary for 75-per-cent-correct detection at three signal bandwidths. The signal duration was 0.25 sec in the second experiment, and the data of the first experiment have been interpolated to allow a comparison at this duration. In the second column of the table the predictions based on the optimum detection model are presented. The difference, once more about 5 db, appears to be about the same for all bandwidths employed and allows us to conclude tentatively that the model accounts, except for an attenuation factor, for the way in which bandwidth influences detection.

TABLE I. COMPARISON OF OBTAINED AND PREDICTED RESULTS FOR VARIATIONS IN SIGNAL BANDWIDTH (DURATION ¼ SEC)

W_s = signal bandwidth	Obtained $10 \log_{10} S_0/N_0$ necessary for 75% correct		Prediction Eq. (7)	Difference (obtained − predicted)
655 cps[a]	Obs 1	−5.8	−11.0	5.7
	Obs 2	−6.5		4.5
3862 cps	Obs 1	−9.5	−14.91	5.4
	Obs 2	−10.0		4.9
5143 cps	Obs 1	−10.0	−15.5	5.5
	Obs 2	− 9.6		5.9

[a] Average over several center frequencies.

COMPARISON OF THE MODEL AND THE EXPERIMENTAL RESULTS

Part I

The comparison of the model and the results may be conveniently divided into two parts. The first part, where the model and data agree, results from considering the data from the standpoint of some constant detectability. If we arbitrarily define the threshold as the signal level necessary for 75 per cent correct and then compare the variation in threshold with the other physical parameters such as bandwidth and duration, we find good agreement between model and data.

For any such arbitrarily defined level of detectability, the model and the obtained data differ by a single constant. There are essentially three principal ways to change a noise signal. We may change the duration, the bandwidth, and the center frequency. All three were investigated in these studies. The model appears to predict, except for a single constant, 5 db, how the signal-to-noise level necessary for 75-per-cent-correct detections is affected by all three variables. Let us consider them, one at a time, and specify the range over which this prediction holds. Signal durations ranging from 3 to 300 msec are consistent with the model (Fig. 5). Signal bandwidths ranging from 600 to 5000 cps are consistent with the model (Table I). Likewise, narrow-band signals (600-cps bandwidth) with center frequencies from 400 to 6000 cps show results consistent with the model (Fig. 9). The limit on the range of prediction for both bandwidth and center frequency is probably due to the width of the critical band. If the signal bandwidth is less than a critical band the model does not apply.[4] Any noise signal with bandwidth larger than a critical band at some center frequency would probably yield results consistent with the model. In short the following equation appears to predict all of the results:

$$d'_{\text{obs}} = ad'_{\text{opt}} = a(WT)^{1/2} \frac{S_0}{N_0} \frac{1}{[\frac{1}{2}(S_0/N_0)^2 + (S_0/N_0) + 1]^{1/2}} \tag{8}$$

where ($d'_{\text{obs}} = ad'_{\text{opt}}$) is the Gaussian transform of the per cent correct actually obtained from the observer and a is a constant which depends on the level of detectability selected and possibly on the individual observer. For d'_{obs} of unity (per cent correct = 75 per cent) a is about 1/4 to 1/3. Using some other constant detectability, the constant ranges from about 1/2 for the 90 per cent level to 1/9 for the 60 per cent level.

Before suggesting any hypothesis to account for this discrepancy, let us note one important implication of this result for the critical-band concept. The most convincing evidence for the critical-band concept comes from an experiment in which the subject is trying to detect a

[4] By assuming that the critical bands at higher frequencies are larger than the noise signal, the discrepancy of the data (Fig. 9) from a horizontal line could be handled. Indeed some people estimate the critical band at 7500 cps to be larger than 600 cps, though this estimate is based on loudness data, not detection data. Besides the obvious post hoc quality of the explanation, it implies in addition that the data for the 6000-cps center-frequency signal should also depart from the expected results; it does not.

sinusoidal signal in a background of noise. By progressively eliminating the background noise at frequencies far removed from the signal frequency, Fletcher (1940) first demonstrated that only the noise in a narrow band around the frequency influenced the detectability of the sinusoidal signal. This narrow band of frequency, which influenced the detection of the signal, was called the critical band.

One interpretation of this result has been to assume that at an early stage in the auditory mechanism there exists some sort of frequency-analysis system which might be likened to a number of narrowly tuned filters. Each filter overlaps with the next and has a bandwidth determined by its center frequency so that, for any particular sinusoidal signal, a filter with the appropriate center frequency is selected, and only that filter is employed in "listening" to the signal.

An important empirical finding was that these bands appeared to increase in width with center frequency. The critical bandwidth at 1000 cps was found to be about 60 cps, while at 4000 cps the critical band had an estimated width of some 200 cps. Since the bandwidth of the filter is wider at higher frequencies, these high-frequency signals should be harder to hear, as indeed they are. In fact, Fletcher suggested that one could determine the bandwidth of the filters, by inference, from measures of the signal-to-noise ratio needed to hear sinusoidal signals. Zwicker, Flottorp, and Stevens (1957) have called this indirect procedure the "critical-ratio method."

Now for sine waves of unlimited duration such as Fletcher used, the narrower the bandwidth of the analyzing filter, the better should be the detection. For a pulsed sinusoidal signal of 1-sec duration the optimum filter bandwidth is about 1 cps. The estimated critical bandwidths of 30 to 500 cps, depending on center frequency, are much larger than the optimum value but are presumably the best the observer can do. Hence the estimated critical bands must be regarded as minimum auditory bandwidths.

But what of the critical bands' maximum width? Or to put the question in another way, can several critical bands be simultaneously combined to provide an effective wide-band auditory analysis? Obviously, to explain the detection of a signal having a wide frequency spectrum, some assumptions concerning this question must be made. Most of the earlier work on the critical-band concept employed narrow-band signals such as sinusoids, and thus there was no explicit discussion of this question.

Recent work appears to have provided two conflicting answers to this question. Green (1958), investigating the detection of complex signals generated by adding two sine waves, suggests that two or more widely separated bands might be used in combination. Such a model appears to be supported by the data he obtained. Marill (1956), investigating a similar problem, obtained data inconsistent with that obtained by Green. Marill's results indicated that a two-component signal was no easier to detect in noise than the single more easily detected component. Tanner, Swets, and Green (1956), investigating a problem where signal frequency was uncertain, obtained data that are more consistent with Marill's results. In general, they suggest the possibility that only one critical band is employed at any instant in time.

The data obtained in the present experiments with noise signals support the view that several bands can be combined. The experiment involving the narrow-band signal at different center frequencies supports this conclusion. If a single critical band is employed, the high frequencies should be easier to hear than the low because detectability should increase with increasing width of the critical band; they are not. Also the data obtained with the wider-band signal support the contention that the auditory bandwidth changes according to the bandwidth of the noise signal. Table I shows that for a change of slightly less than a decade in signal bandwidth the 75-per-cent-correct point changes by about 4 db. This almost exactly parallels the change predicted by the optimum-detection model which, of course, changes the receiver bandwidth to match the signal bandwidth. Such a correspondence is strong presumptive evidence for a similar change in the bandwidth of the auditory mechanism. The most easily envisioned mechanism for such a change would be a linear combination of several critical bands that would effectively broaden the frequency-analysis mechanism of the ear.

Another point should be made concerning the detectability of the narrow-band signal. In effect, the model holds that the width of the band alone determines the detectability of the signal. This band may be distributed around 400 or 4000 cps; only its linear range or width influences detection. The results support such a notion (Fig. 9). The author, at least, was somewhat surprised by this finding. Certainly in other areas —pitch judgment, detection of the change in frequency, musical intervals, etc.—linear frequency does not seem to be the most fundamental scale. Some transformation of the linear-frequency scale, usually logarithmic, provides a more direct or reasonable representation of the psychological effect of this variable. Indeed the phenomenal impression of the 600-cps signal noise centered at 400 and 4000 cps appears quite different. At 400 cps the noise band has the familiar hissing quality of noise and sounds at least similar to wide-band noise. At 4000 cps the band of noise sounds more like a rather poor whistle, shrill and irregular but having a fairly definite pitch character. Despite these perceptual differences, the detection of each noise in wide-band noise was about the same if they were equated in power. The important variable for this particular detection task is linear frequency and not some nonlinear transformation of that variable.

Finally, let us direct our attention to the *constant difference* between the optimum prediction and the results obtained for some arbitrary level of detectability. With only the data discussed thus far, several reasonable theoretical alternatives could be presented to account for the difference. Two suggestions can be rejected by the data just considered. The first might involve some non-optimum filtering. The previous discussion, however, leads to the conclusion that the observer appears to match the frequency-analysis mechanism of the ear to the signal bandwidth. Secondly one might assume that the observer of the signal knows the duration and starting time only *approximately*. The optimum-detection device knows these parameters *exactly*. This difference, then, might account for the discrepancy. It would seem, however, that such temporal uncertainty should be greater for a 10-msec signal than for a signal of 1000 msec. The results (Fig. 5) show that signal duration does not influence the difference between the obtained results and the optimum equation until durations as long as 1000 msec are reached, and then the difference is in the wrong direction. Thus simple uncertainty as to starting time or duration does not appear to explain the difference. Clearly, the difference between the predicted and obtained results for some constant detectability could be due to some constant "internal noise." Alternatively, one can imagine some uncertainty as to which interval contains the larger measure on the decision axis. Perhaps the observer can only imperfectly distinguish which interval contains the largest power or whatever. Thus some random uncertainty in the decision rule might yield the results obtained. There are probably many other suggestions that might be put forth to explain the difference. Before discussing any of these suggestions in detail, let us turn to the second part of the comparison of the data and the model, namely, the variation of percentage correct with the signal power level.

Part II

Figures 2 to 4, 7, and 8 all show the results which are very difficult to account for in terms of the proposed model. These results indicate that the difference between the data obtained and the model's predictions depends upon the signal-to-noise level. Weak signals are much harder to hear relative to the predictions of the model than they should be. This nonlinearity in the basic psychometric function poses a serious theoretical problem.

Neither "internal noise" nor uncertainty as to which interval is larger accounts for this relation. Both suggestions amount to assuming that the model underestimates the actual amount of variance in the samples on which the decision is based. This leads to a correction of the derived equations but a correction of the type which simply shifts the psychometric curve by a constant amount. As was pointed out earlier, the results obtained can be summarized by Eq. (8) but the constant, a, of the equation depends on the value of d'_{opt}. It is interesting to note that this same inconsistency between the optimum equation and the observed psychometric function has been observed in work involving pure-tone signals in noise (Green, Birdsall, and Tanner, 1957). This effect has not been successfully explained. Most attempts to explain this discrepancy involve the *ad hoc* assumption of what amounts to the addition of noise in a nonlinear manner. While such attempts appear promising, the exact mathematics of such a process is uncommonly difficult. Until some more quantitative suggestions are forthcoming, we shall refrain from further speculation.

CONCLUSIONS

In conclusion three points should be stressed. First, if the aim is simply to predict the "threshold" of the noise signal in noise, the present model, with one additional parameter, provides extremely accurate predictions of the obtained data. Variation of signal bandwidth or duration or center frequency and detectability are completely consistent with the optimum-model equations, at least for the major range of bandwidth, center frequency, and duration investigated.

Second, the fact that signal detectability is independent of center frequency, if bandwidth power and duration are held constant, leads to an important substantive inference, namely, that the critical bands are adjustable beyond their minimum widths. That is, this extremely basic parameter of the hearing mechanism appears to be adjustable once it becomes effective to employ more than a minimum critical bandwidth. This inference has important implications for detection situations in which stimuli other than simple sinusoidal stimuli are used as signals.

Finally, the model is not a completely adequate explanation of all the data. The area of particular disagreement is the shape of the psychometric function: the basic relation of signal intensity and the percentage of correct responses. The form of the psychometric function is hardly a new problem in psychophysics. Many different models have been proposed to account for the shape of the psychometric function. Most of the models have several free parameters and unfortunately do not specify, in detail, the physical parameters that should be used in determining the abscissa of the psychometric function. The optimum model used in this paper avoids these difficulties but fails to account for the data. Nevertheless, the nature of the discrepancy between model and data is instructive, and in the light of the other data several seemingly reasonable proposals to account for the discrepancy have been rejected. Certainly this remains as one of the major unsolved problems, both for noise and sinusoidal signals.

SUMMARY

Measurements of the detectability of a noise signal in noise are reported in this paper. Parameters of the noise signal such as the bandwidth, duration, and center frequency are investigated. The results are compared with an optimum-detection model. For some constant detectability the equation generated by the model and one constant, an attenuation factor, closely fit the experimental data over the major range of the experimental parameters. The major area of discrepancy between model and data is the shape of the psychometric function. Implications of the data for the critical-band mechanism are also discussed.

ACKNOWLEDGMENTS

Two laboratories kindly provided the facilities necessary to undertake the research presented in this paper. The writer is indebted to W. P. Tanner, Jr., Head of the Psychophysical Laboratory, Electronic Defense Group, University of Michigan, for his encouragement and cooperation. T. G. Birdsall also provided considerable assistance in mathematical matters. The author wishes to thank Miss Ann Mills for her help in obtaining and analyzing the data. The research at Michigan was carried out with support from the Operational Applications Laboratory of the U. S. Air Force.

The author is equally indebted to John Karlin and the members of his group at the Bell Telephone Laboratories, Murray Hill, New Jersey. Though the author's visit to Bell Telephone Laboratories was short, their kind cooperation and assistance enabled him to complete the experiment conducted there. Miss Nancy Bowles also deserves special mention for her assistance in guiding the data collection and analysis to a speedy conclusion.

This article appeared in J. acoust. Soc. Am., *1960,* **32,** *121–131.*

References

- Fletcher, H. Auditory patterns, *Revs. mod. Phys.*, 1940, **12,** 47–65.
- Green, D. M. Detection of multiple component signals in noise. *J. acoust. Soc. Am.*, 1958, **30,** 904–911. [25]
- Green, D. M., Birdsall, T. G., and Tanner, W. P., Jr. Signal detection as a function of signal intensity and duration. *J. acoust. Soc. Am.*, 1957, **29,** 523–531. [11]
- Hawkins, J. E., and Stevens, S. S. The masking of pure tones and of speech by white noise. *J. acoust. Soc. Am.*, 1950, **22,** 6–13.
- Marill, T. Psychophysics and signal detection theory. Massachusetts Institute of Technology: Research Laboratory of Electronics, 1956, Technical Report No. 319.
- Miller, G. A. Sensitivity to changes in the intensity of white noise and its relation to masking and loudness. *J. acoust. Soc. Am.*, 1947, **19,** 609–619.
- Peterson, W. W., and Birdsall, T. G. The theory of signal detectability. University of Michigan: Electronic Defense Group, 1953, Technical Report No. 13 (also available in 1954 Symposium on Information Theory, IRE Trans., September, 1954).
- Slepian, D. Some comments on the detection of Gaussian signals in Gaussian noise. *Trans. IRE Professional Group on Information Theory*, 1958, **PGIT-4,** 65–68.
- Tanner, W. P., Jr., and Swets, J. A. A decision-making theory of visual detection. *Psychol. Rev.*, 1954, **61,** 401–409.
- Tanner, W. P., Jr., Swets, J. A., and Green, D. M. Some general properties of the hearing mechanism. University of Michigan: Electronic Defense Group, 1956, Technical Report No. 30.
- Zwicker, E., Flottorp, G., and Stevens, S. S. Critical band width in loudness summation. *J. acoust. Soc. Am.*, 1957, **29,** 548–557.

28

Detection of Auditory Sinusoids of Uncertain Frequency

David M. Green

In an auditory detection experiment where the masking stimulus is noise and the signal is a sinusoid, a standard precaution is to make very sure that the observer is aware of the frequency of the signal. The reasons for this precaution are partly intuitive (one seems to listen for a sound of a certain frequency) and partly theoretical. (The concept of a critical band suggests that frequency analysis plays a very important role in this kind of experiment.) Recently, there have been several studies that have investigated the influence of signal-frequency uncertainty on the observer's ability to detect a sinusoidal signal in noise. The results have not been completely clear. One generally finds a decrease in the ability to detect the signal when frequency uncertainty is deliberately introduced, but the amount of this decrease is rather small. Whether this finding indicates that frequency uncertainty has relatively little influence or whether the conditions of the experiments were not sufficient to indicate the full effect of this variable is still in doubt.

The experiments reported in this paper, by employing extreme conditions of signal uncertainty, attempt to clarify this question. The results are in general agreement with the previous data as to the size of the decrease. They are, however, greatly inconsistent with several proposed models for the process, because this decrease was obtained under extreme conditions of frequency uncertainty. We shall first review the previous studies and discuss the inference drawn from these results. The experimental procedure and results of the present study will then be presented. Finally, the implications of these results will be discussed.

PREVIOUS STUDIES

All of the previous studies used the same basic experimental design. The signal is presented with equal probability in either one or the other of two separate time intervals. The subject is asked to detect the signal by selecting the correct interval. The experiment consists in first establishing a base line or standard from which the results of signal uncertainty may be evaluated. Thus several sinusoidal signals are equated in detectability by selecting an amplitude appropriate to each frequency. Once these amplitudes are established, the experimenter proceeds with the uncertain-frequency (or experimental) condition. In an uncertain-frequency condition the subject is told, for example, that one or another of some number of frequencies will be used as the signal on any given trial. Once more the subject's task is simply to detect the signal by selecting the correct temporal interval. The basic datum consists of a comparison of the percentage of correct detections in the known (control) and unknown (experimental) frequency conditions.

The first experimental results were reported by Tanner, Swets, and Green (1956). They noted a decrease in the percentage of correct detections for the condition where the signal might be either of two frequencies as compared with the fixed-frequency condition. The decrease was small but seemed to depend on the frequency separation of the two possible signals.

Veniar (1958*a*, *b*) reported several experiments; some repeated the condition of the Tanner, Swets, and Green study and some extended the number of possible signals in the uncertain-frequency condition. Her results cannot be summarized easily. There is considerable scatter in the data both between subjects and also for the same subject in similar conditions. For three or four subjects, the decrease associated with signal uncertainty increases as the frequency separation of the two signals increases. But it is doubtful that any statistical test would achieve the 5-per-cent level. Likewise, the decrease is greater for four or eight signal frequencies than it is for two. Once again, however, this trend is insufficient to receive statistical support.

Creelman (1960) has recently reported an extensive investigation on the variable of frequency separation when the uncertain-frequency conditions consist of one of two possible sinusoids. Once again, the variability of the data makes any simple conclusion hazardous.

Veniar's data and Creelman's data, while insufficient to establish conclusively the influence of the parameters on the decrease associated with the uncertain-frequency condition, have questioned several models that have been proposed to account for the phenomenon. Since these models have already been discussed in detail and since the data obtained in the present experiment directly clash with these models, they will be discussed only briefly.

The first model, the narrow-band scanning model, was suggested by Tanner, Swets, and Green (1956). This model is an extension of the concept of the critical band. It assumes that the first stage of the auditory process is a narrow-band filter that is adjustable in center frequency. The decrease found in the uncertain-frequency condition is therefore due to the filters' having been adjusted to the wrong frequency region on at least some portion of the trials. The manner of scanning is not specified.

Green (1958), investigating the detection of multiple sinusoidal signals in noise, rejected this model and suggested a multiple-band model. If the signal energy was not concentrated in frequency, it was assumed that the observer used several critical bands. For the multiple-tone experiment, using several critical bands was interpreted as simply adding the outputs of several simple band-pass filters. Thus the observer was sensitive to the frequency ranges that contained signal energy but, if we assume that the bands were added together, also listened to more masking noise. Hence the decrease resulted because the observer now listened to a larger number of critical bands, and, since the signal occurred in only one of these bands, the effective signal-to-noise ratio was decreased.

Creelman (1960) suggested a modification of this model. Instead of simply adding the outputs from several critical bands, he suggested that the decision rule might be based on the maximum output of each band. This modification predicts a higher percentage of correct detections in the uncertain-frequency condition (less decrease) than the model suggested by Green.

None of these models has received consistent support from the experimental data of Creelman and Veniar. But in both experiments one can find particular conditions and subjects for which the results are in close agreement with one of the models. For these restricted conditions of frequency uncertainty, the predictions based on any of the models do not differ greatly. In addition, the nature of the experiment leads to a considerable amount of variability in the results because the basic datum is a comparison of two experimentally determined percentages and is, therefore, subject to two possible sources of error. Unless extreme conditions of signal uncertainty are used, it seems likely that no very strong conclusions can be drawn either about the models or the process itself.

In the present experiment the aim was to establish both the magnitude of the phenomenon and the importance of certain obvious physical variables.

EXPERIMENTAL PROCEDURE

In a typical experimental session, the observer listened to 100 two-alternative forced-choice trials. On each trial he judged in which of the two temporal intervals a sinusoidal signal was presented in a continuous background of masking noise. The noise was presented at a spectrum level of 40 db *re* 0.0002 d/cm^2. The signal was gated for a specific duration without regard to phase. The observers listened binaurally with both headphones in phase.

The two-alternative forced-choice procedure used the following temporal sequence: (1) warning interval, 150 msec; (2) space, 500 msec; (3) first observation interval, duration of the signal; (4) space, 600 msec; (5) second observation interval, duration of the signal; (6) space, 100 msec; (7) answer interval, 1300 msec; (8) feedback interval, informing the observer of the correct answer, 100 msec; (9) space, 350 msec. Hence the total trial duration was 3.3 sec if the signal duration was 100 msec. One hundred such trials constituted a single session, and 8 to 10 such sessions were conducted each day in a two-hour period.

One of two general conditions prevailed in any given experimental session. Either the signal on each trial was a sinusoid of some fixed frequency or the signal was a sinusoid randomly selected on each trial from some range of signal frequencies. The selection of the frequency of the signal in the uncertain-frequency condition was accomplished as follows. A pushbutton oscillator generated the signal. Frequencies were designated within some given range that could be conveniently obtained by selecting buttons on the oscillator. These frequencies were then selected at random to be the signal on any given trial of the session. For example, for the range of 500 cps about the center frequency of 2250 cps, the frequencies were 2000, 2010, 2020, ··· 2480, 2490, 2500 cps. There were 51 such frequencies and each one could be selected, with equal probability, as the signal frequency on any single trial of the session.

Considerable effort was made to clarify the exact conditions of the experiment before each experimental session. When a fixed signal frequency was used, it was presented several times at a high level before the session. In the uncertain-frequency condition the center frequency and both extreme frequencies of the range were presented several times at a high signal level before the actual session began. Before any experimental session began the subjects reported that they understood the task and were ready.

In the main experiment, the center frequency was 2250 cps, and ranges of 100, 300, 500, 1000, and 3500 cps were used in the uncertain-frequency conditions. In addition, signal duration was varied for a range of 1500 cps about a center frequency of 1250 cps. Finally, a small amount of data was collected at a 0.1-sec duration for various center frequencies.

For each experimental condition the signal level was varied in order to trace out a psychometric function. Most of the main results of the experiment are reported as the signal energy to noise-power density necessary for 75-per-cent-correct detections.[1] This value was obtained by fitting the psychometric function by eye with a monotonically increasing curve with asymptotes at 50 per cent and 100 per cent.

Before discussing the experimental results we must outline our method of determining the amplitude of the signal in the uncertain-frequency condition.

Signal level and the signal filter

It is well known that two sinusoids of different frequency and the same amplitude are not generally equally detectable in white noise. In the uncertain-frequency condition, where different frequencies are used for the signal, it would facilitate any comparison we wish to make if somehow we could equate the detectability of these different frequencies. To accomplish this objective we constructed a filter that differentially weighted the amplitudes of the various sinusoids so that they were roughly of equal detectability in white noise. This weighting function was obtained from previous data (Green, McKey, and Licklider, 1959). For all experimental conditions except one noted later, this filter was placed across the oscillator. The signal energy when the signal is of fixed frequency is simply signal energy measured at the headphone. When signal energy is reported for an uncertain-frequency condition, this refers to the signal energy of the center frequency of the range. The higher frequencies of this range were presented at a greater energy and the lower frequencies at a smaller energy. Their detectability, however, is

[1] Signal energy (E) is the square of signal amplitude integrated for the duration of the signal. Noise-power density (N_0) is the average noise power in a one-cycle band. The quantity $10 \log E/N_0$ is denoted by a script $\mathcal{E} - \mathcal{N}_0$ throughout the paper.

roughly the same. This measure is unambiguous, and a certain decibel change in this energy means that all of the frequencies of the range are changed by the same amount. To demonstrate the effectiveness of the attempt to equate the detectability of different frequencies, for the observers in the present experiment, the data of Fig. 1 are presented. The filter characteristic is displayed as the solid line in Fig. 1.

The data points are the logarithm of signal energy to noise-power density necessary for 75 per cent when a fixed signal frequency was used. If the "equal-detectability" filter exactly accomplished its objective for these subjects, we would expect the data points to scatter about the line. The magnitude of the departure is fairly small (about 1 db). Thus in an uncertain-signal-frequency condition the signals of different frequencies will have different energies (as indicated by the solid line of Fig. 1). The detectability of these signals will be approximately the same.[2]

EXPERIMENTAL RESULTS

Detection as a function of the range of uncertainty

In this experiment the main variable is the range of signal-frequency uncertainty. The duration of the signal is 100 msec. The center frequency

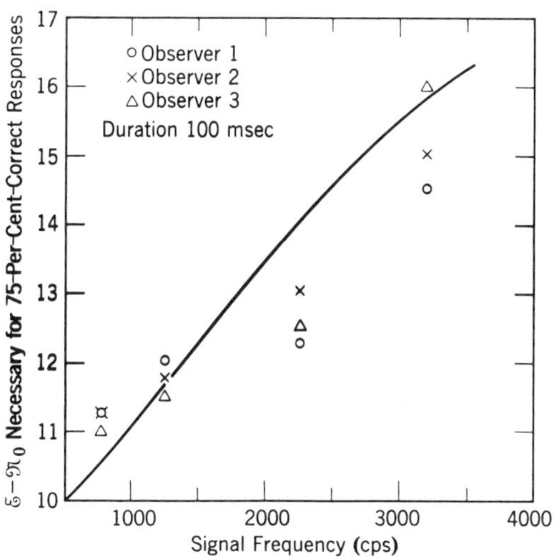

FIG. 1. The points indicate the ratio of signal energy to noise-power density in decibels necessary for the observers to attain 75-per-cent-correct detections. The signal frequency is indicated by the abscissa. The solid line depicts the relative gain in decibels of the "equal-detectability" filter as a function of frequency.

[2] The analysis presented in the Appendix is also relevant here.

of the range is always 2250 cps. Six signal ranges were used: 0 (no uncertainty), 100, 300, 500, 1000, and 3500 cps. We shall present the results by contrasting the signal energy needed in each condition to obtain a certain percentage of correct detections. First, however, let us establish that this comparison is not greatly affected by the particular level of detection that we select.

Figure 2 shows the psychometric functions obtained for a variety of the experimental conditions. For each particular condition the function has been shifted by a number of decibels so that the 75-per-cent point occurs near 5 db on the arbitrary scale of this figure. The collection of points to the left represents all those conditions in which the signal frequency was fixed. The collection of points at the right is a sample of the various ranges of signal uncertainty. The percentage is the proportion of correct responses on 400 trials. The main point to be noted is that the functions appear similar in form. This greatly simplifies the summary of the data, since to compare any two experimental conditions we need only contrast the signal intensity in decibels needed to achieve some arbitrary percentage of correct detections. We shall use the value of 75-per-cent-correct detections because it is probably the most stable point on the function. Any conclusions drawn by contrasting the signal conditions at

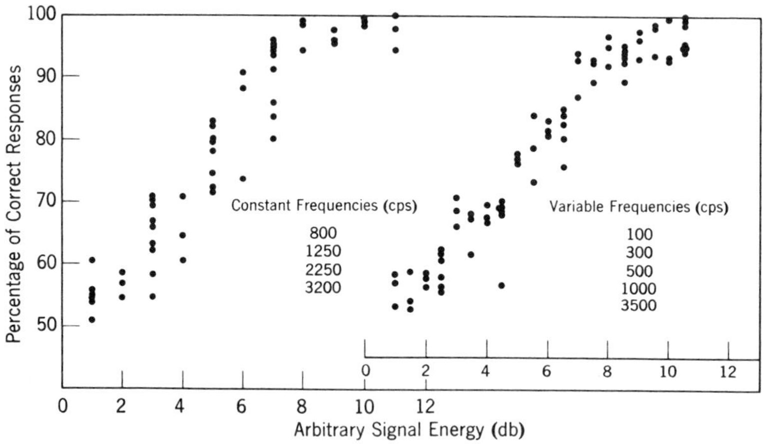

FIG. 2. Several specific psychometric functions obtained in both fixed and variable signal-frequency conditions. Each specific condition relates the signal energy to the percentage of correct detections in a two-interval forced-choice procedure. These functions are plotted together by adjusting each curve so that the 75-per-cent point occurs at about 5 db on the arbitrary scale of signal energy. The main point to note is that the shapes of the functions do not differ markedly.

this value would be approximately the same as for any other value selected.

Figure 3 shows the main experimental results. It shows how one must increase the signal energy to maintain 75-per-cent-correct detection as the signal range is increased. An $\mathcal{E} - \mathfrak{N}_0$ value of approximately 12.5 db was necessary in the fixed-frequency condition. As the range of signal frequency increased up to a range extending from 500 to 4000 cps, the signal level was raised about 3 db in order to achieve the same percentage of detection.[3] The solid line is drawn through the means of the three points. In this experiment, frequency uncertainty is at least an order of magnitude greater than that used in previous experiments, yet the extreme decrease is no more than 3 db. This decrease caused by signal-frequency uncertainty is very small compared with the prediction based on the models we considered earlier. Before discussing this point in detail, however, let us consider two other experimental variables: (1) the duration of the signal and (2) the center frequency of the range.

Duration of signal and center frequency

At a center frequency of 1250 cps we compared the decrease in detectability caused by signal-frequency uncertainty for a fixed range of 1500 cps (500 to 2000 cps). This comparison was carried out at 4 signal dura-

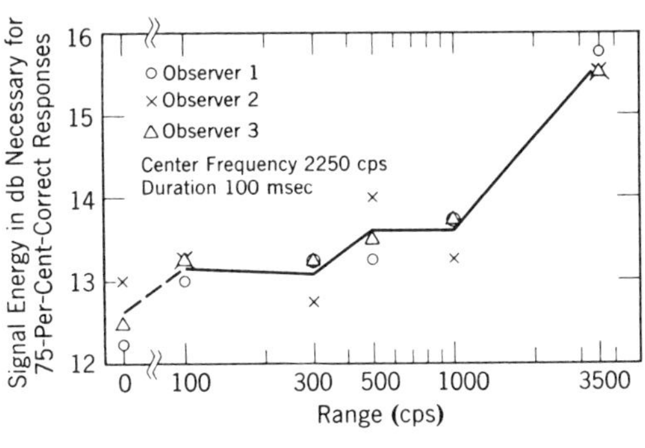

FIG. 3. Graph showing how the signal energy in decibels must be increased to maintain the same percentage of correct detections as the range of signal-frequency uncertainty is increased. For example, using the 3500-cps range, the signal might occur anywhere between 500 and 4000 cps. The signal energy was increased from about 12.5 db in the fixed-frequency condition, 0 range, to about 15.5 db for the 3500-cps range. The ordinate is in fact the quantity $\mathcal{E} - \mathfrak{N}_0$ for the zero-range condition.

[3] This means that the signal level of all frequencies was raised 3 db.

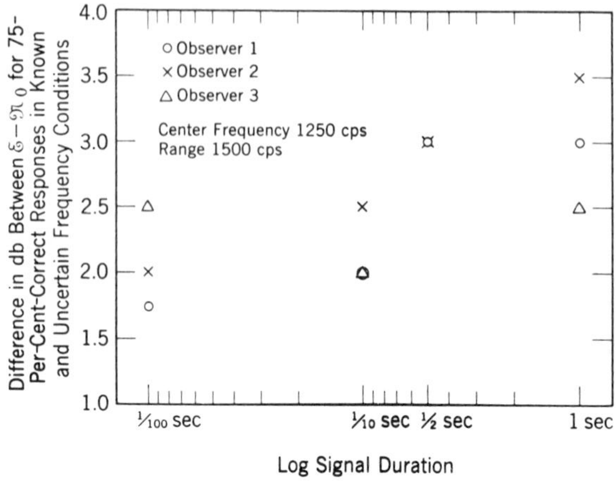

FIG. 4. The ordinate represents the decrease in signal detectability, caused by introducing signal-frequency uncertainty, as a function of signal duration. The ordinate is the signal energy in decibels needed to obtain 75-per-cent-correct responses in the uncertain-frequency condition, minus the signal energy in decibels needed to obtain 75-per-cent-correct responses in the fixed-signal frequency condition.

tions. Figure 4 shows the result of this experiment. Each point is plotted by contrasting the signal energy necessary for 75 per cent, when the signal frequency is fixed, with the signal energy at the same duration when the signal may occur anywhere in a 1500-cps range.[4] The decrease appears to depend on the duration, but the magnitude of this effect is very small (about 1 db for two logarithmic units of signal duration).

One should note, however, that the decrease at 100 msec (about 2 to 2.5 db) is somewhat larger than that obtained for the same duration but at a higher center frequency (Fig. 3). At the higher center frequency, 2250 cps, a decrease of about 1 db for a range of 1000 cps is noted. Table I summarizes the results of different ranges at different center frequencies. Although it is extremely difficult to obtain precise relations with so small a decrease, there is a small but consistent trend indicating that the effects of uncertainty are dependent on center frequency. For example, with a range of about 500 cps, an average decrease of 1.6 db is obtained

[4] For the 10-msec duration no filter was used to equate the detectability of the different frequencies. This procedure was adopted because of the data of Green (1959). Data obtained for three fixed frequencies (500, 1250, 2000 cps) at this duration were not consistent for all observers. Observer 3, in particular, indicated that the highest frequency (2000 cps) was not as easily detectable as the lower two. This may explain why his data point is higher at this duration than at the other two frequencies.

TABLE I. Comparison of Decrease[a] over Range and Center Frequency; Duration: 100 msec

Center frequency (cps)	Range (cps)	Observer	Decrease	Mean decrease
800	600	1	1.25	1.6 db
		2	1.75	
		3	1.75	
2250	500	1	1.00	1.00 db
		2	1.00	
		3	1.00	
2250	1000	1	1.50	1.00 db
		2	0.25	
		3	1.25	
3200	1600	1	0.75	0.32 db
		2	0.50	
		3	0.25	

[a] Decrease is $\mathcal{E} - \mathfrak{N}_0$ for 75 per cent in known-minus-unknown condition.

at a center frequency of 800 cps, whereas at 2250-cps center frequency the value is 1.0 db. Similarly, at a center frequency of 2250 cps the decrease is larger than at the higher center frequency of 3200 cps, where there is an even greater range of frequency uncertainty. The tentative conclusion is that for a given range the decrease in signal detectability caused by frequency uncertainty will be less, the higher the center frequency of the range. One might, of course, take some transformation of frequency and measure the range as the difference between the high and low frequency on this transform scale. The decrease might be nearly independent of center frequency if some convex function such as the logarithm of frequency were used as the transformation.

Implications

Let us consider the largest decrease arising from signal uncertainty observed in any of the experiments. Figure 3 shows that for a 100-msec duration and a center frequency of 2250 cps, a range of signal uncertainty of 3500 cps necessitates an increase of 3 db in signal power to hold detectability constant. The size of the decrease predicted by the narrow-band scanning model is difficult to evaluate because the model is not specific about details of the mode and rate of scan. It seems intuitively clear, however, that the decrease will be a great deal larger than 3 db.[5] Furthermore, such a model would predict that signal duration would play a very critical role. The results indicate that it does not, and the trend of the data is even in the wrong direction for this model.

According to the multiple-band model, the decrease will be 5 times the logarithm of the number of critical bands needed to span the range. Fortunately, we need not worry too much about the exact size of the critical bandwidth or even the number of such bands because the most favorable calculation indicates that the model predicts a decrease of at least 10 db for the extreme range of frequency uncertainty. Hence this model fails by at least 7 db.

Frequency information

Even more damaging to the multiple-band model are the following data. In a separate experiment, in which the range was 3500 cps, the observer was asked to say whether he thought the signal was high or low in frequency. The mid-value of 2250 cps was used as the dividing line, and the subjects were instructed to indicate whether the signal presented was higher or lower in frequency than this value. No detection response was required. The signal occurred randomly in either the first or second observation interval; the subject listened to both and responded "high" or "low." The data are displayed in Fig. 5. The solid-line segments indicate the mean detection data, i.e., responses concerning the temporal occurrence of the signal, independent of frequency. It is clear from Fig. 5 that at any given signal energy the subject has, in addition to information about the presence and absence of the signal, some information about the gross frequency characteristic of the signal. The difference in signal energy required for an identifying response as opposed to a detection response appears to be no greater than 1 to 2 db. This result in itself severely taxes any model that asserts that the observer acts like a broadband energy detector. The data indicate that some frequency information is preserved, but they do not permit one to estimate the exact amount of this information. We can only say that at a given signal intensity, the observers are about as accurate in a two-choice decision about the frequency characteristics of the signal as they are in a two-choice decision about the temporal occurrence of the signal.

[5] If we assume a very simple linear scan model, the decrease caused by frequency uncertainty should be greater than 12 db. See Batten, Jorgensen, Macnee, and Peterson (1952).

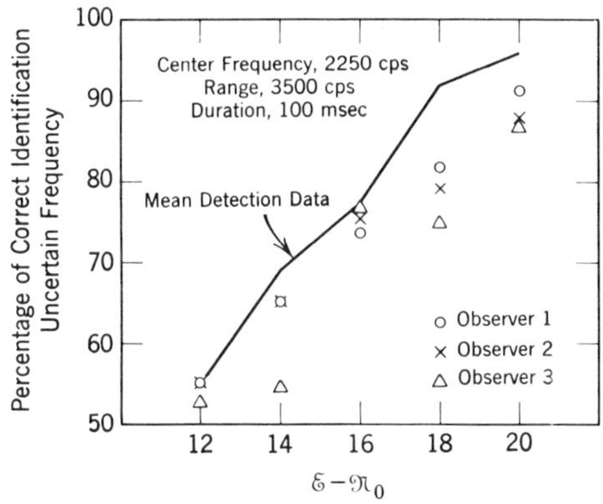

FIG. 5. The ordinate is the percentage of responses that indicated correctly whether the signal frequency on each trial was higher or lower than the mid-value of 2250 cps. The abscissa is the ratio of the signal energy to noise-power density in decibels. The solid line is the mean percentage correct for the three observers in the detection experiment, in which the observers indicated the temporal occurrence of the signal independent of signal frequency.

CONCLUSION

The results of these experiments indicate that there is a relatively small change in the ability of the observers to detect sinusoids in noise caused by the introduction of frequency uncertainty. Even in the most extreme conditions (where the signal might be anywhere between 500 and 4000 cps) an increase in signal power by a factor of two was sufficient to offset the decrease caused by frequency uncertainty. We also know that this result is not confined to the particular mode of stimulus uncertainty used in this study.

Recently, Egan, Schulman, and Greenberg (1959) studied the effects of *temporal* uncertainty on the detectability of a gated sinusoidal signal in noise. In their most extreme condition of uncertainty a signal, 0.25 sec in duration might occur, with equal probability, in any one of 16 non-overlapping segments of a 4.0-sec interval. The effect of such temporal uncertainty was to decrease the signal detectability by about 2 db.

Thus we see that experimentally-introduced uncertainty about the two major signal parameters, frequency and time, affects detectability very little. We must not conclude, however, that signal uncertainty plays a relatively minor role in this detection situation. Rather, we shall now argue that signal uncertainty plays a major role in determining the detectability of sinusoidal signals in noise.

The argument runs as follows. First, we should realize that the effects of signal uncertainty have been evaluated by comparing the detectability of some physically-fixed frequency and time condition. But simply because the physical conditions are fixed and specified, we need not infer that the observer knows these values exactly. The observer may be quite uncertain about both the signal frequency and the precise temporal occurrence of the signal. In fact, if we assume that there is a considerable amount of initial uncertainty about the signal parameters, we can expect comparatively little change in detectability as we introduce experimentally various degrees of signal uncertainty.

Let us consider this point in somewhat greater detail. Assume that we have a detection situation with white Gaussian noise as the masking stimulus. The signal to be detected is not specified exactly; rather, a class of possible signals is specified. On any given trial a signal is presented by a random (equiprobable) selection of one member from this class. Each signal is assumed to have the same energy and each signal is assumed to be orthogonal to all other $(M - 1)$ signals.[6] If $M = 1$ we have, of course, a situation in which the signal is specified exactly: there is no signal uncertainty. If $M = 2$, the signal might be either $s_1(t) = a(\sin wt)$ with $0 < t < T$, or $s_2(t) = a(-\sin wt)$ with $0 < t < T$. Alternatively, we might think of $s_1(t)$ as $a \sin w_1 t$ and $s_2(t)$ as $a \sin w_2 t$, where w_1 and w_2 are such that the integral of the cross-product over the observation interval is zero. For example, if the signal duration is 1.0 sec, the sine wave might have a frequency of either 1000 cps or 1001 cps; this would then represent frequency uncertainty. Similarly, we might consider the observation interval to be 2.0 sec long and think of two orthogonal signals as being a 1.0-sec signal occurring in either the first or second half of the 2.0-sec interval. We would then have a case of temporal uncertainty.

Peterson, Birdsall, and Fox (1954), assuming a particular representation of noise, have determined how the detection of these signals depends on the number M of such signals for an optimum likelihood-ratio detection device. Whatever the mode of uncertainty, whether frequency or time, the degree of uncertainty is measured by the number of possible signals M. As M increases, we find, as we might expect, that the signal energy must be increased in order to hold the detectability of the signal constant. For example, if we increase M from 1 to 10, we must increase

---

[6] Two signals, $s_1(t)$ and $s_2(t)$, which are orthogonal, satisfy the following relation $\int_0^T s_1(t)s_2(t)\,dt = 0$, where T is the duration over which the signals may occur. The assumption of orthogonality is equivalent to an assumption of independence in the statistical treatment of such signals. Though somewhat restrictive, this assumption greatly simplifies the mathematical derivations.

the signal power by approximately 4.5 db in order to maintain 75-per-cent correct detection in a two-interval forced-choice detection task. The important point, however, is that a further increase in uncertainty does not necessitate a corresponding increase in signal power. For example, increasing signal uncertainty of M from 10 to 100 can be offset by an increase in signal power of only about 2.5 db. Thus one soon finds a point of diminishing returns for increases in signal uncertainty.

This general result of a highly nonlinear relation between increases in uncertainty and increases in signal power is not restricted to devices that employ likelihood ratio in the decision procedure. The author has considered a different, less-than-optimum, decision procedure and obtained results that are similar. In this model we might think of a decision based on the cross-correlation of the incoming waveform and the set of stored signals representing the set of possible signals. If the signal might occur in either of two intervals (as in a two-interval forced-choice situation) the decision rule was simply to pick the interval in which the largest normalized correlation occurred. Thus, if M equals 2, there are four correlations: two in the first observation interval and two in the second. The maximum value of these four correlations would occur in either the first or the second observation interval, and that interval would be chosen in the decision. Once again, a highly nonlinear relation between the parameter M and the signal energy necessary to maintain a constant percentage of correct decisions resulted.

Thus we are suggesting that the results obtained in detection experiments, where we introduce uncertainty experimentally, can best be understood by assuming that even in the fixed-signal situation the observer has a considerable amount of initial uncertainty. Another way of expressing this idea is to observe that the models considered earlier in the paper had one common characteristic; they all assumed that the hypothesis tested in the detection task was the presence or absence of a particular signal. All of these models lead one to expect a rather large change in detectability as the class of possible signals increases. The uncertainty models, on the other hand, postulate that even in the single-signal situation the observer is in fact testing for the presence or absence of a large class of signals. Hence the change in detection, as uncertainty is deliberately introduced, is rather small.

Obviously, this hypothesis of large initial uncertainty is not the only possible explanation of the results obtained. One might, for example, claim that two quite separate mechanisms are responsible for the results obtained with fixed and uncertain signal conditions. In addition to appealing to parsimony, I would point out one other virtue of the hypothesis of initial uncertainty: the psychometric functions that might be expected on the basis of a large-uncertainty ($M = 20$) model appear to fit the observed data. Since this point has been presented in a previous paper (Green, 1960) it will not be discussed here.

In summary, the explanation that the author advances is that an observer in a detection task—even with fixed and specified signals—is in large part uncertain about the parameters of these signals. Experimental changes in certain aspects of the signal, such as frequency or time of occurrence of the signal, will increase this uncertainty. This increase will necessitate an increase in the power of the signal in order to maintain the same level of detectability. However, the increase in signal power will be rather small (2 or 3 db) because the signal uncertainty is not initially small but rather large, and a point of diminishing returns has already been reached.

SUMMARY

The decrease in the detectability of a gated sinusoidal signal in noise caused by deliberately introducing uncertainty about the signal's frequency is no greater than 3 db, even in an extreme condition of uncertainty. In this extreme condition the signal duration is 0.1 sec, and the signal frequency is varied between 500 and 4000 cps. This effect is not critically dependent on signal duration. Moreover, the observers not only detect the signal but display at least gross information about the frequency of the signal in the uncertain-frequency conditions.

Several models, suggested in previous studies, are considered. The magnitude of the decrease observed in the data falls far short of the predictions of these models. An interpretation suggested by the data is that the observers in a detection task, even when a signal of fixed frequency is used, are highly uncertain as to the exact physical parameters of the signal. Another way of stating this assumption is to say that the observer never tests for the presence or absence of a signal on the basis of one simple hypothesis. From this assumption we should expect little decrease in detectability from deliberately introducing frequency uncertainty. This interpretation suggests that the same result would be obtained if time were the major experimental variable.

APPENDIX

In each uncertain-frequency condition we have a complete trial-by-trial record of the signal frequency used and whether or not each observer responded correctly. For several conditions we analyzed the proportions of correct responses as a function of signal frequency. For example, with a range of signal frequency from 500 to 4000 cps the proportion of correct responses occurring in ten bands of frequency, each 350 cps wide, was determined. If the observers were prone to listen at one or another frequency region, or if the amplitudes of the signals were such that the signals were not equally detectable, we should expect some of these proportions to be higher than others. A chi-square test was used to determine whether or not the observed differences in these proportions represented anything more than sampling fluctuation. These tests were conducted in sessions in which the observers were obtaining about 75-per-cent-correct detections, since data in which the percentage is much higher or lower would be inappropriate for our purpose. Of a dozen or so analyses, only one achieved the 5-per-cent level of significance. Inspection of this individual's data revealed (it was observer 1 in the range 3500-cps, 0.1-sec experiment) that he obtained more correct decisions on the high-frequency signals (about 80 per cent for signals above 2000 cps) and fewer on the lower-frequency signals (about 70 per cent). This result is consistent with the detection data shown in Fig. 1. For no other condition or observer was a significant chi-square value obtained. It is concluded, therefore, that the "equal-detectability" filter achieved its objective, and the observers showed no striking inclination to attend to any particular frequency range in an uncertain-frequency condition.

ACKNOWLEDGMENTS

This research was conducted in the Research Laboratory of Electronics of the Massachusetts Institute of Technology with support from the U. S. Air Force (Operational Applications Laboratory, and Office of Scientific Research), Signal Corps, and Office of Naval Research. This article appeared as Tech. Rept. No. AFCCDD-TR-61-8, and in J. acoust. Soc. Am., *1961,* **33,** *897–903.*

References

- Batten, H. W., Jorgensen, R. A., Macnee, A. B., and Peterson, W. W. The response of a panoramic receiver to CW and pulse signals. University of Michigan: Electronic Defense Group, 1952, Technical Report No. 3.
- Creelman, C. D. Detection of signals of uncertain frequency. *J. acoust. Soc. Am.,* 1960, **32,** 805–810.
- Egan, J. P., Schulman, A. I., and Greenberg, G. Z. Detection of signals presented at random times. *J. acoust. Soc. Am.,* 1959, **31,** 1579. (Abstract)
- Green, D. M. Detection of multiple component signals in noise. *J. acoust. Soc. Am.,* 1958, **30,** 904–911. [25]

- Green, D. M. Detection of a pulsed auditory signal in noise as a function of duration and frequency. *J. acoust. Soc. Am.*, 1959, **31,** 836. (Abstract)
- Green, D. M. Psychoacoustics and detection theory. *J. acoust. Soc. Am.*, 1960, **32,** 1189–1203. [2]
- Green, D. M., McKey, M. J., and Licklider, J. C. R. Detection of a pulsed sinusoid in noise as a function of frequency. *J. acoust. Soc. Am.*, 1959, **31,** 1446–1452. [26]
- Peterson, W. W., Birdsall, T. G., and Fox, W. C. The theory of signal detectability. *Trans. IRE Professional Group on Information Theory,* 1954, **PGIT-4,** 171–212.
- Tanner, W. P., Jr., Swets, J. A., and Green, D. M. Some general properties of the hearing mechanism. University of Michigan: Electronic Defense Group, 1956, Technical Report No. 30.
- Veniar, F. A. Signal detection as a function of frequency ensemble, I. *J. acoust. Soc. Am.*, 1958*a*, **30,** 1020–1024; II. *J. acoust. Soc. Am.*, 1958*b*, **30,** 1075–1078.

29

Central Factors in Auditory-Frequency Selectivity

John A. Swets

In 1940, Harvey Fletcher reported an experiment that established the psychophysical study of auditory-frequency analysis. His paper introduced the concept of the "critical band," the band of frequencies over which the listener integrates acoustic power, and his experiment provided a basis for quantifying the concept. Fletcher's experiment showed that only noise components in a narrow region about a pure tone are effective in masking the tone. He found, in particular, that the amplitude required for a tone to be just detectable remained constant, despite variations in the width of a band of noise surrounding the tone, if these bands were wider than some critical value. For bands of noise that were narrower than the critical value, the amplitude of the just-detectable tone decreased as the width of the band of noise decreased. He also observed that the width of the critical band increased with its center frequency; the width of the critical band appeared to be approximately 7 per cent of its center frequency over a large range.

Fletcher was concerned with the peripheral aspects of the process of frequency analysis, with the frequency selectivity that is accomplished in the ear. Illustrative of this interest is his suggestion that the critical bandwidths at different center frequencies represent equal distances on the basilar membrane. Other investigations have followed in this tradition, including those of Schafer, Gales, Shewmaker, and Thompson (1950), Hamilton (1957), Zwicker, Flottorp, and Stevens (1957), Greenwood (1961*a*), and Swets, Green, and Tanner (1962). Four of these studies, all those except that of Zwicker et al., confirmed Fletcher's basic result in experiments that were similar to his; two of them (Schafer et al. and Swets et al.) showed close quantitative agreement with Fletcher's estimate of the critical bandwidth. Zwicker et al. showed the existence of a critical band in several different kinds of psychophysical experiments: experiments on masking of noise by tones, on loudness summation, on detection of multiple tones, and on phase sensitivity. Although these different experiments showed a dependence of critical bandwidth on frequency similar to that observed by Fletcher, they have led, along with the replications of Fletcher's experiment by Hamilton and by Greenwood, to substantially greater estimates of the width of the critical band. The estimates of critical bandwidth obtained in these experiments are, on the average, 15 to 20 per cent of the center frequency of the band. Both Zwicker et al. and Greenwood have pursued the suggestion that the critical bandwidth may be simply related to the anatomy of the ear. Greenwood (1961*b*) accepts as valid the larger estimates of critical bandwidth and concludes that each critical band corresponds to one millimeter along the basilar membrane. Scharf (1961) has recently reviewed most of the studies that focus on peripheral frequency analysis.

By the mid-1950's, there became apparent several reasons for considering the role of central, or cognitive, factors in the process of auditory-frequency analysis. In general, it seemed fruitful to view the auditory analysis system as including more than fixed sensory elements, and to examine the way in which adaptive portions of this larger system adjust to different auditory tasks. The approach to the analysis process on this different, but perhaps not entirely independent, level of inquiry originated with the work of Tanner, Swets, and Green (1956). It is exemplified in the studies of Karoly and Isaacson (1956), Tanner (1956), Green (1958, 1960, 1961), Veniar (1958), Swets, Shipley, McKey, and Green (1959), Green, McKey, and Licklider (1959), Creelman (1960), and Swets and Sewall (1961). The following pages review this research effort. After a consideration of the motivation for the research, the two theoretical models that have been proposed to incorporate the action of central factors are discussed, and the experiments conducted to test predictions from these models are described.

THE MOTIVATION FOR AN EXAMINATION OF CENTRAL FACTORS

Not all of the reasons for assuming and investigating adaptive aspects in auditory-frequency analysis are clear for, to some extent, they derive from the spirit of the times. We shall, however, attempt a brief characterization of this spirit, and we shall single out the more important details.

DEVELOPMENTS IN NEUROPHYSIOLOGICAL AND IN PSYCHOLOGICAL THEORY. It is now a commonplace that much of psychological theory rests implicitly on prevailing neurophysiological concepts. Before and for some time after Fletcher's work, the conceptual nervous system was a passive system, in which only those energy changes at the receptor determined what information was conveyed to the brain. In the 1950's neurophysiological theory adapted to the rapidly accumulating evidence that sensory information is fed into a central nervous system that is continuously active and organized, and that extensively modulates the sensory flow, in part through efferent control of receptors (Lashley, 1951; Sperry, 1952; Hebb, 1949, 1955). Experimental results in audition which are illustrative of this newer conception are the finding that a cat's auditory nerve activity in response to a clicking sound can be inhibited by impulses aroused in the brain which pass out to the cochlea (Galambos, 1956), and the finding that the electrical response of the cat's auditory cortex to a click vanishes after a period of habituation, reappears if the click is paired with a noxious stimulus, and disappears again when the click is no longer followed by the noxious stimulus (Galambos, Sheatz, and Vernier, 1956).

Quite independent of the impetus from neurophysiology, several developments within psychology have contributed to the recent concern for central factors in sensory processes. One of particular relevance, noted by Broadbent (1962), is the research on the human operator's ability to process information which has helped to make respectable again the concept of attention. Broadbent's paper describes recent experiments on listening to two voice messages simultaneously. The results of those experiments are in good agreement with the experimental results reviewed in the following pages.

SPECIFICATION OF CENTRAL FACTORS IN THE DETECTION PROCESS. Another circumstance that suggests that central factors play a part in the process of frequency selectivity is the finding that they play a very large part in even the simplest sensory-detection task. In general, the detection of a fixed signal by a practiced observer depends critically on the observer's information about the probability of signal occurrence, on his information about the values and costs associated with the various response outcomes, and on his detection goal (Tanner and Swets, 1954; Swets, 1961). Furthermore, a number of studies have shown that the observer performs better when he has more information about the physical characteristics of the signal, and that this information affects the receptive system rather than the response system. One example comes from an experiment in which the observer was required to detect a tonal signal that could, at random, have either of two specified frequencies. Telling the observer which frequency occurred on a given trial, after the occurrence of the signal, had little, if any, effect; whereas similar frequency information given before the trial improved the detection significantly (Swets and Sewall, 1961). In another experiment, relatively strong and weak tonal signals of constant frequency were presented at random. A higher proportion of correct responses was observed on the trials following a correct response to a strong signal than on the trials following a correct response to a weak signal. This result suggests that strong signals provide better cues to the nature of the signal than do weak signals, and that the observer's perceptual set is correspondingly better after a strong signal (Shipley, 1959). Other studies have demonstrated that the observer's efficiency in detecting a given signal is markedly improved when cues to the nature of the signal, or aids to the observer's memory, are provided along with the signal. Apparently the observer has a residual uncertainty about the signal's frequency even when a single frequency is used throughout a long series of trials. His performance is more efficient when he is required to detect an increment in a continuous, quite audible tone than it is when he is required to detect a tone burst in the absence of an immediate cue to frequency. Similarly, if the audible tone is pulsed, sometimes with the increment that constitutes the signal and sometimes without, this precise cue to the starting time and duration of the signal improves the observer's efficiency. Again, an immediate cue to the signal's amplitude is beneficial. When all of these aids to the observer's memory of the salient characteristics of the signal are present, the human observer's performance falls only about 3 db below that calculated for a mathematically ideal detector with complete knowledge of the signal; without these aids, the observer falls short of the calculated ideal by 12 to 15 db (Swets, 1961).

DIVERSE ESTIMATES OF CRITICAL BANDWIDTH. More specific to the problem at hand, an investigation of central factors in frequency selectivity holds forth a promise of accounting for the large variability exhibited by various estimates of the critical bandwidth. The lack of agreement among the estimates, as noted, has presented a problem. There seems to be no good reason for discarding any of the estimates as unreliable, particularly because each of them has company. The differences, however, have not been reconciled. It is possible, of course, for the estimates to vary while the critical bandwidth underlying them is stable. A fixed critical bandwidth might manifest itself differently as different sensory tasks are posed for the observer; if, for example, the edges of the critical band have a gradual, rather than a steep, slope, then the effect of these edges on the experimental results would depend upon the frequency distribution and the intensity of the stimuli used in the experiment. Furthermore, as Hamilton (1957) has pointed out, small differences in experimental procedure and filter characteristics can lead to large differences in estimated critical-band values, even in experiments of the same type. Still another source of variability in the estimates is the particular shape of the critical band that is assumed in the analysis; Swets et al. (1962) have shown that a single set of data can lead to various estimates of the width of the critical band which correspond to various assumptions about its shape. Thus the variability observed might be attributable to differences in experimental procedure. It is also possible, on the other hand, that some of the variability in the estimates of the critical bandwidth results from variation in the analysis system. Different estimates may accurately reflect what are, in effect, different critical bandwidths, which have been adjusted to suit best the requirements of different auditory tasks.

THE OBVIOUS NEED TO TREAT CERTAIN CENTRAL FACTORS. Besides the *Zeitgeist*, the collateral evidence for central factors in auditory-frequency selectivity, and the possibility of reconciling various estimates of the critical bandwidth, is the clear evidence for the operation of certain central factors in the selection process. If the observer suppresses masking noise outside the critical band, then he must suppress signals outside the band as well. If signal and noise were separable, noise would not be noise. Moreover, if the observer's filter passes only the noise components in a band about 1000 cps when he is expecting a 1000-cps signal, and if only noise components about 2000 cps are effective when he is expecting a 2000-cps signal, then the analysis system is somehow different under these two circumstances. At least one parameter of the system is adjusted in accordance with the observer's expectations. The observer apparently controls in an intelligent way—that is, in accordance with information available to him and his goals—the focus of his attention. Several empirical questions that are relevant to frequency selectivity follow immediately from this statement. How rapidly can the observer adjust the center frequency of the critical band? With what precision? Can he adjust as well other parameters of the analysis system? Can he, for example, control the width of the critical band? Can he control the number of different critical bands that are operative at one time? The answers to questions like these were the aims of the theoretical and experimental work reviewed in the remainder of this paper.

THEORY AND EXPERIMENT

The single-band model of the process

In a first attempt to deal with central factors in the process of frequency selectivity, Tanner et al. (1956) developed what has been termed the single-band model of the process. In this model, as in Fletcher's conception, the observer is viewed at any given time as integrating acoustic power over only a limited range of frequencies. The single-band model goes beyond the original hypothesis of the critical band in making explicit the fact that the observer controls the momentary frequency location of this range. It is further asserted in the model, in order to be specific, that a change in the frequency location of the band of sensitivity is effected by sweeping the band through the intervening frequencies, and that the time required to make a change increases with the extent of the change. It may be noted that this model bears a strong resemblance to the familiar searchlight analogy of the process of attention.

Four different types of experiments were conducted to test various predictions derived from this model. In the various experiments, the observer was required to detect a signal at an unexpected frequency, to detect a signal that was equally likely to be either of two specified frequencies, to recognize which of two specified frequencies was presented, and to detect signals composed of two frequencies.

DETECTION OF A SIGNAL AT AN UNEXPECTED FREQUENCY. In the first experiment, Tanner et al. (1956) gave unpracticed observers several training sessions that employed only a 1000-cps signal, 0.15 sec in duration, in a continuous background of white noise. The four-alternative forced-choice method of response was used; that is, each trial consisted of four time intervals, only one of which contained the signal, and the observer indicated which interval he believed was most likely to have contained the signal. The proportion of correct responses, denoted $P(c)$, was taken as the measure of performance.

After the several practice sessions, unknown to the observers the signal frequency was changed to 1300 cps and presented with the energy that had yielded a $P(c) = 0.65$ for the 1000-cps signal. For the 1300-cps signal, $P(c)$ was very nearly 0.25, the value representing chance success. In later sessions in which the observers expected the signal to be 1300 cps, and after they had heard this frequency without noise, the $P(c)$ at the same signal energy was approximately 0.65. The essentials of this experiment were repeated by Karoly and Isaacson (unpublished) with similar results: unexpected signals of 500 cps and 1500 cps, presented infrequently on randomly selected trials, led to significantly lower values of $P(c)$ than did the expected signal of 1000 cps.

DETECTION OF ONE OF TWO SPECIFIED FREQUENCIES. In another experiment (Tanner et al., 1956) the observer knew that the signal would be either of two specified frequencies, and that the two were equally likely to occur on a given trial. Again, the four-alternative forced-choice method of response was used. The observers chose the interval that they believed contained the signal; they were not asked to identify the frequency that had been presented. The effects of the uncertainty were assessed by comparing the $P(c)$ obtained from groups of trials in which either frequency might occur, denoted $P(c)_{1v2}$, with the average value of $P(c)$ obtained when the observer knew that the signal would have only one of the two frequencies throughout a group of trials, denoted $P(c)_{1,2}$. The signal energies were adjusted so that $P(c)_1$ and $P(c)_2$ were very nearly equal.

According to the single-band model, $P(c)_{1v2}$ decreases as the separation between the two frequencies increases, that is, as it becomes less likely that the band of sensitivity is centered at the signal frequency that is presented. $P(c)_{1v2}$ reaches a minimum when the separation between the two frequencies is sufficiently large that the observer is unable to shift the band of sensitivity from one to the other during the time of the signal. This minimum is specified under the assumption that the observer listens for the frequency that is presented on one-half of the trials, and that, when he listens to the frequency presented, his probability of being correct is equal to what it is with a known frequency; on the other one-half of the trials, when the observer is listening for the wrong frequency, chance determines the probability of a correct detection. Thus the minimum $P(c)_{1v2} = (1/2)P(c)_{1,2} + (1/2)(1/4)$.

We shall reproduce here the results of this experiment, since the publication in which they appear is not generally available. They are shown in Table I. The left-hand column, labeled "Δf," shows the various frequency separations used in the experiment. The second column shows the frequencies used to produce each value of Δf. Each entry in the table under "$P(c)_{1,2}$" is based on 700 trials, 350 at each frequency. Each entry under "$P(c)_{1v2}$" is based on 250 trials. The column headed "Minimum $P(c)_{1v2}$" shows the extreme prediction of the single-band model. The column labeled "Decrement" shows the difference between $P(c)_{1v2}$ and $P(c)_{1,2}$. The right-hand column shows the duration of the signal.

In three of the four cases represented in Table I, $P(c)_{1v2}$ approaches very nearly, at the larger values of Δf, the minimum specified by the single-band model. In the fourth case, Observer 1 at 0.3 sec, there is the possibility that the experiment was not carried far enough, since the decrement from uncertainty has not reached a demonstrated maximum. There is also the suggestion in the data that the signal duration influences the size of the decrement in a direction that is consistent with the model, but, since only one observer participated at both signal durations, this conclusion remains tentative.

RECOGNITION OF TWO SPECIFIED FREQUENCIES. Tanner (1956) applied the single-band model to frequency recognition. In the recognition experiment, a signal having either of two specified frequencies occurred in the single observation interval of each trial, and the subject indicated which frequency he thought had occurred. Along with the presentation of a rationale for the fact that the $P(c)$ increases as the separation between the frequencies increases from a very small to a larger value, Tanner made explicit the prediction from the single-band model that, at some value of frequency separation, $P(c)$ would begin to decrease and would reach a specifiable minimum. The recognition would suffer at large values of Δf because the observer could not, presumably, listen for both frequencies during the time of the signal. The data obtained in the experiment on the detection of one of two frequencies suggested that, for 0.1-sec signals in the vicinity of 1000 cps, $P(c)$ would begin to decrease at a Δf of approximately 100 cps and reach a minimum at Δf = 300 cps.

The results of the recognition experiment were sufficiently variable that no very clear evidence for or against the prediction of the single-band model emerged. In general, the results were consistent with the prediction. For two short signal durations, 0.05 sec and 0.1 sec, $P(c)$ at frequency separations of 300 to 600 cps approached the minimum specified by the model. For durations of 0.5 sec and 1.0 sec, no decrease in $P(c)$ was evident as Δf increased, a result that is consistent with a capability of observing both frequencies, given sufficient time.

DETECTION OF A SIGNAL COMPOSED OF TWO FREQUENCIES. In an instance of the fourth type of experiment relevant to the single-band model, Marill (1956) presented two frequencies together. The observer stated in

TABLE I. DETECTION OF ONE OF TWO SPECIFIED FREQUENCIES COMPARED WITH THE PREDICTION OF THE SINGLE-BAND MODEL

		Observer 1				Observer 2				Observer 3				
Δf	Frequencies	$P(c)_{1,2}$	$P(c)_{1v2}$	Minimum $P(c)_{1v2}$	Decrement	$P(c)_{1,2}$	$P(c)_{1v2}$	Minimum $P(c)_{1v2}$	Decrement	$P(c)_{1,2}$	$P(c)_{1v2}$	Minimum $P(c)_{1v2}$	Decrement	Signal duration
50	1000, 1050	.88	.88	.57	.00	.84	.84	.55	.00					
150	900, 1050	.87	.78	.56	.09									0.3
250	800, 1050	.89	.74	.57	.15	.90	.55	.58	.35					sec
350	700, 1050	.86	.68	.56	.18	.90	.57	.58	.33					
100	900, 1000	.93	.89	.59	.04					.80	.75	.53	.05	
200	800, 1000	.92	.73	.59	.19					.78	.63	.52	.15	0.1
300	700, 1000	.85	.58	.55	.27					.71	.50	.48	.21	sec

which of the two time intervals on each trial he thought the compound signal occurred. Marill found that a compound signal with a Δf of 40 cps led to a significantly higher $P(c)$ than either of the two frequencies taken singly. In fact, this value of Δf produced perfect power summation. He found, also, that a compound signal with Δf = 600 cps showed no summation at all; the pair of frequencies was no more detectable than the more detectable member of the pair. This result is in agreement with the single-band model and with the results of the other three experiments described previously.

The multiband model of the process

A different attempt to deal with central factors in the analysis process is represented in the multiband model proposed by Green (1958). This model was developed specifically for the type of detection task studied by Marill, the detection of a signal composed of two frequencies. According to this model, the observer is capable of listening to any number of frequency bands at the same time. He selects the number and frequency locations of the bands to which he listens and bases his decision on the linear combination of the outputs of the bands he has selected. The model predicts a degree of power summation something less than perfect, even for large separations between the frequencies.

Experimental comparisons of the single-band and multiband models

DETECTION OF A SIGNAL COMPOSED OF TWO FREQUENCIES. The multiband model is inconsistent with the data reported by Marill, which show no summation for large values of Δf. However, Green (1958) reports data that are consistent with the model. He presented compound signals consisting of all possible pairs of 500 cps, 1000 cps, 1832 cps, and 2000 cps, and found very nearly the predicted amount of summation in every case.

The conflict between the results obtained by Marill and those obtained by Green has not been resolved. However, Green's results are in agreement with the earlier results of Schafer and Gales (1949), which also showed a degree of summation at large values of Δf. And in addition, they are in agreement with results that were obtained by Green et al. (1959) in an extension of the study of compound signals to signals composed of 16 frequencies. The frequencies used were all multiples of 250 cps. The use of 16 frequencies makes the difference between the summation and the no-summation predictions very large. The data from this experiment match very closely the predictions of the multiband model.

DETECTION OF ONE OF TWO SPECIFIED FREQUENCIES. The two models can also be compared with data on the detection of one of two specified frequencies. Derivation of the quantitative predictions from the multiband model for this type of experiment would take us too far afield, but it will be intuitively clear that the multiband model predicts that a decrement in $P(c)$ will result from frequency uncertainty. According to the model, the observer who listens to bands at both of the possible frequencies will be listening to more noise power, but not more signal power, than the observer who listens to a single band. Furthermore, the model leads to the prediction that $P(c)_{1v2}$ will decrease as the frequency separation increases, until, in terms of the model, the point of no overlap of the two bands is reached. The multiband model predicts values of $P(c)_{1v2}$ for extreme values of Δf that are somewhat greater than those predicted by the single-band model.

It may be recalled that the results of the detection of one of two frequencies given in Table I show three cases in close agreement with the single-band prediction. We can now observe that the fourth case, Observer 1 at a signal duration of 0.3 sec, agrees more closely with the prediction of the multiband model. (The $P(c)_{1v2}$ predicted from the multiband model for this case, Observer 1 at 0.3 sec, is 0.72. The multiband prediction for Observer 1 at 0.1 sec is 0.70; for Observer 2, 0.76; and for Observer 3, 0.58.) We note again, however, the possibility that the observed $P(c)_{1v2}$ that agrees more nearly with the multiband prediction would have decreased further had the experiment been carried to larger values of Δf.

After the arrival of the multiband model on the scene to compete with the single-band model, other experiments were conducted to compare the predictions of these models for the detection of one of two specified frequencies. Veniar (1958) found that two of her observers matched the multiband prediction while the decrement exhibited by the other two observers was even less than that predicted under the multiband assumption. Unfortunately, this experiment was not carried to large enough values of Δf to establish that the decrement had reached a maximum. Swets et al. (1959) found that two observers matched the single-band prediction and a third observer matched the multiband prediction. Creelman (1960) found that, when the $P(c)$ for the two frequencies taken individually was approximately 0.90, all four of his observers yielded data in close agreement with the multiband prediction; when the $P(c)$ for the individual frequencies was approximately 0.75, data from three of the observers agreed with the multiband prediction and the data from the fourth matched the single-band prediction. The same picture emerged when the experiment was repeated at a higher level of background noise. Swets and Sewall (1961) found that the data from their three observers matched the single-band prediction when the $P(c)$ for the single frequencies was approximately 0.75, and fell in between the two predictions at greater levels of signal strength. Swets (unpublished work), using signals that led to a $P(c)$ of approximately 0.90 when taken individually, found that both of his observers yielded results in good agreement with the predictions of the multiband model.

A different kind of evidence that is relevant to the attempt to distinguish between the two models is provided by an additional analysis of the data of one of the studies cited. Swets et al. (1959) made a contingency analysis of their data to determine the $P(c)$ on a given trial for each of the four conditions that could have held on the previous trial: (*a*) same frequency, correct response, (*b*) same frequency, incorrect response, (*c*) different frequency, correct response, and (*d*) different frequency, incorrect response. It was found that, if the same frequency were presented on two successive trials, the observer was more likely to be correct on the second if he had been correct on the first; the average difference in $P(c)$ between conditions *a* and *b* was 0.06. If different frequencies were presented on two successive trials, the observer was more likely to be correct on the second if he had been *incorrect* on the first; the average difference in $P(c)$ between conditions *c* and *d* was 0.12. This analysis provides support for the single-band model in its indication that the observer is differentially sensitive to the two frequencies at a given point in time, in particular, in the indication that the observer perseveres to some extent in listening to a given frequency band.

Present status of the single-band and multiband models

SUMMARY OF THE FOREGOING RESULTS. Both the single-band and multiband models are consistent with the studies of detection of an unexpected frequency. Concerning the detection of one of two specified frequencies, several studies favor one model and approximately an equal number of studies favor the other. A contingency analysis of the data in this type of experiment, however, offers fairly strong support for the single-band model. Although the results of the study of recognition of two specified frequencies are not entirely clear, they are in general agreement with the single-band model. The single-band model also gains an advantage in this case by default: the multiband model in its present form, with the assumption that a simple linear combination of the outputs of the sensitive bands takes place before the final detection stage, is not applicable to the recognition experiment. With respect to the detection of signals composed of two or more frequencies, there exist again conflicting results, but the general superiority of the multiband model for this type of experiment seems clear.

TASK-SPECIFIC RESULTS. We have compared the two models proposed to date with the results of different types of experiments under the tacit assumption that the models are thoroughly competitive—that experiments will single out one model as generally preferable to the other. This is a reasonable procedure to follow at first, for one of the models may indeed be disclosed as superior to the other for all of the experiments considered. To persist in regarding the models as strong rivals, in the absence of such a clear result, would not be in keeping with the spirit of the exploration of central factors. If central factors play a significant role, if the analysis process is subject to intelligent control, or, to state it still another way, if the observer can vary his strategy of listening to suit the requirements of different tasks, then we should examine the possibility that both of the models are satisfactory, but under different circumstances. From this point of view, a comparison of the models with the results of a variety of experimental tasks is undertaken to accentuate the relative strengths and weaknesses of the two models. We can note, as the outcome of the comparison, a tendency for the models to complement each other with respect to the several tasks we have considered. Let us briefly re-examine the evidence for task-specific results, with an eye toward the possibility that the observer is able to use either of the general strategies represented in the two models.

If we adopt the language of our models, we would say that, if the signal is composed of 16 frequencies separated by 250 cps, the observer listens with as many bands as there are frequencies, or perhaps with a single band that is as wide as the range of frequencies (Green et al., 1959). If the signal is composed of two frequencies, the observer listens, for reasons that are not evident, either with two bands (Green, 1958; Schafer and Gales, 1949) or with just one (Marill, 1956). It appears that if the signal is either of two specified frequencies, in which case the more efficient procedure is not readily apparent to the observer, especially at low signal levels, some observers listen with both bands and others with just one (Tanner et al., 1956; Veniar, 1958; Swets et al., 1959; Creelman, 1960; Swets and Sewall, 1961; Swets, unpublished work).

Green (1960) described another experiment that suggests that the observer can adjust to the demands of the task. In this experiment the signal was a band of noise 650 cps wide. The center frequency of the band was varied, with the observer's knowledge, from one group of trials to another. It was observed that the detectability of the signal was independent of its frequency location. This result would not be obtained if the observer were restricted at any given time to a single, classical critical band whose width is a fixed, increasing function of frequency. If he were, the signal would increase in detectability as its center frequency increased, for he would be listening to a larger part of it. Green inferred from this result that critical bands are adjusted to be larger than their minimum widths when it is effective to adjust them so.

It is also relevant to consider some fragmentary evidence that individual observers tend to show differences in the number of bands or in the width of the band that they employ, which persist from one task to another. Veniar (1958) pointed out that her Observer 1 was superior to her Observer 2 in detecting single frequencies, as if Observer 1 were listening to a narrower band of masking noise. Furthermore, Observer 1 showed a large decrement when asked to detect one of two specified frequencies, while Observer 2 exhibited a very small decrement in this task. Finally, Observer 2 performed significantly better than Observer 1 when the signal was a wide band of noise. Similarly, Swets et al. (1959) found that the one of their three observers who matched the multiband prediction in detecting one of two frequencies (the other two observers matched the single-band prediction) performed very much better than the other two when the signal was composed of 16 frequencies separated by 250 cps.

OTHER STUDIES RELEVANT TO THE TWO MODELS. The results of two additional experiments contribute to an evaluation of the two models that are considered here. One of these experiments, on the reaction time in detecting one of two specified frequencies, is generally supportive for both models. The other, on the detection of one of a large number of frequencies, weighs against the generality of both models.

Swets (unpublished work) conducted an experiment, similar to those previously described on the detection of one of two specified frequencies, in which reaction time was recorded as well as the percentage of correct responses. The analysis of reaction times corroborates the major results observed previously in terms of percentage of correct responses, namely, that a decrement in performance is produced by frequency uncertainty and that this decrement is related to the frequency separation. In particular, as the separation between the two frequencies increased and as $P(c)_{1v2}$ decreased, the reaction time was observed to increase. This outcome is consistent with both of the models under discussion. This result is to be expected, in terms of the single-band model, because it is stated explicitly in this model that more time is required to observe at two frequencies than at one and that the amount of additional time required is a function of the difference between the two frequencies. The prediction for reaction time from the multiband model derives clearly from the model with the aid of an intermediate step. According to the multiband model, the amount of effective noise entering the detection process increases as the critical bands that are adjusted to the two frequencies overlap less and less, and hence the effective signal strength decreases. It is well known that reaction time is inversely related to signal strength.

Green (1961) studied detection under extreme conditions of frequency uncertainty: the signal could have any frequency between 500 and 4000 cps. The decrement that resulted from such extreme uncertainty is only slightly larger than that which results from uncertainty about which of two specified frequencies will occur. Neither model comes close to predicting this result. Specifically, both models would predict a decrement in this case amounting to at least 10 to 12 db of signal power, whereas the observed decrement is approximately 3 db.

ON THE GENERALITY OF THE TWO MODELS. We discussed earlier the particular limitations of each of the two models which indicated that they are, to some extent, complementary. The result of the study of extreme uncertainty reveals that, taken together, they fail to represent adequately the operation of central factors in the analysis process. This result certainly weakens their position. However, to discard the two models because they are deficient in this single instance seems too severe an action. It would seem advisable to retain them for further consideration on a number of counts. They are, for one, still useful in yielding predictions in the range in which they apply. Moreover, a more adequate replacement has not yet appeared. Still more to the point, perhaps, is the fact that it is not yet entirely clear that now is the time to attempt to formulate a more general model that would replace both these models and also account for the wayward result. If we are dealing with a process as versatile as that implied by the assumption of a large contribution from central factors, it would seem reasonable to consider an alternative, deliberately temporizing approach—an approach in which other simple, single-strategy models are formulated to supplement the ones we have—at least until the flow of data gives signs of lessening.

CONCLUSION

There is now considerable evidence for the involvement of central, or cognitive, factors in the process of auditory-frequency selectivity. Although the models proposed so far to deal with the central factors have been found wanting, they have also enjoyed some success, and the experiments that they inspired have demonstrated the extensive adaptability of the process. It seems clear that the number, the frequency locations, and the widths of the critical bands which are operative in a given auditory task reflect to a substantial extent the strategy of listening that is adopted by the observer for that particular task.

Although it is equally clear that fixed elements in the ear accomplish a peripheral analysis, it is conceivable that central modulation of sensory information is extensive enough to make unlikely the discovery, through psychophysical methods, of a unitary peripheral process that remains stable despite changes in the observer's task, his information, and his aims. Psychophysical techniques constitute an ideal way to explore central factors in sensory tasks, or to explore a larger sensory system defined to include central factors, but the value of a psychophysical approach to peripheral sensory mechanisms depends upon the ability to specify, and then on the ability to isolate, the central contribution to the observer's response.

ACKNOWLEDGMENTS

The preparation of this paper was supported in part by the Instituut voor Perceptie Onderzoek, Eindhoven, the Netherlands. The author is indebted to J. F. Schouten, Director of the Instituut, for his encouragement and advice. Support was also obtained from the U. S. Army Signal Corps, the Air Force (Operational Applications Laboratory and Office of Scientific Research), and the Office of Naval Research. This article appeared as Technical Report No. ESD-TDR-62-193, and in Psychol. Bull., *1963,* **60,** *429–440.*

References

- Broadbent, D. E. Attention and the perception of speech. *Sci. Am.,* 1962, **206,** 143–151.
- Creelman, C. D. Detection of signals of uncertain frequency. *J. acoust. Soc. Am.,* 1960, **32,** 805–809.
- Fletcher, H. Auditory patterns. *Revs. mod. Phys.,* 1940, **12,** 47–65.
- Galambos, R. Suppression of auditory nerve activity by stimulation of efferent fibers to cochlea. *J. Neurophysiol.,* 1956, **19,** 424–437.
- Galambos, R., Sheatz, G., and Vernier, V. G. Electrophysiological correlates of a conditioned response in cats. *Science,* 1956, **123,** 376–377.
- Green, D. M. Detection of multiple component signals in noise. *J. acoust. Soc. Am.,* 1958, **30,** 904–911. [25]
- Green, D. M. Auditory detection of a noise signal. *J. acoust. Soc. Am.,* 1960, **32,** 121–131. [27]
- Green, D. M. Detection of auditory sinusoids of uncertain frequency. *J. acoust. Soc. Am.,* 1961, **33,** 879–903. [28]

- Green, D. M., McKey, M. J., and Licklider, J. C. R. Detection of a pulsed sinusoid in noise as a function of frequency. *J. acoust. Soc. Am.*, 1959, **31,** 1446–1452. [26]
- Greenwood, D. D. Auditory masking and the critical band. *J. acoust. Soc. Am.*, 1961*a*, **33,** 484–502.
- Greenwood, D. D. Critical bandwidth and the frequency coordinates of the basilar membrane, *J. acoust. Soc. Am.*, 1961*b*, **33,** 1344–1356.
- Hamilton, P. M. Noise masked thresholds as a function of tonal duration and masking noise bandwith. *J. acoust. Soc. Am.*, 1957, **29,** 506-511.
- Hebb, D. O. *The organization of behavior.* New York: Wiley, 1949.
- Hebb, D. O. Drives and the C. N. S. (Conceptual nervous systems). *Psychol. Rev.*, 1955, **62,** 243–254.
- Lashley, K. S. The problem of serial order in behavior. In L. A. Jeffress (Ed.), *Cerebral mechanisms in behavior.* New York: Wiley, 1951, pp. 112–136.
- Marill, T. Psychophysics and detection theory. Massachusetts Institute of Technology: Research Laboratory of Electronics, 1956, Technical Report No. 319.
- Schafer, T. H., and Gales, R. S. Auditory masking of multiple tones by random noise. *J. acoust. Soc. Am.*, 1949, **21,** 392–398.
- Schafer, T. H., Gales, R. S., Shewmaker, C. A., and Thompson, R. O. Frequency selectivity of the ear as determined by masking experiments. *J. acoust. Soc. Am.*, 1950, **22,** 490–496.
- Scharf, B. Complex sounds and critical bands. *Psychol. Bull.*, 1961, **58,** 205–217.
- Shipley, E. F. Cueing as a determiner of apparent variability in sensitivity. Massachusetts Institute of Technology: Research Laboratory of Electronics, 1959, Quarterly Progress Report No. 53; and *J. acoust. Soc. Am.*, 1959, **31,** 834. (Abstract)
- Sperry, R. W. Neurology and the mind-brain problem. *Am. Sci.*, 1952, **40,** 291–312.
- Swets, J. A. Detection theory and psychophysics: A review. *Psychometrika,* 1961, **26,** 49–63.
- Swets, J. A., Green, D. M., and Tanner, W. P., Jr. On the width of critical bands. *J. acoust. Soc. Am.*, 1962, **34,** 108–113. [23]
- Swets, J. A., and Sewall, S. T. Stimulus versus response uncertainty in recognition. *J. acoust. Soc. Am.*, 1961, **33,** 1586–1592. [20]
- Swets, J. A., Shipley, E. F., McKey, M. J., and Green, D. M. Multiple observations of signals in noise. *J. acoust. Soc. Am.*, 1959, **31,** 514–521. [9]
- Tanner, W. P., Jr. A theory of recognition. *J. acoust. Soc. Am.*, 1956, **28,** 882–888. [19]
- Tanner, W. P., Jr., and Swets, J. A. A decision-making theory of visual detection. *Psychol. Rev.*, 1954, **61,** 401–409.
- Tanner, W. P., Jr., Swets, J. A., and Green, D. M. Some general properties of the hearing mechanism. University of Michigan: Electronic Defense Group, 1956, Technical Report No. 30.
- Veniar, F. A. Signal detection as a function of frequency ensemble, I. *J. acoust. Soc. Am.*, 1958, **30,** 1020–1024; II, *J. acoust. Soc. Am.*, 1958, **30,** 1075–1078.
- Zwicker, E., Flottorp, G., and Stevens, S. S. Critical band width in loudness summation. *J. acoust. Soc. Am.*, 1957, **29,** 548–557.

section seven

SPEECH COMMUNICATION

Many of the experimental procedures that were developed to study performance with simple signals have been used to study speech recognition, including yes-no decisions, confidence ratings, second choices, repetition of items, and deferred decisions. Several analytical techniques supplied by detection theory have also been employed in this context.

Egan and Clarke, in "Source and Receiver Behavior in the Use of a Criterion" [30], extend the conventional articulation test by requiring the receiver to return the message to the source for confirmation, and they compare the source's decision behavior with that of the receiver. Pollack and Decker, in "Confidence Ratings, Message Reception, and the Receiver Operating Characteristic" [31], add a rating scale to the standard articulation test procedure, and they report a more thorough analysis of rating behavior than is available elsewhere.

In "The Effect of Vocabulary Size on Articulation Score" [32], Green and Birdsall show that the detection-theory predictions for d' as a function of signal-to-noise ratio, with the degree of uncertainty as the parameter, provide a method for transforming to a single function the articulation scores obtained from vocabularies of different sizes. Clarke relates "Confidence Ratings, Second-Choice Responses, and Confusion Matrices" [33]. He shows that ratings add a significant amount of information to the identification response whereas second choices do not. He shows also that an analysis of the confusion matrix makes it possible to reduce results with different-sized vocabularies to one function, and that the results of a monitoring task can be predicted from results obtained with an identification-plus-rating task.

30

Source and Receiver Behavior in the Use of a Criterion

James P. Egan and Frank R. Clarke

When a source attempts to communicate with a receiver over a noisy channel, one or both of the operators may be required to confirm or reject each message. In our previous studies of the communication process (Egan, Clarke, and Carterette, 1955, 1956), a message was sent from the source to the receiver, and then the receiver sent his best estimate of the original message back to the source for confirmation. In this situation, the source must accept or reject the returned message according to some criterion, and it is desirable that his behavior be quantitatively described. The source-operating-characteristic, or SOC, curve is the relation, for a constant speech-to-noise ratio, between the conditional probability of a correct confirmation and the conditional probability of an incorrect confirmation. To determine such a relationship, the source adopts various criteria for acceptance on successive tests. This curve describes an important aspect of the source's behavior in the transmission and confirmation of messages.

Clearly, the receiver can also judge whether or not he has correctly heard the message. The receiver can adopt a criterion, and after recording his response he can estimate whether or not that response is correct. The receiver-operating-characteristic, or ROC, curve shows the relation between the probability that the receiver will accept his response when in fact he heard the message correctly and the probability of an acceptance when in fact he recorded the message incorrectly. The curve is generated by requiring the receiver to adopt various criteria for acceptance on successive tests conducted at the same speech-to-noise ratio (Peterson and Birdsall, 1953; Tanner and Swets, 1954).

By using the concept of the ROC curve and of the SOC curve, it is possible to analyze a number of procedures for transmitting messages efficiently in noise. In order to provide this information, two experiments were conducted which compare the behavior of the receiver with that of the source with respect to the process of confirming messages.

PROCEDURE

In the first experiment, a talker (ET) read lists of words over a noisy channel to two listeners (FC and JE). One of the listeners simply wrote down the words he heard as in an articulation test. After recording each word, the listener made a judgment as to whether or not his response was correct, and he indicated his decision after each word on the answer blank. This listener was analogous to a receiver in the "over and back" situation. The other listener was analogous to a source in the "over and back" situation, and he was provided with an answer blank consisting of a list of words, one word for each of the test words read by the talker. For one-half of the test words, the word on the source's answer blank was the same as that on the talker's list. For the other half, the corresponding words were different. These test words, which were different from those on the source's answer blank, simulated "receiver errors" to the corresponding words on the source's list. These particular test words were selected from a confusion matrix based upon previous articulation tests so that, insofar as possible, one-half of these test words were frequent receiver errors and the other half were infrequent receiver errors. Thus, this listener was acting as if he were a source in an "over and back" situation in which the articulation of the receiver was 50 per cent.

It must be mentioned that the validity of a comparison between source and receiver behavior depends upon how closely the "receiver errors" (confusers, or *B* items) are simulated. The difficulty of the source test will depend upon the proportion of "receiver errors" that are high in confusability with respect to the source's list of items. Our opinion, based upon a careful examination of the confusion matrix for the 50 spondees, is that the *source* test used in the present study contains close to the correct proportion of difficult and easy items.

Each test list consisted of 200 highly homogeneous items. Fifty spondees had been selected from a set of 84 on the basis of an item analysis (Egan, Clarke, and Carterette, 1956). These 50 spondees were memorized, and in each test list of 200 items each spondee was represented four times. One measure of homogeneity of a list of items is the slope of the gain function, and during the practice tests this testing crew obtained a slope of nearly 14 per cent per decibel.

Thirty-two such 200-word tests were conducted in such a way that each listener was acting as a source for 16 of the tests and as a receiver for the other 16 tests. Each listener changed his criterion from test to test so that the range from very strict to very lax was covered.

A speech-to-noise ratio of -13 db was used for both the source and the receiver tests so that their behavior in the use of a criterion could be meaningfully compared. The noise had a nearly uniform spectrum level from 60 to 7000 cps, and a VU meter was used to measure the overall levels of speech and of noise. The value of the speech-to-noise ratio was so chosen that the articulation score for the receiver would be nearly 50 per cent. The mean for one listener for the 16 tests during which he acted as a receiver was 51.5 per cent, and for the other listener (16 tests) the mean was 48.9 per cent. The grand mean was 50.2 per cent. Since it was desired to obtain the data for the SOC and the ROC curves under homogeneous conditions, it was decided in advance of the experiment to discard those tests on which the listener who was acting as a receiver obtained an articulation score of less than 35 per cent or greater than 65 per cent. Only one test was discarded and repeated. Considerable care was exercised throughout in order to maintain constant conditions, and the three members of the testing crew were highly experienced. The one-way interphone consisted of high-fidelity components.

It was considered advisable to repeat this experiment using listeners who were much less informed about the nature of the experiment and who were less concerned about its outcome. In this second experiment, six graduate students served as subjects. Each was given the set of 50 spondees to memorize, and then six practice tests of 200 words each were conducted using a progressively lower speech-to-noise ratio from the first to the last test. Six additional practice tests were then conducted in which the listeners had to adopt various criteria in accepting and rejecting the words. Each listener acted as a source for three of these tests and as a receiver for the other three tests. Since the number of tests was necessarily limited, the listeners were asked to avoid the extreme criteria, since such data do not determine the position of the SOC or ROC curve as well as do the data gathered using the intermediate criteria.

The results of these practice tests are not reported, but they are in essential agreement with those obtained in the experiment proper.

For this second experiment, the 200-word lists were recorded on magnetic tape by talker JE, and during playback the electrical signal was mixed with live noise (uniform spectrum level, 60 to 7000 cps). In the experiment, the speech-to-noise ratio (as read on a VU meter) was held constant at -12 db for all tests. Three 200-word tests were conducted during each of four experimental sessions. For two of these sessions the listeners acted as receivers and for the other two sessions they acted as sources. The mean articulation score was 51.2 per cent.

In order to secure a measure of how well the subjects knew the words, the listeners were asked to write down as many of the 50 spondee words as they could recall. Only 10 minutes were allowed for this memory test, and it was conducted after the articulation tests were completed. The mean number recalled was 41 spondees.

RESULTS

The results based upon the two experienced listeners used in the first experiment are shown in Fig. 1. The results for each listener were plotted separately for each condition of listening (as a source or as a receiver), and the position of a theoretical curve was fitted by eye to each set of data. The behavior of the two listeners was so similar that the results were pooled for each of the two conditions of listening. The theoretical curves shown in the figure are based upon a model described in a previous publication (Egan, Clarke, and Carterette, 1956).

The following numerical example illustrates how the various probabilities were computed for the receiver tests. On one of the 200-word tests, the receiver correctly recorded 105 words, giving an articulation score of 52.5 per cent. Of these 105 correct responses, the receiver confirmed 80 of them. Thus, the conditional probability of a correct confirmation was 0.76. For this same test, the listener confirmed 24 of his 95 incorrect responses. Therefore, the conditional probability of an incorrect confirmation was 0.25. A point having the coordinates $p(Y|A_r) = 0.76$ and $p(Y|B_r) = 0.25$ is plotted as a filled circle on Fig. 1.

Figure 1 shows that the confirmation of messages is somewhat more accurate when the listener acts as a source and thus knows the original message than when he acts as a receiver and does not know the original message. That is to say, the source has a higher proportion of "hits" than does the receiver when both operators have the same "false-alarm rate." It should be recalled that the source has to decide only whether

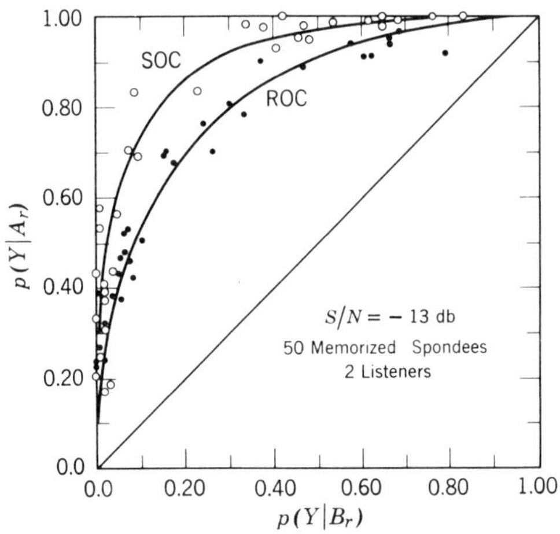

FIG. 1. SOC and ROC curves obtained with the same test materials and with the same speech-to-noise ratio. Each point represents the result of one 200-word test for each listener. The two experienced listeners are not presented separately on the graph since their data were nearly the same. The SOC curve shows the relation between the conditional probability of accepting a correct stimulus and the conditional probability of accepting an incorrect stimulus. The ROC curve defines the relation between the conditional probability of accepting a correct response and the conditional probability of accepting an incorrect response. Thus, the conditional probabilities for the source's behavior are based upon the acceptances of correct and incorrect stimuli presented to the source. The conditional probabilities for the receiver's behavior are based upon the acceptances by the receiver of his own correct and incorrect responses. The data for each relationship are obtained by instructing the listener to adopt different criteria of acceptance from test to test, while the speech-to-noise ratio remains at a constant average value for all tests. The position of the theoretical curves was fitted by eye.

the message he has received is the same as or different from the message on his answer blank, whereas the receiver must select his response from 50 alternatives and then decide whether or not he has made a correct choice. The high performance level of the receiver is probably contingent upon the use of a small, memorized set of messages.

The results of the second experiment are shown in Figs. 2 and 3. These results also show that, although the receiver does not do as well as the source, the receiver can add a considerable amount of information to each response by confirming or rejecting that response.

In order to maintain that the receiver's acceptance or rejection of his responses adds information to the process of the reception of messages, it is necessary to show that the articulation score is not adversely affected by the adoption of a criterion. The differences among the mean articula-

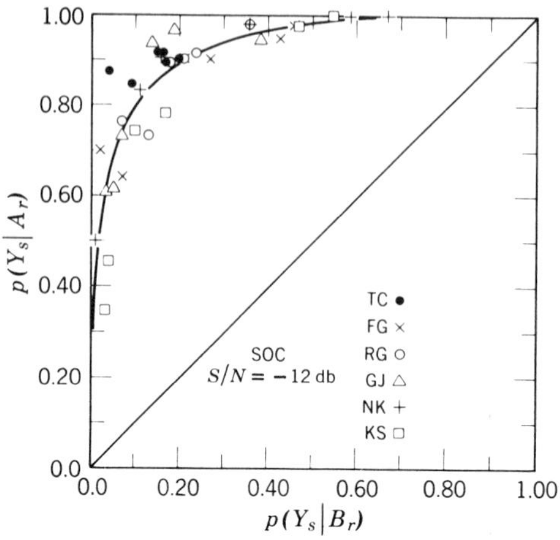

FIG. 2. SOC curve based upon six listeners. Each point represents the result of one 200-word test for one listener.

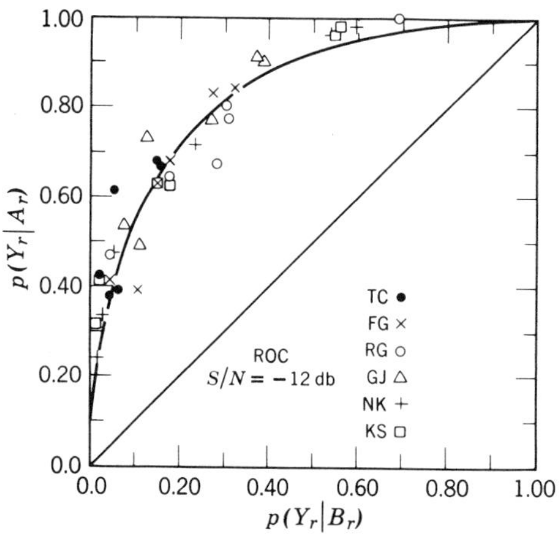

FIG. 3. ROC curve based upon the same six listeners as those used to obtain the data for the previous figure. Each point represents the result of one 200-word test for one listener.

tion scores obtained with and without the use of various criteria were not systematic, and the largest difference was 3.8 percentage units. A statistical analysis of the data of both experiments leads us to conclude that for practical purposes the adoption of a criterion does not affect the probability of correctly receiving a message.

SUMMARY

A listener in an articulation test is confident of some of his responses and dubious about others. On the basis of this fact, it is reasonable to require that a receiver decide whether or not his response is correct. If he adopts various criteria from test to test, a receiver operating characteristic may be obtained which will be one way of describing quantitatively this type of behavior. The curve showing the confirming and rejecting behavior of the receiver is compared to that of the source using the same test materials and the same speech-to-noise ratio.

ACKNOWLEDGMENTS

This research was conducted in the Hearing and Communication Laboratory of Indiana University with support from the Operational Applications Laboratory of the U. S. Air Force. This article appeared as Tech. Rept. No. AFCRC-TN-56-56, and in J. acoust. Soc. Am., *1956,* **28,** *1267–1269.*

References

- Egan, J. P., Clarke, F. R., and Carterette, E. C. On a theory of the transmission and confirmation of messages in noise. Indiana University: Hearing and Communication Laboratory, 1955, Technical Note AFCRC-TN-55-67.
- Egan, J. P., Clarke, F. R., and Carterette, E. C. On the transmission and confirmation of messages in noise. *J. acoust. Soc. Am.*, 1956, **28,** 536–550.
- Peterson, W. W., and Birdsall, T. G. The theory of signal detectability. University of Michigan: Electronic Defense Group, 1953, Technical Report No. 13.
- Tanner, W. P., Jr., and Swets, J. A. A decision-making theory of visual detection. *Psychol. Rev.*, 1954, **61,** 401–409.

31

Confidence Ratings, Message Reception, and the Receiver Operating Characteristic

Irwin Pollack and Louis R. Decker

At the Operational Applications Laboratory, we have been interested in exploring the application of new techniques and procedures to speech communication. In the present study, we shall consider the application of a rating procedure which, in essence, adds a confidence judgment to the standard articulation-test procedure. The additional confidence judgment will be used to obtain independent information about the listener's criterion for message acceptance or rejection.

Recent human-operator studies in signal detection, notably those of the Michigan (Tanner, Swets, and Green, 1956) and Indiana (Egan, 1957) groups, have shown that information about a listener's performance need not be limited to the correctness of his message reception. In these tests, the listener is instructed to establish a given criterion of performance. He is then instructed to reject items which fail to meet the criterion and to accept items which do meet the criterion. By requiring a range of criteria in successive experiments, with the binary-decision procedure, one can obtain an empirical estimate of a receiver's message acceptance.

At first examination, the binary-decision procedure appears inefficient. Often listeners report that they can make finer discriminations than the simple yes-no judgment of message acceptance or message rejection.

These remarks suggested that a finer rating classification might be employed to advantage. Furthermore, it appeared likely that the time spent in the determination of listener's criterion behavior could be sharply reduced with the rating procedure.

In addition, it has been shown that listeners can judge the average intelligibility of a list of words presented in noise.[1] For these and other reasons, the rating procedure seemed to merit consideration for further study.

Specifically, we asked three questions.

First, do message-accuracy ratings interfere with message reception?

Second, does the rating procedure yield criterion relationships of the same type obtained by the binary yes-no decision procedure?

And, third, is there a simple invariant relationship between confidence ratings and message reception over a range of speech-to-noise ratios?

PROCEDURE

The testing procedure employed was identical to standard intelligibility-test procedure with one addition: After the listener recorded each test word, he also recorded his judged accuracy of message reception. The rating scale is presented in Table I. In all, six categories were employed. For example, the listener was instructed to assign a triple-plus

TABLE I. CONFIDENCE RATING SCALE FOR JUDGING ACCURACY OF MESSAGE RECEPTION

+++	Positive I received the message correctly.
++	Fairly certain I received the message correctly.
+	Can't decide, but I think I received the message correctly.
−	Can't decide, but I think I received the message incorrectly.
−−	Fairly certain I received the message incorrectly.
−−−	Positive I received the message incorrectly.

rating when he was positive he received the message correctly. Similarly, he was instructed to assign the double-plus rating when he was fairly certain he received the message correctly. He was instructed to assign a triple-minus rating when his response represented no better than a

[1] M. H. Abrams et al. "Subjective ratings of the intelligibility of talkers in noise," cited by Miller, Wiener, and Stevens (1946).

chance guess. No additional instructions were given to control the manner in which the listeners used the rating scale.[2]

The speech material used consisted of a closed message set of 64 spondee words. Successive shufflings of two lists of 64 words yielded lists of 75 words each. Each list of 75 words was read at a constant speech-to-noise (S/N) ratio. The S/N ratio was varied by introduction of attenuation into the speech channel. The S/N ratio was announced at the beginning of each list. Intelligibility was tested at three S/N ratios in order to study the distribution of accuracy ratings over a wide range of difficulty levels. The average percentage of spondee words correctly received was: 85.2, 59.8, and 31.8 at S/N ratios of -9, -12, and -15 db, respectively. The S/N ratios were counterbalanced upon successive tests within a given test session. Each word was preceded by a 1000-cycle warning tone with a 1-sec delay between the tone and the test word. A 10-sec separation between words permitted sufficient time for each listener to record the received word and to record his accuracy rating.

An experienced male talker, seated in an isolated room, announced each test word into an RCA-88 microphone. No introductory carrier phrase was employed. The talker monitored his vocal output by means of a VU meter. The speech signal was mixed with white noise with an upper cutoff at 7000 cps. The mixed signal was presented over earphones (RCA H-70) mounted in the AIC-10 headset, to three listeners in an adjoining room. Speech levels were expressed in terms of the VU meter readings for the test words. Noise levels were expressed in terms of over-all level, as read on a "true" rms meter (Ballantine model 320). The over-all sound pressure level of the noise, as measured in a 6-cc coupler, was held constant at 86 db *re* 0.0002 dyne/cm^2.

Three university students, selected from a pool of experienced subjects, served as listeners. They were paid for their services. They were required initially to memorize the 64 spondee words. In addition, listeners were provided with an alphabetically arranged list of the 64 spondee words. Fourteen sessions, each lasting approximately two hours, were devoted to preliminary training. At the end of each test list of 75 words the correct key was furnished and the listener corrected his own paper. At the end of each test session, each listener also tabulated his category ratings with respect to correct and incorrect message reception.

---

[2] We have learned that two signal-detection studies have previously employed versions of the rating scale. Specifically, Smith and Wilson (1953) have employed a four-category rating scale; Swets, Tanner, and Birdsall (1955) required their observers to judge the a posteriori probability of a correct detection.

GENERAL APPROACH

"*The Receiver's Operating Characteristic*, or the ROC-curve, shows the relation between the probability that the receiver will confirm his response when in fact he correctly heard the message and the probability of an acceptance when in fact he incorrectly recorded the message. The ROC-curve is investigated by instructing the receiver to adopt various criteria for confirmation on successive tests conducted at the same S/N ratio" (Egan, 1957, p. 68). This excellent description of the ROC concept in message reception also sketches the binary-decision procedure from which the ROC curve is typically obtained.

We now turn to the relation of the rating procedure to the binary-decision procedure by means of which the ROC curves are usually derived. The rating procedure essentially provides a finer grained analysis of the listener's discrimination continuum than that provided by the binary-decision procedure. Moreover, the data of the rating procedure can be compressed to that of the binary-decision procedure. If we start with the six-position rating scale of Table I, we can impose any type of arbitrary slicing to compress the rating data into a binary decision. For example, if a slice is imposed between the single-plus category and the single-minus category, we have two new binary-response categories. One of the binary categories is composed of the three categories containing the plus sign and one is composed of the three categories containing the minus sign. In the same manner, with other slicings along the six-position rating scale, we can create other binary classifications.

Before considering the experimental results, it will be profitable to examine the notation and concepts in Table II and typical calculations in Table III. Table II presents the separate probabilities of occurrence of events associated with message reception and the rating procedure. Table III illustrates the calculation of the separate probability measures. The data of Table III represent the combined results for three listeners, each exposed to 1350 words, under a single S/N ratio (-9 db).

TABLE II. NOTATION FOR THE CLASS OF EVENTS ASSOCIATED WITH MESSAGE RECEPTION AND CONFIDENCE RATINGS

$p(A_r)$	The probability of a correct message reception, irrespective of rating category assigned. The probability that message A was presented to the receiver and message A was received.
$p(B_r)$	The probability of an incorrect message reception, irrespective of rating category assigned. The probability that message A was presented to the receiver, and message B ($A \neq B$) was received.

TABLE II (*Cont.*)

$p(R_j)$	The probability of assignment of a message to rating category j, irrespective of correct or incorrect message reception where rating categories are designated: $R_s \cdots R_j \cdots R_l$, where s is the most strict $(+++)$ and l is the most lax $(---)$ rating category.
$P(R_j) = \sum_s^j p(R_j)$	The cumulative probability of assignment of a message to rating category j, or stricter, irrespective of correct or incorrect message reception.
$p(A_r \cdot R_j)$	The joint probability of a correct message reception and assignment to rating category j.
$p(B_r \cdot R_j)$	The joint probability of occurrence of an incorrect message reception and assignment to rating category j.
$P(A_r \cdot R_j)$	The joint cumulative probability of a correct message reception and assignment to rating category j, or stricter.
$P(B_r \cdot R_j)$	The joint cumulative probability of an incorrect message reception and assignment to rating category j, or stricter.
$p(R_j \vert A_r)$	The conditional probability of an assignment of rating category j, given a correct message reception.
$P(R_j \vert A_r)$	The cumulative conditional probability of an assignment of rating category j, or stricter, given a correct message reception.
$P(R_j \vert B_r)$	The cumulative conditional probability of an assignment of rating category j, or stricter, given an incorrect message reception.
$p(A_r \vert R_j)$	The conditional probability of a correct message reception, given assignment to rating category j.
ROC	The receiver operating characteristic, the relationship between $P(R_j \vert A_r)$, the cumulative probability of a correct confirmation, and $P(R_j \vert B_r)$, the cumulative probability of a false alarm.
$T(m,r)$	Transmitted information, in bits per presentation, common to accuracy of message reception and to rating categories.
$H(m)$	Informational uncertainty of message reception, in bits per presentation.
$H(r)$	Informational uncertainty of rating categories, in bits per presentation.
$H(m,r)$	Joint informational uncertainty of message reception and rating categories, in bits per presentation.

TABLE III. Examples of the Application of Notation of Table II

A. Sample data: (Average of three listeners at -9 db S/N)

Scale category	$A_r \cdot R_j$	$B_r \cdot R_j$	R_j
$+++$	2434	122	2556
$++$	519	48	567
$+$	388	182	570
$-$	100	141	241
$--$	17	65	82
$---$	4	30	34
Totals	3462	588	4050

B. Example of binary classification:

Scale category	A_r	B_r	R_j
$+++$ to $++$	2953	170	3123
$+$ to $---$	509	418	927
Totals	3462	588	4050

C. Typical calculations:

Figures 1 and 2. ROC curves.

$$P(R_{++}|A_r) = \frac{P(A_r \cdot R_{++})}{p(A_r)} = \frac{2953}{4050} \div \frac{3462}{4050} = 0.853$$

$$P(R_{++}|B_j) = \frac{P(B_r \cdot R_{++})}{p(B_r)} = \frac{170}{4050} \div \frac{588}{4050} = 0.289$$

Figure 3. Distribution of confidence ratings.

$$p(R_{++}) = p(A_r \cdot R_{++}) + p(B_r \cdot R_{++}) = \frac{519}{4050} + \frac{48}{4050} = \frac{567}{4050} = 0.140$$

Figure 4. Distribution of confidence ratings for correct message receptions.

$$p(R_{++}|A_r) = \frac{p(A_r \cdot R_{++})}{p(A_r)} = \frac{519}{4050} \div \frac{3462}{4050} = 0.150$$

Figures 5, 6, and 7. Probability of correct message reception within a given confidence rating.

$$p(A_r|R_{++}) = \frac{p(A_r \cdot R_{++})}{p(R_{++})} = \frac{519}{4050} \div \frac{567}{4050} = 0.915$$

Figure 8. Information-transmission scores.

$$H(m) = -\sum_i p(m_j) \log p(m_i)$$

$$\text{where } p(m_j) = \frac{3462}{4050}; \frac{588}{4050} \text{ (for all categories)}$$

TABLE III. (*Cont.*)

$$H(r) = -\sum_j p(r_j) \log p(r_j), \text{ where } p(r_j) =$$

$$\text{2 categories: } \frac{3693}{4050};\ \frac{357}{4050}$$

$$\text{3 categories: } \frac{3123}{4050};\ \frac{811}{4050};\ \frac{116}{4050}$$

$$\text{6 categories: } \frac{2556}{4050};\ \frac{567}{4050};\ \cdots\ \frac{34}{4050}$$

$$H(r,m) = -\sum_i \sum_j p(r_j,m_i) \log p(r_j,m_i) \text{ where } p(r_j,m_i) =$$

$$\text{2 categories: } \frac{3341}{4050};\ \frac{352}{4050};\ \cdots\ \frac{236}{4050}$$

$$\text{3 categories: } \frac{2953}{4050};\ \frac{170}{4050};\ \cdots\ \frac{95}{4050}$$

$$\text{6 categories: } \frac{2434}{4050};\ \frac{122}{4050};\ \cdots\ \frac{30}{4050}$$

$$T = H(m) + H(r) - H(r,m)$$

for 2 categories: $T = 0.598 + 0.430 - 0.925 = 0.103$
for 3 categories: $T = 0.598 + 0.900 - 1.348 = 0.150$
for 6 categories: $T = 0.598 + 1.628 - 2.057 = 0.169$

The first column of Table IIIA presents the rating categories. The second column presents the number of correct message receptions assigned to each rating category (e.g., 519 correct receptions were assigned to the + + category). The third column presents the number of incorrect message receptions assigned to each rating category (e.g., 48 incorrect receptions were assigned to the + + category). The fourth column presents R_j, the total number of messages assigned to each rating category, irrespective of correct or incorrect message reception (e.g., a total of 567 receptions were assigned to the + + category).

It may be noted that the results of the present experiment are expressed in terms of average scores based upon probability transformations imposed upon the data of the individual listeners, and then averaged over individuals. The alternative procedure—namely, pooling responses over listeners, and then performing the probability transformations—yields nearly equivalent calculations. For the entries of Fig. 5, for example, the two procedures yield nearly equivalent results under all conditions with the exception of the specific example selected in Table IIIC (Fig. 5).

RESULTS

Our first question was: *Do message-accuracy ratings interfere with message reception?* Apparently not, at least not under the conditions of the present experiment. Control tests were conducted which were identical to the experimental tests, with the exception that no accuracy ratings were required. In two series of tests with 1200 words, there was only a 3-per-cent difference in scores for the two procedures, and the difference was in the direction of lower error with the accompanying rating procedure.

Our second question was: *Does the rating procedure yield criterion relationships of the same type obtained by the binary yes-no decision procedure?* Apparently, yes. The ROC curves given by the rating procedure exhibit the typical linear function drawn upon double probability axes, which characterizes the results with the binary-decision procedure. These functions are shown in Fig. 1 for a single subject, and in Fig. 2 for the combined results of three subjects.

The ordinate of Figs. 1 and 2 represent, in effect, the probability that the listener was willing to wager (in terms of his confidence judgment) that he had received the message correctly, when in fact he had received it correctly; the abscissa represents the probability that the listener was

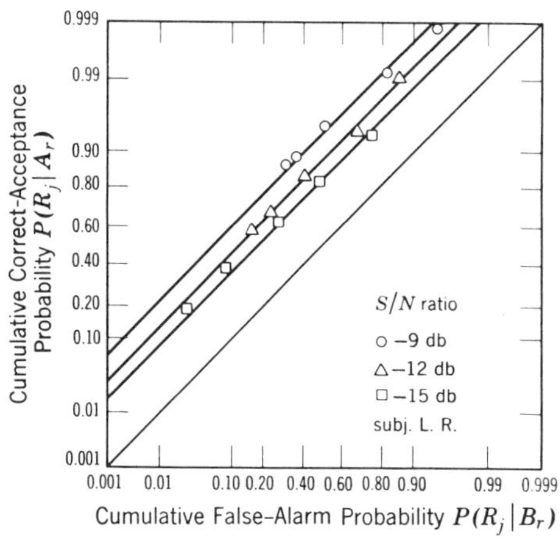

FIG. 1. The receiver operating characteristic for a single listener. The abscissa is the cumulative probability that the listener was willing to state (in terms of his confidence judgment) that the received message was correct, when in fact it was incorrect. The ordinate is the cumulative probability that the listener was willing to state that the received message was correct, when in fact it was correct. The parameter is speech-to-noise ratio. Each curve is based upon 1350 observations with a single experimental subject.

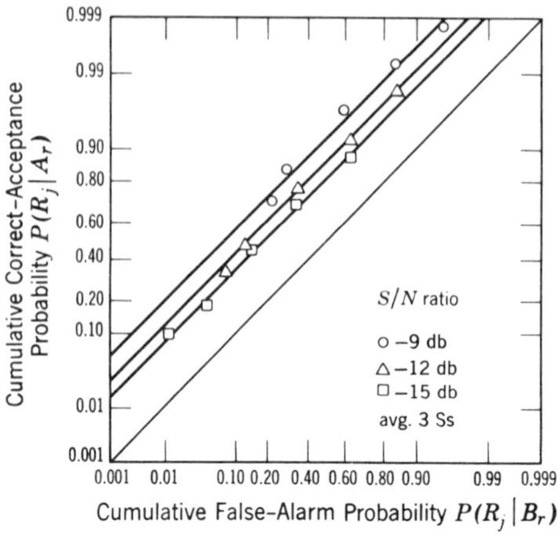

FIG. 2. The receiver operating characteristic, averaged over three listeners, as in Fig. 1, which was for a single listener.

willing to wager that he had received the message correctly, when in fact he had failed to receive it correctly. In these terms, the separate points are conceived as different wagering levels. In signal-detection terminology, the ordinate represents the probability of a correct confirmation; the abscissa represents the probability of a false alarm. The parameter of Figs. 1 and 2 is the S/N ratio under test.

The diagonal 45° line between the corners of the graphs represents chance performance. Distance to the left of the line represents higher detection performance. As the S/N ratio is decreased from -9 db to -15 db, the ROC curve more closely approaches the chance diagonal. A slope of 1.0 (as drawn for the present results) suggests that, in the conceptual decision model of message reception, the variances of the message and noise distributions are equal (Tanner, Swets, and Green, 1956).

An illustration of the application of the rating-scale procedure in the derivation of ROC curves is presented in Table IIIB and Table IIIC (Figs. 1 and 2). In essence, arbitrary binary classifications or slicings were imposed upon the data and the results were compressed upon each side of the slice. For example, Table IIIB is the result of an arbitrary slicing between rating categories + + and + of Table IIIA. Specifically, the first two rows of Table IIIA were combined within each column $(2434 + 519 = 2953; \cdots)$, and the last four rows of Table IIIA were combined within each column $(388 + 100 + 17 + 4 = 509; \cdots)$. The points on the ROC curve were determined by a series of successive slicings at different rating categories, as in Table IIIC, and as plotted in Fig. 2.

Our third question was: *Is there a simple invariant relationship between rating criteria and message reception?* Apparently, yes. The invariant relation is the resultant of two factors:

First, irrespective of correctness of message reception, listeners employ low rating categories (i.e., − − − and − −) more often at lower S/N ratios than at higher S/N ratios. This relationship is demonstrated in Fig. 3. The ordinate of Fig. 3 is $p(R_j)$—the probability of employing a selected response category, irrespective of correctness of message reception. The abscissa of Figs. 3 to 6 is the rating category employed. The parameter of Figs. 3 to 6 is S/N ratio in decibels. Sample calculations upon which Fig. 3 is based are presented in Table IIIC (Fig. 3).

Second, for *correct* message receptions *only*, listeners employ low confidence categories (i.e., − − − and − −) more often at lower S/N ratios. This is demonstrated in Fig. 4. The ordinate of Fig. 4 is $p(R_j|A_r)$, the conditional probability of employing a selected response category, given that the message was received correctly. Sample calculations upon which Fig. 4 is based are presented in Table IIIC (Fig. 4).

The net effect of these two factors yields the invariant relationship of Fig. 5. The ordinate of Fig. 5 is $p(A_r|R_j)$—the probability of receiving

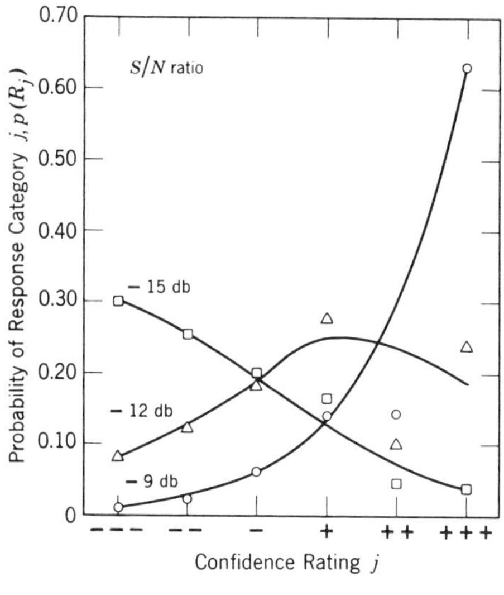

FIG. 3. Confidence ratings assigned at three speech-to-noise ratios. The abscissa is the confidence rating assigned by the listeners. The ordinate is the relative frequency of category assignment, irrespective of correctness of message reception. Average results for three listeners.

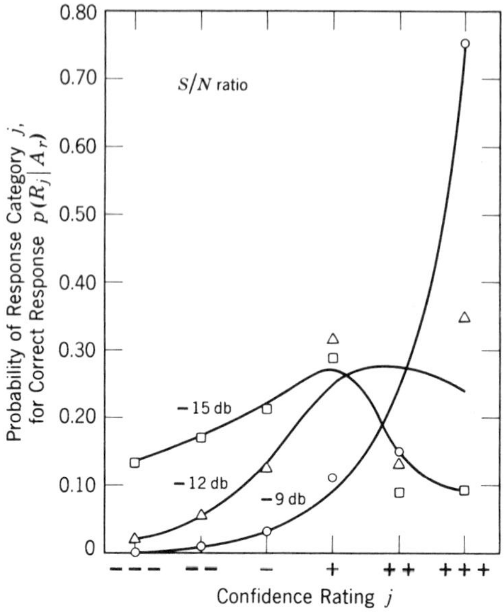

FIG. 4. Confidence ratings assigned to correct message receptions only, at three speech-to-noise ratios. The abscissa is the confidence rating assigned by the listeners. The ordinate is the relative frequency of category assignment among the correct message receptions. Average results for three listeners.

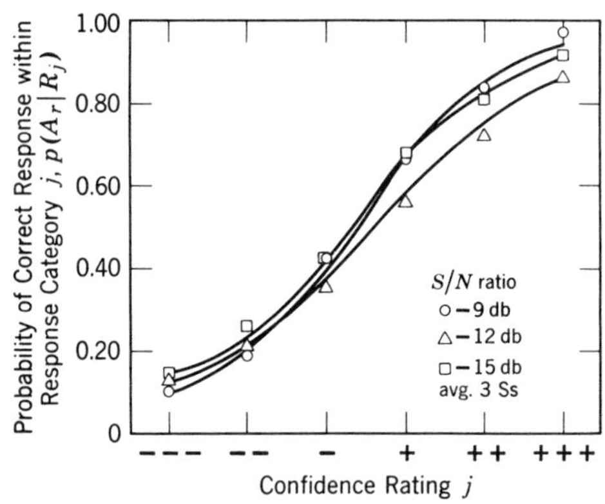

FIG. 5. The probability of a correct message reception within given rating categories at three speech-to-noise ratios. The abscissa is the confidence rating assigned by the listeners. The ordinate is the proportion of correct message receptions of the total number of responses assigned each rating category. Average results for three listeners.

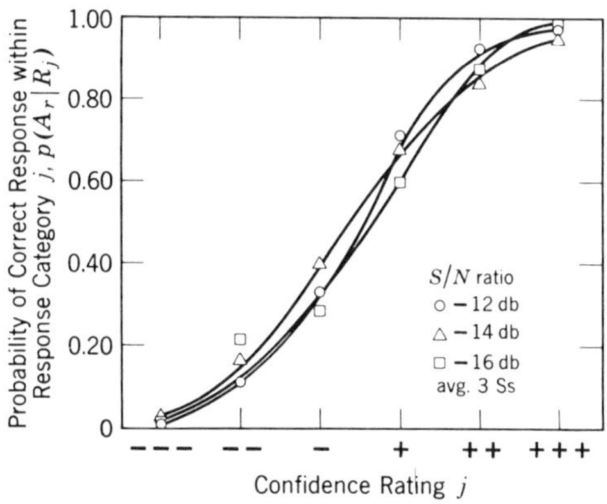

FIG. 6. The probability of a correct response message reception with given rating categories at three speech-to-noise ratios. As in Fig. 5, for an additional experiment with three different listeners and volume-compressed speech. Each speech-to-noise ratio is based upon 600 observations.

a word correctly, given that the words were assigned to a selected rating category. To a good approximation, this proportion is substantially independent of the S/N ratio under test. That is to say, over a range of S/N ratios, subjects apparently employ the strategy of assigning their confidence ratings to achieve fixed *average* levels of message reception. Stated otherwise, listeners make apparently little attempt to readjust their confidence ratings of their correct messages when faced with different S/N ratios. Their strategy is a reasonable one; their confidence rating assignment is related to their message accuracy, irrespective of S/N ratio.

Figure 6 presents the results of a second experiment with an additional group of three subjects under test conditions similar to the present study, with the exception that volume-compressed speech was employed. The major conclusion of Fig. 6 supports that of Fig. 5, although the exact form of the empirical function differs somewhat.

RATING PROCEDURE AND SUBSET SELECTION

An additional analysis was carried out to examine the generality of the ROC curves obtained by the rating procedure. From the tests represented in Fig. 2, a set of the 10 most difficult words (defined over all S/N ratios), a set of the 10 least difficult words, and a set of 10 words of intermediate difficulty were examined. Separate ROC analyses were performed for the individual subsets. The ROC curves were again linear on the double-probability plot with a slope of 1.0. Thus, the rating procedure yields ROC functions for subsets arbitrarily selected from the master set as well as for the master set itself.

However, certain discrepancies arise with respect to the invariant relationships of Figs. 5 and 6, and should be noted. First, consider, for each S/N ratio, the $p(A_r|R_j)$ scores with message subset as the parameter. Here, we badly miss the invariant relationship of Fig. 5. Specifically, over the entire rating scale, the $p(A_r|R_j)$ scores associated with the three subsets rank order with the average difficulty of the subset. Highest $p(A_r|R_j)$ scores are associated with the least difficult words and lowest scores are associated with the most difficult words. We, therefore, cannot replace S/N ratio with word difficulty to obtain the invariant relation of Figs. 5 and 6.

Second, and more important, consider, for each subset of words, the $p(A_r|R_j)$ scores with S/N as the parameter. This evaluation corresponds directly with the analysis presented in Fig. 5, but for restricted subsets from the master set. In general, the $p(A_r|R_j)$ scores for the separate S/N ratios approach an invariant relation of the type shown in Fig. 5, but with some systematic discrepancies. Specifically, for the high confidence criteria, high S/N ratios are associated with systematically higher $p(A_r|R_j)$ scores; and lower S/N ratios are associated with systematically lower scores.

Therefore, we are forced to conclude that the invariant relation of Figs. 5 and 6 may be ascribed to the *average* probability of correct detection, and must be interpreted with caution in generalizing to subsets of the master set.

DISCUSSION

We have answered the initial three questions originally posed. Under conditions of the experiment, the addition of accuracy ratings did not interfere with message reception. The form of the ROC curves yielded by the rating procedure is identical with that yielded by the binary-decision procedure. And, finally, there is an important invariant relationship between ratings and message reception over a range of S/N ratios. This relation is that the accuracy rating defines the *average* percent-correct message reception, irrespective of the S/N ratio. We are now in the process of examining other communication situations to determine the generality of the relationship.

A preliminary look at the application of ratings to another procedure for manipulating the intelligibility of speech in noise is provided by

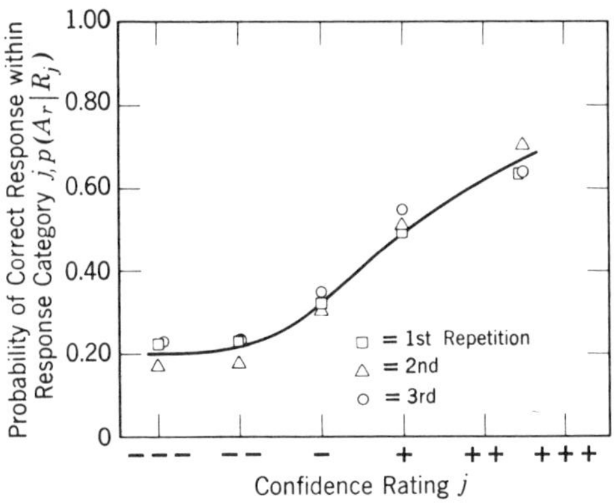

FIG. 7. The probability of a correct response within a given rating category for three successive repetitions of the same message with each repetition requiring individual confidence ratings. Each repetition is based upon the average results of three listeners and a total of 525 observations. The data are presented as in Figs. 5 and 6.

Fig. 7. In these tests, the talker read a given word three times, with each repetition separated by 10 sec. The listener had full knowledge of the restrictions imposed. As in the main tests, the listeners rated their accuracy of message reception after each word was received. The listeners, the test procedure, and the test equipment were those represented in Figs. 2 to 5.

Our initial hypothesis was that message reception scores would change very little with successive repetitions, but that the distribution of rating categories would be markedly affected. In this way, the invariant relationship of Figs. 5 and 6 would fail to be confirmed. As we expected, repetition produced only slight gains in word intelligibility. The average percentage of correct message receptions, $p(A_r)$ increased from 30.3 to 34.8 to 39.4 per cent on successive repetitions. However, we were wrong about the modification in the rating categories. The small gains in speech reception were apparently precisely balanced by proportional shifts in the distribution of rating categories, as evidenced by Fig. 7.

The coordinates of Fig. 7 are identical with Figs. 5 and 6. The parameter of Fig. 7 is the number of successive repetitions. (Because of the small number of responses in the upper two categories, responses in these categories were combined.) To a rough approximation, the relationship between correct message reception and rating categories is independent of the number of presentations of the test word. It may be noted that the empirical function in Fig. 7 diverges from that of Figs. 5 and 6. This finding adds a further caution to the generalization of a single relationship between confidence ratings and message reception. Nevertheless, to the extent that Figs. 5, 6, and 7 are independent examinations of the application of the rating procedure under different conditions, it is tempting to make statements about the generality of the listener's strategy of assigning confidence ratings to message reception. We shall not yield to the temptation until more situations are examined.[3]

There are, of course, many questions about the rating procedure which must be explored before it can be used effectively. For example, we do not know how fine a rating scale is possible or practicable. To obtain a preliminary answer to the question of the proper grain of the rating scale, we have analyzed the six-category rating scale in terms of the amount of transmitted information (Shannon, 1948) common to the confidence ratings and the accuracy of message reception.[4] An example of a typical calculation is presented in Table IIIC (Fig. 8). We also arbitrarily combined responses of successive categories (i.e., + + + and + +, + and −, − − and − − −) to provide a new table of three

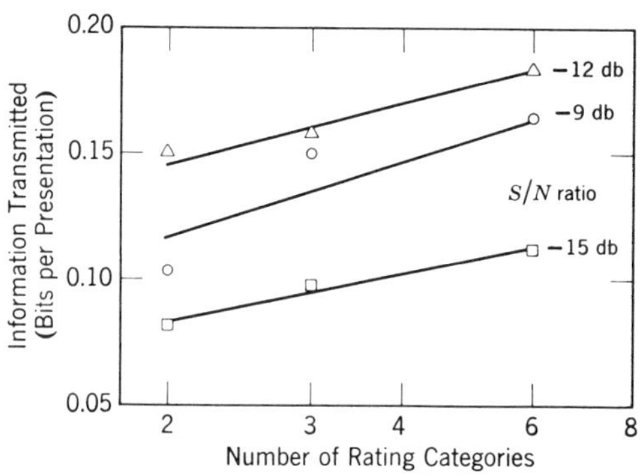

FIG. 8. Average transmitted information common to accuracy of message reception and rating categories at three speech-to-noise ratios. The abscissa represents the number of rating categories employed in the response analysis. The original six-category responses were unaltered. For reduction to three response categories, successive pairs of rating categories were combined. For reduction to two response categories, successive triplets of rating categories were combined.

---

[3] We have preliminary evidence that the single relationship between confidence ratings and message reception is not obtained with different low-pass filtering conditions (Decker and Pollack, 1958).

[4] Smith and Wilson (1953) and Munson and Karlin (1954) have applied an informational analysis to the results of the binary-decision procedure. In addition, Smith and Wilson have applied an informational analysis to the results of a 4-category rating procedure that were collapsed to the form of the binary-decision procedure.

rating categories. And, finally, we arbitrarily combined responses of three successive categories (i.e., + + +, + +, +; and −, − −, − − −) to provide a table of two rating categories. The amount of transmitted information associated with the several response categories is presented in Fig. 8.

Two points may be made with respect to the information analysis of Fig. 8. First, the transmitted scores were disappointingly low (maximum score: 1 bit per response). Second, there appears to be a small, but continued, gain in transmitted information up to at least six rating categories.[5]

We feel that the rating procedure also has important operational applications. It has been shown that a trained observer can adopt near-optimal modes of operation when the values and costs are known to him (Swets, Tanner, and Birdsall, 1955). However, the values and costs are often not known to the observer. The rating procedure permits a completely independent evaluation of values and costs by some external observer, or at some later date. This is a powerful advantage in its favor over the binary-decision procedure.

We have little information on the operational evaluation of the rating procedure. However, since it does everything that a fixed binary-decision procedure does, and preserves the operational data in a form for a later decision, and does it more exactly and more expeditiously, we are betting that it will be a handy procedure in the bag of tricks of the communications engineer in operational evaluation.

SUMMARY

A rating scale was added to the standard articulation-test procedure in order to obtain independent information about a listener's criterion

[5] The latter conclusion must be qualified. It may be shown, in the binary-decision procedure, that maximum transmission scores will be obtained when the rating responses are subdivided into two categories in proportion to the subdivision of correct and incorrect message receptions. However, there are 5 different ways the results of the six response categories can be collapsed to two response categories. And, there are 10 different ways of collapsing to three response categories. In the present experiment, maximum transmission scores were obtained with two response categories: at the −9-db S/N ratio when the subdivision was made between the ++ and + rating categories; at the −12-db S/N ratio when the subdivision was made between the + and − rating categories; and at the −15-db S/N ratio when the subdivision was made between the − and − − rating categories. In each instance, maximum transmission was achieved when the subdivision was made so that $P(R_j)$ most closely equaled $p(A_r)$. When the "optimal" subdivision was made for two response categories, the average transmitted score continued to be somewhat less than the score associated with six response categories.

for message acceptance or rejection. We find that assignment of confidence ratings does not interfere with the accuracy of message reception. The form of the receiver operating characteristic—the relationship between correct confirmations and false alarms—yielded by the rating procedure is similar to that yielded by a binary decision of message acceptance or rejection. In addition, the confidence rating is directly related to the average accuracy of message reception. This relationship is relatively invariant over a range of speech-to-noise ratios.

ACKNOWLEDGMENTS

The writers wish to thank Professor James P. Egan for his comments on notation. This research was conducted in the Operational Applications Laboratory of the U. S. Air Force. This article appeared as Tech. Rept. No. AFCRC-TR-57-11, and in J. acoust. Soc. Am., *1958,* **30,** *286–292.*

References

- Decker, L. R., and Pollack, I. Confidence ratings and message reception for filtered speech. *J. acoust. Soc. Am.,* 1958, **30,** 432–434.
- Egan, J. P. Message repetition, operating characteristics, and confusion matrices in speech communication. Indiana University: Hearing and Communication Laboratory, 1957, Technical Report No. AFCRC-TR-57-50.
- Miller, G. A., Wiener, F. M., and Stevens, S. S. Transmission and reception of sounds under combat conditions. National Defense Research Committee, 1946, Summary Technical Report of Division 17, Vol. 3, Chapter 14.
- Munson, W. A., and Karlin, J. E. The measurement of the human channel transmission characteristics. *J. acoust. Soc. Am.,* 1954, **26,** 542–553.
- Shannon, C. E. A mathematical theory of communication. *Bell System tech. J.,* 1948, **27,** 379–423.
- Smith, M., and Wilson, E. A. A model of the auditory threshold and its application to the problem of the multiple observer. *Psychol. Monogr.,* 1953, **67,** No. 9, Whole No. 359.
- Swets, J. A., Tanner, W. P., Jr., and Birdsall, T. G. The evidence for a decision-making theory of visual detection. University of Michigan: Electronic Defense Group, 1955, Technical Report No. 40. [See 1]
- Tanner, W. P., Jr., Swets, J. A., and Green, D. M. Some general properties of the hearing mechanism. University of Michigan: Electronic Defense Group, 1956, Technical Report No. 30.

32

The Effect of Vocabulary Size on Articulation Score

David M. Green and Theodore G. Birdsall

The dependence of the articulation score upon vocabulary size has been studied empirically by Miller, Heise, and Lichten (1951). In this paper we attempt to account for the data they obtained in terms of a statistical-decision model. The main virtue of the application is that a single set of transformations of the data yields a single function relating an inferred variable, d', to the physical measure of the stimulus employed in the study.

The model is not developed here in full. Rather, one plausible manner of interpreting the model will be explained. The results derived, while encouraging, need confirmation from other studies. The problems involved in checking the model with other data will be discussed.

THE MODEL

Let the set of words be denoted W, and a particular word of the set $W_i(t)$. $W_i(t)$ may be interpreted as the voltage waveform of the ith word. Suppose the receiver cross-correlates the received input $S_i(t)$ (the ith stimulus waveform) with every expected word. $S_i(t)$ may be considered as composed of two parts,

$$S_i(t) = W_i(t) + n(t)$$

where $W_i(t)$ is the ith word and $n(t)$ is random noise. Let us further assume that all words in set W are orthogonal with equal energy,

$$\int_0^T W_i(t)\ W_j(t)\ dt = 0 \qquad \text{for} \quad i \neq j$$

and

$$\int_0^T W_i(t)\ W_j(t)\ dt = E \qquad \text{for} \quad i = j$$

where T is the duration of the word and E is the energy of the word. Note that E is independent of i. All words are assumed to have the same energy. Now if a stimulus word $S_k(t)$ is presented, the receiver will cross-correlate every stored word $W(t)$ with the received input. Suppose that n such words may be presented. There will be n correlations. Of these $n - 1$ will be of the type

$$C_{k \neq j} = \int_0^T S_k(t)\ W_j(t)\ dt = \int_0^T [W_k(t) + n(t)]\ W_j(t)\ dt = \int_0^T n(t)\ W_j(t)\ dt$$

and one will be of the type

$$C_j = \int_0^T n(t)\ W_j(t)\ dt + E \qquad \text{for} \quad j = k.$$

These correlations can be transformed so that the $(n - 1)$ correlations of the type $C_{k \neq j}$ will be normally distributed with zero mean and unit variance, and the one correlation C_j will be normally distributed with a nonzero mean and unit variance.[1] This normalized mean is called d' and increases as E increases.

Let us assume that the receiver selects the largest correlation value and reports the corresponding word as the stimulus received. Then the probability that this response is correct is the probability that the correlation $C_{k=j}$ is larger than the largest of the $(n - 1)$ correlations of the type $C_{k \neq j}$.

Using the transform of these correlations, this is the probability that the largest of $n - 1$ drawings from a normal deviate with mean zero and unit variance is smaller than the drawing from a single normal deviate with mean d' and unit variance. Birdsall and Peterson (1954) have calculated a graphic answer for this problem to provide the relation

[1] That C_k is normally distributed can most easily be seen by considering this integral as a sum using the sampling theorem. It then becomes a linear sum of normal variables. The sum therefore is a normal variable (Peterson, Birdsall, and Fox, 1954).

between d' and the percentage of correct responses for various size vocabularies. The Appendix discusses these calculations in detail.

Figure 1 shows the results of these computations. The graph shows that if there are 32 possible words the mean of the "word-sent" distribution must be 3 times greater than the variance in order to be correctly chosen 80 per cent of the time. For the receiver discussed previously, $d' = \sqrt{2E/N_0}$ where E is the energy in each word and N_0 is the noise power in a 1-cps band.

APPLICATION OF THE MODEL

In Miller, Heise, and Lichten's (1951) study the articulation score is plotted as a function of signal-to-noise ratio (S/N) with vocabulary size as a parameter. From the raw data, we used each per cent correct identi-

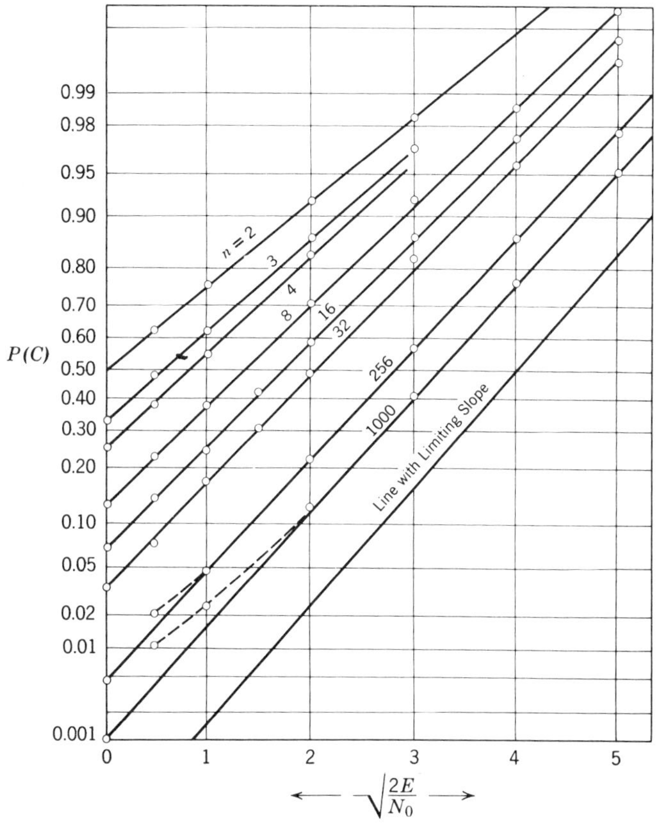

FIG. 1. Maximum probability of a correct forced choice among n orthogonal alternatives.

fication to enter Fig. 1. Using the line appropriate for this vocabulary size, a d' value was obtained. These values for d' were then plotted against the signal-to-noise ratio which was used in the study. Figure 2 shows the result of this work.

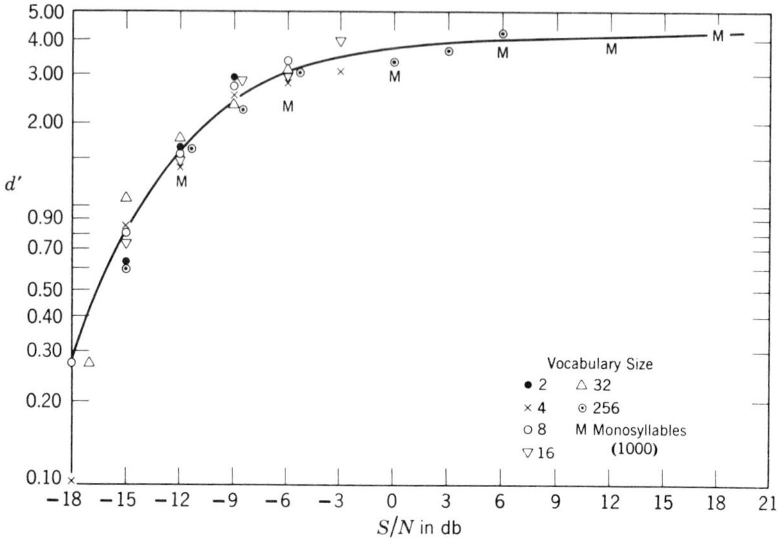

FIG. 2. The model applied to the data of Miller, Heise, and Lichten (1951).

The following examples illustrate this procedure. For a vocabulary size of two, -12 db gave 87 per cent correct; in Fig. 1, 87 per cent corresponds to a $d' = 1.60$ for a 2-word vocabulary. For a vocabulary of size 32, -12 db gives 39 per cent correct; in Fig. 1, 39 per cent yields d' of 1.73 for a 32-word vocabulary. The actual data obtained in the experiment, not the smoothed curves, were used to construct Fig. 2. In Fig. 2 a smooth line was drawn by eye through the cluster of points. The line drawn is presented in Table 1.

In order to evaluate the fit of the line to the data, the following procedure was employed. For each value of S/N the d' given in the table was assumed. This was used to re-enter Fig. 1 and to predict the articulation score. We have thus a set of per-cent-correct values as inferred from the line and the set obtained in the experiment. These two values (of predicted and obtained per cent correct) are displayed in Fig. 3. As can be seen, the line drawn in Fig. 2 appears to fit the data fairly well. Several data points do not appear on the graph. For a vocabulary of size 2, the points obtained with the smallest signal-to-noise ratio were

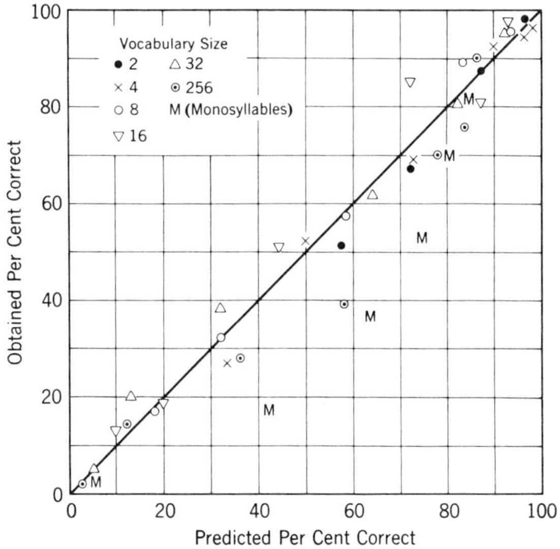

FIG. 3. Predicted versus obtained data.

49 per cent and 51 per cent. These led to estimates of d' which are too small to appear on Fig. 2. Only one is displayed in Fig. 3, since the other would have about the same value.

TABLE I. VALUES FROM THE CURVE OF FIG. 1

S/N (in db)	d'	S/N (in db)	d'
−18	.27	3	3.8
−15	.80	6	3.9
−12	1.55	9	4.0
−9	2.40	12	4.1
−6	3.00	15	4.2
−3	3.4	18	4.3
0	3.6	21	4.4

The points obtained with the monosyllables (M) depart considerably from the predicted value. One reason for this divergence is that the condition under which these data were collected is different from the procedure used with the other vocabulary sizes. The monosyllables were selected from a list of 1000 words, but the subject had no list of the 1000 words. Therefore, he could not possibly perform the operations assumed for the model. If one assumes that the apparent vocabulary size is between 2000 to 4000 words, a better prediction of these data is obtained.

We now arrive at the knotty problem of what the measure (S/N in db) means. According to Miller, Heise, and Lichten (1951), "A S/N of zero db means, therefore, that the electrical measurements indicated the two voltages, speech and noise, were equal in magnitude." A consideration of the time waveform of speech and noise leads us to believe that these voltages were not equal in magnitude for any period of time. What was done was the familiar monitoring of the speech by a volume indicator (VU). The carrier phrase "You will write . . . " was held constant by this method and the words spoken in their natural manner. The peak deflection of the meter were used to measure the individual words, and the average, therefore, gives us a definition of S in decibels. The noise was then measured on the same meter and this gives us a definition of N in decibels.

If one interprets the S/N in db as varying linearly with $\log 2E/N_0$, then one might well expect $\log d'$ to vary linearly with S/N in db. Hence, in Fig. 2, if the observer acts as an ideal receiver, one would expect a single straight line to fit the data. It must be remembered, however, that two assumptions were made in deriving the equation for the ideal receiver. First, the words were assumed to be orthogonal, and second, they were assumed to be equal in energy. Both assumptions appear unlikely, especially for the larger vocabulary sizes.

The exact manner in which a violation of these assumptions affects the expected percentage of correct detections is hard to evaluate. We can say with some certainty that a violation of either assumption will decrease the expected percentage correct. Beyond this trivial statement, little of a concrete nature can be stated. The equations for percentage of correct answers with correlated words or words of quite different energies are rather complex, and no simplifying forms have been discovered.

CONCLUSION

Although the assumptions made by the model are obviously too strong, the present analysis provides a logical way of transforming the articulation score with different vocabulary sizes to a single function. The single function was derived empirically from the data, and hence the main question remains: will the function work in other experiments? It is rather difficult to apply the functions to other experiments when the measure of the noise is dependent on the bandwidth of the system employed in the experiment. Also, until some relation is determined between "the peak VU meter deflection" and the energy in a word, it remains impossible to test the model in any detailed way.

APPENDIX: PROBABILITY OF BEING CORRECT IN A CHOICE OF n ORTHOGONAL SIGNALS

Figure 1 displays the probability of a correct choice among n orthogonal alternatives. Mathematically this is equivalent to the probability that a single drawing from a normal deviate with mean d' and unit variance will be larger than the largest of $n - 1$ drawings from a normal deviate with mean zero and variance 1. Let this probability be denoted $P_n(d')$.

The original computations for this problem were carried out by Birdsall and Peterson (1954). They used an approximate integration technique which had an error no greater than about 2 per cent. Table A1 shows the results of these computations.

Their results indicated that $P_n(d')$ could be approximated by a rather simple form

$$P_n(d') = \Phi(a_n d' - b_n) \tag{1}$$

where Φ is the (area) normal distribution function, i.e.,

$$\Phi(x) = \int_{-\infty}^{x} \frac{1}{\sqrt{2\pi}} e^{-t^2/2}\, dt$$

The value b_n is obtained by setting $d' = 0$; then $P_n(0) = \Phi(-b_n) = 1/n$. The value a_n was computed for several values of n and is listed in Table A2. For values of n between those listed, a_n may be obtained by graphic interpolation.

Tippett's (1925) tables have the distribution function for the largest of n drawings from a normal deviate with mean zero and unit variance. By convoluting this distribution function with the normal density function having mean d' and unit variance, it is possible to obtain $P_n(d')$. That is,

$$P_n(d') = \int_{-\infty}^{+\infty} T_{n-1}(x)\, \phi(x - d')\, dx \tag{2}$$

where $T_{n-1}(x)$ is Tippett's distribution and $\phi(x - d')$ is the normal density function with mean d' and unit variance. Table A3 shows the values obtained by convolution and those obtained from the report of Birdsall and Peterson (1954).

TABLE A1. COMPUTED PROBABILITY OF BEING CORRECT[a] IN A FORCED CHOICE AMONG n ORTHOGONAL ALTERNATIVES

N \ d'	0	0.5	1.0	1.5	2	3	4	5	6
Exact[b] 2	.5000	.6381	.7602	—	.9198	.9830	—	—	—
2	.5000	.6385	.7601	—	.9213	.9831	—	—	—
3	.3333	.4827	.6336	—	.8658	.9689	—	—	—
4	.2500	.3893	.5522	—	.8321	.9573	—	—	—
8	.1250	.2375	.3853	—	.7110	.9220	.9865	.9988	—
16	.0625	.1417	.2585	.4218	.5952	.8660	.9750	.9974	—
32	.03125	.0844	.1747	.3126	.4840	.8029	.9571	.9954	—
256	.00391	.0206	.0488	—	.2249	.5691	.8658	.9787	.9984
1000	.00010	.0106	.0224	—	.1247	.4118	.7645	.9509	.9950

[a] When $d' = 0$, all the variables have zero mean and unit variance. The probability that any one will be the greatest is $1/n$, and hence $P(c) = 1/n$. For the sake of clarity it must be pointed out that these P(Correct) curves are not "corrected for chance" or normalized in any manner except for that occurring from the definition of d'.

[b] These computations are exact since the greatest of one drawing from a normal deviate is simply the normal deviate. The computations listed in the line below are those obtained using the approximation formula.

TABLE A2. a_n FOR SEVERAL VALUES OF n

n	2	4	8	16	32	256	1000
a_n	.707	.827	.855	.884	.890	.916	.964

TABLE A3. COMPARISON OF TWO METHODS OF ESTIMATION

d'	0	1	3.5	
$P_{31}(d')$	.03225	.174974	.903456	Convolution with Tippett's function
$P_{32}(d')$	.03125	.1747	.89480	Birdsall and Peterson

d'	0	2	3.5	5	6	
$P_{1001}(d')$	.000999	.120231	.59818	.950594	.99484	Convolution with Tippett's function
$P_{1000}(d')$	.001	.1247	.61179	.9506	.9948	Birdsall and Peterson

If one is not satisfied with a graphic interpolation for the values of a_n, a second method may be suggested which perhaps is somewhat more accurate. To obtain $P_n(d')$ for $n \geq 30$, Tippett's distribution may be approximated by a normal distribution function, for values of $.01 \leq T_n(x) \leq .99$. That is,

$$T_n(x) \approx \Phi\left(\frac{x - m_n}{\sigma_n}\right) \tag{3}$$

where

$$m_n = \lim_{b\to\infty} [b - \int_0^b T_n(x)\,dx] \qquad n > 30 \tag{4}$$

and

$$\sigma_n^2 = \lim_{b\to\infty} [b^2 - 2\int_0^b x\,T_n(x)\,dx] - m_n^2 \qquad n > 30 \tag{5}$$

Then

$$P_{n+1}(d') = \int_{-\infty}^{\infty} \Phi\left(\frac{x - m_n}{\sigma_n}\right) \phi\,(x - d')\,dx \tag{6}$$

$$= \Phi\left(\frac{d' - m_n}{\sqrt{1 + \sigma_n^2}}\right)$$

Note that $m_n/\sqrt{1 + \sigma_n^2}$ plays a role like b_n in Eq. (1) and $1/\sqrt{1 + \sigma_n^2}$ is like a_n in Eq. (1).

For larger n ($n > 1000$) the approximations suggested by the Bureau of Standards (1953) are useful. They suggest that

$$T_n(x) = \Phi\left(\frac{x - m_n}{\sigma_n}\right) \tag{7}$$

where $m_n = U_n + \dfrac{.57722}{\alpha_n}$, and U_n is such that $\Phi(U_n) = 1 - \dfrac{1}{n}$ and

$$\alpha_n = n\phi(U_n) \text{ and } \sigma_n = \frac{\pi}{\sqrt{6}\,\alpha_n} = \frac{1.28255}{\alpha_n}$$

Since for large x ($x \geq 4$)

$$\Phi(x) = 1 - \Phi(-x) \doteq 1 - \frac{1}{x}\phi(x)$$

$$\frac{1}{U_n}\phi(U_n) \doteq \frac{1}{n}$$

$$n\,\phi(U_n) \doteq U_n$$

$$\alpha_n \doteq U_n \quad \text{for} \quad n > 10^3$$

Using the Bureau of Standards' approximations as the constants in Eq. (1),

$$\text{if } n = 10^6, \text{ then } P_n(d') = \Phi(.96796\,d' - 4.71416)$$
$$\text{if } n = 10^9, \text{ then } P_n(d') = \Phi(.97885\,d' - 5.96303)$$
$$\text{if } n = 10^{12}, \text{ then } P_n(d') = \Phi(.98434\,d' - 7.00358)$$

The term a_n approaches unity for very large n, that is, the variance of the extreme value distribution (Tippett's distribution) approaches zero for very large n.

To summarize, Birdsall and Peterson's calculations provide good approximations to the probability $P_n(d')$ for moderate values of n, $n \leq 1000$, and for practical ranges of d' (Eq. 1). Better accuracy is guaranteed using convolutions with Tippett's tables (Eq. 2). Another method similar to Birdsall and Peterson's, but employing Tippett's table is demonstrated (Eq. 6). Finally, for large n ($n > 1000$), the Bureau of Standards' approximations are useful (Eq. 7).

SUMMARY

A statistical-decision model is applied to the recognition of voice signals in noise. Certain strong simplifying assumptions are made to make the mathematics of the model manageable. The model is compared with the data of Miller, Heise, and Lichten (1951). The main problem considered is how the size of the vocabulary affects the articulation score. A discussion is included of the physical parameters involved in such tests. An appendix presents various approximations to the problem involved in predicting the percentage of correct recognition for the conditions considered by the model.

ACKNOWLEDGMENTS

The application of the one-of-n-orthogonal-signal computations to the problem of vocabulary size has been made earlier by W. P. Tanner, Jr. The particular form expressed in this paper is the responsibility of the authors. This research was conducted in the laboratories of the Electronic Defense Group of the University of Michigan with support from the Operational Applications Laboratory of the U. S. Air Force. This article appeared as Tech. Repts. No. 81 and No. AFCRC-TR-57-58.

References

• Birdsall, T. G., and Peterson, W. W. Probability of correct decision in a forced choice among m alternatives. University of Michigan: Electronic Defense Group, 1954, Quarterly Progress Report No. 10. [See Appendix 1]

• Miller, G. A., Heise, G. A., and Lichten, W. The intelligibility of speech as a function of the context of the test materials. *J. exp. Psychol.,* 1951, **41,** 329–335.

• Peterson, W. W., Birdsall, T. G., and Fox, W. C. The theory of signal detectability. *Trans. IRE Professional Group on Information Theory,* 1954, **PGIT-4,** 171–212.

• Tippett, L. H. C. On the extreme individuals and the range of samples taken from a normal population. *Biometrika,* 1925, **17,** 364–387.

• U. S. Dept of Commerce, National Bureau of Standards: Probability tables for the analysis of extreme-value data. Applied Mathematics Series 22, 1953.

33

Confidence Ratings, Second-Choice Responses, and Confusion Matrices in Intelligibility Tests

Frank R. Clarke

In the standard intelligibility test, words (or some other message units) are read in random order over a noisy channel and the listener attempts to identify each stimulus item on the basis of the degraded signal available to him. The typical measure of the listener's performance is the percentage of stimuli correctly identified. Aside from many clinical and engineering applications, this dependent variable, the intelligibility score, has been of great use in the study of speech perception. However, without extending the listener's task, it is possible to get a more complete description of his performance. By the use of small closed message sets it becomes feasible to construct confusion matrices which show the proportion of instances in which any given response is made to any given stimulus. This detailed analysis of the listener's identification responses has been used profitably in an analysis of perceptual confusions among English consonants (Miller and Nicely, 1955), and in the development of a rule for predicting the confusion matrix for any subset of items, given the confusion matrix for its master set (Clarke, 1957; Clarke and Anderson, 1957).

As we attempt to extend our knowledge of the behavior of a listener in identifying degraded speech signals, it is apparent that the listener's task in the intelligibility test, i.e., writing down a single response to each stimulus item, is such that some of the information about the stimulus which is available to him is discarded. For example, we know that on some occasions the listener is quite certain that his response is correct, and on others, he is fairly uncertain of his response. It has been shown that the listener can assign ratings of confidence to his identification responses in a nonchance manner, and thus such ratings carry additional information about the stimulus items transmitted.

Still another possible information-bearing response of the listener has had little study. This is the listener's second-choice response. Often, after making his best guess as to the identity of the stimulus, the listener feels that he can make a reasonable second choice, with some confidence that this second choice would be correct in the event that his first choice were incorrect.

The experiments to be reported in this paper were designed to investigate certain aspects of a listener's ratings of confidence and of his second-choice responses.

CONFIDENCE RATINGS APPLIED TO IDENTIFICATION RESPONSES

The experiment in this section will be used to provide the framework for the explanation of some of the concepts to be used throughout this paper. The data from this experiment will serve for making predictions and comparisons in later sections. This experiment deals with the use of a confidence rating by a listener to estimate the probability that his attempted identification of a transmitted message is, in fact, correct. The nature of these data is best understood by considering the manner in which they were obtained.

Procedure

Five highly trained listeners participated in this experiment. A closed set of stimulus words was used in intelligibility tests. This set consisted of the five spondees: *duckpond*, *eggplant*, *greyhound*, *stairway*, and *vampire*. Each of these words was represented equally often in a deck of 75 cards, and test lists containing these 75 items were constructed by shuffling the deck of cards. Each of these test lists was read by one talker (FC). The speech signals were mixed electrically with white noise (uniform spectrum level, 100 cps to 7000 cps), and then they were presented to the listeners over binaural headsets (PDR-10 earphones). The speech level was defined by the average (over all items read in the tests) of the peak deflections on a Daven VU meter of the signals, as measured in the speech channel. The noise level was observed on a Daven VU meter placed across the noise channel. The speech-to-noise ratio was computed using these values, with suitable corrections for attenuators in the circuit and correction for the reduction in the bandwidth of the noise at the earphones. A speech-to-noise ratio of approximately -16.5 db was chosen, with the aim of achieving an average articulation score of about 60 per cent. The overall level of the noise was approximately 82 db *re* 0.0002 dyne/cm^2. Items were read at the rate of one every 10 sec. On each stimulus presentation the listeners made two responses: (1) they attempted to identify the word read by the talker by writing down one of the five possible responses; and (2) they assigned a rating of 1, 2, 3, 4, or 5 to indicate how confident they were that their attempted identification of the stimulus item was, in fact, correct. The listeners were instructed to use the rating 1 in such a way that responses given this rating would have a probability of being correct lying within the range 0.90 to 1.00. Ratings of 2 through 5 were to indicate estimates of a posteriori probabilities within the ranges 0.75 to 0.90, 0.55 to 0.75, 0.35 to 0.55, and 0.00 to 0.35, respectively. After each test of 75 items, the listeners scored and tabulated their own responses, and thus had constant feedback to aid them in their attempt to use the ratings as instructed to. Before the tests for which data are here reported, the listeners had taken 299 intelligibility tests of typical length, 90 of which involved the use of the previously mentioned set of spondees presented at the speech-to-noise ratio of -16.5 db. Twelve of these tests provided practice in the use of ratings. Twenty-two of the subsequent 24 tests met a pre-established criterion that the average articulation score for the group be between 50 per cent and 70 per cent. These tests provided the data for the following discussion.

Results and discussion

The proportions obtained in this and the following experiments will be taken as estimates of underlying probabilities. The data for any individual listener may be presented in complete detail (except for any time-dependent effects) in a 5×25 matrix—5 rows for each of the stimuli and 25 columns for each of the response pairs (one of 5 identification responses followed by one of 5 ratings). By summing entries in this table over rating categories, we may obtain a typical confusion matrix with rows corresponding to stimuli and the 5 columns corresponding to identification responses. For certain of the conclusions to be presented, it is assumed that this latter matrix does not differ systematically from the one that would have been obtained if the listener had made a single identification response and had not followed this response with a confidence rating. Intuitively this seems reasonable, and from previous studies (Egan and Clarke, 1956; Pollack and Decker, 1958) it is known that the added confidence rating does not depress the listener's articulation score.

One concern of this study is the extent to which the additional rating response adds information over and above the information transmitted by the identification response. Implicitly, at least, we will be considering this in a general sense throughout the rest of this section. However, first let us examine the data in terms of the technical meaning of the term "information," using Shannon's (1949) measure of information transmitted. To calculate the amount of information added by the rating response to that already transmitted by the identification response, it is necessary to determine the amount of information transmitted when both responses are considered jointly, and subtract from this the information transmitted when only the identification response is considered. Since the degrees of freedom for the two tables differ, it is first necessary to apply the Miller-Madow correction for bias (Miller, 1955) to the calculated values of information transmitted (I_t).

Table I summarizes the results for each listener in terms of calculated rates of information transmission. On the average, the rating response added 0.127 bit per item to the rate of information transmission for the identification response alone. Of the information carried by the identification response and the rating response considered jointly, 16.5 per cent was contributed uniquely by the ratings.

TABLE I. Analysis of Rate of Information Transmitted for Each of the Five Listeners in This Experiment. Column A Shows Information Transmitted per Stimulus Item When Identification Responses and Rating Responses Are Considered Jointly. Column B Shows Information Transmitted per Stimulus Item When Only Identification Responses Are Considered. Columns C and D Are Self-explanatory. Column E Gives the Percentage of Correct Responses for Each Listener.

	A $I_t(S \times I \cdot R)$	B $I_t(S \times I)$	C $A - B$	D B/A	E $p(C)$
*L*1	0.689	0.553	0.136	0.803	0.566
*L*2	0.994	0.889	0.105	0.894	0.697
*L*3	1.063	0.905	0.158	0.851	0.696
*L*4	0.547	0.471	0.076	0.861	0.520
*L*5	0.686	0.527	0.159	0.768	0.566
Mean	0.796	0.669	0.127	0.835	0.609
Mdn.	0.689	0.553	0.136	0.851	0.566

In many communication situations the listener could easily utilize the additional information provided by the ratings. For example, if the listener is provided with a back-channel and is allowed to trade speed of transmission for accuracy, then he could accept only those messages which he rated with a rating R_k or stricter, and ask for repeats on all others (Egan, Clarke, and Carterette, 1956; Carterette, 1958). In Table I we see that the articulation score, $p(C)$, for $L1$ is 0.566. Now, if the listener decided to accept his identification response only when his confidence rating was a 1 or a 2, and if whenever his confidence rating was a 3, 4, or 5 he were to ask the speaker to repeat the message, then, $L1$ would be expected to identify correctly 0.769 of the messages in the set; but it would take 4.5 times as long as needed to attain 0.566 identification. Note that this method of increasing accuracy of message reception only involves trading speed for accuracy; it does not depend on the listener's having a knowledge of his confusion matrix. Of course, the articulation score may be improved without the use of ratings merely by repeating each message several times before moving on to the next message. At the end of each series of transmitted messages, the listener may then make a single response in attempting to identify the transmitted message. However, the addition of ratings in this situation also results in a marked improvement. (See Egan, 1957, for details; especially Case 2 in Chap. 3 and in Chap. 5, and Appendix D.)

The ability of the receiver to assign ratings in accordance with a posteriori probabilities is indicated in Fig. 1. The points in this figure show the obtained a posteriori probabilities associated with each of the rating categories, while the bars show the probability with which the listener used each category. The obtained a posteriori probabilities were calculated by dividing the number of times a listener assigned a given rating to a correct identification response by the total number of times that the listener used that particular rating. It will be noted that all listeners did a fairly good job of using the rating categories as directed. However, these are averages over the five stimulus items, and a more detailed analysis of the data indicated that the listeners tended to overestimate a posteriori probabilities for items of relatively low intelligibility and to underestimate these probabilities for items of relatively high intelligibility. This supports a similar finding by Pollack and Decker (1958).

The results of much of the recent work dealing with the confirming behavior of a receiver have been reported in terms of the Type II ROC curve (Clarke, Birdsall, and Tanner, 1959; Pollack, 1959). This curve, the receiver operating characteristic, is a plot of the probability that the receiver will confirm his identification response, given that it is correct,

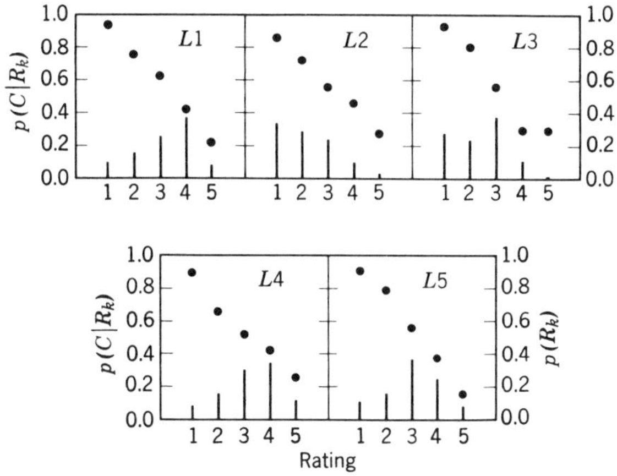

FIG. 1. The bars in this figure show the probability, $p(R_k)$, that the listener assigned the rating R_k to his identification response. The points indicate the probability that the listener was correct, given that he assigned the rating R_k to his identification response. The data for each listener are shown separately.

against the probability that he will confirm his identification response, given that it is incorrect. Where ratings are used, rather than a binary decision, the assumption is made that under some particular criterion, the receiver would accept as correct all identification responses to which a confidence of R_k or stricter had been given and would reject all responses in which he had less confidence. Figure 2 shows the data for the five listeners plotted as a receiver operating characteristic of Type II. In this figure the proportions are plotted on a linear scale. The solid curve drawn through the data points fits very nicely, and since it is a straight line when plotted on normal-normal probability paper, as in Fig. 3, a listener's performance may be specified by two parameters. The two parameters chosen to represent the line are $(d_e)^{1/2}$ and s, the slope of the line (Clarke, Birdsall, and Tanner, 1959). For each listener's data, the straight line which minimized the sum of the squares of the perpendicular distances from the points to the line was obtained. The average value of $(d_e)^{1/2}$ and the average value of s were used to construct the single line plotted in Fig. 2.

THE USE OF TWO IDENTIFICATION RESPONSES

We have seen in the previous section that requiring a listener to rate his confidence in his identification response is one method of recovering some of the information which is available to the listener but which is

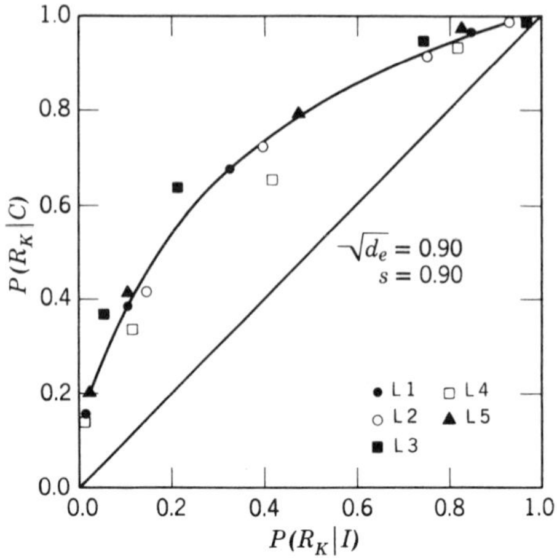

FIG. 2. A Type II ROC curve for five listeners obtained with a set of five spondees read at a speech-to-noise ratio of -16.5 db. The ordinate shows the probability of a listener's accepting his identification response as correct, given that his identification response is, in fact, correct. The abscissa indicates the probability of a listener's accepting his identification response as correct, given that it was incorrect. Here, $P(R_k|C) = \sum_{k=1,K} p(R_k|C)$ and $P(R_K|I) = \sum_{k=1,K} p(R_k|I)$. The two parameters describing the solid curve drawn through the data are $(d_e)^{1/2}$ and s.

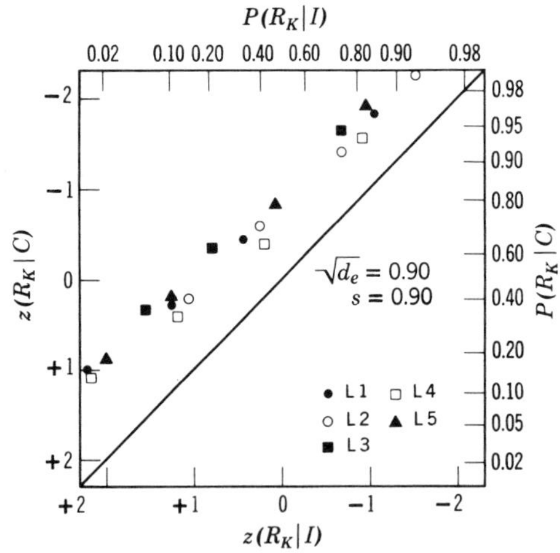

FIG. 3. The data of Fig. 2 plotted on normal-normal probability paper.

normally lost when he makes a single identification response. Another method of attempting to tap this additional information is to require the listener to respond to each stimulus presentation with his best estimate of what item was transmitted and to follow this with his second-best estimate.

Little research has been carried out concerning a subject's second-choice behavior. Shannon (1951) required subjects to use first, second, and additional "guesses" as a technique for estimating the entropy of printed English. Blank and Quastler (1954) have used this technique to estimate information transmitted by visual displays. In neither of these instances was the emphasis on the analysis of the subject's second and subsequent choice behavior per se.

Swets, Tanner, and Birdsall (1955) investigated the second-choice behavior of a viewer attempting to determine in which of four short intervals of time an increment in the intensity of a light occurred. They found the viewer's second-choice performance to be significantly better than that predicted by chance, and, in fact, they were able to make fairly good predictions of the obtained data, using their "decision-making theory of visual detection."

Pollack (1952), in a verbal learning context, investigated the information content of the subjects' second, third, and fourth choices. Here, when a subject made an error in attempting to recall an item, he was so informed and required to make another guess. Bricker and Chapanis (1953) carried out a similar experiment with tachistoscopically presented stimuli. In both of these studies, the information transmitted by the subject's second choice was compared with the information to be expected under the simplest of threshold models. Both studies purported to demonstrate that considerable information is transmitted by the subject's second and later choices. However, they did not analyze their data in such a way as to determine to what degree the information contained in the second choice (for example) is independent of that contained in the first choice. The fact that the second choice contains a considerable amount of information about the stimulus does not permit the conclusion that the second choice adds information to that already contained in the first choice. Certainly, one cannot conclude that the information transmitted by the first and second responses considered jointly is equal to the information transmitted by the first choice plus the information transmitted by the second choice. The present study will attempt to determine to what extent the information contained in the second choice does, in fact, add to that contained in the first choice.

The study reported in this section is largely empirical. Because of the paucity of data concerning second-choice behavior, as well as the complexity of the speech signal, there is no adequate theory which leads to the prediction of a listener's stimulus-by-second-choice confusion matrix given only his stimulus-by-first-choice matrix. A simple threshold model fails to account for the obtained data. An extension of the constant-ratio rule suggests that the listener would make his second-choice response as though he were responding to the stimulus item with a set of response alternatives limited by removing his first choice from his original set of alternatives. However, in this study, this model also fails to account for the obtained data. A simplified version of the theory of signal detectability also fails to account for the observed data.

Procedure

The procedure for obtaining the data to be reported in this section was essentially the same as that described in the previous section, the only basic change being in the instructions to the listeners. Here, the listeners were instructed to make their best attempt to identify the stimulus item, and to follow this with their next best choice. Thus, after the stimulus item was spoken only once, the listeners made two identification responses. Both choices could not be the same. The same talker and listeners were used here as in obtaining the rating data reported in the previous section. Two additional listeners were used for some of these second-choice tests. Two sets of five spondees each were used: Set 1, *cupcake*, *padlock*, *pancake*, *starlight*, and *wildcat;* and Set 2, *duckpond*, *eggplant*, *greyhound*, *stairway*, and *vampire*. Listeners were highly practiced on the second-choice task with these message sets before data were obtained. It will be noted that Set 2 is identical to that used to obtain the rating data; thus, direct comparisons between the two types of second responses are possible. The data in this section were obtained prior to those reported in the previous section.

Results and discussion

Before examining data of more general interest, it is necessary to consider the possibility that any information transmitted by a listener's second choice is gained at the expense of information in his first choice. That is, when a listener's task is to give two responses to each stimulus item he might distribute the information available to him over both responses; yet, if he were limited to a single response he might well be able to convey the same amount of information in this single response. If this were occurring, it would almost certainly have the effect that the listener's articulation score for his best estimate of the stimulus item when he was required to make two responses would be lower than the articulation score for his best estimate when required to make only one response to each stimulus item. The equivalence of a listener's first-choice behavior when required to make only one response to each transmitted message and when required to make two responses to each message was investigated by comparing first-choice articulation scores obtained by each of the two procedures. Carefully controlled tests were conducted using a set of five items. On one-half of the tests the five listeners responded with a single best estimate of the transmitted message. On the remaining tests they responded with their best estimate followed by a second choice. Tests were counterbalanced, and talker variables were eliminated through the use of recorded tests. (Recorded speech was mixed with "live" noise.) Twelve tests were conducted under each condition. The mean and median articulation scores of the single-choice tests were 0.617 and 0.640, respectively. Corresponding mean and median articulation scores for the listener's first choice in the two-response tests were 0.631 and 0.640. Clearly, this observed difference is not statistically significant. It would appear safe to conclude that requiring a listener to make a second-choice response does not depress his first-choice performance (Swets, Tanner, and Birdsall, 1955).

For the information analysis we will first look at some of the data obtained using Set 2. As there were five stimulus items in this set, on any given trial a listener could respond with any one of the five items as his first identification response and with any one of the four remaining items as his second identification response. Thus, the data for each listener may be presented in a 5×20 matrix having entries which show the proportion of instances in which a particular response pair occurred, given that a particular stimulus item was read. By appropriately collapsing this large matrix, we may obtain for each listener two separate matrices: (1) a stimulus-by-first-identification-response matrix, and (2) a stimulus-by-second-identification-response matrix. For each of these three matrices, we may calculate the corresponding rate of information transmission. These are (1) the information transmitted by the listener's first and second responses considered jointly, $I_t(S \times 1 \cdot 2)$; (2) the information transmitted by the listener's first identification response, $I_t(S \times 1)$; and (3) the information transmitted by the listener's second choice, $I_t(S \times 2)$. The information transmitted by the listener's second identification response which is independent of that transmitted by his first response is given by $I_t(S \times 1 \cdot 2)$ minus $I_t(S \times 1)$.

Table II summarizes the results obtained in this experiment using stimulus Set 2, the same set of items for which rating results were reported in the previous section. As all conditions except the listener's

TABLE II. Analysis of the Rate of Information Transmitted for Each of the Listeners in the Second-Choice Experiment Utilizing Message Set 2. Column A Shows the Rate of Information Transmission When the Listener's First and Second Identification Responses Are Considered Jointly. Column B Shows the Rate of Information Transmission When Only the Listener's First Identification Response Is Considered. Column C Shows the Rate of Information Transmission When Only the Listener's Second Identification Response Is Considered. Columns D, E, and F Are Self-explanatory. Column G Shows the Probability That the Listener's First Identification Response Is Correct. Column H Shows the Probability That the Listener's Second Identification Response Is Correct, Given That His First Identification Response Was Incorrect.

	A	B	C	D	E	F	G	H
	$I(S \times 1 \cdot 2)$	$I(S \times 1)$	$I(S \times 2)$	$A - B$	$(A - B)/C$	B/A	$p(C_1)$	$p(C_2 \mid I_1)$
L1	0.556	0.527	0.100	0.029	0.290	0.948	0.559	0.376
L2	0.852	0.830	0.113	0.022	0.195	0.974	0.667	0.331
L3	1.002	0.950	0.461	0.052	0.113	0.948	0.713	0.495
L4	0.393	0.383	0.136	0.010	0.074	0.975	0.487	0.348
L5	0.562	0.548	0.227	0.014	0.062	0.975	0.567	0.404
Mean	0.673	0.648	0.207	0.025	0.147	0.964	0.599	0.391
Median	0.562	0.548	0.136	0.022	0.113	0.974	0.567	0.376
L6	0.638	0.597	0.286	0.041	0.143	0.936	0.580	0.475

second-response task are as similar as possible to the conditions reported in the previous section, Table II may be directly compared with Table I. Comparison of the two sets of data shows that the average articulation scores for the group differ by only 1 per cent; furthermore, for the two sets of data the average rates of information transmission for the stimulus-by-first-response matrix differ by only 0.021 bit per item. Thus, comparison of the information-carrying capacity of the two types of additional responses, ratings and second identification responses, appears justifiable. In Table I, we see that the rating response carried on the average 0.127 bit per item over and above that carried by the identification response. In Table II, we see that the second identification response averages only 0.025 bit per item which is independent of the information carried by the first identification response. Thus, on the average, only 14.5 per cent of the information carried by the second response was independent of that carried by the first response. Furthermore, unlike the case with the rating response, there is no simple way in which the listener can utilize the additional information carried by the second identification response, and in most cases it would be of no practical use.

From column H of Table II, we see, given that the listener's first identification response was incorrect, the probability of his being correct on his second response is 0.391. Comparing this figure with the one that would be expected by "chance," 0.250, we see that the subject's performance may seem paradoxically "good," considering the small amount of information which the second identification response adds to that transmitted by the first identification response. However, it must be realized that the fact that the listener's second choices are considerably better than "chance," when measured in terms of percentage correct, in no way implies that the second choice carries any information about the stimulus which is not already carried by the first response. For example, given a set of words with a nonhomogeneous confusion matrix, we could read the words in a background of noise to a listener who makes a single identification response. He could then pass his response on to a second subject who was not allowed to listen to the stimulus item when it was read. This second subject could be required to make the second identification response, that is, attempt to identify the stimulus on the assumption that the listener's identification was incorrect. If the stimulus items had varying degrees of interconfusibility, and if the second subject had some knowledge of the various factors leading to confusions among items, we would expect him to make identification considerably better than "chance expectation" even though he did not hear the stimulus item. Clearly in this case the second subject is making his response to a stimulus which is the response of the listener, and even though this second response may contain considerable information about the stimulus, it cannot contain any information independent of that contained in the listener's response.

In order to give some meaning, in terms of percentage correct, to the average of 0.025 bit per symbol added by the listener's second identification response, the listener's actual performance will be compared with that which might be expected on the assumption that the listener's second response was, in fact, a response made to his first response, and that it was not otherwise influenced by the stimulus. For this purpose, let us look only at those instances in which the listener's first response was incorrect. Then, for each listener we may construct a stimulus-by-first-choice matrix, given that the first choice was incorrect as well as a first-choice-by-second-choice matrix for those instances in which the first choice was incorrect. As these are tables of conditional probabilities, we may treat them as transition matrices for a Markov chain; therefore, the product of these two matrices gives the expected stimulus-by-second-choice matrix for the listener under the assumption that the second response is made solely to the first response, and otherwise is uninfluenced by the transmitted stimulus item. By way of example, Table III compares the obtained stimulus-by-second-choice matrix for *L*1 with that computed by taking the product of these matrices. It will be noted that

TABLE III. The Upper Entries in the Table Indicate the Obtained Stimulus-by-Second-Choice Matrix for *L*1. The Lower, Parenthetical Entries Resulted from Taking the Product of This Listener's Stimulus-by-First-Choice Matrix, Given That the First Choice Was Incorrect and His First-Choice-by-Second-Choice Matrix, Given That the First Choice Was Incorrect.

	Second response when first incorrect				
Stimulus	*DP*	*EP*	*GH*	*SW*	*VP*
DP	0.558	0.115	0.182	0.079	0.067
	(0.440)	(0.157)	(0.218)	(0.094)	(0.091)
EP	0.230	0.390	0.198	0.037	0.144
	(0.225)	(0.299)	(0.232)	(0.054)	(0.191)
GH	0.281	0.248	0.318	0.073	0.080
	(0.319)	(0.242)	(0.257)	(0.067)	(0.116)
SW	0.301	0.145	0.120	0.241	0.193
	(0.426)	(0.134)	(0.110)	(0.133)	(0.198)
VP	0.212	0.217	0.179	0.043	0.348
	(0.212)	(0.287)	(0.207)	(0.071)	(0.223)

the matrix computed on the Markov assumption looks very different from a "chance matrix." Figure 4 indicates the relationship between the entries of the obtained stimulus-by-second-choice matrix and those computed by the Markov assumption for all listeners. Although a more restricted definition of "information" than Shannon's is utilized, the fact that 22 out of 25 of the obtained diagonal entries are higher than the computed diagonal entries implies that the 0.025 bit per item added by the listener's second response is highly significant in a statistical sense.

The data for *L*6 which are included in Table II, but not otherwise referred to thus far, are included as a check on the training and motivation of the other five listeners. This listener (the author) was an experienced and highly motivated subject and comparison of his data with those of the other listeners would imply that their training and motivation were sufficient to result in a meaningful test of the information-carrying capacity of the second identification response.

The preceding analysis was based upon the results obtained with stimulus Set 2. Table IV summarizes the results for these listeners with stimulus Set 1. These data clearly support those reported in Table II.

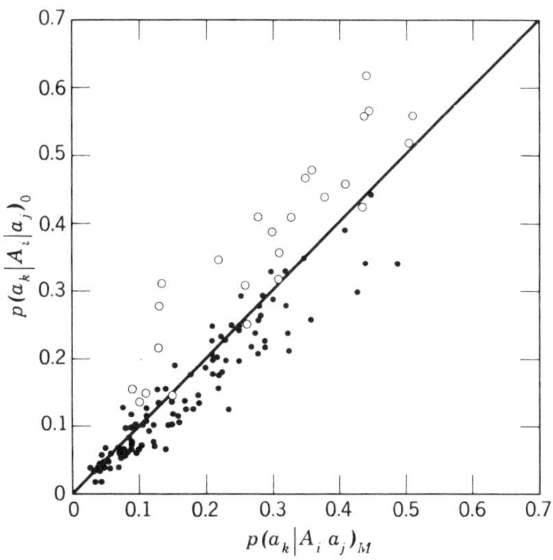

FIG. 4. The obtained probability of a second-choice response, given that the first identification response was incorrect, plotted against the corresponding predicted probability under a Markov assumption. The open circles indicated obtained and predicted probabilities of correct responses on the listener's second choice. The solid points show obtained and predicted probabilities of incorrect responses on the listener's second choice.

TABLE IV. Analysis of the Rate of Information Transmitted for Each of the Listeners in the Second-Choice Experiment Utilizing Message Set 1. All Entries Are to Be Interpreted in the Same Way as Those in Table II.

	A	B	C	D	E	F	G	H
	$I(S \times 1 \cdot 2)$	$I(S \times 1)$	$I(S \times 2)$	$A - B$	$(A - B)/C$	B/A	$p(C_1)$	$p(C_2 \mid I_1)$
*L*1	0.526	0.516	0.295	0.010	0.034	0.981	0.569	0.386
*L*2	0.720	0.719	0.223	0.001	0.004	0.999	0.628	0.367
*L*3	0.970	0.911	0.367	0.059	0.161	0.939	0.701	0.452
*L*4	0.381	0.388	0.192	−0.007	−0.036	1.018	0.504	0.345
*L*5	0.555	0.537	0.255	0.018	0.071	0.968	0.570	0.412
*L*7	0.664	0.650	0.305	0.014	0.046	0.979	0.619	0.379
Mean	0.636	0.620	0.273	0.016	0.047	0.981	0.598	0.390
Mdn.	0.610	0.594	0.275	0.012	0.040	0.980	0.594	0.082

The data reported in this section may be summarized by making the following points: (1) On the average, of the information carried by the listener's second identification response, only about 7 per cent is independent of information carried by the listener's first-choice response. (2) On the average, of the information carried by the first and second responses considered jointly, over 97 per cent is carried by the first choice alone. (3) If the second response is a rating response, it will add about six times as much information to that carried by a first identification response as will a second identification response. Furthermore, the additional information in the ratings is easily utilized by the listener, whereas that in the second identification response cannot easily be used in most situations.

It must be pointed out that the generality of these results may be limited. It is clear that the information content of the listener's second identification response will depend upon both the size of the message set and upon the signal-to-noise ratio at the listener's ear. If sets of only two items are used, the subject's second-identification response will contain as much information as his first choice, but the second choice can contain no information independent of that contained in his first. As the size of the message set is increased, it becomes possible for the second choice to contain less information than the first choice (though probably not more), but some of this information may now be independent of that contained in the first choice. As the signal-to-noise ratio is varied from minus infinity to plus infinity, the information in the second choice which is independent of that in the first choice would be expected to range from zero through a maximum and then back to zero again.

In order to make calculations of I_t, the number of probabilities to be estimated grows as the cube of the size of the message set. It was this consideration which limited the size of the message set investigated. The speech-to-noise ratio was chosen in an attempt to come near to maximizing the independent information content of the second response.

A POSTERIORI PROBABILITIES AND THE RECEIVER OPERATING CHARACTERISTIC

We have seen that, for a given message set at a particular speech-to-noise ratio, the listeners can be trained to give fairly accurate estimates of the probability that their identification response is correct. There is the question of whether or not the listeners can make accurate estimates of a posteriori probabilities when the speech-to-noise ratio and the size of the message set change from test to test. The data presented in this section deal with this question. These data will also serve to give some indication of how the parameters of the receiver operating characteristic vary as a function of the size of the message set and the speech-to-noise ratio.

Procedure

In general, the procedure for obtaining these data was the same as that described previously. The listener always made two responses to each item: an identification response, and a rating that indicated his degree of confidence in the correctness of his identification response. Five rating categories were used to indicate estimates of a posteriori probabilities in the following ranges: (1) .90–1.00; (2) .70–.90; (3) .50–.70; (4) .30–.50; and (5) .00–.30. Speech-to-noise ratios for the various tests ranged from -9 db to -18 db in 3-db steps. Closed message sets of two sizes were used: $m = 4$, and $m = 16$. Sixteen four-word message sets and four sixteen-word message sets were selected randomly from a list of 1000 monosyllabic words (Egan, 1944). On each test, the listeners had copies of the message set before them, and they were required to respond to each item with a word from this list. The talker and five listeners had served in the experiments reported in the earlier sections of this paper. After two days of practice, which covered all message sets and all speech-to-noise ratios to be used in this experiment, the following basic design was replicated (using different sets of words) four times. On each of three consecutive days there were two 80-item intelligibility tests utilizing a single message set of 16 words. There were also two intelligibility tests of 20 items with each of four of the message sets containing four words. The first day of each three-day period was considered as practice, and the results on the following two days were taken as data. Over these two days, for each message set there was one test at each of the four speech-to-noise ratios. The order of the tests was counterbalanced over the entire experiment. After each presentation of 80 stimuli (either a single test with $m = 16$ or four tests with $m = 4$), the listeners scored the tests, and they calculated their a posteriori probability for each rating.

Results

Figure 5 indicates the degree to which the listeners were able to estimate a posteriori probabilities. In constructing this figure, all data were treated as though from a single listener. This was necessary in order that the conditional probabilities for some of the less-used ratings could be based on a large enough sample to assure a reasonable degree of reliability. Inherent in this averaging procedure is the danger of misrepresenting data for individuals. However, each listener's data were also analyzed separately and the average data are representative of their performance. Proportions having a denominator of less than 100 are not plotted in Fig. 5.

Despite changing speech-to-noise ratios and changing size of message sets from test to test, the listeners were able to do a fairly good job of partitioning their identification responses as instructed. By and large, the points for the various rating categories tend to fall within or very close to the boundaries which the listeners were instructed to use. These boundaries are represented by the solid horizontal lines in Fig. 5. However, comparison of their data with those reported in Fig. 1 shows that the listeners were able to do much better when speech-to-noise ratio and size of message set were not varied. As would be expected, at the high speech-to-noise ratios the listeners limited themselves primarily to high estimates of a posteriori probabilities and for low speech-to-noise ratios their estimates of a posteriori probabilities were generally low. This is clear from Fig. 5, when it is recalled that points are only plotted when the denominator is equal to or greater than 100.

It has been shown by many investigators that for many types of psychophysical judgments observers have a tendency to make their judg-

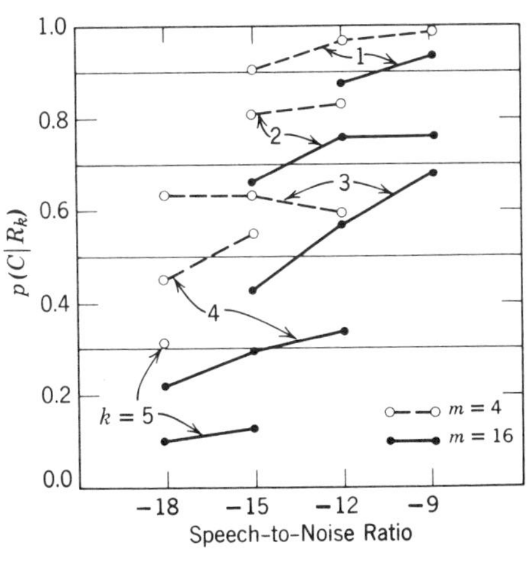

FIG. 5. Average a posteriori probabilities obtained for identification responses given confidence ratings of 1 through 5, as a function of size of message set and speech-to-noise ratio. The solid horizontal lines indicate the ranges of a posteriori probabilities for which the observers were instructed to use the rating categories.

ments relative to the range of stimuli encountered in the experiment (Helson, 1947). In view of this fact it is reasonable to expect that the listeners would tend to rate the "intelligibility" of any given item relative to the range of "intelligibilities" encountered within any particular test. Such a tendency would account for the fact that the curves showing the relation between $p(C|R_k)$ and speech-to-noise ratio have, for the most part, positive slopes. This "adaptation-level" factor would also be consistent with the observed fact that, for the larger message set relative to the smaller, the listeners overestimate their probability of being correct on their identification response. Apparently, there is an interaction between estimated a posteriori probabilities and both speech-to-noise ratio and size of message set. This interaction should not obscure the main finding that the listeners were fairly capable of estimating a posteriori probabilities over the entire range of conditions tested. It should be noted that Pollack and Decker (1958) did not find an interaction between the a posteriori probabilities associated with the listeners' ratings and speech-to-noise ratio.

Figures 6 and 7 show the Type-II receiver operating characteristics obtained. The curves passing through the data would be straight lines if plotted on normal-normal probability paper. Thus, these curves may be characterized by the two parameters $(d_e)^{1/2}$ and s. There was no systematic variation in the slopes of these lines as a function of either message size or speech-to-noise ratio, and a slope of 0.9 was taken as representative of all of the data. However, $(d_e)^{1/2}$ appears to be a function of both

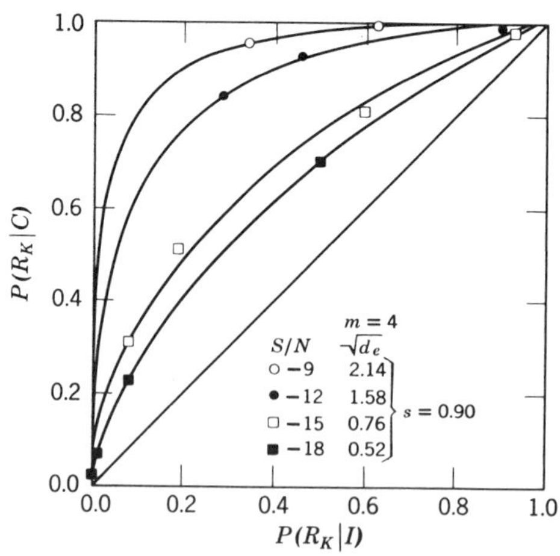

FIG. 6. Type-II ROC curves for message sets of four items.

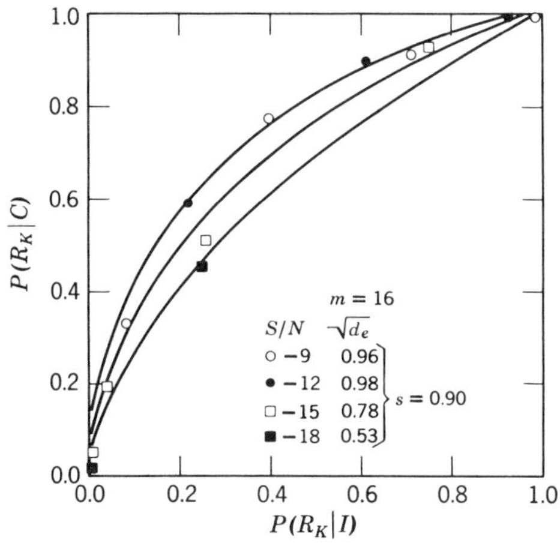

FIG. 7. Type-II ROC curves for message sets of sixteen items.

of these variables, as is seen most clearly in Fig. 8. These data suggest that at the lower speech-to-noise ratios the size of the message set is not an important variable in affecting $(d_e)^{1/2}$. Of course, when the speech-to-noise ratio is equal to minus infinity, $(d_e)^{1/2}$ must equal zero, and the curves of Fig. 8 must converge. Thus, the data suggest that as the speech-to-noise ratio increases the curves relating $(d_e)^{1/2}$ to speech-to-noise ratio for all sizes of message set climb together and then fan out at higher speech-to-noise ratios.

THE *P*-10 INDEX

It has been shown (Egan and Clarke, 1956; Miller, Heise, and Lichten, 1951) that the intelligibility score is markedly affected by the number of

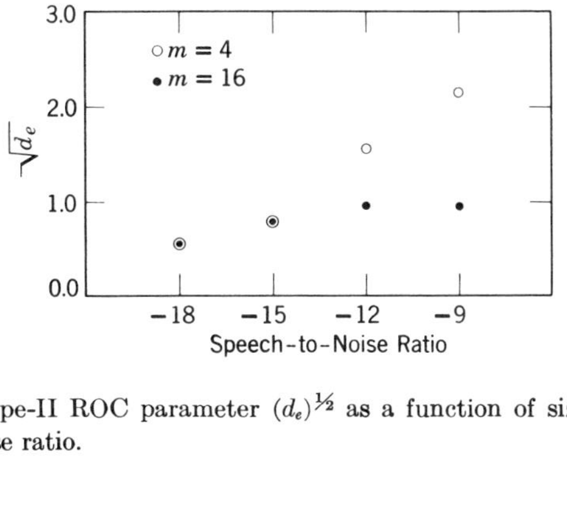

FIG. 8. The Type-II ROC parameter $(d_e)^{1/2}$ as a function of size of message set and speech-to-noise ratio.

alternatives from which the listener must choose his response on each stimulus presentation. This section will discuss some transformations of $p(C)$ which were selected in an attempt to describe a family of intelligibility gain functions (with m as a parameter) by a single function. The P-10 index is suggested as a transformed score which shows promise of fulfilling this aim.

Because of its common use it is first necessary to examine the long-used "correction for guessing." As its name implies (and its formula verifies), this transformation of obtained proportions is based on a threshold model. This model states that a listener either "hears an item," in which case he identifies it correctly, or he "hears nothing," in which case he merely guesses at the identity of the item. It is further assumed that if the listener must guess, each of the m alternatives in the set has the probability $1/m$ of being selected. With this model, the obtained proportion of correct responses with a set of size m, p_m, may be transformed to p_T, the proportion of instances in which the listener "heard the item." This transformation is accomplished by the formula

$$p_T = \frac{mp_m - 1}{m - 1} \tag{1}$$

The degree to which this formula leads to a transformation of p_m which is independent of m may be evaluated by considering the intelligibility gain functions obtained from the experiment reported in the previous section. Figure 9 shows these gain functions. Scores were averaged over all five listeners; the curve for $m = 16$ represents data pooled for the four message sets of 16 words each, while the curve for $m = 4$ is based on averages over the 16 message sets of 4 words each. When the obtained

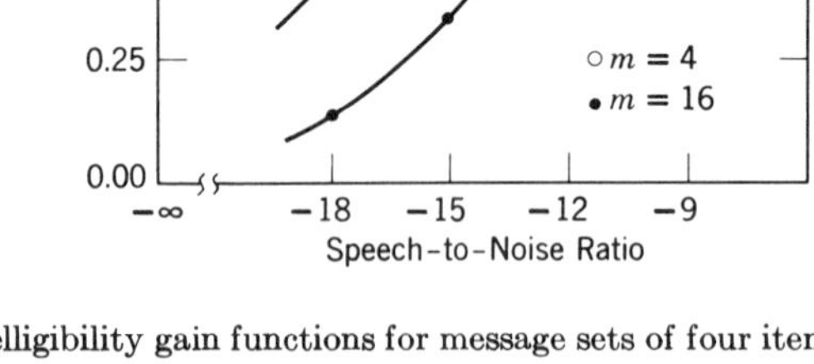

FIG. 9. Intelligibility gain functions for message sets of four items and for message sets of sixteen items.

proportions of Fig. 9 are transformed by Eq. (1), the functions illustrated in Fig. 10 are obtained. Although the "correction for guessing" does reduce the separation between the functions of Fig. 9, it is clear that the two sets of points cannot be described by a single curve.

The constant-ratio rule (Clarke, 1957; Clarke and Anderson, 1957) is an empirical rule which states that when a subject is attempting to identify unordered stimuli in a background of noise, the ratio between any pair of entries in a row of the confusion matrix for some particular set of items will equal the ratio between the corresponding pair of entries in the confusion matrix for any subset of these items. Thus, for a message set of size m_1 whose confusion matrix is known, it is possible to predict the confusion matrix (which yields the intelligibility score) for any subset of items. Egan (1957*b*) has suggested that the *average* intelligibility score for a number of possible subsets of size m_2 drawn from a master set of size m_1 may be approximated without having detailed knowledge of the confusion matrix for the master set. This is accomplished by assuming a uniform confusion matrix for the master set of items. This assumed uniform matrix has all diagonal entries equal to the articulation score for the master set, $p_{m_1}(C)$, and all of the off-diagonal entries equal to $(1 - P_{m_1})/(m_1 - 1)$. Then, with such a matrix, regardless of the particular subset of size m_2 chosen from this master set, the constant-ratio rule predicts that the sub-set will have an articulation score given by the formula

$$p_{m_2} = \frac{(m_1 - 1)p_{m_1}}{m_2 - 1 + (m_1 - m_2)p_{m_1}} \tag{2}$$

Egan pointed out that this approximation may be very poor for predict-

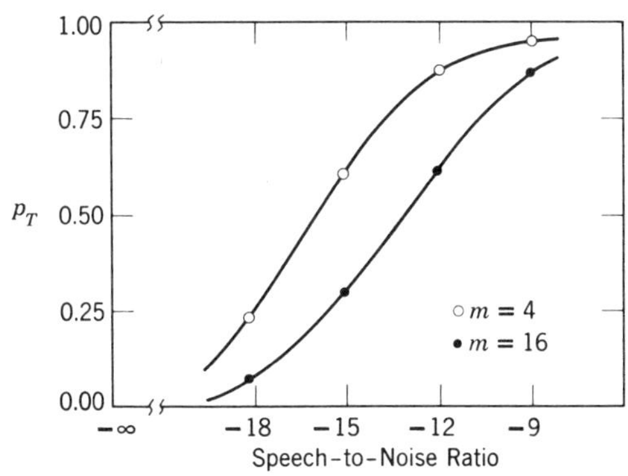

FIG. 10. The intelligibility gain functions of Fig. 9 after application of the "correction for guessing" based on a simple threshold model.

ing the articulation score for any particular subset of size m_2. However, he has presented calculations which suggest that it may be an excellent estimate of the average articulation score for a large sample of subsets of size m_2.

This suggests that average articulation scores for various sizes of message sets could be equated by computing the articulation score that would have been expected had message sets of some particular size, say $m = 10$, been used. We shall denote this transformed score as P-10. Thus from Eq. (2) we obtain

$$P\text{-}10 = \frac{(m - 1)p_m}{9 + (m - 10)p_m} \tag{3}$$

In this formula m may take any value; it need not be less than 10. The term p_m is the average articulation score obtained with a large sample of message sets, each of size m. P-10 is assumed to be the average articulation score which would have been obtained had a large sample of message sets of size $m = 10$ been drawn from the same population of messages.

Applying this transformation to the intelligibility scores of Fig. 9, we obtain the single function seen in Fig. 11. Although this result looks very promising, a note of caution must be expressed. When applied to the data obtained by Miller, Heise, and Lichten (1951), the P-10 index does not do such an excellent job of reducing their family of curves to a single function. As the constant-ratio rule has been tested primarily with listeners who were highly practiced with the particular sets of messages under test, it may be that the P-10 index is applicable only when these conditions prevail.

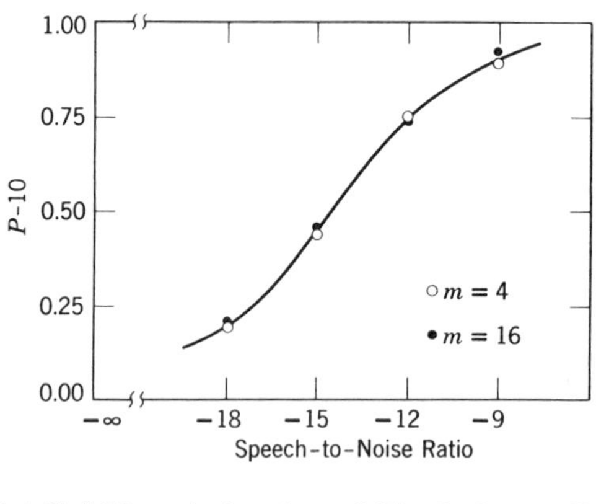

FIG. 11. The intelligibility gain functions of Fig. 9 after application of a transformation based on the constant-ratio rule.

Green and Birdsall (1958), on the basis of a theory of signal detectability, have proposed a set of transformations of the obtained data designed to yield a single function relating an inferred variable, d', to speech-to-noise ratio. For a detailed discussion of this model, the reader is referred to their report. The theory of signal detectability incorporating their simplifying assumptions does a somewhat less adequate job of reducing the data of Fig. 9 to a single function than does the P-10 index, but it does a somewhat better job of handling the Miller, Heise, and Lichten data.

Prediction of MOC curves from ROC data

The monitoring task may be defined as follows (Egan, 1957*a*). A listener is provided with a subset of messages drawn from a known set of messages. On each stimulus presentation the listener's task is to state whether or not the transmitted item is one of the messages in the subset to be monitored. As defined here, the monitor's task is not to identify specifically the transmitted item; he must merely state whether the transmitted message is a member of the subset to be monitored, or whether it is a member of the complementary subset. Here, as in the identification task, the listener may vary the criterion under which he will accept a transmitted message as a message of the subset to be monitored.

Clearly, the identification task and the monitoring task are closely related. If a listener is willing to accept his identification response as being correct and is very confident that he is correct, then, if this message is one of the subset to be monitored, he should be very confident that the transmitted message was, in fact, a message of the subset to be monitored. Thus, in this instance the listener should be willing to accept, with a high degree of confidence, the hypothesis that the transmitted message was a monitored message. If, on the other hand, the identification response made with a high degree of confidence is not of the subset to be monitored, then the listener should accept the hypothesis that the transmitted item was of the set to be monitored only with a very low degree of confidence. This reasoning provides a mechanism for predicting a monitor's (MOC) curve from an ROC curve. That this argument is an oversimplified one is made clear by the following example. Suppose that the subset of messages to be monitored consists of two messages A_1 and A_2. In the identification task, the listener on some particular stimulus presentation may not have much confidence in his identification response because, although he has great confidence that the message was either

A_1 or A_2, he may not have the necessary information to decide which of the two was in fact transmitted. In this instance, then, the listener would have relatively low confidence in his identification response but high confidence in assigning the transmitted stimulus to the subset to be monitored. The previously described method of moving from the ROC curve to the MOC curve does not take account of such occurrences.

Procedure

Five listeners were used in this experiment. None of these observers had served in any of the experiments previously described. The general experimental conditions matched those already described as closely as possible. The same message set of five spondees and the same talker were used for both experiments. In this experiment the listener's task on each stimulus presentation was to accept or reject the hypothesis that the transmitted message was a message of the set to be monitored. On each test of 100 items the listeners attempted to maintain a constant criterion. Tests were run at four different criterion levels which were merely described by the labels "very strict," "strict," "medium," and "lax." Data were obtained following 33 practice tests. The listeners always scored their own tests. On any given monitor test, the subset of items to be monitored consisted of two words: either *greyhound* and *stairway*, or *eggplant* and *vampire*. These will be called MI tests and MII tests, respectively. Data were obtained on twelve MI tests and twelve MII tests, three of each conducted at each of the four criterion levels. Twelve standard intelligibility tests were also conducted. The various types of tests were presented in a counterbalanced manner in a period of six days. In all test lists, each of the items occurred twenty times. The method of prediction was as follows. Consider the MI tests. The two items GH and SW are to be monitored. The data reported in the second section of this chapter can be used to plot theoretical MOC curves for these two M items. Consider the data for $L1$ in Table I. Utilizing the assumptions mentioned, we can compute for each level of confidence the proportion of instances in which $L1$ responded with GH or SW, given that the transmitted stimulus was either GH or SW. We may also compute the proportion of instances in which $L1$ responded with either GH or SW, given that one of the other three messages was transmitted. These proportions may then be cumulated from the strictest to the most lax confidence level. These cumulated proportions for the various confidence levels may serve as estimates of $p(Y|M)$ and $p(Y|S)$. Here, $p(Y|M)$ is the probability of the listener's accepting the hypothesis that the transmitted message was one from the subset to be monitored, given that it was from this subset, and $p(Y|S)$ is the probability of the listener's accepting the hypothesis that the transmitted message was one from the subset to be monitored when it was one of the secondary messages.

The derived points for these theoretical MOC curves were plotted on normal-normal probability paper for each of the listeners in the experiment described at the beginning of this paper. A single straight line (fit visually) was drawn through these points. These two curves, one for each of the two subsets to be monitored, serve as the predicted MOC curves for the experiment reported here. As pointed out, these predicted curves were based upon a different crew of listeners from those used in the present experiment.

Results

Figures 12 and 13 show the predicted curves and the obtained data points (solid dots). In both cases the obtained value of s differs from the predicted value. In Fig. 12 the obtained value of s is 1.02 while the predicted value is 0.73. In Fig. 13 the obtained and predicted values of s are 0.84 and 1.06, respectively. The predicted MOC curve in Fig. 12 has a $(d_e)^{1/2}$ of 1.68 while the obtained $(d_e)^{1/2}$ is 1.45. The fit is somewhat better in Fig. 13 where the predicted and obtained values of $(d_e)^{1/2}$ are 1.24 and 1.22, respectively.

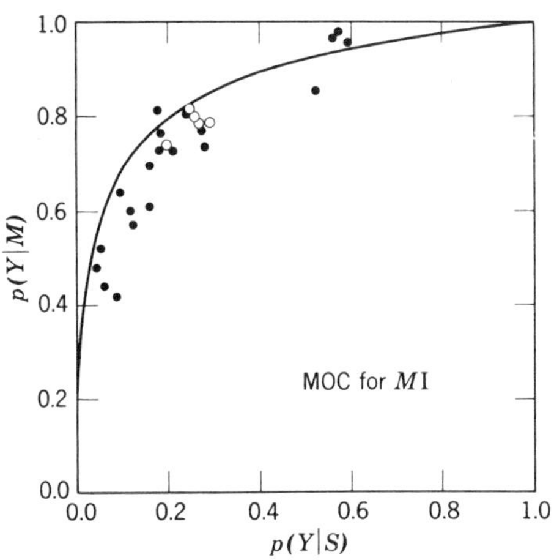

FIG. 12. The solid line shows the predicted MOC curve for the MI monitoring tests. This predicted curve is based on an earlier experiment. The solid points show the obtained data. The open circles are points predicted from articulation tests given in this experiment.

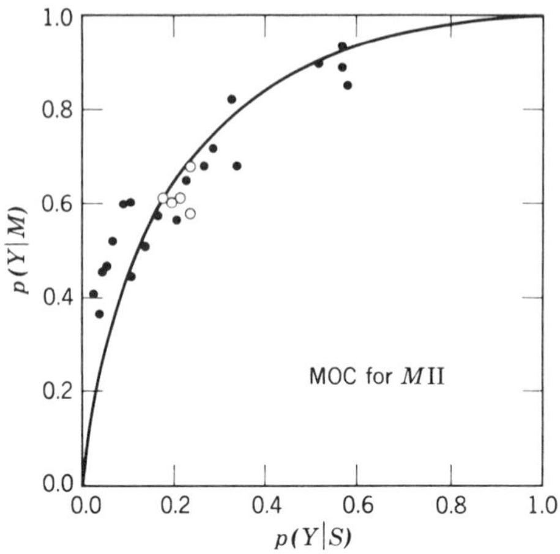

FIG. 13. The predicted MOC curve and obtained data for the MII monitoring tests.

The discrepancies observed do not necessarily mean that the suggested model is inadequate. It could be that other differences between the two experiments (different sets of listeners employed, slight changes in the talker's manner of pronouncing the words, etc.) led to the discrepancies. This problem of interpreting discrepant results was anticipated, and the articulation tests were conducted to provide some discrimination between these two possibilities. The confusion matrices obtained by these articulation tests enable us to predict a single point on the MOC curve for each subject. If these points fall on or near the MOC curves predicted from data of the previous experiment, then it would appear that the proposed method of predicting MOC curves from ROC data is inadequate. If, on the other hand, these points fall in with the obtained MOC data, it would appear that the method of prediction is adequate at least for predicting $(d_e)^{1/2}$ though possibly not for s. The open circles in Figs. 12 and 13 are MOC points predicted from the articulation tests of the current experiment. These lead us to the conclusion that the method of prediction is fairly adequate [at least for predicting $(d_e)^{1/2}$] but that uncontrolled differences in the two experiments led to the failure of prediction from one to the other. The most notable difference (one which it was impractical to control) is the very different level of training for the two groups of listeners.

SUMMARY

The studies reported in this paper have dealt with the responses of human observers to speech stimuli transmitted in a background of white

Gaussian noise. In all cases the listeners attempted to identify the transmitted items and then made a second response in an attempt to convey additional information. It was found that when the listeners were allowed a second-choice identification response, very little information was contained in these responses which was not already contained in the listeners' first identification response. When the second response was a confidence rating, a significant amount of information was added to what was carried by the identification response.

The rating which followed each identification response was assigned by the observers in an attempt to estimate the probability that their identification response was, in fact, correct. For message sets of four items and for sets of sixteen items, it was found that the observers were quite capable of making such estimates over a wide range of speech-to-noise ratios. Their estimates did appear to be affected to some extent by the size of the message set and by the speech-to-noise ratio, but this interaction was slight.

The observers' rating responses were used to generate ROC curves. These curves were adequately fitted by straight lines when the data were plotted on normal-normal probability paper. Regardless of the size of the message set, all curves for all speech-to-noise ratios were fitted by a single slope. However, the point at which these curves intersected the abscissa was a function of both variables.

Data from one set of observers in the rating experiments were used in an attempt to predict the performance of a different group of observers whose task was to monitor subsets of messages. While predictions were fairly good, discrepancies were noted. An internal check in the monitoring experiment strongly suggests that these discrepancies arose because of differences between the two groups of observers.

ACKNOWLEDGMENTS

This research was conducted in the Hearing and Communication Laboratory of Indiana University with support from the Operational Applications Laboratory of the U.S. Air Force. This article appeared as Tech. Rept. No. AFCRC-TR-58-54, and in J. acoust. Soc. Am., *1960,* **32,** *35–46.*

References

- Blank, A. A., and Quastler, H. Notes on the estimation of information measures. University of Illinois: Control Systems Laboratory, 1954, R-56.
- Bricker, P. D., and Chapanis, A. Do incorrectly perceived tachistoscopic stimuli convey some information? *Psychol. Rev.*, 1953, **60,** 181–188.
- Carterette, E. C. Message repetition and receiver confirmation of messages in noise. *J. acoust. Soc. Am.*, 1958, **30,** 846–855.

- Clarke, F. R. Constant-ratio rule for confusion matrices in speech communication. *J. acoust. Soc. Am.,* 1957, **29,** 715–720.
- Clarke, F. R., and Anderson, C. D. Further test of the constant-ratio rule in speech communication. *J. acoust. Soc. Am.,* 1957, **29,** 1318–1320.
- Clarke, F. R., Birdsall, T. G., and Tanner, W. P., Jr. Two types of ROC curves and definitions of parameters. *J. acoust. Soc. Am.,* 1959, **31,** 629–630.
- Egan, J. P. Articulation testing methods II. Harvard University: Psycho-Acoustic Laboratory, 1944, OSRD No. 3802.
- Egan, J. P. Monitoring task in speech communication. *J. acoust. Soc. Am.,* 1957*a*, **29,** 482–489.
- Egan, J. P. Message repetition, operating characteristics, and confusion matrices in speech communication. Indiana University: Hearing and Communication Laboratory, 1957*b*, Technical Report No. AFCRC-TR-57-50.
- Egan, J. P., and Clarke, F. R. Source and receiver behavior in the use of a criterion. *J. acoust. Soc. Am.,* 1956, **28,** 1267–1269. [30]
- Egan, J. P., Clarke, F. R., and Carterette, E. C. On the transmission and confirmation of messages in noise. *J. acoust. Soc. Am.,* 1956, **28,** 536–550.
- Green, D. M., and Birdsall, T. G. The effect of vocabulary size on articulation score. University of Michigan: Electronic Defense Group, 1958, Technical Memorandum No. 81. [32]
- Helson, H. Adaptation-level as frame of reference for prediction of psychophysical data. *Am. J. Psychol.,* 1947, **60,** 1–29.
- Miller, G. A. Note on the bias of information estimates. In H. Quastler (Ed.), *Information theory in psychology.* Glencoe, Ill.: Free Press, 1955.
- Miller, G. A., Heise, G. A., and Lichten, W. The intelligibility of speech as a function of the context of the test materials. *J. exp. Psychol.,* 1951, **41,** 329–335.
- Miller, G. A., and Nicely, P. E. Analysis of perceptual confusions among some English consonants.. *J. acoust. Soc. Am.,* 1955, **27,** 338–352.
- Pollack, I. Assimilation of sequentially-encoded information: IV. Washington, D. C.: Human Resources Research Laboratory, 1952, Memorandum Report No. 25.
- Pollack, I. On indices of signal and response discriminability. *J. acoust. Soc. Am.,* 1959, **31,** 1031.
- Pollack, I., and Decker, L. R. Confidence ratings, message reception, and the receiver operating characteristic. *J. acoust. Soc. Am.,* 1958, **30,** 286–292. [31]
- Shannon, C. E. Prediction and entropy of printed English. *Bell System Tech. J.,* 1951, **30,** 50–64.
- Shannon, C. E., and Weaver, W. *The mathematical theory of communication.* Urbana, Ill.: University of Illinois Press, 1949.
- Swets, J. A., Tanner, W. P., Jr., and Birdsall, T. G. The evidence for a decision-making theory of visual detection. University of Michigan: Electronic Defense Group, 1955. Technical Report No. 40. [see 1]

APPENDICES

Appendix 1 contains "Tables of d′" for the yes-no task and for forced-choice tasks with different numbers of alternatives, calculated by Patricia Elliott. She also discusses the assumptions underlying the calculations. Appendix 2 consists of a "Bibliography: Applications of Detection Theory in Psychophysics" prepared by J. A. Swets. Part A lists published papers; Part B lists technical reports printed as separates, doctoral dissertations, and printed meeting papers.

Appendix 1—Tables of d'

Patricia B. Elliott

YES-NO TABLES

These tables were compiled for use in a specific type of experiment in signal detectability. A single signal with fixed probability of occurrence is transmitted over a channel in which band-limited white Gaussian noise is added. At the end of a fixed observation interval the receiver must make a "yes-no" decision indicating whether signal plus noise or noise alone was present. Repetition of the task yields the data necessary to establish a value of d'. The statistic d' is not merely descriptive; it incorporates a comparison of obtained performance with "ideal" performance. "Ideal" implies that optimum use is made of the information available; however, because of the noise present in the channel, even an ideal receiver will not achieve perfect detection. In terms of the signal-to-noise energy ratio in the channel, a value of d' represents the minimum value of $\sqrt{2E/N_0}$ necessary to lead to the performance obtained if an ideal receiver had been used in place of the receiver under study.

In the type of experiments for which the theory of signal detectability provides an appropriate model, d' has certain advantages over other measures such as the percentage of correct responses. To illustrate, d' is not a function of the a priori probability that a signal is present. Neither is d' affected by altering the values and costs of a correct answer.

Whereas other measures are sensitive to both the receiver's specific criterion and the instructions given by the experimenter, changes in these parameters leave d' relatively invariant. In addition to these evidences of stability, d' is a tool for isolating aspects of the signal information which are utilized by the receiver. These ideas are discussed more fully by Tanner and Birdsall (1956).

Before considering the way in which a specific signal-to-noise energy ratio can be described as ideal, or as associated with certain probabilities in the ideal case, it is useful to introduce some notation. The data necessary to establish a value of d' come from the detection rate and false-alarm rate recorded during an experiment. The detection rate and the false-alarm rate serve as estimates of the desired detection probability, $P_{SN}(A)$, and false-alarm probability, $P_N(A)$.

SN —There is signal plus noise.
N —There is noise alone.
A —The receiver says there is signal plus noise.
CA —The receiver says there is noise alone.
$P_{SN}(A)$—The probability that the receiver reports SN when SN was present.
$P_N(A)$—The probability that the receiver reports SN when N was present.

	A	CA
SN	w	x
N	y	z

$$P_{SN}(A) = \frac{w}{w+x}$$

$$P_N(A) = \frac{y}{y+z}$$

By means of the computed values of $P_{SN}(A)$ and $P_N(A)$, the appropriate value of d' may be read from the table.

For the case of the signal known exactly, d' is defined as equal to $\sqrt{2E/N_0}$. This definition arises from consideration of a signal of known waveform. T denotes the waveform duration and W its bandwidth. The waveform has associated with it a signal voltage, s, and a noise voltage, n, so that the input voltage to the receiver is

$$x(t) = n(t) + s(t) \text{ when the signal is present} \tag{1}$$

or

$$x(t) = n(t) \text{ when noise alone is present.} \tag{2}$$

Therefore at an arbitrary sample point, t_i,

$$x_i = n_i + s_i \tag{3}$$

Considering the ith sample point, the probability density of the noise voltage for white Gaussian noise of power N is

$$f_N(x_i) = f_N(n_i) = \sqrt{\frac{1}{2\pi N}} \exp\left(-\frac{x_i^2}{2N}\right) \tag{4}$$

This equation represents a normal curve with zero mean and variance N. If, however, the signal is also present at the ith point, the effect on the probability density distribution of x_i is to shift its mean from zero to s_i because the signal at any instantaneous point is simply a constant (see Fig. 1).

The two equations are

$$f_N(x_i) = \sqrt{\frac{1}{2\pi N}} \exp\left(-\frac{x_i^2}{2N}\right) \tag{4}$$

and

$$f_{SN}(x_i) = \sqrt{\frac{1}{2\pi N}} \exp\left[-\frac{(x_i - s_i)^2}{2N}\right] \tag{5}$$

For any given observation the receiver's decision is based on the ratio of the likelihood that the observed waveform occurred, if signal plus noise were present, to the likelihood of the occurrence of the waveform if noise alone were present (Tanner and Birdsall, 1956). This likelihood ratio, $l[x(t)]$, refers to the entire observation interval $0 < t < T$, so Eqs. (4) and (5) must first be extended over the interval before they are used to form a likelihood ratio.

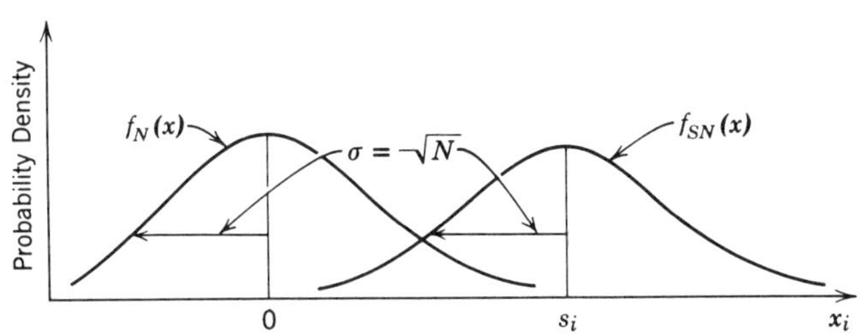

FIG. 1. Probability densities for x at an arbitrary sample point conditional on noise alone and on signal plus noise.

Since the probability density function of the total waveform is the product of the individual probability densities at each independent sampling point (spaced ½W apart), Eqs. (4) and (5) become

$$f_N(x) = \prod_{i=1}^{2WT} f_N(x_i) = \left(\frac{1}{2\pi N}\right)^{WT} \exp\left(-\frac{1}{2N}\sum_{i=1}^{2WT} x_i^2\right) \tag{6}$$

and

$$f_{SN}(x) = \prod_{i=1}^{2WT} f_{SN}(x_i) = \left(\frac{1}{2\pi N}\right)^{WT} \exp\left[-\frac{1}{2N}\sum_{i=1}^{2WT} (x_i - s_i)^2\right] \tag{7}$$

Forming the ratio we have

$$l(x) = \frac{f_{SN}(x)}{f_N(x)} = \frac{\exp\left[-\frac{1}{2N}\sum_{i=1}^{2WT}(x_i - s_i)^2\right]}{\exp\left(-\frac{1}{2N}\sum_{i=1}^{2WT} x_i^2\right)}$$

$$= \exp\left(\frac{1}{N}\sum_{i=1}^{2WT} x_i s_i - \frac{1}{2N}\sum_{i=1}^{2WT} s_i^2\right) \tag{8}$$

The natural logarithm of the likelihood ratio is equally useful in the decision task because it is the result of a monotonic transformation, and, in addition, its probability density functions are normally distributed. Thus, we have

$$\log_e l(x) = \frac{1}{N}\sum_{i=1}^{2WT} x_i s_i - \frac{1}{2N}\sum_{i=1}^{2WT} s_i^2 \tag{9}$$

Before determining the distribution of $\log_e l(x)$ it is convenient to state the sampling theorem (Peterson and Birdsall, 1953):

$$\frac{1}{2W}\sum_{i=1}^{2WT} s_i^2 = \int_0^T [s(t)]^2\,dt = E(s) \tag{10}$$

where $E(s)$ refers to the signal energy. Using this theorem,

$$\frac{1}{2N}\sum_{i=1}^{2WT} s_i^2 = \frac{1}{N_0}\cdot\frac{1}{2W}\sum_{i=1}^{2WT} s_i^2 = \frac{1}{N_0}\int_0^T [s(t)]^2\,dt = \frac{E(s)}{N_0} \tag{11}$$

The noise power N is converted to N_0, the noise power per unit bandwidth, by the relation $N_0 = N/W$.

To find the distribution of $\log_e l(x)$ it is necessary to know the mean and the variance for noise alone and for signal plus noise. Considering the situation in which noise alone is present during the observation interval, to find the mean and variance of $\log_e l(x)$ it should be observed that the x_i's are independent and that each x_i has the probability density function of Eq. (4). Since Eq. (4) represents a normal distribution with zero mean and variance N, the mean of $\log_e l(x)$ is the sum of the means, and the variance is the sum of the variances. Because the signal is a constant at the ith point, working with Eq. (9),

$$\mu_N(x_i s_i) = s_i \mu_N(x_i) = s_i \cdot 0 = 0 \tag{12}$$

This implies that

$$\mu_N\left(\frac{1}{N}\sum_{i=1}^{2WT} x_i s_i\right) = 0 \tag{13}$$

Utilizing Eqs. (13) and (11), Eq. (9) indicates that

$$\mu_N[\log_e l(x)] = -\frac{E(s)}{N_0} \tag{14}$$

This same procedure is used to find the mean when the signal is present. Thus

$$\mu_{SN}(x_i s_i) = s_i \mu_{SN}(x_i) = s_i^2 \tag{15}$$

$$\mu_{SN}\left(\frac{1}{N}\sum_{i=1}^{2WT} x_i s_i\right) = \frac{1}{N}\sum_{i=1}^{2WT} s_i^2 = \frac{2E(s)}{N_0} \tag{16}$$

and

$$\mu_{SN}[\log_e l(x)] = \frac{2E(s)}{N_0} - \frac{E(s)}{N_0} = +\frac{E(s)}{N_0} \tag{17}$$

In Eq. (9) the only term which contributes to the variance is

$$\frac{1}{N}\sum_{i=1}^{2WT} x_i s_i$$

and therefore

$$\sigma^2{}_{SN}[\log_e l(x)] = \sigma^2{}_N[\log_e l(x)] = \sigma^2\left(\frac{1}{N}\sum_{i=1}^{2WT} x_i s_i\right) \tag{18}$$

Applying the fact that the variance of the product of a constant and a random variable is equal to the product of the constant squared and the variance of the variable, at the ith point

$$\sigma^2(x_i s_i) = s_i^2 \sigma^2(x_i) = s_i^2 N \tag{19}$$

By the same rule,

$$\sigma^2\left(\frac{1}{N}\sum_{i=1}^{2WT} x_i s_i\right) = \frac{1}{N^2}\sigma^2\left(\sum_{i=1}^{2WT} x_i s_i\right) \tag{20}$$

The combination of Eqs. (19) and (20) and the use of the sampling theorem show the variance to be

$$\sigma^2[\log_e l(x)] = \frac{1}{N^2}\sum_{i=1}^{2WT} N s_i^2 = \frac{1}{N}\sum_{i=1}^{2WT} s_i^2 = \frac{2E(s)}{N_0} \tag{21}$$

To conclude the discussion of the definition of d' as based on the consideration of a waveform, it is only necessary to divide the difference between the means for the two conditions by the standard deviation to arrive at d':

$$\frac{\mu_{SN} - \mu_N}{\sigma} = \frac{\dfrac{E}{N_0} - \left(-\dfrac{E}{N_0}\right)}{\sqrt{\dfrac{2E}{N_0}}} = \sqrt{\frac{2E}{N_0}}$$

The two distributions are shown in Fig. 2.

Figure 2 leads directly to an interpretation of d' in terms of an ROC (receiver-operating-characteristic) curve. Whenever $\log_e l(x)$ is greater than a certain critical number, an optimum receiver will consistently choose to accept the observation as resulting from signal plus noise. The area under the noise curve to the right of the given value of $\log_e l(x)$ is the probability, $P_N(A)$, that if noise alone is present the receiver will say there is signal plus noise. Similarly, the area to the right of $\log_e l(x)$ under the signal-plus-noise curve is $P_{SN}(A)$. The coordinates $[P_N(A), P_{SN}(A)]$ locate a point on the ROC curve. Thus each point on the abscissa of Fig. 2 considered as a critical number in the decision process determines a point on the associated ROC curve. For the ideal receiver each value of d' yields a separate ROC curve. An example for $d' = 1.00$ is given in Fig. 3*a*. When a transformation of the axis is made from linear to probability scales, the same ROC curve

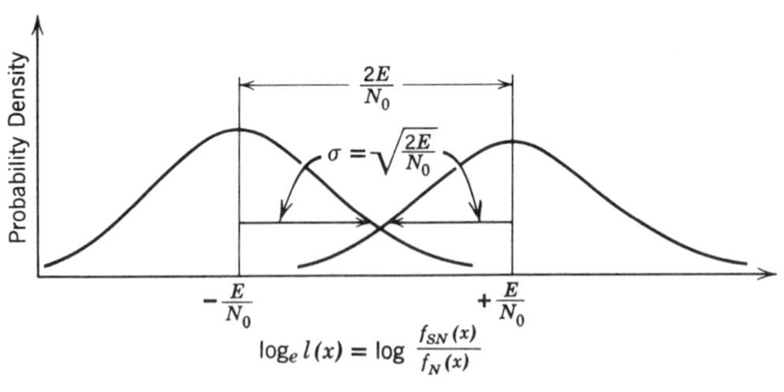

FIG. 2. Probability densities for $\log_e l(x)$ conditional on noise alone and on signal plus noise.

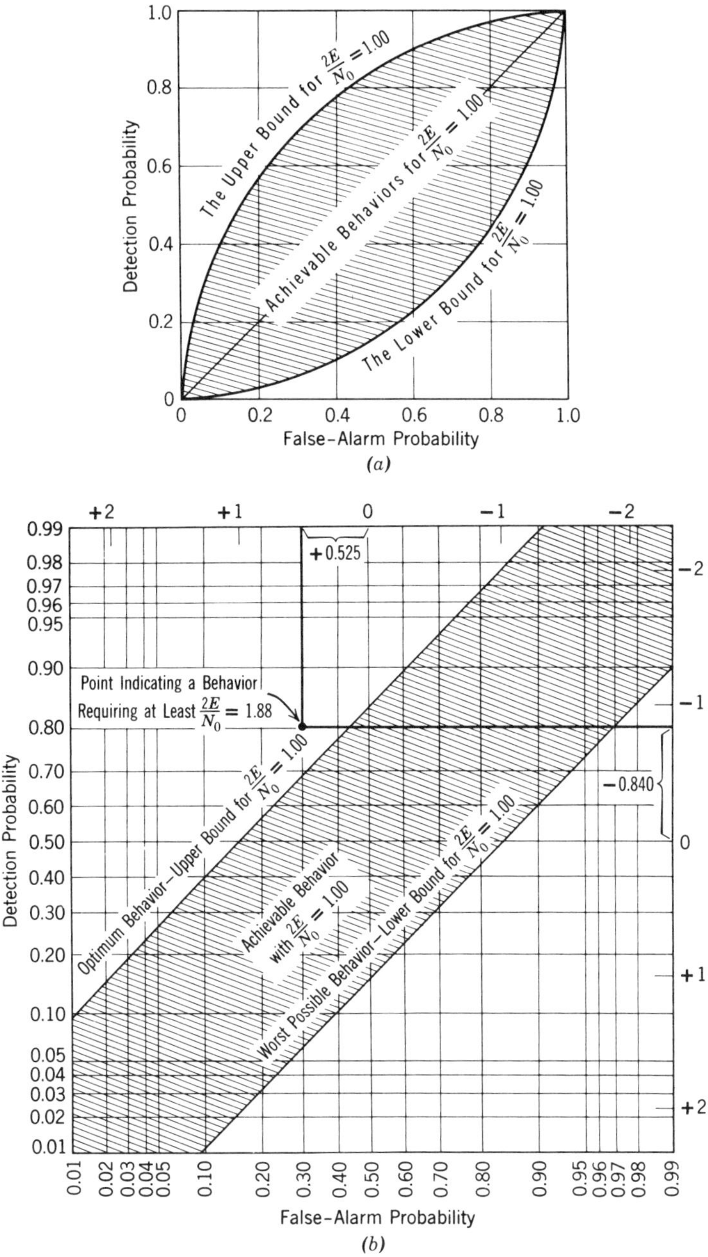

FIG. 3. (*a*) Receiver operating characteristic (ROC) for the ideal receiver when $2E/N_0 = 1.0$. (*b*) Transformation to double probability paper for the ROC curve of (*a*).

appears as in Fig. 3*b*. With the double probability paper, it is then possible to read off the signal-to-noise energy ratio which an ideal receiver would have needed to achieve any combination of $P_{SN}(A)$ and $P_N(A)$. Referring to the point on Fig. 3*b*, if a receiver gave a detection rate of .80 when its false-alarm rate was .30, the ideal receiver would have required a $\sqrt{2E/N_0}$ of 1.365 to attain this performance. To avoid repeating this procedure for each experimental value, Table I has been drawn up. The table facilitates the process of determining d' in the situation where a signal known exactly is presented during a fixed observation interval.

TABLE I. VALUES OF d' FOR THE YES-NO PROCEDURE

$P_{SN}(A)$ \ $P_N(A)$	.01	.02	.03	.04	.05	.06	.07	.08	.09	.10
.01	0	−.27	−.44	−.57	−.68	−.77	−.85	−.92	−.98	−1.04
.02	.27	0	−.17	−.30	−.41	−.50	−.58	−.65	−.71	−.77
.03	.44	.17	0	−.13	−.24	−.33	−.41	−.48	−.54	−.60
.04	.57	.30	.13	0	−.11	−.20	−.28	−.35	−.41	−.47
.05	.68	.41	.24	.11	0	−.09	−.17	−.24	−.30	−.36
.06	.77	.50	.33	.20	.09	0	−.08	−.15	−.21	−.27
.07	.85	.58	.41	.28	.17	.08	0	−.07	−.13	−.19
.08	.92	.65	.48	.35	.24	.15	.07	0	−.06	−.12
.09	.98	.71	.54	.41	.30	.21	.13	.06	0	−.06
.10	1.04	.77	.60	.47	.36	.27	.19	.12	.06	0
.11	1.09	.82	.65	.52	.41	.32	.24	.17	.11	.05
.12	1.14	.88	.70	.58	.46	.38	.30	.22	.16	.10
.13	1.19	.92	.75	.62	.51	.42	.34	.27	.21	.15
.14	1.24	.97	.80	.67	.56	.47	.39	.32	.26	.20
.15	1.28	1.01	.84	.71	.60	.51	.43	.36	.30	.24
.16	1.33	1.06	.89	.76	.65	.56	.48	.41	.35	.29
.17	1.37	1.10	.93	.80	.69	.60	.52	.45	.39	.33
.18	1.40	1.14	.96	.84	.72	.64	.56	.48	.42	.36
.19	1.44	1.17	1.00	.87	.76	.67	.59	.52	.46	.40
.20	1.48	1.21	1.04	.91	.80	.71	.63	.56	.50	.44
.21	1.52	1.24	1.08	.94	.84	.74	.66	.60	.54	.48
.22	1.55	1.28	1.11	.98	.87	.78	.70	.63	.57	.51
.23	1.58	1.31	1.14	1.01	.90	.81	.73	.66	.60	.54
.24	1.62	1.34	1.18	1.04	.94	.84	.76	.70	.64	.58
.25	1.64	1.38	1.20	1.08	.96	.88	.80	.72	.66	.60
.26	1.68	1.41	1.24	1.11	1.00	.91	.83	.76	.70	.64
.27	1.71	1.44	1.27	1.14	1.03	.94	.86	.79	.73	.67
.28	1.74	1.47	1.30	1.17	1.06	.97	.89	.82	.76	.70
.29	1.76	1.50	1.32	1.20	1.08	1.00	.92	.84	.78	.72
.30	1.80	1.52	1.36	1.22	1.12	1.02	.94	.88	.82	.76
.31	1.82	1.54	1.38	1.24	1.14	1.04	.96	.90	.84	.78
.32	1.85	1.58	1.41	1.28	1.17	1.08	1.00	.93	.87	.81
.33	1.88	1.61	1.44	1.31	1.20	1.11	1.03	.96	.90	.84
.34	1.91	1.64	1.47	1.34	1.23	1.14	1.06	.99	.93	.87
.35	1.94	1.66	1.50	1.36	1.26	1.16	1.08	1.02	.96	.90
.36	1.96	1.69	1.52	1.39	1.28	1.19	1.11	1.04	.98	.92
.37	1.99	1.72	1.55	1.42	1.31	1.22	1.14	1.07	1.01	.95
.38	2.02	1.74	1.58	1.44	1.34	1.24	1.16	1.10	1.04	.98
.39	2.04	1.77	1.60	1.47	1.36	1.27	1.19	1.12	1.06	1.00
.40	2.06	1.80	1.62	1.50	1.38	1.30	1.22	1.14	1.08	1.02
.41	2.09	1.82	1.65	1.52	1.41	1.32	1.24	1.17	1.11	1.05
.42	2.12	1.85	1.68	1.55	1.44	1.35	1.27	1.20	1.14	1.08
.43	2.14	1.87	1.70	1.57	1.46	1.37	1.29	1.22	1.16	1.10
.44	2.17	1.90	1.73	1.60	1.49	1.40	1.32	1.25	1.19	1.13
.45	2.19	1.92	1.75	1.62	1.51	1.42	1.34	1.27	1.21	1.15
.46	2.22	1.95	1.78	1.65	1.54	1.45	1.37	1.30	1.24	1.18
.47	2.24	1.98	1.80	1.68	1.56	1.48	1.40	1.32	1.26	1.20
.48	2.27	2.00	1.83	1.70	1.59	1.50	1.42	1.35	1.29	1.23
.49	2.30	2.02	1.86	1.72	1.62	1.52	1.44	1.38	1.32	1.26
.50	2.32	2.05	1.88	1.75	1.64	1.55	1.47	1.40	1.34	1.28

TABLE I. *(Continued)*

$P_{SN}(A)$ \ $P_N(A)$	.01	.02	.03	.04	.05	.06	.07	.08	.09	.10
.51	2.34	1.08	1.90	1.78	1.66	1.58	1.50	1.42	1.36	1.30
.52	2.37	2.10	1.93	1.80	1.69	1.60	1.52	1.45	1.39	1.33
.53	2.40	2.12	1.96	1.82	1.72	1.62	1.54	1.48	1.42	1.36
.54	2.42	2.15	1.98	1.85	1.74	1.65	1.57	1.50	1.44	1.38
.55	2.45	2.18	2.01	1.88	1.77	1.68	1.60	1.53	1.47	1.41
.56	2.47	2.20	2.03	1.90	1.79	1.70	1.62	1.55	1.49	1.43
.57	2.50	2.23	2.06	1.93	1.82	1.73	1.65	1.58	1.52	1.46
.58	2.52	2.25	2.08	1.95	1.84	1.75	1.67	1.60	1.54	1.48
.59	2.55	2.28	2.11	1.98	1.87	1.78	1.70	1.63	1.57	1.51
.60	2.58	2.30	2.14	2.00	1.90	1.80	1.72	1.66	1.60	1.54
.61	2.60	2.33	2.16	2.03	1.92	1.83	1.75	1.68	1.62	1.56
.62	2.62	2.36	2.18	2.06	1.94	1.86	1.78	1.70	1.64	1.58
.63	2.65	2.38	2.21	2.08	1.97	1.88	1.80	1.73	1.67	1.61
.64	2.68	2.41	2.24	2.11	2.00	1.91	1.83	1.76	1.70	1.64
.65	2.70	2.44	2.26	2.14	2.02	1.94	1.86	1.78	1.72	1.66
.66	2.73	2.46	2.29	2.16	2.05	1.96	1.88	1.81	1.75	1.69
.67	2.76	2.49	2.32	2.19	2.08	1.99	1.91	1.84	1.78	1.72
.68	2.79	2.52	2.35	2.22	2.11	2.02	1.94	1.87	1.81	1.75
.69	2.82	2.56	2.38	2.26	2.14	2.06	1.98	1.90	1.84	1.78
.70	2.84	2.58	2.40	2.28	2.16	2.08	2.00	1.92	1.86	1.80
.71	2.88	2.60	2.44	2.30	2.20	2.10	2.02	1.96	1.90	1.84
.72	2.90	2.63	2.46	2.33	2.22	2.13	2.05	1.98	1.92	1.86
.73	2.93	2.66	2.49	2.36	2.25	2.16	2.08	2.01	1.95	1.89
.74	2.96	2.69	2.52	2.39	2.28	2.19	2.11	2.04	1.98	1.92
.75	3.00	2.72	2.56	2.42	2.32	2.22	2.14	2.08	2.02	1.96
.76	3.02	2.76	2.58	2.46	2.34	2.26	2.18	2.10	2.04	1.98
.77	3.06	2.79	2.62	2.49	2.38	2.29	2.21	2.14	2.08	2.02
.78	3.09	2.82	2.65	2.52	2.41	2.32	2.24	2.17	2.11	2.05
.79	3.12	2.86	2.68	2.56	2.44	2.36	2.28	2.20	2.14	2.08
.80	3.16	2.89	2.72	2.59	2.48	2.39	2.31	2.24	2.18	2.12
.81	3.20	2.93	2.76	2.63	2.52	2.43	2.35	2.28	2.22	2.16
.82	3.24	2.96	2.80	2.66	2.56	2.46	2.38	2.32	2.26	2.20
.83	3.27	3.00	2.83	2.70	2.59	2.50	2.42	2.35	2.29	2.23
.84	3.31	3.04	2.87	2.74	2.63	2.54	2.46	2.39	2.33	2.27
.85	3.36	3.09	2.92	2.79	2.68	2.59	2.51	2.44	2.38	2.32
.86	3.40	3.13	2.96	2.83	2.72	2.63	2.55	2.48	2.42	2.36
.87	3.45	3.18	3.01	2.88	2.77	2.68	2.60	2.53	2.47	2.41
.88	3.50	3.22	3.06	2.92	2.82	2.72	2.64	2.58	2.52	2.46
.89	3.55	3.28	3.11	2.98	2.87	2.78	2.70	2.63	2.58	2.51
.90	3.60	3.33	3.16	3.03	2.92	2.83	2.75	2.68	2.62	2.56
.91	3.66	3.39	3.22	3.09	2.98	2.89	2.81	2.74	2.68	2.62
.92	3.72	3.45	3.28	3.15	3.04	2.95	2.87	2.80	2.74	2.68
.93	3.79	3.52	3.35	3.22	3.11	3.02	2.94	2.87	2.81	2.75
.94	3.87	3.60	3.43	3.30	3.19	3.10	3.02	2.95	2.89	2.83
.95	3.96	3.69	3.52	3.39	3.28	3.19	3.11	3.04	2.98	2.92
.96	4.07	3.80	3.63	3.50	3.39	3.30	3.22	3.15	3.09	3.03
.97	4.20	3.93	3.76	3.63	3.52	3.43	3.35	3.28	3.22	3.16
.98	4.37	4.10	3.93	3.80	3.69	3.60	3.52	3.45	3.39	3.33
.99	4.64	4.37	4.20	4.07	3.96	3.87	3.79	3.72	3.66	3.60

TABLE I. *(Continued)*

$P_{SN}(A)$ \ $P_N(A)$	.11	.12	.13	.14	.15	.16	.17	.18	.19	.20
.01	−1.09	−1.14	−1.19	−1.24	−1.28	−1.33	−1.37	−1.40	−1.44	−1.48
.02	− .82	− .88	− .92	− .97	−1.01	−1.06	−1.10	−1.14	−1.17	−1.21
.03	− .65	− .70	− .75	− .80	− .84	− .89	− .93	− .96	−1.00	−1.04
.04	− .52	− .58	− .62	− .67	− .71	− .76	− .80	− .84	− .87	− .91
.05	− .41	− .46	− .51	− .56	− .60	− .65	− .69	− .72	− .76	− .80
.06	− .32	− .38	− .42	− .47	− .51	− .56	− .60	− .64	− .67	− .71
.07	− .24	− .30	− .34	− .39	− .43	− .48	− .52	− .56	− .59	− .63
.08	− .17	− .22	− .27	− .32	− .36	− .41	− .45	− .48	− .52	− .56
.09	− .11	− .16	− .21	− .26	− .30	− .35	− .39	− .42	− .46	− .50
.10	− .05	− .10	− .15	− .20	− .24	− .29	− .33	− .36	− .40	− .44
.11	0	− .06	− .10	− .15	− .19	− .24	− .28	− .32	− .35	− .39
.12	.06	0	− .04	− .10	− .14	− .18	− .22	− .26	− .30	− .34
.13	.10	.04	0	− .05	− .09	− .14	− .18	− .22	− .25	− .29
.14	.15	.10	.05	0	− .04	− .09	− .13	− .16	− .20	− .24
.15	.19	.14	.09	.04	0	− .05	− .09	− .12	− .16	− .20
.16	.24	.18	.14	.09	.05	0	− .04	− .08	− .11	− .15
.17	.28	.22	.18	.13	.09	.04	0	− .04	− .07	− .11
.18	.32	.26	.22	.16	.12	.08	.04	0	− .04	− .08
.19	.35	.30	.25	.20	.16	.11	.07	.04	0	− .04
.20	.39	.34	.29	.24	.20	.15	.11	.08	.04	0
.21	.42	.37	.32	.28	.24	.18	.14	.11	.08	.04
.22	.46	.40	.36	.31	.27	.22	.18	.14	.11	.07
.23	.49	.44	.39	.34	.30	.25	.21	.18	.14	.10
.24	.52	.47	.42	.38	.34	.28	.24	.21	.18	.14
.25	.56	.50	.46	.40	.36	.32	.28	.24	.20	.16
.26	.59	.54	.49	.44	.40	.35	.31	.28	.24	.20
.27	.62	.56	.52	.47	.43	.38	.34	.30	.27	.23
.28	.65	.60	.55	.50	.46	.41	.37	.34	.30	.26
.29	.68	.62	.58	.52	.48	.44	.40	.36	.32	.28
.30	.70	.65	.60	.56	.52	.46	.42	.39	.36	.32
.31	.72	.67	.62	.58	.54	.48	.44	.41	.38	.34
.32	.76	.70	.66	.61	.57	.52	.48	.44	.41	.37
.33	.79	.74	.69	.64	.60	.55	.51	.48	.44	.40
.34	.82	.76	.72	.67	.63	.58	.54	.50	.47	.43
.35	.84	.79	.74	.70	.66	.60	.56	.53	.50	.46
.36	.87	.82	.77	.72	.68	.63	.59	.56	.52	.48
.37	.90	.84	.80	.75	.71	.66	.62	.58	.55	.51
.38	.92	.87	.72	.78	.74	.68	.64	.61	.58	.54
.39	.95	.90	.85	.80	.76	.71	.67	.64	.60	.56
.40	.98	.92	.88	.82	.78	.74	.70	.66	.62	.58
.41	1.00	.94	.90	.85	.81	.76	.72	.68	.65	.61
.42	1.03	.98	.93	.88	.84	.79	.75	.72	.68	.64
.43	1.05	1.00	.95	.90	.86	.81	.77	.74	.70	.66
.44	1.08	1.02	.98	.93	.89	.84	.80	.76	.73	.69
.45	1.10	1.04	1.00	.95	.91	.86	.82	.78	.75	.71
.46	1.13	1.08	1.03	.98	.94	.89	.85	.82	.78	.74
.47	1.16	1.10	1.06	1.00	.96	.92	.88	.84	.80	.76
.48	1.18	1.12	1.08	1.03	.99	.94	.90	.86	.83	.79
.49	1.20	1.15	1.10	1.06	1.02	.96	.92	.89	.86	.82
.50	1.23	1.18	1.13	1.08	1.04	.99	.95	.92	.88	.84

TABLE I. *(Continued)*

$P_{SN}(A)$ \ $P_N(A)$	.11	.12	.13	.14	.15	.16	.17	.18	.19	.20
.51	1.26	1.20	1.16	1.10	1.06	1.02	.98	.94	.90	.86
.52	1.28	1.22	1.18	1.13	1.09	1.04	1.00	.96	.93	.89
.53	1.30	1.25	1.20	1.16	1.12	1.06	1.02	.99	.96	.92
.54	1.33	1.28	1.23	1.18	1.14	1.09	1.05	1.02	.98	.94
.55	1.36	1.30	1.26	1.21	1.17	1.12	1.08	1.04	1.01	.97
.56	1.38	1.32	1.28	1.23	1.19	1.14	1.10	1.06	1.03	.99
.57	1.41	1.36	1.31	1.26	1.22	1.17	1.13	1.10	1.06	1.02
.58	1.43	1.38	1.33	1.28	1.24	1.19	1.15	1.12	1.08	1.04
.59	1.46	1.40	1.36	1.31	1.27	1.22	1.18	1.14	1.11	1.07
.60	1.48	1.43	1.38	1.34	1.30	1.24	1.20	1.17	1.14	1.10
.61	1.51	1.46	1.41	1.36	1.32	1.27	1.23	1.20	1.16	1.12
.62	1.54	1.48	1.44	1.38	1.34	1.30	1.26	1.22	1.18	1.14
.63	1.56	1.50	1.46	1.41	1.37	1.32	1.28	1.24	1.21	1.17
.64	1.59	1.54	1.49	1.44	1.40	1.35	1.31	1.28	1.24	1.20
.65	1.62	1.56	1.52	1.46	1.42	1.38	1.34	1.30	1.26	1.22
.66	1.64	1.58	1.54	1.49	1.45	1.40	1.36	1.32	1.29	1.25
.67	1.67	1.62	1.57	1.52	1.48	1.43	1.39	1.36	1.32	1.28
.68	1.70	1.64	1.60	1.55	1.51	1.46	1.42	1.38	1.35	1.31
.69	1.74	1.68	1.64	1.58	1.54	1.50	1.46	1.42	1.38	1.34
.70	1.76	1.70	1.66	1.60	1.56	1.52	1.48	1.44	1.40	1.36
.71	1.78	1.73	1.68	1.64	1.60	1.54	1.50	1.47	1.44	1.40
.72	1.81	1.76	1.71	1.66	1.62	1.57	1.53	1.50	1.46	1.42
.73	1.84	1.78	1.74	1.69	1.65	1.60	1.56	1.52	1.49	1.45
.74	1.87	1.82	1.77	1.72	1.68	1.63	1.59	1.56	1.52	1.48
.75	1.90	1.85	1.80	1.76	1.72	1.66	1.62	1.59	1.56	1.52
.76	1.94	1.88	1.84	1.78	1.74	1.70	1.66	1.62	1.58	1.54
.77	1.97	1.92	1.87	1.82	1.78	1.73	1.69	1.66	1.62	1.58
.78	2.00	1.94	1.90	1.85	1.81	1.76	1.72	1.68	1.65	1.61
.79	2.04	1.98	1.94	1.88	1.84	1.80	1.76	1.72	1.68	1.64
.80	2.07	2.02	1.97	1.92	1.88	1.83	1.79	1.76	1.72	1.68
.81	2.11	2.06	2.01	1.96	1.92	1.87	1.83	1.80	1.76	1.72
.82	2.14	2.09	2.04	2.00	1.96	1.90	1.86	1.83	1.80	1.76
.83	2.18	2.12	2.08	2.03	1.99	1.94	1.90	1.86	1.83	1.79
.84	2.22	2.16	2.12	2.07	2.03	1.98	1.94	1.90	1.87	1.83
.85	2.27	2.22	2.17	2.12	2.08	2.03	1.99	1.96	1.92	1.88
.86	2.31	2.26	2.21	2.16	2.12	2.07	2.03	2.00	1.96	1.92
.87	2.36	2.30	2.26	2.21	2.17	2.12	2.08	2.04	2.01	1.97
.88	2.40	2.35	2.30	2.26	2.22	2.16	2.12	2.09	2.06	2.02
.89	2.46	2.40	2.36	2.31	2.27	2.22	2.18	2.14	2.11	2.07
.90	2.51	2.46	2.41	2.36	2.32	2.27	2.23	2.20	2.16	2.12
.91	2.57	2.52	2.47	2.42	2.38	2.33	2.29	2.26	2.22	2.18
.92	2.63	2.58	2.53	2.48	2.44	2.39	2.35	2.32	2.28	2.24
.93	2.70	2.64	2.60	2.55	2.51	2.46	2.42	2.38	2.35	2.31
.94	2.78	2.72	2.68	2.63	2.59	2.54	2.50	2.46	2.43	2.39
.95	2.87	2.82	2.77	2.72	2.68	2.63	2.59	2.56	2.52	2.48
.96	2.98	2.92	2.88	2.83	2.79	2.74	2.70	2.66	2.63	2.59
.97	3.11	3.06	3.01	2.96	2.92	2.87	2.83	2.80	2.76	2.72
.98	3.28	3.22	3.18	3.13	3.09	3.04	3.00	2.96	2.93	2.89
.99	3.55	3.50	3.45	3.40	3.36	3.31	3.27	3.24	3.20	3.16

TABLE I. *(Continued)*

$P_{SN}(A)$ \ $P_N(A)$	.21	.22	.23	.24	.25	.26	.27	.28	.29	.30
.01	−1.52	−1.55	−1.58	−1.62	−1.64	−1.68	−1.71	−1.74	−1.76	−1.80
.02	−1.24	−1.28	−1.31	−1.34	−1.38	−1.41	−1.44	−1.47	−1.50	−1.52
.03	−1.08	−1.11	−1.14	−1.18	−1.20	−1.24	−1.27	−1.30	−1.32	−1.36
.04	−.94	−.98	−1.01	−1.04	−1.08	−1.11	−1.14	−1.17	−1.20	−1.22
.05	−.84	−.87	−.90	−.94	−.96	−1.00	−1.03	−1.06	−1.08	−1.12
.06	−.74	−.78	−.81	−.84	−.88	−.91	−.94	−.97	−1.00	−1.02
.07	−.66	−.70	−.73	−.76	−.80	−.83	−.86	−.89	−.92	−.94
.08	−.60	−.63	−.66	−.70	−.72	−.76	−.79	−.82	−.84	−.88
.09	−.54	−.57	−.60	−.64	−.66	−.70	−.73	−.76	−.78	−.82
.10	−.48	−.51	−.54	−.58	−.60	−.64	−.67	−.70	−.72	−.76
.11	−.42	−.46	−.49	−.52	−.56	−.59	−.62	−.65	−.68	−.70
.12	−.37	−.40	−.44	−.47	−.50	−.54	−.56	−.60	−.62	−.65
.13	−.32	−.36	−.39	−.42	−.46	−.49	−.52	−.55	−.58	−.60
.14	−.28	−.31	−.34	−.38	−.40	−.44	−.47	−.50	−.52	−.56
.15	−.24	−.27	−.30	−.34	−.36	−.40	−.43	−.46	−.48	−.52
.16	−.18	−.22	−.25	−.28	−.32	−.35	−.38	−.41	−.44	−.46
.17	−.14	−.18	−.21	−.24	−.28	−.31	−.34	−.37	−.40	−.42
.18	−.11	−.14	−.18	−.21	−.24	−.28	−.30	−.34	−.36	−.39
.19	−.08	−.11	−.14	−.18	−.20	−.24	−.27	−.30	−.32	−.36
.20	−.04	−.07	−.10	−.14	−.16	−.20	−.23	−.26	−.28	−.32
.21	0	−.04	−.06	−.10	−.13	−.16	−.20	−.22	−.25	−.28
.22	.04	0	−.03	−.06	−.10	−.13	−.16	−.19	−.22	−.24
.23	.06	.03	0	−.04	−.06	−.10	−.13	−.16	−.18	−.22
.24	.10	.06	.04	0	−.03	−.06	−.10	−.12	−.15	−.18
.25	.13	.10	.06	.03	0	−.04	−.06	−.10	−.12	−.15
.26	.16	.13	.10	.06	.04	0	−.03	−.06	−.08	−.12
.27	.20	.16	.13	.10	.06	.03	0	−.03	−.06	−.08
.28	.22	.19	.16	.12	.10	.06	.03	0	−.02	−.06
.29	.25	.20	.18	.15	.12	.08	.06	.02	0	−.03
.30	.28	.24	.22	.18	.15	.12	.08	.06	.03	0
.31	.30	.26	.24	.20	.17	.14	.10	.08	.05	.02
.32	.34	.30	.27	.24	.20	.17	.14	.11	.08	.06
.33	.36	.33	.30	.26	.24	.20	.17	.14	.12	.08
.34	.40	.36	.33	.30	.26	.23	.20	.17	.14	.12
.35	.42	.38	.36	.32	.29	.26	.22	.20	.17	.14
.36	.44	.41	.38	.34	.32	.28	.25	.22	.20	.16
.37	.48	.44	.41	.38	.34	.31	.28	.25	.22	.20
.38	.50	.46	.44	.40	.37	.34	.30	.28	.25	.22
.39	.52	.49	.46	.42	.40	.36	.33	.30	.28	.24
.40	.55	.52	.48	.45	.42	.38	.36	.32	.30	.27
.41	.58	.54	.51	.48	.44	.41	.38	.35	.32	.30
.42	.60	.57	.54	.50	.48	.44	.41	.38	.36	.32
.43	.62	.59	.56	.52	.50	.46	.43	.40	.38	.34
.44	.66	.62	.59	.56	.52	.49	.46	.43	.40	.38
.45	.68	.64	.61	.58	.54	.51	.48	.45	.42	.40
.46	.70	.67	.64	.60	.58	.54	.51	.48	.46	.42
.47	.73	.70	.66	.63	.60	.56	.54	.50	.48	.45
.48	.76	.72	.69	.66	.62	.59	.56	.53	.50	.48
.49	.78	.74	.72	.68	.65	.62	.58	.56	.53	.50
.50	.80	.77	.74	.70	.68	.64	.61	.58	.56	.52

TABLE I. *(Continued)*

$P_{SN}(A)$ \ $P_N(A)$	.21	.22	.23	.24	.25	.26	.27	.28	.29	.30
.51	.83	.80	.76	.73	.70	.66	.64	.60	.58	.55
.52	.86	.82	.79	.76	.72	.69	.66	.63	.60	.58
.53	.88	.84	.82	.78	.75	.72	.68	.66	.63	.60
.54	.90	.87	.84	.80	.78	.74	.71	.68	.66	.62
.55	.94	.90	.87	.84	.80	.77	.74	.71	.68	.66
.56	.96	.92	.89	.86	.82	.79	.76	.73	.70	.68
.57	.98	.95	.92	.88	.86	.82	.79	.76	.74	.70
.58	1.00	.97	.94	.90	.88	.84	.81	.78	.76	.72
.59	1.04	1.00	.97	.94	.90	.87	.84	.81	.78	.76
.60	1.06	1.02	1.00	.96	.93	.90	.86	.84	.81	.78
.61	1.08	1.05	1.02	.98	.96	.92	.89	.86	.84	.80
.62	1.11	1.08	1.04	1.01	.98	.94	.92	.88	.86	.83
.63	1.14	1.10	1.07	1.04	1.00	.97	.94	.91	.88	.86
.64	1.16	1.13	1.10	1.06	1.04	1.00	.97	.94	.92	.88
.65	1.19	1.16	1.12	1.09	1.06	1.02	1.00	.96	.94	.91
.66	1.22	1.18	1.15	1.12	1.08	1.05	1.02	.99	.96	.94
.67	1.24	1.21	1.18	1.14	1.12	1.08	1.05	1.02	1.00	.96
.68	1.28	1.24	1.21	1.18	1.14	1.11	1.08	1.05	1.02	1.00
.69	1.31	1.28	1.24	1.21	1.18	1.14	1.12	1.08	1.06	1.03
.70	1.33	1.30	1.26	1.23	1.20	1.16	1.14	1.10	1.08	1.05
.71	1.36	1.32	1.30	1.26	1.23	1.20	1.16	1.14	1.11	1.08
.72	1.38	1.35	1.32	1.28	1.26	1.22	1.19	1.16	1.14	1.10
.73	1.42	1.38	1.35	1.32	1.28	1.25	1.22	1.19	1.16	1.14
.74	1.44	1.41	1.38	1.34	1.32	1.28	1.25	1.22	1.20	1.16
.75	1.48	1.44	1.42	1.38	1.35	1.32	1.28	1.26	1.23	1.20
.76	1.51	1.48	1.44	1.41	1.38	1.34	1.32	1.28	1.26	1.23
.77	1.54	1.51	1.48	1.44	1.42	1.38	1.35	1.32	1.30	1.26
.78	1.58	1.54	1.51	1.48	1.44	1.41	1.38	1.35	1.32	1.30
.79	1.61	1.58	1.54	1.51	1.48	1.44	1.42	1.38	1.36	1.33
.80	1.64	1.61	1.58	1.54	1.52	1.48	1.45	1.42	1.40	1.36
.81	1.68	1.65	1.62	1.58	1.56	1.52	1.49	1.46	1.44	1.40
.82	1.72	1.68	1.66	1.62	1.59	1.56	1.52	1.50	1.47	1.44
.83	1.76	1.72	1.69	1.66	1.62	1.59	1.56	1.53	1.50	1.48
.84	1.80	1.76	1.73	1.70	1.66	1.63	1.60	1.57	1.54	1.52
.85	1.84	1.81	1.78	1.74	1.72	1.68	1.65	1.62	1.60	1.56
.86	1.88	1.85	1.82	1.78	1.76	1.72	1.69	1.66	1.64	1.60
.87	1.94	1.90	1.87	1.84	1.80	1.77	1.74	1.71	1.68	1.66
.88	1.98	1.94	1.92	1.88	1.85	1.82	1.78	1.76	1.73	1.70
.89	2.04	2.00	1.97	1.94	1.90	1.87	1.84	1.81	1.78	1.76
.90	2.08	2.05	2.02	1.98	1.96	1.92	1.89	1.86	1.84	1.80
.91	2.14	2.11	2.08	2.04	2.02	1.98	1.95	1.92	1.90	1.86
.92	2.20	2.17	2.14	2.10	2.08	2.04	2.01	1.98	1.96	1.92
.93	2.28	2.24	2.21	2.18	2.14	2.11	2.08	2.05	2.02	2.00
.94	2.36	2.32	2.29	2.26	2.22	2.19	2.16	2.13	2.10	2.08
.95	2.44	2.41	2.38	2.34	2.32	2.28	2.25	2.22	2.20	2.16
.96	2.56	2.52	2.49	2.46	2.42	2.39	2.36	2.33	2.30	2.28
.97	2.68	2.65	2.62	2.58	2.56	2.52	2.49	2.46	2.44	2.40
.98	2.86	2.82	2.79	2.76	2.72	2.69	2.66	2.63	2.60	2.58
.99	3.12	3.09	3.06	3.02	3.00	2.96	2.93	2.90	2.88	2.84

TABLE I. *(Continued)*

$P_{SN}(A)$ \ $P_N(A)$	.31	.32	.33	.34	.35	.36	.37	.38	.39	.40
.01	-1.82	-1.85	-1.88	-1.91	-1.94	-1.96	-1.99	-2.02	-2.04	-2.06
.02	-1.54	-1.58	-1.61	-1.64	-1.66	-1.69	-1.72	-1.74	-1.77	-1.80
.03	-1.38	-1.41	-1.44	-1.47	-1.50	-1.52	-1.55	-1.58	-1.60	-1.62
.04	-1.24	-1.28	-1.31	-1.33	-1.36	-1.39	-1.42	-1.44	-1.47	-1.50
.05	-1.14	-1.17	-1.20	-1.23	-1.26	-1.28	-1.31	-1.34	-1.36	-1.38
.06	-1.04	-1.08	-1.11	-1.14	-1.16	-1.19	-1.22	-1.24	-1.27	-1.30
.07	-.96	-1.00	-1.03	-1.06	-1.08	-1.11	-1.14	-1.16	-1.19	-1.22
.08	-.90	-.93	-.96	-.99	-1.02	-1.04	-1.07	-1.10	-1.12	-1.14
.09	-.84	-.87	-.90	-.93	-.96	-.98	-1.01	-1.04	-1.06	-1.08
.10	-.78	-.81	-.84	-.87	-.90	-.92	-.95	-.98	-1.00	-1.02
.11	-.72	-.76	-.79	-.82	-.84	-.87	-.90	-.92	-.95	-.98
.12	-.67	-.70	-.74	-.76	-.79	-.82	-.84	-.87	-.90	-.92
.13	-.62	-.66	-.69	-.72	-.74	-.77	-.80	-.82	-.85	-.88
.14	-.58	-.61	-.64	-.67	-.70	-.72	-.75	-.78	-.80	-.82
.15	-.54	-.57	-.60	-.63	-.66	-.68	-.71	-.74	-.76	-.78
.16	-.48	-.52	-.55	-.58	-.60	-.63	-.66	-.68	-.71	-.74
.17	-.44	-.48	-.51	-.54	-.56	-.59	-.62	-.64	-.67	-.70
.18	-.41	-.44	-.48	-.50	-.53	-.56	-.58	-.61	-.64	-.66
.19	-.38	-.41	-.44	-.47	-.50	-.52	-.55	-.58	-.60	-.62
.20	-.34	-.37	-.40	-.43	-.46	-.48	-.51	-.54	-.56	-.58
.21	-.30	-.34	-.36	-.40	-.42	-.44	-.48	-.50	-.52	-.55
.22	-.26	-.30	-.33	-.36	-.38	-.41	-.44	-.46	-.49	-.52
.23	-.24	-.27	-.30	-.33	-.36	-.38	-.41	-.44	-.46	-.48
.24	-.20	-.24	-.26	-.30	-.32	-.34	-.38	-.40	-.42	-.45
.25	-.17	-.20	-.24	-.26	-.29	-.32	-.34	-.37	-.40	-.42
.26	-.14	-.17	-.20	-.23	-.26	-.28	-.31	-.34	-.36	-.38
.27	-.10	-.14	-.17	-.20	-.22	-.25	-.28	-.30	-.33	-.36
.28	-.08	-.11	-.14	-.17	-.20	-.22	-.25	-.28	-.30	-.32
.29	-.05	-.08	-.12	-.14	-.17	-.20	-.22	-.25	-.28	-.30
.30	-.02	-.06	-.08	-.12	-.14	-.16	-.20	-.22	-.24	-.27
.31	0	-.04	-.06	-.10	-.12	-.14	-.18	-.20	-.22	-.25
.32	.04	0	-.03	-.06	-.08	-.11	-.14	-.16	-.19	-.22
.33	.06	.03	0	-.03	-.06	-.08	-.11	-.14	-.16	-.18
.34	.10	.06	.03	0	-.02	-.05	-.08	-.10	-.13	-.16
.35	.12	.08	.06	.02	0	-.02	-.06	-.08	-.10	-.13
.36	.14	.11	.08	.05	.02	0	-.03	-.06	-.08	-.10
.37	.18	.14	.11	.08	.06	.03	0	-.02	-.05	-.08
.38	.20	.16	.14	.10	.08	.06	.02	0	-.02	-.05
.39	.22	.19	.16	.13	.10	.08	.05	.02	0	-.02
.40	.25	.22	.18	.16	.13	.10	.08	.05	.02	0
.41	.28	.24	.21	.18	.16	.13	.10	.08	.05	.02
.42	.30	.27	.24	.21	.18	.16	.13	.10	.08	.06
.43	.32	.29	.26	.23	.20	.18	.15	.12	.10	.08
.44	.36	.32	.29	.26	.24	.21	.18	.16	.13	.10
.45	.38	.34	.31	.28	.26	.23	.20	.18	.15	.12
.46	.40	.37	.34	.31	.28	.26	.23	.20	.18	.16
.47	.43	.40	.36	.34	.31	.28	.26	.23	.20	.18
.48	.46	.42	.39	.36	.34	.31	.28	.26	.23	.20
.49	.48	.44	.42	.38	.36	.34	.30	.28	.26	.23
.50	.50	.47	.44	.41	.38	.36	.33	.30	.28	.26

TABLE I. *(Continued)*

$P_{SN}(A)$ \ $P_N(A)$	.31	.32	.33	.34	.35	.36	.37	.38	.39	.40
.51	.53	.50	.46	.44	.41	.38	.36	.33	.30	.28
.52	.56	.52	.49	.46	.44	.41	.38	.36	.33	.30
.53	.58	.54	.52	.48	.46	.44	.40	.38	.36	.33
.54	.60	.57	.54	.51	.48	.46	.43	.40	.38	.36
.55	.64	.60	.57	.54	.52	.49	.46	.44	.41	.38
.56	.66	.62	.59	.56	.54	.51	.48	.46	.43	.40
.57	.68	.65	.62	.59	.56	.54	.51	.48	.46	.44
.58	.70	.67	.64	.61	.58	.56	.53	.50	.48	.46
.59	.74	.70	.67	.64	.62	.59	.56	.54	.51	.48
.60	.76	.72	.70	.66	.64	.62	.58	.56	.54	.51
.61	.78	.75	.72	.69	.66	.64	.61	.58	.56	.54
.62	.81	.78	.74	.72	.69	.66	.64	.61	.58	.56
.63	.84	.80	.77	.74	.72	.69	.66	.64	.61	.58
.64	.86	.83	.80	.77	.74	.72	.69	.66	.64	.62
.65	.89	.86	.82	.80	.77	.74	.72	.69	.66	.64
.66	.92	.88	.85	.82	.80	.77	.74	.72	.69	.66
.67	.94	.91	.88	.85	.82	.80	.77	.74	.72	.70
.68	.98	.94	.91	.88	.86	.83	.80	.78	.75	.72
.69	1.01	.98	.94	.92	.89	.86	.84	.81	.78	.76
.70	1.03	1.00	.96	.94	.91	.88	.86	.83	.80	.78
.71	1.06	1.02	1.00	.96	.94	.92	.88	.86	.84	.81
.72	1.08	1.05	1.02	.99	.96	.94	.91	.88	.86	.84
.73	1.12	1.08	1.05	1.02	1.00	.97	.94	.92	.89	.86
.74	1.14	1.11	1.08	1.05	1.02	1.00	.97	.94	.92	.90
.75	1.18	1.14	1.12	1.08	1.06	1.04	1.00	.98	.96	.93
.76	1.21	1.18	1.14	1.12	1.09	1.06	1.04	1.01	.98	.96
.77	1.24	1.21	1.18	1.15	1.12	1.10	1.07	1.04	1.02	1.00
.78	1.28	1.24	1.21	1.18	1.16	1.13	1.10	1.08	1.05	1.02
.79	1.31	1.28	1.24	1.22	1.19	1.16	1.14	1.11	1.08	1.06
.80	1.34	1.31	1.28	1.25	1.22	1.20	1.17	1.14	1.12	1.10
.81	1.38	1.35	1.32	1.29	1.26	1.24	1.21	1.18	1.16	1.14
.82	1.42	1.38	1.36	1.32	1.30	1.28	1.24	1.22	1.20	1.17
.83	1.46	1.42	1.39	1.36	1.34	1.31	1.28	1.26	1.23	1.20
.84	1.50	1.46	1.43	1.40	1.38	1.35	1.32	1.30	1.27	1.24
.85	1.54	1.51	1.48	1.45	1.42	1.40	1.37	1.34	1.32	1.30
.86	1.58	1.55	1.52	1.49	1.46	1.44	1.41	1.38	1.36	1.34
.87	1.64	1.60	1.57	1.54	1.52	1.49	1.46	1.44	1.41	1.38
.88	1.68	1.64	1.62	1.58	1.56	1.54	1.50	1.48	1.46	1.43
.89	1.74	1.70	1.67	1.64	1.62	1.59	1.56	1.54	1.51	1.48
.90	1.78	1.75	1.72	1.69	1.66	1.64	1.61	1.58	1.56	1.54
.91	1.84	1.81	1.78	1.75	1.72	1.70	1.67	1.64	1.62	1.60
.92	1.90	1.87	1.84	1.81	1.78	1.76	1.73	1.70	1.68	1.66
.93	1.98	1.94	1.91	1.88	1.86	1.83	1.80	1.78	1.75	1.72
.94	2.06	2.02	1.99	1.96	1.94	1.91	1.88	1.86	1.83	1.80
.95	2.14	2.11	2.08	2.05	2.02	2.00	1.97	1.94	1.92	1.90
.96	2.26	2.22	2.19	2.16	2.14	2.11	2.08	2.06	2.03	2.00
.97	2.38	2.35	2.32	2.29	2.26	2.24	2.21	2.18	2.16	2.14
.98	2.56	2.52	2.49	2.46	2.44	2.41	2.38	2.36	2.33	2.30
.99	2.82	2.79	2.76	2.73	2.70	2.68	2.65	2.62	2.60	2.58

TABLE I. *(Continued)*

$P_{SN}(A)$ \ $P_N(A)$	.41	.42	.43	.44	.45	.46	.47	.48	.49	.50
.01	−2.09	−2.12	−2.14	−2.17	−2.19	−2.22	−2.24	−2.27	−2.30	−2.32
.02	−1.82	−1.85	−1.87	−1.90	−1.92	−1.95	−1.98	−2.00	−2.02	−2.05
.03	−1.65	−1.68	−1.70	−1.73	−1.75	−1.78	−1.80	−1.83	−1.86	−1.88
.04	−1.52	−1.55	−1.57	−1.60	−1.62	−1.65	−1.68	−1.70	−1.72	−1.75
.05	−1.41	−1.44	−1.46	−1.49	−1.51	−1.54	−1.56	−1.59	−1.62	−1.64
.06	−1.32	−1.35	−1.37	−1.40	−1.42	−1.45	−1.48	−1.50	−1.52	−1.55
.07	−1.24	−1.27	−1.29	−1.32	−1.34	−1.37	−1.40	−1.42	−1.44	−1.47
.08	−1.17	−1.20	−1.22	−1.25	−1.27	−1.30	−1.32	−1.35	−1.38	−1.40
.09	−1.11	−1.14	−1.16	−1.19	−1.21	−1.24	−1.26	−1.29	−1.32	−1.34
.10	−1.05	−1.08	−1.10	−1.13	−1.15	−1.18	−1.20	−1.23	−1.26	−1.28
.11	−1.00	−1.03	−1.05	−1.08	−1.10	−1.13	−1.16	−1.18	−1.20	−1.23
.12	− .94	− .98	−1.00	−1.02	−1.04	−1.08	−1.10	−1.12	−1.15	−1.18
.13	− .90	− .93	− .95	− .98	−1.00	−1.03	−1.06	−1.08	−1.10	−1.13
.14	− .85	− .88	− .90	− .93	− .95	− .98	−1.00	−1.03	−1.06	−1.08
.15	− .81	− .84	− .86	− .89	− .91	− .94	− .96	− .99	−1.02	−1.04
.16	− .76	− .79	− .81	− .84	− .86	− .89	− .92	− .94	− .96	− .99
.17	− .72	− .75	− .77	− .80	− .82	− .85	− .88	− .90	− .92	− .95
.18	− .68	− .72	− .74	− .76	− .78	− .82	− .84	− .86	− .89	− .92
.19	− .65	− .68	− .70	− .73	− .75	− .78	− .80	− .83	− .86	− .88
.20	− .61	− .64	− .66	− .69	− .71	− .74	− .76	− .79	− .82	− .84
.21	− .58	− .60	− .62	− .66	− .68	− .70	− .73	− .76	− .78	− .80
.22	− .54	− .57	− .59	− .62	− .64	− .67	− .70	− .72	− .74	− .77
.23	− .51	− .54	− .56	− .59	− .61	− .64	− .66	− .69	− .72	− .74
.24	− .48	− .50	− .52	− .56	− .58	− .60	− .63	− .66	− .68	− .70
.25	− .44	− .48	− .50	− .52	− .54	− .58	− .60	− .62	− .65	− .68
.26	− .41	− .44	− .46	− .49	− .51	− .54	− .56	− .59	− .62	− .64
.27	− .38	− .41	− .43	− .46	− .48	− .51	− .54	− .56	− .58	− .61
.28	− .35	− .38	− .40	− .43	− .45	− .48	− .50	− .53	− .56	− .58
.29	− .32	− .36	− .38	− .40	− .42	− .46	− .48	− .50	− .53	− .56
.30	− .30	− .32	− .34	− .38	− .40	− .42	− .45	− .48	− .50	− .52
.31	− .28	− .30	− .32	− .36	− .38	− .40	− .43	− .46	− .48	− .50
.32	− .24	− .27	− .29	− .32	− .34	− .37	− .40	− .42	− .44	− .47
.33	− .21	− .24	− .26	− .29	− .31	− .34	− .36	− .39	− .42	− .44
.34	− .18	− .21	− .23	− .26	− .28	− .31	− .34	− .36	− .38	− .41
.35	− .16	− .18	− .20	− .24	− .26	− .28	− .31	− .34	− .36	− .38
.36	− .13	− .16	− .18	− .21	− .23	− .26	− .28	− .31	− .34	− .36
.37	− .10	− .13	− .15	− .18	− .20	− .23	− .26	− .28	− .30	− .33
.38	− .08	− .10	− .12	− .16	− .18	− .20	− .23	− .26	− .28	− .30
.39	− .05	− .08	− .10	− .13	− .15	− .18	− .20	− .23	− .26	− .28
.40	− .02	− .06	− .08	− .10	− .12	− .16	− .18	− .20	− .23	− .26
.41	0	− .03	− .05	− .08	− .10	− .13	− .16	− .18	− .20	− .23
.42	.03	0	− .02	− .05	− .07	− .10	− .12	− .15	− .18	− .20
.43	.05	.02	0	− .03	− .05	− .08	− .10	− .13	− .16	− .18
.44	.08	.05	.03	0	− .02	− .05	− .08	− .10	− .13	− .15
.45	.10	.07	.05	.02	0	− .03	− .06	− .08	− .10	− .13
.46	.13	.10	.08	.05	.03	0	− .02	− .05	− .08	− .10
.47	.16	.12	.10	.08	.06	.02	0	− .02	− .05	− .08
.48	.18	.15	.13	.10	.08	.05	.02	0	− .02	− .05
.49	.20	.18	.16	.13	.10	.08	.05	.02	0	− .02
.50	.23	.20	.18	.15	.13	.10	.08	.05	.02	0

TABLE I. *(Continued)*

$P_{SN}(A)$ \ $P_N(A)$	.41	.42	.43	.44	.45	.46	.47	.48	.49	.50
.51	.26	.22	.20	.18	.16	.12	.10	.08	.05	.02
.52	.28	.25	.23	.20	.18	.15	.12	.10	.08	.05
.53	.30	.28	.26	.22	.20	.18	.15	.12	.10	.08
.54	.33	.30	.28	.25	.23	.20	.18	.15	.12	.10
.55	.36	.33	.31	.28	.26	.23	.20	.18	.16	.13
.56	.38	.35	.33	.30	.28	.25	.22	.20	.18	.15
.57	.41	.38	.36	.33	.31	.28	.26	.23	.20	.18
.58	.43	.40	.38	.35	.33	.30	.28	.25	.22	.20
.59	.46	.43	.41	.38	.36	.33	.30	.28	.26	.23
.60	.48	.46	.44	.40	.38	.36	.33	.30	.28	.26
.61	.51	.48	.46	.43	.41	.38	.36	.33	.30	.28
.62	.54	.50	.48	.46	.44	.40	.38	.36	.33	.30
.63	.56	.53	.51	.48	.46	.43	.40	.38	.36	.33
.64	.59	.56	.54	.51	.49	.46	.44	.41	.38	.36
.65	.62	.58	.56	.54	.52	.48	.46	.44	.41	.38
.66	.64	.61	.59	.56	.54	.51	.48	.46	.44	.41
.67	.67	.64	.62	.59	.57	.54	.52	.49	.46	.44
.68	.70	.67	.65	.62	.60	.57	.54	.52	.50	.47
.69	.74	.70	.68	.66	.64	.60	.58	.56	.53	.50
.70	.76	.72	.70	.68	.66	.62	.60	.58	.55	.52
.71	.78	.76	.74	.70	.68	.66	.63	.60	.58	.56
.72	.81	.78	.76	.73	.71	.68	.66	.63	.60	.58
.73	.84	.81	.79	.76	.74	.71	.68	.66	.64	.61
.74	.87	.84	.82	.79	.77	.74	.72	.69	.66	.64
.75	.90	.88	.86	.82	.80	.78	.75	.72	.70	.68
.76	.94	.90	.88	.86	.84	.80	.78	.76	.73	.70
.77	.97	.94	.92	.89	.87	.84	.82	.79	.76	.74
.78	1.00	.97	.95	.92	.90	.87	.84	.82	.80	.77
.79	1.04	1.00	.98	.96	.94	.90	.88	.86	.83	.80
.80	1.07	1.04	1.02	.99	.97	.94	.92	.89	.86	.84
.81	1.11	1.08	1.06	1.03	1.01	.98	.96	.93	.90	.88
.82	1.14	1.12	1.10	1.06	1.04	1.02	.99	.96	.94	.92
.83	1.18	1.15	1.13	1.10	1.08	1.05	1.02	1.00	.98	.95
.84	1.22	1.19	1.17	1.14	1.12	1.09	1.06	1.04	1.02	.99
.85	1.27	1.24	1.22	1.19	1.17	1.14	1.12	1.09	1.06	1.04
.86	1.31	1.28	1.26	1.23	1.21	1.18	1.16	1.13	1.10	1.08
.87	1.36	1.33	1.31	1.28	1.26	1.23	1.20	1.18	1.16	1.13
.88	1.40	1.38	1.36	1.32	1.30	1.28	1.25	1.22	1.20	1.18
.89	1.46	1.43	1.41	1.38	1.36	1.33	1.30	1.28	1.26	1.23
.90	1.51	1.48	1.46	1.43	1.41	1.38	1.36	1.33	1.30	1.28
.91	1.57	1.54	1.52	1.49	1.47	1.44	1.42	1.39	1.36	1.34
.92	1.63	1.60	1.58	1.55	1.53	1.50	1.48	1.45	1.42	1.40
.93	1.70	1.67	1.65	1.62	1.60	1.57	1.54	1.52	1.50	1.47
.94	1.78	1.75	1.73	1.70	1.68	1.65	1.62	1.60	1.58	1.55
.95	1.87	1.84	1.82	1.79	1.77	1.74	1.72	1.69	1.66	1.64
.96	1.98	1.95	1.93	1.90	1.88	1.85	1.82	1.80	1.78	1.75
.97	2.11	2.08	2.06	2.03	2.01	1.98	1.96	1.93	1.90	1.88
.98	2.28	2.25	2.23	2.20	2.18	2.15	2.12	2.10	2.08	2.05
.99	2.55	2.52	2.50	2.47	2.45	2.42	2.48	2.37	2.34	2.32

TABLE I. *(Continued)*

$P_{SN}(A)$ \ $P_N(A)$	.51	.52	.53	.54	.55	.56	.57	.58	.59	.60
.01	−2.34	−2.37	−2.40	−2.42	−2.45	−2.47	−2.50	−2.52	−2.55	−2.58
.02	−2.08	−2.10	−2.12	−2.15	−2.18	−2.20	−2.23	−2.25	−2.28	−2.30
.03	−1.90	−1.93	−1.96	−1.98	−2.01	−2.03	−2.06	−2.08	−2.11	−2.14
.04	−1.78	−1.80	−1.82	−1.85	−1.88	−1.90	−1.93	−1.95	−1.98	−2.00
.05	−1.66	−1.69	−1.72	−1.74	−1.77	−1.79	−1.82	−1.84	−1.87	−1.90
.06	−1.58	−1.60	−1.62	−1.65	−1.68	−1.70	−1.73	−1.75	−1.78	−1.80
.07	−1.50	−1.52	−1.54	−1.57	−1.60	−1.62	−1.65	−1.67	−1.70	−1.72
.08	−1.42	−1.45	−1.48	−1.50	−1.53	−1.55	−1.58	−1.60	−1.63	−1.66
.09	−1.36	−1.39	−1.42	−1.44	−1.47	−1.49	−1.52	−1.54	−1.57	−1.60
.10	−1.30	−1.33	−1.36	−1.38	−1.41	−1.43	−1.46	−1.48	−1.51	−1.54
.11	−1.26	−1.28	−1.30	−1.33	−1.36	−1.38	−1.41	−1.43	−1.46	−1.48
.12	−1.20	−1.22	−1.25	−1.28	−1.30	−1.32	−1.36	−1.38	−1.40	−1.43
.13	−1.16	−1.18	−1.20	−1.23	−1.26	−1.28	−1.31	−1.33	−1.36	−1.38
.14	−1.10	−1.13	−1.16	−1.18	−1.21	−1.23	−1.26	−1.28	−1.31	−1.34
.15	−1.06	−1.09	−1.12	−1.14	−1.17	−1.19	−1.22	−1.24	−1.27	−1.30
.16	−1.02	−1.04	−1.06	−1.09	−1.12	−1.14	−1.17	−1.19	−1.22	−1.24
.17	− .98	−1.00	−1.02	−1.05	−1.08	−1.10	−1.13	−1.15	−1.18	−1.20
.18	− .94	− .96	− .99	−1.02	−1.04	−1.06	−1.10	−1.12	−1.14	−1.17
.19	− .90	− .93	− .96	− .98	−1.01	−1.03	−1.06	−1.08	−1.11	−1.14
.20	− .86	− .89	− .92	− .94	− .97	− .99	−1.02	−1.04	−1.07	−1.10
.21	− .83	− .86	− .88	− .90	− .94	− .96	− .98	−1.00	−1.04	−1.06
.22	− .80	− .82	− .84	− .87	− .90	− .92	− .95	− .97	−1.00	−1.02
.23	− .76	− .79	− .82	− .84	− .87	− .89	− .92	− .94	− .97	−1.00
.24	− .73	− .76	− .78	− .80	− .84	− .86	− .88	− .90	− .94	− .96
.25	− .70	− .72	− .75	− .78	− .80	− .82	− .86	− .88	− .90	− .93
.26	− .66	− .69	− .72	− .74	− .77	− .79	− .82	− .84	− .87	− .90
.27	− .64	− .66	− .68	− .71	− .74	− .76	− .79	− .81	− .84	− .86
.28	− .60	− .63	− .66	− .68	− .71	− .73	− .76	− .78	− .81	− .84
.29	− .58	− .60	− .63	− .66	− .68	− .70	− .74	− .76	− .78	− .81
.30	− .55	− .58	− .60	− .62	− .66	− .68	− .70	− .72	− .76	− .78
.31	− .53	− .56	− .58	− .60	− .64	− .66	− .68	− .70	− .74	− .76
.32	− .50	− .52	− .54	− .57	− .60	− .62	− .65	− .67	− .70	− .72
.33	− .46	− .49	− .52	− .54	− .57	− .59	− .62	− .64	− .67	− .70
.34	− .44	− .46	− .48	− .51	− .54	− .56	− .59	− .61	− .64	− .66
.35	− .41	− .44	− .46	− .48	− .52	− .54	− .56	− .58	− .62	− .64
.36	− .38	− .41	− .44	− .46	− .49	− .51	− .54	− .56	− .59	− .62
.37	− .36	− .38	− .40	− .43	− .46	− .48	− .51	− .53	− .56	− .58
.38	− .33	− .36	− .38	− .40	− .44	− .46	− .48	− .50	− .54	− .56
.39	− .30	− .33	− .36	− .38	− .41	− .43	− .46	− .48	− .51	− .54
.40	− .28	− .30	− .33	− .36	− .38	− .40	− .44	− .46	− .48	− .51
.41	− .26	− .28	− .30	− .33	− .36	− .38	− .41	− .43	− .46	− .48
.42	− .22	− .25	− .28	− .30	− .33	− .35	− .38	− .40	− .43	− .46
.43	− .20	− .23	− .26	− .28	− .31	− .33	− .36	− .38	− .41	− .44
.44	− .18	− .20	− .22	− .25	− .28	− .30	− .33	− .35	− .38	− .40
.45	− .16	− .18	− .20	− .23	− .26	− .28	− .31	− .33	− .36	− .38
.46	− .12	− .15	− .18	− .20	− .23	− .25	− .28	− .30	− .33	− .36
.47	− .10	− .12	− .15	− .18	− .20	− .22	− .26	− .28	− .30	− .33
.48	− .08	− .10	− .12	− .15	− .18	− .20	− .23	− .25	− .28	− .30
.49	− .05	− .08	− .10	− .12	− .16	− .18	− .20	− .22	− .26	− .28
.50	− .02	− .05	− .08	− .10	− .13	− .15	− .18	− .20	− .23	− .26

TABLE I. *(Continued)*

$P_{SN}(A)$ \ $P_N(A)$	.51	.52	.53	.54	.55	.56	.57	.58	.59	.60
.51	0	−.02	−.05	−.08	−.10	−.12	−.16	−.18	−.20	−.23
.52	.02	0	−.02	−.05	−.08	−.10	−.13	−.15	−.18	−.20
.53	.05	.02	0	−.02	−.06	−.08	−.10	−.12	−.16	−.18
.54	.08	.05	.02	0	−.03	−.05	−.08	−.10	−.13	−.16
.55	.10	.08	.06	.03	0	−.02	−.05	−.07	−.10	−.12
.56	.12	.10	.08	.05	.02	0	−.03	−.05	−.08	−.10
.57	.16	.13	.10	.08	.05	.03	0	−.02	−.05	−.08
.58	.18	.15	.12	.10	.07	.05	.02	0	−.03	−.06
.59	.20	.18	.16	.13	.10	.08	.05	.03	0	−.02
.60	.23	.20	.18	.16	.12	.10	.08	.06	.02	0
.61	.26	.23	.20	.18	.15	.13	.10	.08	.05	.02
.62	.28	.26	.23	.20	.18	.16	.12	.10	.08	.05
.63	.30	.28	.26	.23	.20	.18	.15	.13	.10	.08
.64	.34	.31	.28	.26	.23	.21	.18	.16	.13	.10
.65	.36	.34	.31	.28	.26	.24	.20	.18	.16	.13
.66	.38	.36	.34	.31	.28	.26	.23	.21	.18	.16
.67	.42	.39	.36	.34	.31	.29	.26	.24	.21	.18
.68	.44	.42	.40	.37	.34	.32	.29	.27	.24	.22
.69	.48	.46	.43	.40	.38	.36	.32	.30	.28	.25
.70	.50	.48	.45	.42	.40	.38	.34	.32	.30	.27
.71	.53	.50	.48	.46	.42	.40	.38	.36	.32	.30
.72	.56	.53	.50	.48	.45	.43	.40	.38	.35	.32
.73	.58	.56	.54	.51	.48	.46	.43	.41	.38	.36
.74	.62	.59	.56	.54	.51	.49	.46	.44	.41	.38
.75	.65	.62	.60	.58	.54	.52	.50	.48	.44	.42
.76	.68	.66	.63	.60	.58	.56	.52	.50	.48	.45
.77	.72	.69	.66	.64	.61	.59	.56	.54	.51	.48
.78	.74	.72	.70	.67	.64	.62	.59	.57	.54	.52
.79	.78	.76	.73	.70	.68	.66	.62	.60	.58	.55
.80	.82	.79	.76	.74	.71	.69	.66	.64	.61	.58
.81	.86	.83	.80	.78	.75	.73	.70	.68	.65	.62
.82	.89	.86	.84	.82	.78	.76	.74	.72	.68	.66
.83	.92	.90	.88	.85	.82	.80	.77	.75	.72	.70
.84	.96	.94	.92	.89	.86	.84	.81	.79	.76	.74
.85	1.02	.99	.96	.94	.91	.89	.86	.84	.81	.78
.86	1.06	1.03	1.00	.98	.95	.93	.90	.88	.85	.82
.87	1.10	1.08	1.06	1.03	1.00	.98	.95	.93	.90	.88
.88	1.15	1.12	1.10	1.08	1.04	1.02	1.00	.98	.94	.92
.89	1.20	1.18	1.16	1.13	1.10	1.08	1.05	1.03	1.00	.98
.90	1.26	1.23	1.20	1.18	1.15	1.13	1.10	1.08	1.05	1.02
.91	1.32	1.29	1.26	1.24	1.21	1.19	1.16	1.14	1.11	1.08
.92	1.38	1.35	1.32	1.30	1.27	1.25	1.22	1.20	1.17	1.14
.93	1.44	1.42	1.40	1.37	1.34	1.32	1.29	1.27	1.24	1.22
.94	1.52	1.50	1.48	1.45	1.42	1.40	1.37	1.35	1.32	1.30
.95	1.62	1.59	1.56	1.54	1.51	1.49	1.46	1.44	1.41	1.38
.96	1.72	1.70	1.68	1.65	1.62	1.60	1.57	1.55	1.52	1.50
.97	1.86	1.83	1.80	1.78	1.75	1.73	1.70	1.68	1.65	1.62
.98	2.02	2.00	1.98	1.95	1.92	1.90	1.87	1.85	1.82	1.80
.99	2.30	2.27	2.24	2.22	2.19	2.17	2.14	2.12	2.09	2.06

TABLE I. *(Continued)*

$P_{SN}(A)$ \ $P_N(A)$	.61	.62	.63	.64	.65	.66	.67	.68	.69	.70
.01	−2.60	−2.62	−2.65	−2.68	−2.70	−2.73	−2.76	−2.79	−2.82	−2.84
.02	−2.33	−2.36	−2.38	−2.41	−2.44	−2.46	−2.49	−2.52	−2.56	−2.58
.03	−2.16	−2.18	−2.21	−2.24	−2.26	−2.29	−2.32	−2.35	−2.38	−2.40
.04	−2.03	−2.06	−2.08	−2.11	−2.14	−2.16	−2.19	−2.22	−2.26	−2.28
.05	−1.92	−1.94	−1.97	−2.00	−2.02	−2.05	−2.08	−2.11	−2.14	−2.16
.06	−1.83	−1.86	−1.88	−1.91	−1.94	−1.96	−1.99	−2.02	−2.06	−2.08
.07	−1.75	−1.78	−1.80	−1.83	−1.86	−1.88	−1.91	−1.94	−1.98	−2.00
.08	−1.68	−1.70	−1.73	−1.76	−1.78	−1.81	−1.84	−1.87	−1.90	−1.92
.09	−1.62	−1.64	−1.67	−1.70	−1.72	−1.75	−1.78	−1.81	−1.84	−1.86
.10	−1.56	−1.58	−1.61	−1.64	−1.66	−1.69	−1.72	−1.75	−1.78	−1.80
.11	−1.51	−1.54	−1.56	−1.59	−1.62	−1.64	−1.67	−1.70	−1.74	−1.76
.12	−1.46	−1.48	−1.50	−1.54	−1.56	−1.58	−1.62	−1.64	−1.68	−1.70
.13	−1.41	−1.44	−1.46	−1.49	−1.52	−1.54	−1.57	−1.60	−1.64	−1.66
.14	−1.36	−1.38	−1.41	−1.44	−1.46	−1.49	−1.52	−1.55	−1.58	−1.60
.15	−1.32	−1.34	−1.37	−1.40	−1.42	−1.45	−1.48	−1.51	−1.54	−1.56
.16	−1.27	−1.30	−1.32	−1.35	−1.38	−1.40	−1.43	−1.46	−1.50	−1.52
.17	−1.23	−1.26	−1.28	−1.31	−1.34	−1.36	−1.39	−1.42	−1.46	−1.48
.18	−1.20	−1.22	−1.24	−1.28	−1.30	−1.32	−1.36	−1.38	−1.42	−1.44
.19	−1.16	−1.18	−1.21	−1.24	−1.26	−1.29	−1.32	−1.35	−1.38	−1.40
.20	−1.12	−1.14	−1.17	−1.20	−1.22	−1.25	−1.28	−1.31	−1.34	−1.36
.21	−1.08	−1.11	−1.14	−1.16	−1.19	−1.22	−1.24	−1.28	−1.31	−1.33
.22	−1.05	−1.08	−1.10	−1.13	−1.16	−1.18	−1.21	−1.24	−1.28	−1.30
.23	−1.02	−1.04	−1.07	−1.10	−1.12	−1.15	−1.18	−1.21	−1.24	−1.26
.24	− .98	−1.01	−1.04	−1.06	−1.09	−1.12	−1.14	−1.18	−1.21	−1.23
.25	− .96	− .98	−1.00	−1.04	−1.06	−1.08	−1.12	−1.14	−1.18	−1.20
.26	− .92	− .94	− .97	−1.00	−1.02	−1.05	−1.08	−1.11	−1.14	−1.16
.27	− .89	− .92	− .94	− .97	−1.00	−1.02	−1.05	−1.08	−1.12	−1.14
.28	− .86	− .88	− .91	− .94	− .96	− .99	−1.02	−1.05	−1.08	−1.10
.29	− .84	− .86	− .88	− .92	− .94	− .96	−1.00	−1.02	−1.06	−1.08
.30	− .80	− .83	− .86	− .88	− .91	− .94	− .96	−1.00	−1.03	−1.05
.31	− .78	− .81	− .84	− .86	− .89	− .92	− .94	− .98	−1.01	−1.03
.32	− .75	− .78	− .80	− .83	− .86	− .88	− .91	− .94	− .98	−1.00
.33	− .72	− .74	− .77	− .80	− .82	− .85	− .88	− .91	− .94	− .96
.34	− .69	− .72	− .74	− .77	− .80	− .82	− .85	− .88	− .92	− .94
.35	− .66	− .69	− .72	− .74	− .77	− .80	− .82	− .86	− .89	− .91
.36	− .64	− .66	− .69	− .72	− .74	− .77	− .80	− .83	− .86	− .88
.37	− .61	− .64	− .66	− .69	− .72	− .74	− .77	− .80	− .84	− .86
.38	− .58	− .61	− .64	− .66	− .69	− .72	− .74	− .78	− .81	− .83
.39	− .56	− .58	− .61	− .64	− .66	− .69	− .72	− .75	− .78	− .80
.40	− .54	− .56	− .58	− .62	− .64	− .66	− .70	− .72	− .76	− .78
.41	− .51	− .54	− .56	− .59	− .62	− .64	− .67	− .70	− .74	− .76
.42	− .48	− .50	− .53	− .56	− .58	− .61	− .64	− .67	− .70	− .72
.43	− .46	− .48	− .51	− .54	− .56	− .59	− .62	− .65	− .68	− .70
.44	− .43	− .46	− .48	− .51	− .54	− .56	− .59	− .62	− .66	− .68
.45	− .41	− .44	− .46	− .49	− .52	− .54	− .57	− .60	− .64	− .66
.46	− .38	− .40	− .43	− .46	− .48	− .51	− .54	− .57	− .60	− .62
.47	− .36	− .38	− .40	− .44	− .46	− .48	− .52	− .54	− .58	− .60
.48	− .33	− .36	− .38	− .41	− .44	− .46	− .49	− .52	− .56	− .58
.49	− .30	− .33	− .36	− .38	− .41	− .44	− .46	− .50	− .53	− .55
.50	− .28	− .30	− .33	− .36	− .38	− .41	− .44	− .47	− .50	− .52

TABLE I. *(Continued)*

$P_{SN}(A)$ \ $P_N(A)$	.61	.62	.63	.64	.65	.66	.67	.68	.69	.70
.51	− .26	− .28	− .30	− .34	− .36	− .38	− .42	− .44	− .48	− .50
.52	− .23	− .26	− .28	− .31	− .34	− .36	− .39	− .42	− .46	− .48
.53	− .20	− .23	− .26	− .28	− .31	− .34	− .36	− .40	− .43	− .45
.54	− .18	− .20	− .23	− .26	− .28	− .31	− .34	− .37	− .40	− .42
.55	− .15	− .18	− .20	− .23	− .26	− .28	− .31	− .34	− .38	− .40
.56	− .13	− .14	− .18	− .21	− .24	− .26	− .29	− .32	− .36	− .38
.57	− .10	− .12	− .15	− .18	− .20	− .23	− .26	− .29	− .32	− .34
.58	− .08	− .10	− .13	− .16	− .18	− .21	− .24	− .27	− .30	− .32
.59	− .05	− .08	− .10	− .13	− .16	− .18	− .21	− .24	− .28	− .30
.60	− .02	− .05	− .08	− .10	− .13	− .16	− .18	− .22	− .25	− .27
.61	0	− .02	− .05	− .08	− .10	− .13	− .16	− .19	− .22	− .24
.62	.02	0	− .02	− .06	− .08	− .10	− .14	− .16	− .20	− .22
.63	.05	.02	0	− .03	− .06	− .08	− .11	− .14	− .18	− .20
.64	.08	.06	.03	0	− .02	− .05	− .08	− .11	− .14	− .16
.65	.10	.08	.06	.02	0	− .02	− .06	− .08	− .12	− .14
.66	.13	.10	.08	.05	.02	0	− .03	− .06	− .10	− .12
.67	.16	.14	.11	.08	.06	.03	0	− .03	− .06	− .08
.68	.19	.16	.14	.11	.08	.06	.03	0	− .04	− .06
.69	.22	.20	.18	.14	.12	.10	.06	.04	0	− .02
.70	.24	.22	.20	.16	.14	.12	.08	.06	.02	0
.71	.28	.25	.22	.20	.17	.14	.12	.08	.05	.03
.72	.30	.28	.25	.22	.20	.17	.14	.11	.08	.06
.73	.33	.30	.28	.25	.22	.20	.17	.14	.10	.08
.74	.36	.34	.31	.28	.26	.23	.20	.17	.14	.12
.75	.40	.37	.34	.32	.29	.26	.24	.20	.17	.15
.76	.42	.40	.38	.34	.32	.30	.26	.24	.20	.18
.77	.46	.44	.41	.38	.36	.33	.30	.27	.24	.22
.78	.49	.46	.44	.41	.38	.36	.33	.30	.26	.24
.79	.52	.50	.48	.44	.42	.40	.36	.34	.30	.28
.80	.56	.54	.51	.48	.46	.43	.40	.37	.34	.32
.81	.60	.58	.55	.52	.50	.47	.44	.41	.38	.36
.82	.64	.61	.58	.56	.53	.50	.48	.44	.41	.39
.83	.67	.64	.62	.59	.56	.54	.51	.48	.44	.42
.84	.71	.68	.66	.63	.60	.58	.55	.52	.48	.46
.85	.76	.74	.71	.68	.66	.63	.60	.57	.54	.52
.86	.80	.78	.75	.72	.70	.67	.64	.61	.58	.56
.87	.85	.82	.80	.77	.74	.72	.69	.66	.62	.60
.88	.90	.87	.84	.82	.79	.76	.74	.70	.67	.65
.89	.95	.92	.90	.87	.84	.82	.79	.76	.72	.70
.90	1.00	.98	.95	.92	.90	.87	.84	.81	.78	.76
.91	1.06	1.04	1.01	.98	.96	.93	.90	.87	.84	.82
.92	1.12	1.10	1.07	1.04	1.02	.99	.96	.93	.90	.88
.93	1.19	1.16	1.14	1.11	1.08	1.06	1.03	1.00	.96	.94
.94	1.27	1.24	1.22	1.19	1.16	1.14	1.11	1.08	1.04	1.02
.95	1.36	1.34	1.31	1.28	1.26	1.23	1.20	1.17	1.14	1.12
.96	1.47	1.44	1.42	1.39	1.36	1.34	1.31	1.28	1.24	1.22
.97	1.60	1.58	1.55	1.52	1.50	1.47	1.44	1.41	1.38	1.36
.98	1.77	1.74	1.72	1.69	1.66	1.64	1.61	1.58	1.54	1.52
.99	2.04	2.02	1.99	1.96	1.94	1.91	1.88	1.85	1.82	1.80

TABLE I. *(Continued)*

$P_{SN}(A)$ \ $P_N(A)$	.71	.72	.73	.74	.75	.76	.77	.78	.79	.80
.01	−2.88	−2.90	−2.93	−2.96	−3.00	−3.02	−3.06	−3.09	−3.12	−3.16
.02	−2.60	−2.63	−2.66	−2.69	−2.72	−2.76	−2.79	−2.82	−2.86	−2.89
.03	−2.44	−2.46	−2.49	−2.52	−2.56	−2.58	−2.62	−2.65	−2.68	−2.72
.04	−2.30	−2.33	−2.36	−2.39	−2.42	−2.46	−2.49	−2.52	−2.56	−2.59
.05	−2.20	−2.22	−2.25	−2.28	−2.32	−2.34	−2.38	−2.41	−2.44	−2.48
.06	−2.10	−2.13	−2.16	−2.19	−2.22	−2.26	−2.29	−2.32	−2.36	−2.39
.07	−2.02	−2.05	−2.08	−2.11	−2.14	−2.18	−2.21	−2.24	−2.28	−2.31
.08	−1.96	−1.98	−2.01	−2.04	−2.08	−2.10	−2.14	−2.17	−2.20	−2.24
.09	−1.90	−1.92	−1.95	−1.98	−2.02	−2.04	−2.08	−2.11	−2.14	−2.18
.10	−1.84	−1.86	−1.89	−1.92	−1.96	−1.98	−2.02	−2.05	−2.08	−2.12
.11	−1.78	−1.81	−1.84	−1.87	−1.90	−1.94	−1.97	−2.00	−2.04	−2.07
.12	−1.73	−1.76	−1.78	−1.82	−1.85	−1.88	−1.92	−1.94	−1.98	−2.02
.13	−1.68	−1.71	−1.74	−1.77	−1.80	−1.84	−1.87	−1.90	−1.94	−1.97
.14	−1.64	−1.66	−1.69	−1.72	−1.76	−1.78	−1.82	−1.85	−1.88	−1.92
.15	−1.60	−1.62	−1.65	−1.68	−1.72	−1.74	−1.78	−1.81	−1.84	−1.88
.16	−1.54	−1.57	−1.60	−1.63	−1.66	−1.70	−1.73	−1.76	−1.80	−1.83
.17	−1.50	−1.53	−1.56	−1.59	−1.62	−1.66	−1.69	−1.72	−1.76	−1.79
.18	−1.47	−1.50	−1.52	−1.56	−1.59	−1.62	−1.66	−1.68	−1.72	−1.76
.19	−1.44	−1.46	−1.49	−1.52	−1.56	−1.58	−1.62	−1.65	−1.68	−1.72
.20	−1.40	−1.42	−1.45	−1.48	−1.52	−1.54	−1.58	−1.61	−1.64	−1.68
.21	−1.36	−1.38	−1.42	−1.44	−1.48	−1.51	−1.54	−1.58	−1.61	−1.64
.22	−1.32	−1.35	−1.38	−1.41	−1.44	−1.48	−1.51	−1.54	−1.58	−1.61
.23	−1.30	−1.32	−1.35	−1.38	−1.42	−1.44	−1.48	−1.51	−1.54	−1.58
.24	−1.26	−1.28	−1.32	−1.34	−1.38	−1.41	−1.44	−1.48	−1.51	−1.54
.25	−1.23	−1.26	−1.28	−1.32	−1.35	−1.38	−1.42	−1.44	−1.48	−1.52
.26	−1.20	−1.22	−1.25	−1.28	−1.32	−1.34	−1.38	−1.41	−1.44	−1.48
.27	−1.16	−1.19	−1.22	−1.25	−1.28	−1.32	−1.35	−1.38	−1.42	−1.45
.28	−1.14	−1.16	−1.19	−1.22	−1.26	−1.28	−1.32	−1.35	−1.38	−1.42
.29	−1.11	−1.14	−1.16	−1.20	−1.23	−1.26	−1.30	−1.32	−1.36	−1.40
.30	−1.08	−1.10	−1.14	−1.16	−1.20	−1.23	−1.26	−1.30	−1.33	−1.36
.31	−1.06	−1.08	−1.12	−1.14	−1.18	−1.21	−1.24	−1.28	−1.31	−1.34
.32	−1.02	−1.05	−1.08	−1.11	−1.14	−1.18	−1.21	−1.24	−1.28	−1.31
.33	−1.00	−1.02	−1.05	−1.08	−1.12	−1.14	−1.18	−1.21	−1.24	−1.28
.34	− .96	− .99	−1.02	−1.05	−1.08	−1.12	−1.15	−1.18	−1.22	−1.25
.35	− .94	− .96	−1.00	−1.02	−1.06	−1.09	−1.12	−1.16	−1.19	−1.22
.36	− .92	− .94	− .97	−1.00	−1.04	−1.06	−1.10	−1.13	−1.16	−1.20
.37	− .88	− .91	− .94	− .97	−1.00	−1.04	−1.07	−1.10	−1.14	−1.17
.38	− .86	− .88	− .92	− .94	− .98	−1.01	−1.04	−1.08	−1.11	−1.14
.39	− .84	− .86	− .89	− .92	− .96	− .98	−1.02	−1.05	−1.08	−1.12
.40	− .81	− .84	− .86	− .90	− .93	− .96	−1.00	−1.02	−1.06	−1.10
.41	− .78	− .81	− .84	− .87	− .90	− .94	− .97	−1.00	−1.04	−1.07
.42	− .76	− .78	− .81	− .84	− .88	− .90	− .94	− .97	−1.00	−1.04
.43	− .74	− .76	− .79	− .82	− .86	− .88	− .92	− .95	− .98	−1.02
.44	− .70	− .73	− .76	− .79	− .82	− .86	− .89	− .92	− .96	− .99
.45	− .68	− .71	− .74	− .77	− .80	− .84	− .87	− .90	− .94	− .97
.46	− .66	− .68	− .71	− .74	− .78	− .80	− .84	− .87	− .90	− .94
.47	− .63	− .66	− .68	− .72	− .75	− .78	− .82	− .84	− .88	− .92
.48	− .60	− .63	− .66	− .69	− .72	− .76	− .79	− .82	− .86	− .89
.49	− .58	− .60	− .64	− .66	− .70	− .73	− .76	− .80	− .83	− .86
.50	− .56	− .58	− .61	− .64	− .68	− .70	− .74	− .77	− .80	− .84

TABLE I. *(Continued)*

$P_{SN}(A)$ \ $P_N(A)$	.71	.72	.73	.74	.75	.76	.77	.78	.79	.80
.51	− .53	− .56	− .58	− .62	− .65	− .68	− .72	− .74	− .78	− .82
.52	− .50	− .53	− .56	− .59	− .62	− .66	− .69	− .72	− .76	− .79
.53	− .48	− .50	− .54	− .56	− .60	− .63	− .66	− .70	− .73	− .76
.54	− .46	− .48	− .51	− .54	− .58	− .60	− .64	− .67	− .70	− .74
.55	− .42	− .45	− .48	− .51	− .54	− .58	− .61	− .64	− .68	− .71
.56	− .40	− .43	− .46	− .49	− .52	− .56	− .59	− .62	− .66	− .69
.57	− .38	− .40	− .43	− .46	− .50	− .52	− .56	− .59	− .62	− .66
.58	− .36	− .38	− .41	− .44	− .48	− .50	− .54	− .57	− .60	− .64
.59	− .32	− .35	− .38	− .41	− .44	− .48	− .51	− .54	− .58	− .61
.60	− .30	− .32	− .36	− .38	− .42	− .45	− .48	− .52	− .55	− .58
.61	− .28	− .30	− .33	− .36	− .40	− .42	− .46	− .49	− .52	− .56
.62	− .25	− .28	− .30	− .34	− .37	− .40	− .44	− .46	− .50	− .54
.63	− .22	− .25	− .28	− .31	− .34	− .38	− .41	− .44	− .48	− .51
.64	− .20	− .22	− .25	− .28	− .32	− .34	− .38	− .41	− .44	− .48
.65	− .17	− .20	− .22	− .26	− .29	− .32	− .36	− .38	− .42	− .46
.66	− .14	− .17	− .20	− .23	− .26	− .30	− .33	− .36	− .40	− .43
.67	− .12	− .14	− .17	− .20	− .24	− .26	− .30	− .33	− .36	− .40
.68	− .08	− .11	− .14	− .17	− .20	− .24	− .27	− .30	− .34	− .37
.69	− .05	− .08	− .10	− .14	− .17	− .20	− .24	− .26	− .30	− .34
.70	− .03	− .06	− .08	− .12	− .15	− .18	− .22	− .24	− .28	− .32
.71	0	− .02	− .06	− .08	− .12	− .15	− .18	− .22	− .25	− .28
.72	.02	0	− .03	− .06	− .10	− .12	− .16	− .19	− .22	− .26
.73	.06	.03	0	− .03	− .06	− .10	− .13	− .16	− .20	− .23
.74	.08	.06	.03	0	− .04	− .06	− .10	− .13	− .16	− .20
.75	.12	.10	.06	.04	0	− .03	− .06	− .10	− .13	− .16
.76	.15	.12	.10	.06	.03	0	− .04	− .06	− .10	− .14
.77	.18	.16	.13	.10	.06	.04	0	− .03	− .06	− .10
.78	.22	.19	.16	.13	.10	.06	.03	0	− .04	− .07
.79	.25	.22	.20	.16	.13	.10	.06	.04	0	− .04
.80	.28	.26	.23	.20	.16	.14	.10	.07	.04	0
.81	.32	.30	.27	.24	.20	.18	.14	.11	.08	.04
.82	.36	.34	.30	.28	.24	.21	.18	.14	.11	.08
.83	.40	.37	.34	.31	.28	.24	.21	.18	.14	.11
.84	.44	.41	.38	.35	.32	.28	.25	.22	.18	.15
.85	.48	.46	.43	.40	.36	.34	.30	.27	.24	.20
.86	.52	.50	.47	.44	.40	.38	.34	.31	.28	.24
.87	.58	.55	.52	.49	.46	.42	.39	.36	.32	.29
.88	.62	.60	.56	.54	.50	.47	.44	.40	.37	.34
.89	.68	.65	.62	.59	.56	.52	.49	.46	.42	.39
.90	.72	.70	.67	.64	.60	.58	.54	.51	.48	.44
.91	.78	.76	.73	.70	.66	.64	.60	.57	.54	.50
.92	.84	.82	.79	.76	.72	.70	.66	.63	.60	.56
.93	.92	.89	.86	.83	.80	.76	.73	.70	.66	.63
.94	1.00	.97	.94	.91	.88	.84	.81	.78	.74	.71
.95	1.08	1.06	1.03	1.00	.96	.94	.90	.87	.84	.80
.96	1.20	1.17	1.14	1.11	1.08	1.04	1.01	.98	.94	.91
.97	1.32	1.30	1.27	1.24	1.20	1.18	1.14	1.11	1.08	1.04
.98	1.50	1.47	1.44	1.41	1.38	1.34	1.31	1.28	1.24	1.21
.99	1.76	1.74	1.71	1.68	1.64	1.62	1.58	1.55	1.52	1.48

TABLE I. *(Continued)*

$P_{SN}(A)$ \ $P_N(A)$	.81	.82	.83	.84	.85	.86	.87	.88	.89	.90
.01	−3.20	−3.24	−3.27	−3.31	−3.36	−3.40	−3.45	−3.50	−3.55	−3.60
.02	−2.93	−2.96	−3.00	−3.04	−3.09	−3.13	−3.18	−3.22	−3.28	−3.33
.03	−2.76	−2.80	−2.83	−2.87	−2.92	−2.96	−3.01	−3.06	−3.11	−3.16
.04	−2.63	−2.66	−2.70	−2.74	−2.79	−2.83	−2.88	−2.92	−2.98	−3.03
.05	−2.52	−2.56	−2.59	−2.63	−2.68	−2.72	−2.77	−2.82	−2.87	−2.92
.06	−2.43	−2.46	−2.50	−2.54	−2.59	−2.63	−2.68	−2.72	−2.78	−2.83
.07	−2.35	−2.38	−2.42	−2.46	−2.51	−2.55	−2.60	−2.64	−2.70	−2.75
.08	−2.28	−2.32	−2.35	−2.39	−2.44	−2.48	−2.53	−2.58	−2.63	−2.68
.09	−2.22	−2.26	−2.29	−2.33	−2.38	−2.42	−2.47	−2.52	−2.57	−2.62
.10	−2.16	−2.20	−2.23	−2.27	−2.32	−2.36	−2.41	−2.46	−2.51	−2.56
.11	−2.11	−2.14	−2.18	−2.22	−2.27	−2.31	−2.36	−2.40	−2.46	−2.51
.12	−2.06	−2.09	−2.12	−2.16	−2.22	−2.26	−2.30	−2.35	−2.40	−2.46
.13	−2.01	−2.04	−2.08	−2.12	−2.17	−2.21	−2.26	−2.30	−2.36	−2.41
.14	−1.96	−2.00	−2.03	−2.07	−2.12	−2.16	−2.21	−2.26	−2.31	−2.36
.15	−1.92	−1.96	−1.99	−2.03	−2.08	−2.12	−2.17	−2.22	−2.27	−2.32
.16	−1.87	−1.90	−1.94	−1.98	−2.03	−2.07	−2.12	−2.16	−2.22	−2.27
.17	−1.83	−1.86	−1.90	−1.94	−1.99	−2.03	−2.08	−2.12	−2.18	−2.23
.18	−1.80	−1.83	−1.86	−1.90	−1.96	−2.00	−2.04	−2.09	−2.14	−2.20
.19	−1.76	−1.80	−1.83	−1.87	−1.92	−1.96	−2.01	−2.06	−2.11	−2.16
.20	−1.72	−1.76	−1.79	−1.83	−1.88	−1.92	−1.97	−2.02	−2.07	−2.12
.21	−1.68	−1.72	−1.76	−1.80	−1.84	−1.88	−1.94	−1.98	−2.04	−2.08
.22	−1.65	−1.68	−1.72	−1.76	−1.81	−1.85	−1.90	−1.94	−2.00	−2.05
.23	−1.62	−1.66	−1.69	−1.73	−1.78	−1.82	−1.87	−1.92	−1.97	−2.02
.24	−1.58	−1.62	−1.66	−1.70	−1.74	−1.78	−1.84	−1.88	−1.94	−1.98
.25	−1.56	−1.59	−1.62	−1.66	−1.72	−1.76	−1.80	−1.85	−1.90	−1.96
.26	−1.52	−1.56	−1.59	−1.63	−1.68	−1.72	−1.77	−1.82	−1.87	−1.92
.27	−1.49	−1.52	−1.56	−1.60	−1.65	−1.69	−1.74	−1.78	−1.84	−1.89
.28	−1.46	−1.50	−1.53	−1.57	−1.62	−1.66	−1.71	−1.76	−1.81	−1.86
.29	−1.44	−1.47	−1.50	−1.54	−1.60	−1.64	−1.68	−1.73	−1.78	−1.84
.30	−1.40	−1.44	−1.48	−1.52	−1.56	−1.60	−1.66	−1.70	−1.76	−1.80
.31	−1.38	−1.42	−1.46	−1.50	−1.54	−1.58	−1.64	−1.68	−1.74	−1.78
.32	−1.35	−1.38	−1.42	−1.46	−1.51	−1.55	−1.60	−1.64	−1.70	−1.75
.33	−1.32	−1.36	−1.39	−1.43	−1.48	−1.52	−1.57	−1.62	−1.67	−1.72
.34	−1.29	−1.32	−1.36	−1.40	−1.45	−1.49	−1.54	−1.58	−1.64	−1.69
.35	−1.26	−1.30	−1.34	−1.38	−1.42	−1.46	−1.52	−1.56	−1.62	−1.66
.36	−1.24	−1.28	−1.31	−1.35	−1.40	−1.44	−1.49	−1.54	−1.59	−1.64
.37	−1.21	−1.24	−1.28	−1.32	−1.37	−1.41	−1.46	−1.50	−1.56	−1.61
.38	−1.18	−1.22	−1.26	−1.30	−1.34	−1.38	−1.44	−1.48	−1.54	−1.58
.39	−1.16	−1.20	−1.23	−1.27	−1.32	−1.36	−1.41	−1.46	−1.51	−1.56
.40	−1.14	−1.17	−1.20	−1.24	−1.30	−1.34	−1.38	−1.43	−1.48	−1.54
.41	−1.11	−1.14	−1.18	−1.22	−1.27	−1.31	−1.36	−1.40	−1.46	−1.51
.42	−1.08	−1.12	−1.15	−1.19	−1.24	−1.28	−1.33	−1.38	−1.43	−1.48
.43	−1.06	−1.10	−1.13	−1.17	−1.22	−1.26	−1.31	−1.36	−1.41	−1.46
.44	−1.03	−1.06	−1.10	−1.14	−1.19	−1.23	−1.28	−1.32	−1.38	−1.43
.45	−1.01	−1.04	−1.08	−1.12	−1.17	−1.21	−1.26	−1.30	−1.36	−1.41
.46	− .98	−1.02	−1.05	−1.09	−1.14	−1.18	−1.23	−1.28	−1.33	−1.38
.47	− .96	− .99	−1.02	−1.06	−1.12	−1.16	−1.20	−1.25	−1.30	−1.36
.48	− .93	− .96	−1.00	−1.04	−1.09	−1.13	−1.18	−1.22	−1.28	−1.33
.49	− .90	− .94	− .98	−1.02	−1.06	−1.10	−1.16	−1.20	−1.26	−1.30
.50	− .88	− .92	− .95	− .99	−1.04	−1.08	−1.13	−1.18	−1.23	−1.28

TABLE I. *(Continued)*

$P_{SN}(A)$ \ $P_N(A)$	.81	.82	.83	.84	.85	.86	.87	.88	.89	.90
.51	−.86	−.89	−.92	−.96	−1.02	−1.06	−1.10	−1.15	−1.20	−1.26
.52	−.83	−.86	−.90	−.94	−.99	−1.03	−1.08	−1.12	−1.18	−1.23
.53	−.80	−.84	−.88	−.92	−.96	−1.00	−1.06	−1.10	−1.16	−1.20
.54	−.78	−.82	−.85	−.89	−.94	−.98	−1.03	−1.08	−1.13	−1.18
.55	−.75	−.78	−.82	−.86	−.91	−.95	−1.00	−1.04	−1.10	−1.15
.56	−.73	−.76	−.80	−.84	−.89	−.93	−.98	−1.02	−1.08	−1.13
.57	−.70	−.74	−.77	−.81	−.86	−.90	−.95	−1.00	−1.05	−1.10
.58	−.68	−.72	−.75	−.79	−.84	−.88	−.93	−.98	−1.03	−1.08
.59	−.65	−.68	−.72	−.76	−.81	−.85	−.90	−.94	−1.00	−1.05
.60	−.62	−.66	−.70	−.74	−.78	−.82	−.88	−.92	−.98	−1.02
.61	−.60	−.64	−.67	−.71	−.76	−.80	−.85	−.90	−.95	−1.00
.62	−.58	−.61	−.64	−.68	−.74	−.78	−.82	−.87	−.92	−.98
.63	−.55	−.58	−.62	−.66	−.71	−.75	−.80	−.84	−.90	−.95
.64	−.52	−.56	−.59	−.63	−.68	−.72	−.77	−.82	−.87	−.92
.65	−.50	−.53	−.56	−.60	−.66	−.70	−.74	−.79	−.84	−.90
.66	−.47	−.50	−.54	−.58	−.63	−.67	−.72	−.76	−.82	−.87
.67	−.44	−.48	−.51	−.55	−.60	−.64	−.69	−.74	−.79	−.84
.68	−.41	−.44	−.48	−.52	−.57	−.61	−.66	−.70	−.76	−.81
.69	−.38	−.41	−.44	−.48	−.54	−.58	−.62	−.67	−.72	−.78
.70	−.36	−.39	−.42	−.46	−.52	−.56	−.60	−.65	−.70	−.76
.71	−.32	−.36	−.40	−.44	−.48	−.52	−.58	−.62	−.68	−.72
.72	−.30	−.34	−.37	−.41	−.46	−.50	−.55	−.60	−.65	−.70
.73	−.27	−.30	−.34	−.38	−.43	−.47	−.52	−.56	−.62	−.67
.74	−.24	−.28	−.31	−.35	−.40	−.44	−.49	−.54	−.59	−.64
.75	−.20	−.24	−.28	−.32	−.36	−.40	−.46	−.50	−.56	−.60
.76	−.18	−.21	−.24	−.28	−.34	−.38	−.42	−.47	−.52	−.58
.77	−.14	−.18	−.21	−.25	−.30	−.34	−.39	−.44	−.49	−.54
.78	−.11	−.14	−.18	−.22	−.27	−.31	−.36	−.40	−.46	−.51
.79	−.08	−.11	−.14	−.18	−.24	−.28	−.32	−.37	−.42	−.48
.80	−.04	−.08	−.11	−.15	−.20	−.24	−.29	−.34	−.39	−.44
.81	0	−.04	−.07	−.11	−.16	−.20	−.25	−.30	−.35	−.40
.82	.04	0	−.04	−.08	−.12	−.16	−.22	−.26	−.32	−.36
.83	.07	.04	0	−.04	−.09	−.13	−.18	−.22	−.28	−.33
.84	.11	.08	.04	0	−.05	−.09	−.14	−.18	−.24	−.29
.85	.16	.12	.09	.05	0	−.04	−.09	−.14	−.19	−.24
.86	.20	.16	.13	.09	.04	0	−.05	−.10	−.15	−.20
.87	.25	.22	.18	.14	.09	.05	0	−.04	−.10	−.15
.88	.30	.26	.22	.18	.14	.10	.04	0	−.06	−.10
.89	.35	.32	.28	.24	.19	.15	.10	.06	0	−.05
.90	.40	.36	.33	.29	.24	.20	.15	.10	.05	0
.91	.46	.42	.39	.35	.30	.26	.21	.16	.11	.06
.92	.52	.48	.45	.41	.36	.32	.27	.22	.17	.12
.93	.59	.56	.52	.48	.43	.39	.34	.30	.24	.19
.94	.67	.64	.60	.56	.51	.47	.42	.38	.32	.27
.95	.76	.72	.69	.65	.60	.56	.51	.46	.41	.36
.96	.87	.84	.80	.76	.71	.67	.62	.58	.52	.47
.97	1.00	.96	.93	.89	.84	.80	.75	.70	.65	.60
.98	1.17	1.14	1.10	1.06	1.01	.97	.92	.88	.82	.77
.99	1.44	1.40	1.37	1.33	1.28	1.24	1.19	1.14	1.09	1.04

TABLE I. *(Continued)*

$P_{SN}(A)$ \ $P_N(A)$	.91	.92	.93	.94	.95	.96	.97	.98	.99
.01	−3.66	−3.72	−3.79	−3.87	−3.96	−4.07	−4.20	−4.37	−4.64
.02	−3.39	−3.45	−3.52	−3.60	−3.69	−3.80	−3.93	−4.10	−4.37
.03	−3.22	−3.28	−3.35	−3.43	−3.52	−3.63	−3.76	−3.93	−4.20
.04	−3.09	−3.15	−3.22	−3.30	−3.39	−3.50	−3.63	−3.80	−4.07
.05	−2.98	−3.04	−3.11	−3.19	−3.28	−3.39	−3.52	−3.69	−3.96
.06	−2.89	−2.95	−3.02	−3.10	−3.19	−3.30	−3.43	−3.60	−3.87
.07	−2.81	−2.87	−2.94	−3.02	−3.11	−3.22	−3.35	−3.52	−3.79
.08	−2.74	−2.80	−2.87	−2.95	−3.04	−3.15	−3.28	−3.45	−3.72
.09	−2.68	−2.74	−2.81	−2.89	−2.98	−3.09	−3.22	−3.39	−3.66
.10	−2.62	−2.68	−2.75	−2.83	−2.92	−3.03	−3.16	−3.33	−3.60
.11	−2.57	−2.63	−2.70	−2.78	−2.87	−2.98	−3.11	−3.28	−3.55
.12	−2.52	−2.58	−2.64	−2.72	−2.82	−2.92	−3.06	−3.22	−3.50
.13	−2.47	−2.53	−2.60	−2.68	−2.77	−2.88	−3.01	−3.18	−3.45
.14	−2.42	−2.48	−2.55	−2.63	−2.72	−2.83	−2.96	−3.13	−3.40
.15	−2.38	−2.44	−2.51	−2.59	−2.68	−2.79	−2.92	−3.09	−3.36
.16	−2.33	−2.39	−2.46	−2.54	−2.63	−2.74	−2.87	−3.04	−3.31
.17	−2.29	−2.35	−2.42	−2.50	−2.59	−2.70	−2.83	−3.00	−3.27
.18	−2.26	−2.32	−2.38	−2.46	−2.56	−2.66	−2.80	−2.96	−3.24
.19	−2.22	−2.28	−2.35	−2.43	−2.52	−2.63	−2.76	−2.93	−3.20
.20	−2.18	−2.24	−2.31	−2.39	−2.48	−2.59	−2.72	−2.89	−3.16
.21	−2.14	−2.20	−2.28	−2.36	−2.44	−2.56	−2.68	−2.86	−3.12
.22	−2.11	−2.17	−2.24	−2.32	−2.41	−2.52	−2.65	−2.82	−3.09
.23	−2.08	−2.14	−2.21	−2.29	−2.38	−2.49	−2.62	−2.79	−3.06
.24	−2.04	−2.10	−2.18	−2.26	−2.34	−2.46	−2.58	−2.76	−3.02
.25	−2.02	−2.08	−2.14	−2.22	−2.32	−2.42	−2.56	−2.72	−3.00
.26	−1.98	−2.04	−2.11	−2.19	−2.28	−2.39	−2.52	−2.69	−2.96
.27	−1.95	−2.01	−2.08	−2.16	−2.25	−2.36	−2.49	−2.66	−2.93
.28	−1.92	−1.98	−2.05	−2.13	−2.22	−2.33	−2.46	−2.63	−2.90
.29	−1.90	−1.96	−2.02	−2.10	−2.20	−2.30	−2.44	−2.60	−2.88
.30	−1.86	−1.92	−2.00	−2.08	−2.16	−2.28	−2.40	−2.58	−2.84
.31	−1.84	−1.90	−1.98	−2.06	−2.14	−2.26	−2.38	−2.56	−2.82
.32	−1.81	−1.87	−1.94	−2.02	−2.11	−2.22	−2.35	−2.52	−2.79
.33	−1.78	−1.84	−1.91	−1.99	−2.08	−2.19	−2.32	−2.49	−2.76
.34	−1.75	−1.81	−1.88	−1.96	−2.05	−2.16	−2.29	−2.46	−2.73
.35	−1.72	−1.78	−1.86	−1.94	−2.02	−2.14	−2.26	−2.44	−2.70
.36	−1.70	−1.76	−1.83	−1.91	−2.00	−2.11	−2.24	−2.41	−2.68
.37	−1.67	−1.73	−1.80	−1.88	−1.97	−2.08	−2.21	−2.38	−2.65
.38	−1.64	−1.70	−1.78	−1.86	−1.94	−2.06	−2.18	−2.36	−2.62
.39	−1.62	−1.68	−1.75	−1.83	−1.92	−2.03	−2.16	−2.33	−2.60
.40	−1.60	−1.66	−1.72	−1.80	−1.90	−2.00	−2.14	−2.30	−2.58
.41	−1.57	−1.63	−1.70	−1.78	−1.87	−1.98	−2.11	−2.28	−2.55
.42	−1.54	−1.60	−1.67	−1.75	−1.84	−1.95	−2.08	−2.25	−2.52
.43	−1.52	−1.58	−1.65	−1.73	−1.82	−1.93	−2.06	−2.23	−2.50
.44	−1.49	−1.55	−1.62	−1.70	−1.79	−1.90	−2.03	−2.20	−2.47
.45	−1.47	−1.53	−1.60	−1.68	−1.77	−1.88	−2.01	−2.18	−2.45
.46	−1.44	−1.50	−1.57	−1.65	−1.74	−1.85	−1.98	−2.15	−2.42
.47	−1.42	−1.48	−1.54	−1.62	−1.72	−1.82	−1.96	−2.12	−2.48
.48	−1.39	−1.45	−1.52	−1.60	−1.69	−1.80	−1.93	−2.10	−2.37
.49	−1.36	−1.42	−1.50	−1.58	−1.66	−1.78	−1.90	−2.08	−2.34
.50	−1.34	−1.40	−1.47	−1.55	−1.64	−1.75	−1.88	−2.05	−2.32

TABLE I. *(Continued)*

$P_{SN}(A)$ \ $P_N(A)$	.91	.92	.93	.94	.95	.96	.97	.98	.99
.51	−1.32	−1.38	−1.44	−1.52	−1.62	−1.72	−1.86	−2.02	−2.30
.52	−1.29	−1.35	−1.42	−1.50	−1.59	−1.70	−1.83	−2.00	−2.27
.53	−1.26	−1.32	−1.40	−1.48	−1.56	−1.68	−1.80	−1.98	−2.24
.54	−1.24	−1.30	−1.37	−1.45	−1.54	−1.65	−1.78	−1.95	−2.22
.55	−1.21	−1.27	−1.34	−1.42	−1.51	−1.62	−1.75	−1.92	−2.19
.56	−1.19	−1.25	−1.32	−1.40	−1.49	−1.60	−1.73	−1.90	−2.17
.57	−1.16	−1.22	−1.29	−1.37	−1.46	−1.57	−1.70	−1.87	−2.14
.58	−1.14	−1.20	−1.27	−1.35	−1.44	−1.55	−1.68	−1.85	−2.12
.59	−1.11	−1.17	−1.24	−1.32	−1.41	−1.52	−1.65	−1.82	−2.09
.60	−1.08	−1.14	−1.22	−1.30	−1.38	−1.50	−1.62	−1.80	−2.06
.61	−1.06	−1.12	−1.19	−1.27	−1.36	−1.47	−1.60	−1.77	−2.04
.62	−1.04	−1.10	−1.16	−1.24	−1.34	−1.44	−1.58	−1.74	−2.02
.63	−1.01	−1.07	−1.14	−1.22	−1.31	−1.42	−1.55	−1.72	−1.99
.64	−.98	−1.04	−1.11	−1.19	−1.28	−1.39	−1.52	−1.69	−1.96
.65	−.96	−1.02	−1.08	−1.16	−1.26	−1.36	−1.50	−1.66	−1.94
.66	−.93	−.99	−1.06	−1.14	−1.23	−1.34	−1.47	−1.64	−1.91
.67	−.90	−.96	−1.03	−1.11	−1.20	−1.31	−1.44	−1.61	−1.88
.68	−.87	−.93	−1.00	−1.08	−1.17	−1.28	−1.41	−1.58	−1.85
.69	−.84	−.90	−.96	−1.04	−1.14	−1.24	−1.38	−1.54	−1.82
.70	−.82	−.88	−.94	−1.02	−1.12	−1.22	−1.36	−1.52	−1.80
.71	−.78	−.84	−.92	−1.00	−1.08	−1.20	−1.32	−1.50	−1.76
.72	−.76	−.82	−.89	−.97	−1.06	−1.17	−1.30	−1.47	−1.74
.73	−.73	−.79	−.86	−.94	−1.03	−1.14	−1.27	−1.44	−1.71
.74	−.70	−.76	−.83	−.91	−1.00	−1.11	−1.24	−1.41	−1.68
.75	−.66	−.72	−.80	−.88	−.96	−1.08	−1.20	−1.38	−1.64
.76	−.64	−.70	−.76	−.84	−.94	−1.04	−1.18	−1.34	−1.62
.77	−.60	−.66	−.73	−.81	−.90	−1.01	−1.14	−1.31	−1.58
.78	−.57	−.63	−.70	−.78	−.87	−.98	−1.11	−1.28	−1.55
.79	−.54	−.60	−.66	−.74	−.84	−.94	−1.08	−1.24	−1.52
.80	−.50	−.56	−.63	−.71	−.80	−.91	−1.04	−1.21	−1.48
.81	−.46	−.52	−.59	−.67	−.76	−.87	−1.00	−1.17	−1.44
.82	−.42	−.48	−.56	−.64	−.72	−.84	−.96	−1.14	−1.40
.83	−.39	−.45	−.52	−.60	−.69	−.80	−.93	−1.10	−1.37
.84	−.35	−.41	−.48	−.56	−.65	−.76	−.89	−1.06	−1.33
.85	−.30	−.36	−.43	−.51	−.60	−.71	−.84	−1.01	−1.28
.86	−.26	−.32	−.39	−.47	−.56	−.67	−.80	−.97	−1.24
.87	−.21	−.27	−.34	−.42	−.51	−.62	−.75	−.92	−1.19
.88	−.16	−.22	−.30	−.38	−.46	−.58	−.70	−.88	−1.14
.89	−.11	−.17	−.24	−.32	−.41	−.52	−.65	−.82	−1.09
.90	−.06	−.12	−.19	−.27	−.36	−.47	−.60	−.77	−1.04
.91	0	−.06	−.13	−.21	−.30	−.41	−.54	−.71	−.98
.92	.06	0	−.07	−.15	−.24	−.35	−.48	−.65	−.92
.93	.13	.07	0	−.08	−.17	−.28	−.41	−.58	−.85
.94	.21	.15	.08	0	−.09	−.20	−.33	−.50	−.77
.95	.30	.24	.17	.09	0	−.11	−.24	−.41	−.68
.96	.41	.35	.28	.20	.11	0	−.13	−.30	−.57
.97	.54	.48	.41	.33	.24	.13	0	−.17	−.44
.98	.71	.65	.33	.50	.41	.30	.17	0	−.27
.99	.98	.92	.85	.77	.68	.57	.44	.27	0

FORCED-CHOICE TABLES

In M-alternative forced-choice experiments, the percentage of correct responses $P(c)$ is usually obtained as the measure of performance. Table II converts $P(c)$ to d′ as a function of the number of alternatives. For the computation of d', $P(c)$ is used as an estimate of the probability of a correct decision.

Since Table II is an extension of a table prepared previously by Birdsall and Peterson (1954), the original introduction is reprinted here.

Optimum forced-choice performance

It is assumed in this discussion that the information which the observer has is equivalent to knowledge of the values for a given trial of M independent normal variables, of which $M - 1$ have mean zero, one has mean d', and all have unit variance. The normal variable with mean d' is the signal plus noise, while the others are noise alone. The observer does not know which variable is signal plus noise, and all are equally likely candidates.

This case can be considered an approximation to many forced-choice psychological tests, in which the signals are orthogonal, equally likely, and have the same energy, and the noise is white Gaussian noise over the bandwidth of the signals. One such set of signals is any set of similar but nonoverlapping (in time or space) pulses, another consists of tones of different frequencies.

The optimum choice is the variable which takes on the highest value. Thus, $P(c)$ is the probability that a Gaussian random variable with mean d' and unit variance will be simultaneously greater than $M - 1$ other independent Gaussian variables with zero mean and the unit variance.

For computation it is more convenient to observe that the probability of an incorrect decision is the probability that the greatest of the zero-mean variables is greater than the variable with mean d', or $M - 1$ times the probability that any particular zero-mean variable will be the greatest of all. If $A(t)$ stands for the area under the normal distribution from minus infinity to t, and $0(t)$ is the ordinate of the normal density (or frequency) function, then the probability of an incorrect decision is

$$P(\text{Incorrect}) = (M-1)\int_{-\infty}^{\infty} A^{M-2}(t)\, A(t - d')\, 0(t)\, dt \qquad (22)$$

The integrand is the probability density that a particular zero-mean variable will have value t (i.e., $0(t)$) times the probability that $(M - 2)$ zero-mean variables and the one variable with mean d' will be below that value t.

This integration was done numerically by the use of Simpson's approximate integration rule after a change of variable of integration. Letting

$$Z^2 = -2(M-1) \ln A(t) \tag{23}$$

the integral becomes

$P(\text{Incorrect}) =$

$$\int_0^\infty Z \exp\left(-\frac{Z^2}{2}\right) A\left\{A^{-1}\left[\exp\left(-\frac{Z^2}{2M-2}\right) - d'\right]\right\} dZ \tag{24}$$

Because $A \leqq 1$, and because the integral of $Z \exp(-Z^2/2)$ from 3.2 to infinity is less than .006, the upper limit can be replaced by 3.2 with less than .6 per cent error. Simpson's rule was used with subdivision points at $Z = 0$, .1, .2, .3, .4, .6, .8, 1.0, 1.2, 1.4, 1.6, 2.0, 2.4, 2.8, and 3.2, guaranteeing an error of less than .014 for a total bound on the error of .02.

Using these approximations, computations were performed for $M =$ 2, 3, 4, 8, 16, 32, 256, and 1000. For $M = 2$, $P(c)$ is the probability that the difference of two independent normal variables is greater than d', and hence is the normal curve, $P(c) = A(d'/\sqrt{2})$. These values as well as the computed values are plotted on probability paper in Fig. 4.

The curves of Fig. 4 are very nearly straight lines, and hence it is possible to represent the results empirically by the following formula:

$$P(c) = A(a_M d' - b_M) \tag{25}$$

where A is the (area) normal distribution function, a_M is determined from the slope of the computed $P(c)$ curves (and is plotted in Fig. 5), and b_M is chosen so that $P(c) = 1/M$ when $d' = 0$. Equation (25) is accurate to within 2 per cent for $M = 8$. For $M = 2$, $P(c)$ has the form of the normal distribution, and hence Equation (25) is exact, with $a_M = 1/\sqrt{2}$ and $b_M = 0$. It can be shown that as M approaches infinity $P(c)$ becomes normal again and a_M approaches 1.

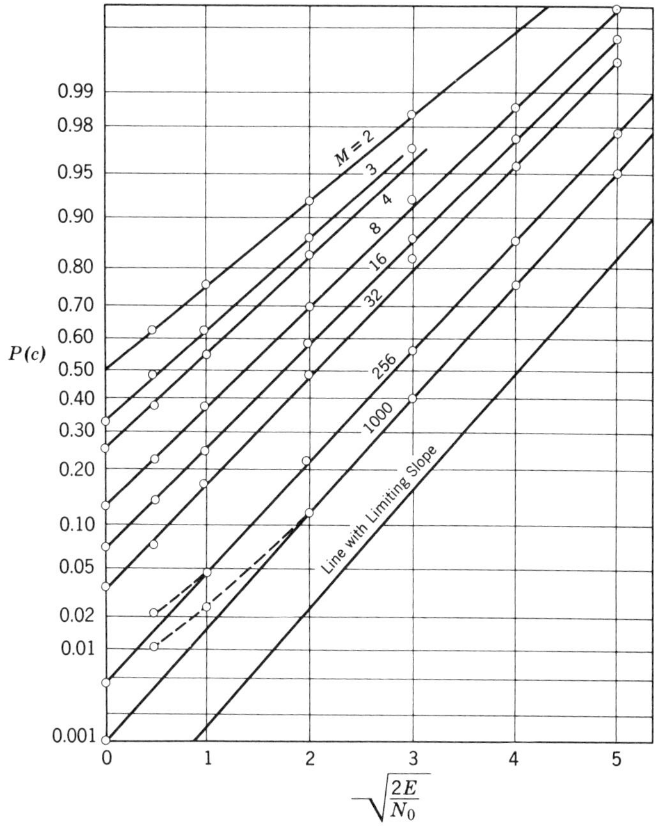

FIG. 4. Maximum probability of a correct forced choice among M orthogonal alternatives.

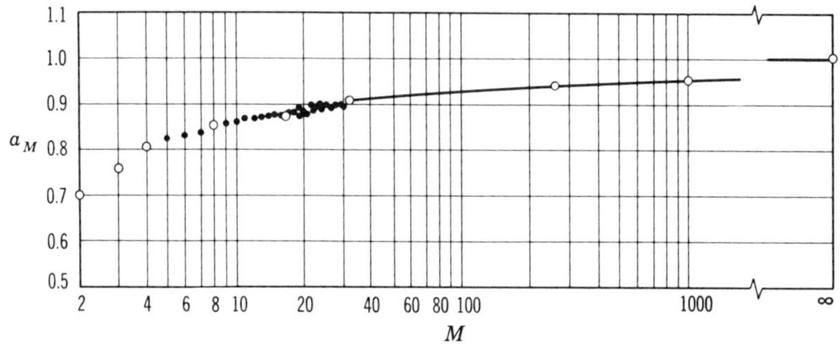

FIG. 5. The constant a_M for the approximation

$$P(c) = \frac{1}{\sqrt{2\pi}} \int_{-\infty}^{a_M d' - b_M} e^{-x^2/2}\, dx.$$

TABLE II. Values of d' for Forced Choice among M Orthogonal Alternatives

$P(c)$ \ M	2	4	8	16	32	256	1000
.01	−3.28	−1.99	−1.37	− .89	− .51	.37	.80
.02	−2.90	−1.66	−1.05	− .58	− .21	.66	1.08
.03	−2.66	−1.46	− .85	− .39	− .02	.85	1.26
.04	−2.48	−1.30	− .70	− .24	.13	.99	1.39
.05	−2.32	−1.17	− .57	− .12	.25	1.11	1.50
.06	−2.19	−1.06	− .47	− .02	.35	1.21	1.60
.07	−2.08	− .96	− .37	.07	.44	1.30	1.68
.08	−1.98	− .88	− .29	.15	.52	1.37	1.75
.09	−1.90	− .80	− .22	.22	.58	1.44	1.82
.10	−1.81	− .73	− .15	.29	.66	1.50	1.88
.11	−1.74	− .67	− .09	.34	.71	1.56	1.93
.12	−1.66	− .60	− .03	.41	.77	1.62	1.99
.13	−1.60	− .55	.02	.46	.82	1.67	2.03
.14	−1.53	− .49	.08	.51	.88	1.72	2.08
.15	−1.47	− .44	.13	.56	.92	1.77	2.13
.16	−1.40	− .38	.19	.62	.98	1.82	2.18
.17	−1.34	− .33	.23	.66	1.02	1.86	2.22
.18	−1.29	− .29	.27	.70	1.06	1.90	2.26
.19	−1.24	− .25	.32	.74	1.10	1.94	2.29
.20	−1.19	− .20	.36	.78	1.15	1.98	2.33
.21	−1.14	− .16	.40	.82	1.19	2.02	2.37
.22	−1.09	− .12	.44	.86	1.23	2.06	2.41
.23	−1.05	− .08	.48	.90	1.26	2.09	2.44
.24	−1.00	− .04	.52	.94	1.30	2.13	2.47
.25	− .95	0	.56	.97	1.33	2.16	2.50
.26	− .90	.04	.60	1.01	1.37	2.20	2.54
.27	− .86	.08	.63	1.04	1.41	2.24	2.57
.28	− .82	.11	.67	1.08	1.44	2.27	2.60
.29	− .78	.14	.70	1.11	1.47	2.30	2.63
.30	− .74	.18	.73	1.14	1.50	2.33	2.66
.31	− .71	.20	.75	1.16	1.52	2.35	2.68
.32	− .66	.25	.80	1.20	1.56	2.39	2.72
.33	− .62	.28	.83	1.24	1.60	2.42	2.75
.34	− .60	.32	.86	1.27	1.63	2.46	2.78
.35	− .54	.35	.89	1.30	1.66	2.48	2.81
.36	− .51	.38	.92	1.33	1.69	2.51	2.83
.37	− .47	.42	.96	1.36	1.72	2.54	2.86
.38	− .43	.45	.99	1.39	1.75	2.57	2.89
.39	− .40	.48	1.02	1.42	1.78	2.60	2.91
.40	− .36	.51	1.05	1.45	1.81	2.62	2.94
.41	− .32	.54	1.08	1.48	1.83	2.65	2.97
.42	− .28	.57	1.11	1.51	1.87	2.68	3.00
.43	− .25	.60	1.13	1.53	1.89	2.71	3.02
.44	− .21	.63	1.17	1.56	1.92	2.74	3.05
.45	− .18	.66	1.19	1.59	1.95	2.76	3.07
.46	− .14	.69	1.23	1.62	1.98	2.79	3.10
.47	− .11	.72	1.26	1.65	2.01	2.82	3.13
.48	− .07	.75	1.29	1.68	2.04	2.85	3.15
.49	− .04	.78	1.32	1.71	2.06	2.88	3.18
.50	0	.81	1.34	1.74	2.09	2.90	3.20

TABLE II. *(Continued)*

$P(c)$ \ M	2	4	8	16	32	256	1000
.51	.04	.84	1.37	1.76	2.12	2.93	3.23
.52	.07	.88	1.40	1.79	2.15	2.96	3.26
.53	.11	.90	1.43	1.82	2.18	2.98	3.28
.54	.14	.94	1.46	1.85	2.20	3.01	3.31
.55	.18	.97	1.50	1.88	2.24	3.04	3.34
.56	.21	1.00	1.52	1.90	2.26	3.07	3.36
.57	.25	1.03	1.56	1.94	2.30	3.10	3.39
.58	.28	1.06	1.58	1.96	2.32	3.12	3.41
.59	.32	1.09	1.61	2.00	2.35	3.15	3.44
.60	.36	1.12	1.64	2.02	2.38	3.18	3.47
.61	.40	1.15	1.67	2.05	2.41	3.21	3.50
.62	.43	1.18	1.70	2.08	2.44	3.24	3.52
.63	.47	1.21	1.73	2.11	2.46	3.26	3.55
.64	.51	1.25	1.77	2.14	2.50	3.30	3.58
.65	.54	1.28	1.80	2.17	2.52	3.32	3.60
.66	.60	1.31	1.82	2.20	2.55	3.35	3.63
.67	.62	1.35	1.86	2.23	2.59	3.38	3.66
.68	.66	1.38	1.89	2.27	2.62	3.42	3.69
.69	.71	1.42	1.94	2.31	2.66	3.45	3.73
.70	.74	1.45	1.96	2.33	2.68	3.48	3.75
.71	.78	1.49	1.99	2.36	2.74	3.51	3.78
.72	.82	1.52	2.02	2.39	2.77	3.54	3.81
.73	.86	1.55	2.06	2.42	2.78	3.57	3.84
.74	.90	1.59	2.09	2.46	2.81	3.60	3.87
.75	.95	1.63	2.13	2.50	2.85	3.64	3.90
.76	1.00	1.67	2.17	2.53	2.88	3.67	3.94
.77	1.05	1.71	2.21	2.57	2.92	3.71	3.97
.78	1.09	1.75	2.24	2.61	2.96	3.74	4.00
.79	1.14	1.79	2.29	2.64	2.98	3.78	4.04
.80	1.19	1.83	2.33	2.68	3.04	3.82	4.08
.81	1.24	1.88	2.37	2.73	3.08	3.86	4.12
.82	1.29	1.92	2.42	2.77	3.12	3.90	4.15
.83	1.34	1.96	2.46	2.81	3.16	3.94	4.19
.84	1.40	2.01	2.50	2.86	3.20	3.98	4.23
.85	1.47	2.07	2.56	2.91	3.26	4.04	4.28
.86	1.53	2.12	2.61	2.96	3.31	4.08	4.32
.87	1.60	2.18	2.67	3.01	3.36	4.14	4.38
.88	1.66	2.24	2.72	3.06	3.41	4.18	4.42
.89	1.74	2.30	2.78	3.13	3.48	4.24	4.48
.90	1.81	2.36	2.84	3.18	3.53	4.30	4.53
.91	1.90	2.44	2.91	3.25	3.60	4.36	4.60
.92	1.98	2.51	2.98	3.32	3.67	4.43	4.66
.93	2.08	2.59	3.06	3.40	3.74	4.51	4.73
.94	2.19	2.69	3.16	3.49	3.83	4.59	4.81
.95	2.32	2.80	3.26	3.59	3.94	4.69	4.91
.96	2.48	2.93	3.39	3.71	4.06	4.81	5.02
.97	2.66	3.09	3.54	3.86	4.20	4.96	5.16
.98	2.90	3.29	3.74	4.05	4.40	5.14	5.33
.99	3.28	3.62	4.06	4.36	4.70	5.44	5.61

ACKNOWLEDGMENTS

These tables and the accompanying discussion appeared in 1959 as Tech. Rept. No. 97 (and as Tech. Rept. No. AFCRC-TR-59-55) of the Electronic Defense Group of the University of Michigan. They were prepared with support from the Operational Applications Laboratory of the U. S. Air Force.

References

- Birdsall, T. G., and Peterson, W. W. Probability of a correct decision in a choice among *m* alternatives. University of Michigan: Electronic Defense Group, 1954, Quarterly Progress Report No. 10.
- Peterson, H. W., and Birdsall, T. G. The theory of signal detectability. University of Michigan: Electronic Defense Group, 1953, Technical Report No. 13.
- Tanner, W. P., Jr., and Birdsall, T. G. Definitions of d' and η as psychophysical measures. University of Michigan Research Institute: Electronic Defense Group, 1956, Technical Report No. 80. [See 5]

Appendix 2—Bibliography: Applications of Detection Theory in Psychophysics

A. Published Papers

1. Atkinson, R. C. A variable sensitivity theory of signal detection. *Psychol. Rev.*, 1963, **70**, 91–106.
2. Barlow, H. B. Retinal noise and the absolute threshold. *J. opt. Soc. Am.*, 1956, **46**, 634–639.
3. Carterette, E. C. Message repetition and receiver confirmation of messages in noise. *J. acoust. Soc. Am.*, 1958, **30**, 846–855.
4. Carterette, E. C., and Cole, M. Comparison of the receiver-operating characteristics received by ear and by eye. *J. acoust. Soc. Am.*, 1962, **34**, 172–178.
5. Clarke, F. R. Confidence ratings, second-choice responses and confusion matrices in intelligibility tests. *J. acoust. Soc. Am.*, 1960, **32**, 35–46.
6. Clarke, F. R., and Bilger, R. C. The theory of signal detectability and the measurement of hearing. In Jerger, J. F. (Ed.), *Modern developments in audiology*. New York: Academic Press, 1963.
7. Clarke, F. R., Birdsall, T. G., and Tanner, W. P., Jr. Two types of ROC curves and definitions of parameters. *J. acoust. Soc. Am.*, 1959, **31**, 629–630.
8. Creelman, C. D. Detection of signals of uncertain frequency. *J. acoust. Soc. Am.*, 1960, **32**, 805–810.
9. Creelman, C. D. Detection of complex signals as a function of signal bandwidth and duration. *J. acoust. Soc. Am.*, 1961, **33**, 89–94.
10. Creelman, C. D. Human discrimination of auditory duration. *J. acoust. Soc. Am.*, 1962, **34**, 582–593.
11. Decker, L. R., and Pollack, I. Confidence ratings and message reception for filtered speech. *J. acoust. Soc. Am.*, 1958, **30**, 432–434.
12. Decker, L. R., and Pollack, I. Multiple observers, message reception, and rating scales. *J. acoust. Soc. Am.*, 1959, **31**, 1327–1328.
13. Edwards, W. Behavioral decision theory. *Ann. Rev. Psychol.* Palo Alto: Annual Reviews, Inc., 1961, pp. 473–498.
14. Egan, J. P. Monitoring task in speech communication. *J. acoust. Soc. Am.*, 1957, **29**, 482–489.
15. Egan, J. P., and Clarke, F. R. Source and receiver behavior in the use of a criterion. *J. acoust. Soc. Am.*, 1956, **28**, 1267–1269.
16. Egan, J. P., and Clarke, F. R. Psychophysics and signal detection. In Sidowski, J. B. (Ed.), *Experimental methods and instrumentation in psychology*. New York: McGraw-Hill, 1963.
17. Egan, J. P., Clarke, F. R., and Carterette, E. C. On the transmission and confirmation of messages in noise. *J. acoust. Soc. Am.*, 1956, **28**, 536–550.
18. Egan, J. P., Greenberg, G. Z., and Schulman, A. I. Interval of the time uncertainty in auditory detection. *J. acoust. Soc. Am.*, 1961, **33**, 771–778.

19. Egan, J. P., Greenberg, G. Z., and Schulman, A. I. Operating characteristics, signal detectability and the method of free response. *J. acoust. Soc. Am.,* 1961, **33,** 993–1007.
20. Egan, J. P., Schulman, A. I., and Greenberg, G. Z. Operating characteristics determined by binary decisions and by ratings. *J. acoust. Soc. Am.,* 1959, **31,** 768–773.
21. Egan, J. P., Schulman, A. I., and Greenberg, G. Z. Memory for waveform and time uncertainty in auditory detection. *J. acoust. Soc. Am.,* 1961, **33,** 779–781.
22. Eijkman, E., and Vendrik, A. J. H. Detection theory applied to the absolute sensitivity of sensory systems. *Biophys. J.,* 1963, **3,** 65–77.
23. Eriksen, C. Discrimination and learning without awareness: A methodological survey and evaluation. *Psychol. Rev.,* 1960, **67,** 279–300.
24. Estes, W. K. Learning theory. *Ann Rev. Psychol.* Palo Alto: Annual Reviews, Inc., 1962, pp. 107–144.
25. Fairbanks, G., House, A. S., and Melrose, J. Auditory detection of the presence and absence of signals in noise. *J. acoust. Soc. Am.,* 1956, **28,** 614–616.
26. FitzHugh, R. The statistical detection of threshold signals in the retina. *J. gen. Physiol.,* 1957, **40,** 925–948.
27. Galanter, E. Contemporary psychophysics. In *New directions in psychology.* New York: Holt, Rinehart, and Winston, 1962, pp. 87–156.
28. Goldiamond, I. Indicators of perception: I. Subliminal perception, subception, unconscious perception: An analysis in terms of psychophysical indicator methodology. *Psychol. Bull.,* 1958, **55,** 373–411.
29. Goldiamond, I. Perception. In Bachrach, A. (Ed.), *The experimental foundations of clinical psychology.* New York: Basic Books, Inc., 1963.
30. Green, B. F., Wolf, A. K., and White, B. W. The detection of statistically defined patterns in a matrix of dots. *Am. J. Psychol.,* 1959, **72,** 503–520.
31. Green, D. M. Detection of multiple component signals in noise. *J. acoust. Soc. Am.,* 1958, **30,** 904–911.
32. Green, D. M. Auditory detection of a noise signal. *J. acoust. Soc. Am.,* 1960, **32,** 121–131.
33. Green, D. M. Psychoacoustics and detection theory. *J. acoust. Soc. Am.,* 1960, **32,** 1189–1203.
34. Green, D. M. Detection of auditory sinusoids of uncertain frequency. *J. acoust. Soc. Am.,* 1961, **33,** 897–903.
35. Green, D. M., Birdsall, T. G., and Tanner, W. P., Jr. Signal detection as a function of signal intensity and duration. *J. acoust. Soc. Am.,* 1957, **29,** 523–531.
36. Green, D. M., McKey, M. J., and Licklider, J. C. R. Detection of a pulsed sinusoid in noise as a function of frequency. *J. acoust. Soc. Am.,* 1959, **31,** 1446–1452.
37. Green, D. M., and Sewall, S. T. Effects of background noise on auditory detection of noise burst. *J. acoust. Soc. Am.,* 1962, **34,** 1207–1216.
38. Gundy, R. F. Auditory detection of an unspecified signal. *J. acoust. Soc. Am.,* 1961, **33,** 1008–1012.
39. Hack, M. H. Signal detection in the rat. *Science,* 1963, **139,** 758–759.
40. Hake, H. W. Perception. *Ann. Rev. Psychol.* Palo Alto: Annual Reviews, Inc., 1962, pp. 145–170.

41. Kuffler, S. W., FitzHugh, R., and Barlow, H. B. Maintained activity in the cat's retina in light and darkness. *J. gen. Physiol.*, 1957, **40,** 683–702.
42. Lee, W. Choosing among confusably distributed stimuli with specified likelihood ratios. *Percept. Motor Skills*, 1963, **16,** 445–467.
43. Licklider, J. C. R. Three auditory theories. In Koch, S. (Ed.), *Psychology: A study of a science,* Vol. 1. New York: McGraw-Hill, 1958.
44. Licklider, J. C. R., and Green, D. M. Aural detection of complex signals in random noise. *Proc. Third Int. Congr. on Acoust.*, 1960, pp. 114–118.
45. Luce, R. D. *Individual choice behavior.* New York: Wiley, 1959, pp 58–67.
46. Luce, R. D. A threshold theory for simple detection experiments. *Psychol. Rev.,* 1963, **70,** 61–79.
47. Lyon, R. H. On the prediction of forced-choice and phenomenal report thresholds by statistical detection theory. *J. acoust. Soc. Am.,* 1960, **32,** 508.
48. Mackworth, J. F. The effect of signal frequency on the detection of two kinds of signals. *Canad. J. Psychol.* (in press).
49. McGill, W. J. Stochastic latency mechanisms. In Bush, R. R., Galanter, E., and Luce, R. D. (Eds.), *Handbook of mathematical psychology,* Vol. I. New York: Wiley, 1963, pp. 309–360.
50. McPherson, R. R. Inapplicability of the threshold concept for the detection of signals in noise. *J. acoust. Soc. Am.*, 1957, **29,** 151.
51. McPherson, R. R. Auditory threshold. *J. acoust. Soc. Am.*, 1957, **29,** 393–394.
52. Munson, W. A., and Karlin, J. E. The measurement of the human channel transmission characteristics. *J. acoust. Soc. Am.,* 1956, **26,** 542–553.
53. Pollack, I. On indices of signal and response discriminability. *J. acoust. Soc. Am.*, 1959, **31,** 1031.
54. Pollack, I. Identification of elementary auditory displays and the method of recognition memory. *J. acoust. Soc. Am.,* 1959, **31,** 1126–1128.
55. Pollack, I. Message uncertainty and message reception. *J. acoust. Soc. Am.,* 1959, **31,** 1500–1508.
56. Pollack, I. Message repetition and message reception. *J. acoust. Soc. Am.*. 1959, **31,** 1509–1515.
57. Pollack, I. Hearing. *Ann. Rev. Psychol.* Palo Alto: Annual Reviews, Inc., 1961, pp. 335–362.
58. Pollack, I., and Decker, L. R. Confidence ratings, message reception, and the receiver operating characteristic. *J. acoust. Soc. Am.,* 1958, **30,** 286–292.
59. Restle, F. *Psychology of judgment and choice.* New York: Wiley, 1961, pp. 135–163.
60. Sherwin, C. W., Kodman, F., Jr., Kovaly, J. J., Prothe, W. C., and Melrose, J. Detection of signals in noise: A comparison between the human detector and an electronic detector. *J. acoust. Soc. Am.,* 1956, **28,** 417–422.
61. Shipley, E. F. A model for detection and recognition with signal uncertainty. *Psychometrika,* 1960, **25,** 273–289.
62. Shipley, E. F. Dependence of successive judgments in detection tasks: Correctness of response. *J. acoust. Soc. Am.,* 1961, **33,** 1142–1143.
63. Smith, M., and Wilson, E. A. A model for the auditory threshold and its application to the multiple observer. *Psychol. Monogr.,* 1953, **67,** No. 9, Whole No. 359.
64. Sorkin, R. D. Extension of the theory of signal detectability to matching procedures in psychoacoustics. *J. acoust. Soc. Am.,* 1962, **34,** 1745–1751.

65. Speeth, S. D., and Mathews, M. V. Sequential effects in the signal-detection situation. *J. acoust. Soc. Am.,* 1961, **33,** 1046–1054.

66. Swets, J. A. Indices of signal detectability obtained with various psychophysical procedures. *J. acoust. Soc. Am.,* 1959, **31,** 511–513.

67. Swets, J. A. Detection theory and psychophysics: A review. *Psychometrika,* 1961, **26,** 49–63.

68. Swets, J. A. Is there a sensory threshold? *Science,* 1961, **134,** 168–177.

69. Swets, J. A. Central factors in auditory frequency selectivity. *Psychol. Bull.,* 1963, **60,** 429–440.

70. Swets, J. A., and Birdsall, T. G. The human use of information: III. Decision making in signal detection and recognition situations involving multiple alternatives. *Trans. IRE Information Theory,* 1956, **IT-2,** 138–165.

71. Swets, J. A., and Green, D. M. Sequential observations by human observers of signals in noise. In Cherry, C. (Ed.), *Information theory.* London: Butterworths, 1961.

72. Swets, J. A., Green. D. M., and Tanner, W. P., Jr. On the width of critical bands. *J. acoust. Soc. Am.,* 1962, **34,** 108–113.

73. Swets, J. A., Millman, S. H., Fletcher, W. E., and Green, D. M. Learning to identify nonverbal sounds: An application of a computer as a teaching machine. *J. acoust. Soc. Am.,* 1962, **34,** 928–935.

74. Swets, J. A., and Sewall, S. T. Stimulus versus response uncertainty in recognition. *J. acoust. Soc. Am.,* 1961, **33,** 1586–1592.

75. Swets, J. A. and Sewall, S. T. The invariance of signal detectability over stages of practice and levels of motivation. *J. exp. Psychol.,* 1963, **66,** 120–126.

76. Swets, J. A., Shipley, E. F., McKey, M. J., and Green, D. M. Multiple observations of signals in noise. *J. acoust. Soc. Am.,* 1959, **31,** 514–521.

77. Swets, J. A., Tanner, W. P., Jr., and Birdsall, T. G. Decision processes in perception. *Psychol. Rev.,* 1961, **68,** 301–340.

78. Tanner, W. P., Jr. On the design of psychophysical experiments. In Quastler, H. (Ed.), *Information theory in psychology.* Glencoe, Ill.: Free Press, 1954.

79. Tanner, W. P., Jr. Theory of recognition. *J. acoust. Soc. Am.,* 1956, **28,** 882–888.

80. Tanner, W. P., Jr. What is masking? *J. acoust. Soc. Am.,* 1958, **30,** 919–921.

81. Tanner, W. P., Jr. Graphical presentation of data in the framework of the theory of signal detectability. *J. acoust. Soc. Am.,* 1959, **31,** 243–244.

82. Tanner, W. P., Jr. Theory of signal detectability as an interpretive tool for psychophysical data. *J. acoust. Soc. Am.,* 1960, **32,** 1140–1147.

83. Tanner, W. P., Jr. Application of the theory of signal detectability to amplitude discrimination. *J. acoust. Soc. Am.,* 1961, **33,** 1233–1244.

84. Tanner, W. P., Jr. Physiological implications of psychophysical data. *Ann. N. Y. Acad. Sci.,* 1961, **89,** 752–765.

85. Tanner, W. P., Jr., and Birdsall, T. G. Definitions of d' and η as psychophysical measures. *J. acoust. Soc. Am.,* 1958, **30,** 922–928.

86. Tanner, W. P., Jr., and Norman, R. The human use of information: II. Signal detection for the case of an unknown signal parameter. *Trans. IRE Professional Group on Information Theory,* 1954, **PGIT-4,** 222–227.

87. Tanner, W. P., Jr., and Swets, J. A. A decision-making theory of visual detection. *Psychol. Rev.,* 1954, **61,** 401–409.

88. Tanner, W. P., Jr., and Swets, J. A. The human use of information: I. Signal detection for the case of the signal known exactly. *Trans. IRE Professional Group on Information Theory,* 1954, **PGIT-4,** 213–221.

89. Taylor, M. M. Figural after-effects: A psychophysical theory of the displacement effect. *Canad. J. Psychol.,* 1962, **16,** 247–277.

90. Taylor, M. M. The geometry of a visual illusion. *J. opt. Soc. Am.,* 1962, **52,** 565–569.

91. Torgerson, W. S. Scaling and test theory. *Ann. Rev. Psychol.* Palo Alto: Annual Reviews, Inc., 1961, pp. 51–70.

92. Veniar, F. A. Effect of auditory cue on discrimination of auditory stimuli. *J. acoust. Soc. Am.,* 1958, **30,** 1079–1081.

93. Veniar, F. A. Signal detection as a function of frequency ensemble, I. *J. acoust. Soc. Am.,* 1958, **30,** 1020–1024.

94. Veniar, F. A. Signal detection as a function of frequency ensemble, II. *J. acoust. Soc. Am.,* 1958, **30,** 1075–1078.

95. Voelcker, H. B. A decision-theory approach to sound lateralization. In Cherry, C. (Ed.), *Information theory.* London: Butterworths, 1961.

96. Weintraub, D. J., and Hake, H. W. Visual discrimination, an interpretation in terms of detectability theory. *J. opt. Soc. Am.,* 1962, **52,** 1179–1184.

*B. Unpublished Papers**

97. Atkinson, R. C. A variable sensitivity theory of signal detection. Stanford University: Applied Mathematics and Statistics Laboratories, 1962. [Technical Report No. 47]

98. Atkinson, R. C., Carterette, E. C., and Kinchla, R. A. Sequential phenomena in psychophysical judgments: A theoretical analysis. Stanford University: Applied Mathematics and Statistics Laboratories, 1962. [Technical Report No. 46]

99. Bilger, R. C. Laboratory facilities employed in psychophysical memory experiments. University of Michigan: Electronic Defense Group, 1959. [Technical Memorandum No. 72]

100. Carterette, E. C., and Cole, M. A comparison of the receiver operating characteristic for messages received by ear and by eye. University of California at Los Angeles: Department of Psychology, 1959. [Technical Report No. 2]

101. Carterette, E. C., and Cole, M. Repetition and confirmation of messages received by ear and by eye. University of California at Los Angeles: Department of Psychology, 1959. [Technical Report No. 3]

102. Clarke, F. R. The theory of signal detectability. In *Signal detection and psychophysics.* University of Michigan Engineering Summer Conferences, 1960.

103. Creelman, C. D. Detection of signals of uncertain frequency. University of Michigan: Electronic Defense Group, 1959. [Technical Memorandum No. 71]

* This section of the bibliography contains all technical reports printed as separates, including those later published as journal articles, doctoral dissertations, and printed meeting papers.

104. Creelman, C. D. The effects of signal duration and bandwidth on detection of complex signals. University of Michigan: Electronic Defense Group, 1959. [Technical Report No. 99]

105. Creelman, C. D. Applications of signal detectability theory to psychophysical research: A bibliography. University of Michigan: Electronic Defense Group, 1960. [Technical Memorandum No. 79]

106. Creelman, C. D. Human discrimination of auditory duration. Doctoral dissertation, University of Michigan, 1960.

107. Creelman, C. D. Human discrimination of auditory duration. University of Michigan: Cooley Electronic Laboratory, 1960. [Technical Report No. 114]

108. Cron, B. F., and Martin, R. L. Statistical-decision observer tests. New London, Conn.: U. S. Navy Underwater Sound Laboratoy, Fort Trumbull, 1958. [USL Research Report No. 400, NE–051600–22A]

109. Egan, J. P. Message repetition, operating characteristics, and confusion matrices in speech communication. Indiana University: Hearing and Communciation Laboratory, 1957. [Technical Report No. AFCRC–TR–57–50]

110. Egan, J. P. Recognition memory and the operating characteristic. Indiana University: Hearing and Communication Laboratory, 1958. [Technical Note AFCRC–TN–58–51]

111. Egan, J. P., Clarke, F. R., and Carterette, E. C. On a theory of the transmission and confirmation of messages in noise. Indiana University: Hearing and Communication Laboratory, 1955. [Technical Note AFCRC–TN–55–67]

112. Egan, J. P., Greenberg, G. Z., and Schulman, A. I. Operating characteristics, signal detectability, and the method of free response. Indiana University: Hearing and Communication Laboratory, 1959. [Technical Report No. AFCRC–TR–59–58]

113. Eijkman, E. G. J. Adaptation of the senses of temperature and touch. Doctoral dissertation, R. C. University, Nijmegen, the Netherlands, 1959.

114. Elliott, P. B. Tables of *d'*. University of Michigan: Electronic Defense Group, 1959. [Technical Report No. 97]

115. Green, D. M. Detection of complex auditory signals in noise. Doctoral dissertation, University of Michigan, 1958.

116. Green, D. M. Detection of signals in noise and the critical band concept. University of Michigan: Electronic Defense Group, 1958. [Technical Report No. 82]

117. Green, D. M., and Birdsall, T. G. The effect of vocabulary size on articulation scores. University of Michigan: Electronic Defense Group, 1958. [Technical Memorandum No. 81]

118. Green, D. M., Birdsall, T. G., and Tanner, W. P., Jr. Signal detection as a function of signal intensity and duration. University of Michigan: Electronic Defense Group, 1957. [Technical Report No. 42]

119. Greenberg, G. Z. Cueing signals and frequency uncertainty in auditory detection. Indiana University: Hearing and Communication Laboratory, 1962. [Technical Report No. ESD–TDR–6238]

120. Licklider, J. C. R. Studies in aural presentation of information. Massachusetts Institute of Technology: Research Laboratory of Electronics, 1957. [Technical Report No. AFCRC–TR–58–53]

121. Marill, T. Detection theory and psychophysics. Massachusetts Institute of Technology: Research Laboratory of Electronics, 1956. [Technical Report No. 319]

122. Swets, J. A. An experimental comparison of two theories of visual detection. Doctoral dissertation, University of Michigan, 1954.

123. Swets, J. A., Tanner, W. P., Jr., and Birdsall, T. G. The evidence for a decision-making theory of visual detection. University of Michigan: Electronic Defense Group, 1955. [Technical Report No. 40]

124. Tanner, W. P., Jr. Visual detection when location is not known exactly. In Proceedings of the Armed-Forces-NRC Vision Committee, held at Toronto, Ontario, Canada, November, 1954.

125. Tanner, W. P., Jr. Theory of recognition. University of Michigan: Electronic Defense Group, 1955. [Technical Report No. 50]

126. Tanner, W. P., Jr. Information theory and form discrimination. In Wulfeck, J. W., and Taylor, J. H. (Eds.), *Form discrimination as related to military problems.* Proceedings of Armed-Forces-NRC Vision Committee Symposium, 1957, Publication 561, National Academy of Sciences, National Research Council, Washington, D. C.

127. Tanner, W. P., Jr. A re-evaluation of Weber's law as applied to pure tones. University of Michigan: Electronic Defense Group, 1958. [Technical Report No. 47]

128. Tanner, W. P., Jr. What is masking? University of Michigan: Electronic Defense Group, 1958. [Technical Memorandum No. 52]

129. Tanner, W. P., Jr. Application of the theory of signal detectability to amplitude discrimination. Doctoral dissertation, University of Michigan, 1959.

130. Tanner, W. P., Jr. The theory of signal detectability as an interpretive tool for psychophysical data. University of Michigan: Electronic Defense Group, 1960. [Technical Memorandum No. 78]

131. Tanner, W. P., Jr. Mathematical models in sensory perception. In Proceedings of Bionics Symposium. Dayton, Ohio: Wright Air Development Division, 1960. [Technical Report No. 60-600]

132. Tanner, W. P., Jr., and Birdsall, T. G. Definitions of d' and η as psychophysical measures. University of Michigan: Electronic Defense Group, 1958. [Technical Report No. 80]

133. Tanner, W. P., Jr., Clarke, F. R., and Birdsall, T. G. The concept of the ideal observer in psychophysics. University of Michigan: Electronic Defense Group, 1960. [Technical Report No. 98]

134. Tanner, W. P., Jr., and Jones, R. C. The ideal sensor system as approached through statistical decision theory and the theory of signal detectability. In Proceedings of the Armed-Forces-NRC Vision Committee, held at Washington, D. C., November, 1959.

135. Tanner, W. P., Jr., and Swets, J. A. A new theory of visual detection. University of Michigan: Electronic Defense Group, 1953. [Technical Report No. 18]

136. Tanner, W. P., Jr., and Swets, J. A. Psychophysical application of the theory of signal detectability. University of Michigan: Electronic Defense Group, 1954. [Report No. 1950-5-S] (Reprinted from Proceedings of Armed-Forces-NRC Vision Committee, held at Fort Knox, Kentucky, November, 1953)

137. Tanner, W. P., Jr., Swets, J. A., and Green, D. M. Some general properties of the hearing mechanism. University of Michigan: Electronic Defense Group, 1956. [Technical Report No. 30]

138. Veniar, F. A. Signal detection as a function of frequency ensemble. University of Michigan: Electronic Defense Group, 1958. [Technical Report No. 86]

Topical Bibliography (1967–1988)

ALTERNATIVE THEORIES

Auerbach, C., and Leventhal, G. Evidence for all-or-none preperceptual processing in perceptual set. *Perception and Psychophysics,* 14, 24–30, 1973.

Baron, J. Perceptual dependence: Evidence for an internal threshold. *Perception and Psychophysics,* 13, 527–533, 1973.

Bamber, D. State-trace analysis: A method of testing simple theories of causation. *Journal of Mathematical Psychology,* 19, (2), 137–181, 1979.

Bartosiewicz, Z., and Falkowski, M. Some corrections of concept of ROC-curve in TSD. Unpublished paper, 1981.

Broadbent, D. E. The two-state threshold model, and rating scale experiments. *Journal of the Acoustical Society of America,* 40, 244, 1966.

Collyer, C. E. Applications of signal detection theory: Can we separate sensory and judgmental aspects of performance? Unpublished paper. University of Rhode Island, 1978.

Doherty, M. E., and Keeley, S. M. A Bayesian prediction of four-look recognition performance from one-look data. *Perception and Psychophysics,* 5, 362–364, 1969.

Dorfman, D. D. Probability matching in signal detection. *Psychonomic Science,* 17, 103, 1969.

Emerson, P. L. Measurement of low-signal suppression and other parameters of the forced-choice psychometric function. *Perception and Psychophysics,* 5, 2–6, 1969.

Green, D. M., and Luce, R. D. Detection of auditory signals presented at random times. *Perception and Psychophysics,* 2, 441–450, 1967.

Green, D. M., and Luce, R. D. Detection of auditory signals presented at random times: III. *Perception and Psychophysics,* 9, 257–268, 1971.

Keeley, S. M., Doherty, M. E., and Bachman, S. P. A Bayesian prediction of four-look recognition performance from one-look data: II. *Perception and Psychophysics,* 7, 218–220, 1970.

Krantz, D. H. Threshold theories of signal detection. *Psychological Review,* 76, 308–324, 1969.

Kubovy, M., Rapoport, A., and Tversky, A. Deterministic vs probabilistic strategies in detection. *Perception and Psychophysics,* 9, 427–429, 1971.

Kubovy, M., and Healy, A. F. Process models of probabilistic categorization. In *Cognitive Processes in Choice and Decision Behavior.,* T. S. Wallsten (ed.), Hillsdale, New Jersey: Lawrence Erlbaum, 1979.

Lee, W. Detection theory, micromatching, and the constant-ratio rule. *Perception and Psychophysics,* 4, 217–219, 1968.

Lee, W., and Janke, M. Categorizing externally distributed stimulus samples for three continua. *Journal of Experimental Psychology*, 68, 376–382, 1964.

Lee, W., and Zentall, T. R. Factorial effects in the categorization of externally distributed stimulus samples. *Perception and Psychophysics*, 1, 120–124, 1966.

Luce, R. D., and Green, D. M. Detection of auditory signals presented at random times, II. *Perception and Psychophysics*, 7, 1–14, 1970.

Massaro, D. W. The role of the decision system in sensory and memory experiments using confidence judgments. *Perception and Psychophysics*, 5, 270–272, 1969.

Meudell, P. R. Two-state threshold theory and the multiple-look k-alternative forced-choice experiment. *Journal of the Acoustical Society of America*, 44, 1139–1140, 1968.

Munsinger, H., and Gummerman, K. Simultaneous visual detection and recognition. *Perception and Psychophysics*, 3, 383–386, 1968.

Norman, D. A. Neural quantum controversy in sensory psychology. *Science*, 181, 467–469, 1973.

Parducci, A., and Sandusky, A. J. Limits on the applicability of signal detection theories. *Perception and Psychophysics*, 7, 63–64, 1970.

Tanner, T. A., Jr., Haller, R. W., and Atkinson, R. C. Signal recognition as influenced by presentation schedules. *Perception and Psychophysics*, 2, 349–358, 1967.

Thomas, E. A. C., and Legge, D. Probability matching as a basis for detection and recognition decision. *Psychological Review*, 77, 65–72, 1970.

Thomas, E. A. C. Criterion adjustment and probability matching *Perception and Psychophysics, 18*, (2), 158–162, 1975.

Wender, K. F. Signal identification: The comparison of two competitive theories. *Perception and Psychophysics, 18*, (4), 250–254, 1975.

Wickelgren, W. A. A test of Luce's two-state decision rule. *Psychonomic Science*, 9, 91–92, 1967.

Wickelgren, W. A. Testing two-state theories with operating characteristics and a posteriori probabilities. *Psychological Bulletin*, 69, 126–131, 1968.

Yellott, J. I., Jr. Correction for fast guessing and the speed-accuracy tradeoff in choice reaction time. *Journal of Mathematical Psychology*, 8, 159–199, 1971.

ANIMAL OBSERVERS

Au, W. W. L., and Penner, R. H. Target detection in noise by echolocating Atlantic bottlenose dolphins. *Journal of the Acoustical Society of America*, 70, (3), 687–693, 1981.

Blough, D. S. Stimulus generalization as signal detection in pigeons. *Science*, 1958, 940–941, 1967.

Boneau, C. A., and Cole, J. L. Decision theory, the pigeon, and the psychophysical function. *Psychological Review*, 74, 123–135, 1967.

Clopton, B. M. Detection of increments in noise intensity by monkeys. *Journal of the Experimental Analysis of Behavior*, 17, 473–481, 1972.

Coltheart, M., and Irvine, D. The slope of ROCs in the rat. *Journal of Auditory Research*, 8, 167–170, 1968.

Dykstra, L. A., and Appel, J. B. Effects of LSD on auditory percpetion: A signal detection approach. *Psychopharmocologia*, 34, 289–307, 1974.

Eijkman, E. G. Learning and fluctuating behavior experiments with goldfish. *Journal of Theoretical Biology*, 26, 251–264, 1970.

Elsmore, T. F. Duration discrimination: effects of probability of stimulus presentation. *Journal of the Experimental Analysis of Behavior*, 18, 465–469, 1972.

Grilly, D. M., and Genovese, R. F. Assessment of shock discrimination in rats with signal detection theory. *Perception and Psychophysics*, 25, (6), 466–472, 1979.

Heinemann, E. G., and Avin, E. On the development of stimulus control. *Journal of the Experimental Analysis of Behavior*, 20, (2), 183–195, 1973.

Heinemann, E. G., Avin, E., Sullivan, M. A., and Chase, S. Analysis of stimulus generalization with a psychophysical method. *Journal of Experimental Psychology*, 80, (2), 215–224, 1969.

Hobson, S. L. Discriminability of fixed-ratio schedules for pigeons: Effects of absolute ratio size. *Journal of the Experimental Analysis of Behavior*, (23), (1), 25–35, 1975.

Hobson, S. L. Discriminability of fixed-ratio schedules for pigeons: Effects of payoff values. *Journal of the Experimental Analysis of Behavior*, 30, (1), 69–81, 1978.

Hodos, W., and Bonbright, J. S., Jr. The detection of visual intensity differences by pigeons. *Journal of the Experimental Analysis of Behavior*, 18, 471–479, 1972.

Irwin, R. J., and Terman, M. Detection of brief tones in noise by rates. *Journal of the Experimental Analysis of Behavior*, 13, 135–143, 1970.

Killeen, P. R. Superstition: A matter of bias, not detectability. *Science*, 199, 88–90, 1978.

Kinchla, J. Discrimination of two auditory durations by pigeons. *Perception and Psychophysics*, 8, 299–307, 1970.

Morrison, G., and Norrison, W. Taste detection in the rat. *Canadian Journal of Psychology*, 20, 208–217, 1966.

Nevin, J. A. On the form of the relation between response rates in a multiple schedule. *Journal of the Experimental Analysis of Behavior*, 21, (2), 237–248, 1974.

Nevin, J. A., Olson, K., Mandell, C., and Yarensky, P. Differential reinforcement and signal detection. *Journal of the Experimental Analysis of Behavior*, 24, (3), 355–367, 1975.

Nevin, J. A. On differential stimulation and differential reinforcement. In *Animal Psychophysics*, W. C. Stebbins (Ed.), Appleton-Century-Crofts, New York, 401–427, 1970.

Schusterman, R. J. California sea lion underwater auditory detection and variation of reinforcement schedules. *Journal of the Acoustical Society of America*, 59, (4), 997–1000, 1976.

Schusterman, R. J. Low false-alarm rates in signal detection by marine mammals. *Journal of the Acoustical Society of America*, 55, (4), 845–858, 1974.

Schusterman, R. J., and Barrett, B. Detection of underwater signals by a California sea lion and a bottlenose porpoise: Variation in the payoff matrix. *Journal of the Acoustical Society of America*, 57, (6), 1526–1532, 1975.

Terman, M. Discrimination of auditory intensities by rats. *Journal of the Experimental Analysis of Behavior*, 13, 145–160, 1970.

Terman, M., and Terman, J. S. Concurrent variation of response and sensitivity in an operant-psychophysical test. *Perception and Psychophysics*, 11, 428–432, 1972.

Treisman, M. Predation and the evolution of gregariousness. I. Models for concealment and evasion. *Animal Behavior*, 23, 779–800, 1975.

Wright, A. A. Psychometric and psychophysical theory within a framework of response bias. *Psychological Review*, 81, (4), 322–347, 1974.

Wright A. A. Psychometric and psychophysical hue discrimination functions for the pigeon. *Vision Research*, 12, 1447–1464, 1972.

Yager, D., and Duncan, I. Signal-detection analysis of luminance generalization in goldfish using latency as a graded response measure. *Perception and Psychophysics*, 9, 353–355, 1971.

ATTENTION

Ahroon, W. A., Jr., Pastore, R. E., and Woltz, J. P. Selective attention. I. Two-channel simultaneous frequency difference limen. *Journal of the Acoustical Society of America*, 61, (3), 811–815, 1977.

Ball, K., and Sekuler, R. Adaptive processing of visual motion. *Journal of Experimental Psychology: Human Perception and Performance*, 7, (4), 780–794, 1981.

Ball, K., and Sekuler, R. Cues reduce direction uncertainty and enhance motion detection. *Perception and Psychophysics*, 30, (2), 119–128, 1981.

Ball, K., and Sekuler, R. Masking of motion by broadband and filtered directional noise. *Perception and Psychophysics*, 26, (3), 206–214, 1979.

Ball, K., and Sekuler, R. Models of stimulus uncertainty in motion perception. *Psychological Review*, 80, (5), 435–469, 1980.

Baron, J. Division of attention in successiveness discrimination. In *Attention and Performance IV*, S. Kornblum (Ed.), Academic Press, New York, 703–711, 1973.

Bashinski, H. S., and Bacharach, V. R. Enhancement of perceptual sensitivity as the result of selectively attending to spatial locations. *Perception and Psychophysics*, 28, (3), 241–248, 1980.

Clement, D. E., and Hosking, K. E. Scanning strategies and differential sensitivity in a visual signal detection task: Intrasubject reliability. *Psychonomic Science*, 22, (6), 323–324, 1971.

Cohn, T. E., Lasley, D. J. Detectability of a luminance increment: Effect of spatial uncertainty. *Journal of the Optical Society of America*, 64, 12, 1715–1719, 1974.

Davis, E. T. Allocation of attention: Uncertainty effects when monitoring one or two visual gratings of noncontiguous spatial frequencies. *Perception and Psychophysics*, 29, (6), 618–622, 1981.

Davis, E. T., and Graham, N. Spatial frequency uncertainty effects in the detection of sinusoidal gratings. *Vision Research*, 21, 705–712, 1980.

Davis, E. T., Kramer, P., and Graham, N. Uncertainty about spatial frequency, spatial position, or contrast of visual patterns. *Perception and Psychophysics*, 33, (1), 20–28, 1983.

Duncan, J. The locus of interference in the perception of simultaneous stimuli. *Psychological Review*, 87, (3), 272–300, 1980.

Eijkman, E., and Vendrik, A. J. H. Can a sensory system be specified by its internal noise? *Journal of the Acoustical Society of America*, 37, (6), 1102–1109, 1965.

Eriksen, C. W., and Spencer, T. Rate of information processing in visual perception: Some results and methodological considerations. *Journal of Experimental Psychology Monograph*, 79, (2), 1–16, 1969.

Forbes, S. M., Taylor, M. M., and Lindsay, P. H. Cue timing in a multi-dimensional detection task. *Perceptual and Motor Skills*, 25, 113–120, 1967.

Franzén, O., Markowitz, J., and Swets, J. A. Spatially-limited attention to vibrotactile stimulation. *Perception and Psychophysics*, 7, 193–196, 1970.

Gardner, G. T. Evidence for independent parallel channels in tachistoscopic perception. *Cognitive Psychology*, 4, 130–155, 1973.

Gilliom, J. D., and Mills, W. M. Information extraction from contralateral cues in the detection of signals of uncertain frequency. *Journal of the Acoustical Society of America*, 59, (6), 1428–1433, 1976.

Gilliom, J. D., and Sorkin, R. D. Sequential vs simultaneous two-channel signal detection: More evidence for a high-level interrupt theory. *Journal of the Acoustical Society of America,* 56, (1), 157–164, 1974.

Green, D. M., and Weber, D. L. Detection of temporally uncertain signals. *Journal of the Acoustical Society of America,* 67, (4), 1304–1311, 1980.

Greenberg, G. Z. Frequency-selective detection at three signal amplitudes. *Perception and Psychophysics,* 6, 297–301, 1969.

Greenberg, G. Z. Frequency selectivity during amplitude discrimination of signals in noise. *Journal of the Acoustical Society of America,* 45, 1438–1442, 1969.

Greenberg, G. Z., and Larkin, W. D. Frequency response characteristic of auditory observers detecting signals of a signal frequency in noise: The probe-signal method. *Journal of the Acoustical Society of America,* 44, 1513–1523, 1968.

Greenhouse, D. S., and Cohn, T. E. Effect of chromatic uncertainty on detectability of a visual stimulus. *Journal of the Optical Society of America,* 68, (2), 266–267, 1978.

Hoffman, J. E. A two-stage model of visual search. *Perception and Psychophysics, 25,* (4), 319–327, 1979.

Hoffman, J. Search through a sequentially presented visual display. *Perception and Psychophysics,* 23, (1), 1–11, 1978.

Howard, J. H., Jr., O'Toole, A. J., Parasuraman, R., and Bennett, K. B. Pattern-directed attention in uncertain-frequency detection. *Perception and Psychophysics,* 35, (3), 256–264, 1984.

Johnson, D. M., and Hafter, E. R. Uncertain-frequency detection: Cueing and condition of observation. *Perception and Psychophysics,* 28, (2), 143–149, 1980.

Kinchla, R. A. Detecting target elements in multielement arrays: A confusability model. *Perception and Psychophysics,* 15, (1), 149–158, 1974.

Kinchla, R. A. "Figure-ground" processing in vision: An organizational operating characteristic. Princeton University Research Report Series, Report No. 22, 1978.

Kinchla, R. A. The measurement of attention. In R. S. Nickerson (ed.), *Attention and Performance VIII.* Hillsdale, New Jersey: Lawrence Erlbaum Associates, 213–237, 1980.

Kinchla, R. A. The role of structural redundancy in the perception of visual targets. *Perception and Psychophysics,* 22, (1), 19–30, 1977.

Kinchla, R. A., and Collyer, C. E. Detecting a target letter in briefly presented arrays: A confidence rating analysis in terms of a weighted additive effects model. *Perception and Psychophysics,* 16, (1), 117–122, 1974.

Kinchla, R. A., and Solis-Macias, V. Attending to different levels of structure in a visual image. *Perception and Psychophysics,* 33, (1), 1–10, 1983.

Kinchla, R. A. Temporal and channel uncertainty in detection: A multiple-observation analysis. *Perception and Psychophysics,* 5, 129–136, 1969.

Kinchla, R. A. An attention operating characteristic in vision. Technical Report No. 29, Department of Psychology, McMaster University, Hamilton, Ontario, 1969.

Kleiss, J. A., and Lane, D. M. Locus and persistence of capacity limitations in visual information processing. *Journal of Experimental Psychology: Human Perception and Performance,* 12, (2), 200–210, 1986.

Kristofferson, A. B., and Allan, L. G. Successiveness and duration discrimination. Technical Report No. 45, Department of Psychology, McMaster University, Hamilton, Ontario, 1971.

Lack, L. C. Selective attention and the control of binocular rivalry. *Perception and Psychophysics,* 15, (1), 193–200, 1974.

Lindsay, P. H., Taylor, M. M., and Forbes, S. M. Attention and multidimensional discrimination. *Perception and Psychophysics*, 4, 113–117, 1968.

Long, J. Division of attention between non-verbal signals: All-or-none or shared processing? *Quarterly Journal of Experimental Psychology*, 28, 47–69, 1976.

Long, J. Reduced efficiency and capacity limitations in multi-dimension signal recognition. *Quarterly Journal of Experimental Psychology*, 27, 599–614, 1975.

Luce, R. D., and Green, D. M. Two tests of a neural attention hypothesis for auditory psychophysics. *Perception and Psychophysics*, 23, (5), 363–371, 1978.

Lupker, S. J., and Massaro, D. W. Selective perception without confounding contributions of decision and memory. *Perception and Psychophysics*, 25, (1), 60–69, 1979.

Macmillan, N. A., and Schwartz, M. A probe-signal investigation of uncertain-frequency detection. *Journal of the Acoustical Society of America*, 58, (5), 1051–1058, 1975.

Moray, N. Attention, control, and sampling behavior. Presented at NATO Conference on "Monitoring Behavior and Supervisory Control," Berchtesgaden, (F. R.) Germany, March 8–12, 160–182, 1976.

Moray, N., Fitter, M., Ostry, D., Favreau, D., and Nagy, V. Attention to pure tones. *Quarterly Journal of Experimental Psychology*, 28, 271–283, 1976.

Moray, B. Time sharing in auditory perception: Effect of stimulus duration. *Journal of the Acoustical Society of America*, 47, 660–661, 1970.

Moray, N., and Fitter, M. A theory and the measurement of attention: tutorial review. In *Attention and Performance IV*, S. Kornblum (Ed.), Academic Press, New York, 3–19, 1973.

Moray, N., and O'Brien, T. Signal-detection theory applied to selective listening. *Journal of the Acoustical Society of America*, 42, 765–772, 1967.

Muller, N. J., and Findlay, J. M. Sensitivity and criterion effects in the spatial cuing of visual attention. *Perception and Psychophysics*, 42, (4), 383–399, 1987.

Navon, D. Resources—A theoretical soup stone? *Psychological Review*, 91, (2), 216–234, 1984.

Nosofsky, R. M. Shifts of attention in the identification and discrimination of intensity. *Perception and Psychophysics*, 33, (2), 103–112, 1983.

Nuechterlein, K. H., Parasuraman, R., and Jiang Q. Visual sustained attention: Image degradation produces rapid sensitivity decrement over time. *Science*, 220, 327–329, 1983.

Ostry, D., Moray, N., and Marks, G. Attention, practice, and semantic targets. *Journal of Experimental Psychology: Human Perception and Performance*, 2, (3), 326–336, 1976.

Pastore, R. E., and Sorkin, R. D. Adaptive auditory signal processing. *Psychonomic Science*, 58, (5), 1051–1058, 1971.

Pastore, R. E., and Sorkin, R. D. Simultaneous two-channel signal detection. I. Simple binaural stimuli. *Journal of the Acoustical Society of America*, 51, 544–551, 1972.

Patterson, R. D. Auditory filter shape. *Journal of the Acoustical Society of America*, 55, (4), 802–809, 1974.

Patterson, R. D. Auditory filter shapes derived with noise stimuli. *Journal of the Acoustical Society of America*, 59, (3), 640–654, 1976.

Patterson, R. D., and Henning, G. B. Stimulus variability and auditory filter shape. *Journal of the Acoustical Society of America*, 62, (3), 649–664, 1977.

Pohlman, L. D., and Sorkin, R. D. Simultaneous three-channel signal detection: Performance and criterion as a function of order of report. *Perception and Psychophysics,* 20, (3), 179–186, 1976.

Posner, M. I., Snyder, C. R. R., and Davidson, B. J. Attention and the detection of signals. *Journal of Experimental Psychology: General,* 109, (2), 160–174, 1980.

Puleo, J. S., and Pastore, R. E. Critical-band effects in two-channel auditory signal detection. *Journal of Experimental Psychology: Human Perception and Performance,* 4, (1), 153–163, 1978.

Puleo, J. S., and Pastore, R. E. Contralateral cueing effects in backward masking. *Journal of the Acoustical Society of America,* 67, (3), 947–951, 1980.

Scharf, B., Quigley, S., Aoki, C., Peachey, N., and Reeves, A. Focused auditory attention and frequency selectivity. *Perception and Psychophysics,* 42, (3), 215–223, 1987.

Sekuler, R., and Ball, K. Mental set alters visibility of moving targets. *Science,* 198, 60–62, 1977.

Shaw, M. L. Attending to multiple sources of information: I. The integration of information in decision making. *Cognitive Psychology,* 14, 353–409, 1982.

Shaw, M. L. Division of attention among spatial locations: A fundamental difference between detection of letters and detection of luminance increments. In R. S. Nickerson (ed.), *Attention and Performance VIII.* New Jersey: Lawrence Erlbaum Associates, 109–121, 1980.

Shaw, M. L. Identifying attentional and decision-making components in information processing. In R. S. Nickerson (ed.), *Attention and Performance VIII.* New Jersey: Lawrence Erlbaum Associates, 277–295, 1980.

Shaw, M. L., Mulligan, R. M., and Stone, L. D. Two-state versus continuous-state stimulus representations: A test based on attentional constraints. *Perception and Psychophysics,* 33, (4), 338–354, 1983.

Shaw, M. L., and Shaw, P. Optimal allocation of cognitive resources to spatial locations. *Journal of Experimental Psychology: Human Perception and Performance,* 3, (2), 201–211, 1977.

Shefsky, M. W., Stenson, H. H., and Miller, L. K. Visual laterality effects: A signal detection analysis. *Perception and Psychophysics,* 30, (2), 175–180, 1981.

Shiffrin, R. M., Gardner, G. T., and Allmeyer, D. H. On the degree of attention and capacity limitations in visual processing. *Perception and Psychophysics,* 14, (2), 231–236, 1973.

Shiffrin, R. M., and Geisler, W. S. Visual recognition in a theory of information processing. In R. L. Solso (ed.), *Contemporary Issues in Cognitive Psychology: The Loyola Symposium.* Washington, D.C.: V. H. Winston & Sons, 53–101, 1973.

Shiffrin, R. M., and Grantham, D. W. Can attention be allocated to sensory modalities? *Perception and Psychophysics,* 15, (3), 460–474, 1974.

Shiffrin, R. M., McKay, D. P., and Shaffer, W. O. Attending to forty-nine spatial positions at once. *Journal of Experimental Psychology: Human Perception and Performance,* 2, (1), 14–22, 1976.

Shiffrin, R. M., Craig, J. C., and Cohen, E. On the degree of attention and capacity limitation in tactile processing. *Perception and Psychophysics,* 13, 328–336.

Shulman, H. G., and Fisher, R. P. Expected value as a determinant of the distribution of attention. *Journal of Experimental Psychology,* 93, (2), 343–348, 1972.

Sorkin, R. D., and Pastore, R. E. Simultaneous binaural signal detection: Comments on "Time sharing in auditory perception: Effect of stimulus duration." *Journal of the Acoustical Society of America,* 49, (4), 1319, 1971.

Sorkin, R. D., Pohlmann, L. D., and Woods, D. D. Decision interaction between auditory channels. *Perception and Psychophysics,* 19, (4), 290–295, 1976.

Sorkin, R. D., and Pastore, R. E. Simultaneous binaural signal detection: Comments on "Time sharing in auditory perception: Effect of stimulus duration" [Journal of the Acoustical Society of America, 47, 660–661, 1970], *Journal of the Acoustical Society of America,* 49, 1319, 1971.

Sorkin, R. S., Pastore, R. E., and Gilliom, J. D. Signal probability and the listening band. *Perception and Psychophysics,* 4, 10–12, 1968.

Sorkin, R. D., Pastore, R. E., and Pohlmann, L. D. Simultaneous two-channel signal detection. II. Correlated and uncorrelated signals. *Journal of the Acoustical Society of America,* 51, 1960–1965, 1972.

Sorkin, R. D., and Pohlmann, L. D. Some models of observer behavior in two-channel auditory signal detection. *Perception and Psychophysics,* 14, 101–109, 1973.

Sorkin, R. D., Pohlmann, L. D., and Gilliom, J. D. Simultaneous two-channel signal detection. III. 630- and 1400-Hz signals. *Journal of the Acoustical Society of America,* 53, 1045–1050, 1973.

Sperling, G., and Melchner, M. J. The attention operating characteristic: Examples from visual search. *Science,* 202, 315–318, 1978.

Sperling, G., and Melchner, M. J. Visual search, visual attention, and the attention operating characteristic. In J. Requin (ed.), *Attention and Performance, VII.* New Jersey: Erlbaum, 675–686, 1978.

Selective attention and learning under various levels of stimulus uncertainty. *Journal of the Acoustical Society of America,* 60, (5), 1176–1186, 1976.

Swets, J. A., and Kristofferson, A. B. Attention. *Annual Review of Psychology,* 21, 339–366, 1970.

Taylor, M. M., Lindsay, P. H., and Forbes, S. M. Quantification of shared-capacity processing in auditory and visual discrimination. *Acta Psychologica,* 27, 223–232, 1967.

Treisman, M. Detection of binaural tone stimuli: time sharing or criterion change? *Journal of the Acoustical Society of America,* 51, 625–629, 1972.

Treisman, A., and Geffen, G. Selective attention: Perception or response? *Quarterly Journal of Experimental Psychology,* 19, 1–17, 1967.

Treisman, A. M. Verbal cues, language, and meaning in selective attention. *Journal of Experimental Psychology,* 206–219, 1962.

Wickens, C. D. The effects of divided time on information processing in manual tracking. *Journal of Experimental Psychology,* 2, (1), 1–13, 1976.

Wickens, C. D. The effect of time sharing on the performance of information processing tasks: A feedback control analysis. Technical Report No. 51, Human Performance Center, University of Michigan, August, 1974.

Wickens, C. D., Mountford, S. J., and Schreiner, W. Multiple resources, task-hemispheric integrity, and individual differences in time-sharing. *Human Factors,* 23, (2), 211–229, 1981.

AUDITION

Abel, S. M. Duration discrimination of noise and tone bursts. *Journal of the Acoustical Society of America,* 51, 1219–1223, 1972.

Ahumada, A., Jr., and Lovell, J. Stimulus features in signal detection. *Journal of the Acoustical Society of America,* 49, 1751–1756, 1971.

Bell, D. W., and Nixon, J. C. Reliability of ratings in an auditory signal-detection experiment. *Journal of the Acoustical Society of America,* 49, 435–439, 1971.

Bourbon, W. T., Evans, T. R., and Deatherage, B. H. Effects of intensity on "critical bands" for tonal stimuli as determined by band limiting. *Journal of the Acoustical Society of America*, 43, 56–59, 1968.

Cuddy, L. L. Training the absolute identification of pitch. *Perception and Psychophysics*, 8, 265–269, 1970.

Doehring, D. G., and Ling, D. Matching to sample of three-tone simultaneous and successive sounds by musical and nonmusical subjects. *Psychonomic Science*, 25, 103–105, 1971.

Egan, J. P. Auditory masking and signal detection theory. *Audiology*, 10, 41–47, 1971.

Egan, J. P., Lindner, W. A., and McFadden, D. Masking-level differences and the form of psychometric function. *Perception and Psychophysics*, 4, 209–215, 1969.

Emmerich, D. S. Receiver operating characteristics determined under several interaural conditions of listening. *Journal of the Acoustical Society of America*, 43, 298–307, 1968.

Emmerich, D. S. Cueing signals in auditory detection and frequency discrimination experiments. *Perception and Psychophysics*, 9, 129–134, 1971.

Fidell, S., Pearsons, K. S., and Bennett, R. Prediction of aural detectability of noise signals. *Human Factors*, 16, (4), 373–383, 1974.

Foyle, C. C., and Watson, C. S. Stimulus-based versus performance-based measurement of auditory backward recognition masking. *Perception and Psychophysics*, 36, (6), 515–522, 1984.

Green, D. M. Additivity of masking. *Journal of the Acoustical Society of America*, 41, 1517–1525, 1967.

Green, D. M. Sine and cosine masking. *Journal of the Acoustical Society of America*, 44, 168–175, 1968.

Green, D. M. Masking with continuous and pulsed sinusoids. *Journal of the Acoustical Society of America*, 46, 939–946, 1969.

Hafter, E. R., Bourbon, W. T., Blocker, A. S., and Tucker, A. Direct comparison between lateralization and detection under conditions of antiphasic masking. *Journal of the Acoustical Society of America*, 46, 1452, 1969.

Hafter, E. R., and Carrier, S. C. Masking-level differences obtained with a pulsed tonal masker. *Journal of the Acoustical Society of America*, 47, 1041–1047, 1970.

Hafter, E. R., and Dye, R. H., Jr. Detection of interaural differences of time in trains of high-frequency clicks as a function of interclick interval and number. *Journal of the Acoustical Society of America*, 73, (2), 644–651, 1983.

Henning, B. G. Frequency discrimination in noise. *Journal of the Acoustical Society of America*, 41, 774–777, 1967.

Henning, B. G. A model for auditory discrimination and detection. *Journal of the Acoustical Society of America*, 42, 1325–1334, 1967.

Henning, B. G. Amplitude discrimination in noise, pedestal experiments, and additivity of masking. *Journal of the Acoustical Society of America*, 45, 426–435, 1969.

Henning, B. G., and Bleiwas, S. L. Amplitude discrimination in noise. *Journal of the Acoustical Society of America*, 41, 1365, 1967.

Henning, G. B., and Psotka, J. An extension of some observations of Leshowitz and Raab. *Journal of the Acoustical Society of America*, 45, 785–786, 1969.

Howard, J. H., Jr., O'Toole, A. J., Rice, S. E. The role of frequency versus informational cues in uncertain frequency detection. *Journal of the Acoustical Society of America*, 79, (3), 788–791, 1986.

Idson, W. L., and Massaro, D. W. Cross-octave masking of single tones and musical sequences: The effects of structure on auditory recognition. *Perception and Psychophysics*, 19, (2), 155–175, 1976.

Jeffress, L. A. Masking. In *Foundations of Modern Auditory Theory*, J. V. Tobias (Ed.), Academic Press, Inc., New York, 85–114, 1972.

Johnson, D. M., Watson, C. S., and Jensen, J. K. Individual differences in auditory capabilities. I. *Journal of the Acoustical Society of America*, 82, (2), 427–438, 1987.

Kinchla, J. Duration discrimination of acoustically defined intervals in the 1- to 8-sec range. *Perception and Psychophysics*, 12, 318–320, 1972.

Kristofferson, A. B., Allan, L. G., and Campbell, F. A. On the detection of stepwise changes in a constant signal level. *Perception and Psychophysics*, 30, (4), 362–371, 1981.

Leshowitz, B., and Cudahy, E. Masking with continuous and gated sinusoids. *Journal of the Acoustical Society of America*, 51, 1921–1929, 1972.

Leshowitz, B., and Raab, D. H. Effects of stimulus duration on the detection of sinusoids added to continuous pedestals. *Journal of the Acoustical Society of America*, 41, 489–496, 1967.

Leshowitz, B., and Wightman, F. L. On-frequency masking with continuous sinusoids. *Journal of the Acoustical Society of America*, 49, 1180–1190, 1971.

Long, Glenis R. The role of the standard in an auditory amplitude discrimination experiment. *Perception and Psychophysics*, 13, 49–59, 1973.

McGill, W. J., and Goldberg, J. P. Pure-tone intensity discrimination and energy detection. *Journal of the Acoustical Society of America*, 44, 576–581, 1968.

Mulligan, B. E., and Adams, J. C. Effect of sound on subsequent detection. *Journal of the Acoustical Society of America*, 44, 1401–1408, 1968.

Mulligan, B. E., Adams, J. C., Mulligan, M. J., and Burwinkle, R. E. Prediction of monaural detection. *Journal of the Acoustical Society of America*, 43, 481–486, 1968.

Nabelek, I., and Hirsh, I. J. On the discrimination of frequency transitions. *Journal of the Acoustical Society of America*, 45, 1510–1519, 1969.

Nosofsky, R. N. Information integration and the identification of stimulus noise and criterial noise in absolute judgment. *Journal of Experimental Psychology: Human Perception and Performance*, 9, (2), 299–309.

Offutt, G. C. Integration of the energy in repeated tone pulses by man and the goldfish. *Journal of the Acoustical Society of America*, 41, 7–12, 1967.

Osman, E., Schacknow, P. N., and Tzuo, P. L. Psychometric functions and a correlation model of binaural detection. *Perception and Psychophysics*, 15, (2), 371–374, 1973.

Osman, E., Tzuo, P. L., and Tzuo, H-Y. On the detection of a brief signal in the temporal center of a noise masker of varying duration. *Perception and Psychophysics*, 30, (4), 372–374, 1981.

Pastore, R. E., and MacLatchy, C. S. Some nonmasking auditory post-signal effects. *Perception and Psychophysics*, 17, (5), 355–359, 1975.

Pastore, R. E., and Sorkin, R. D. Adaptive auditory signal processing. *Psychonomic Science*, 23, (4), 259–260, 1971.

Patterson, J. H. Masking of tones by transient signals having identical energy spectra. *Journal of the Acoustical Society of America*, 50, 1126–1132, 1971.

Pfafflin, S. M. Detection of auditory signal in restricted sets of reproducible noise. *Journal of the Acoustical Society of America*, 43, 487–490, 1968.

Pollack, I. On the combination of intensity and frequency differences in auditory discrimination. *Journal of the Acoustical Society of America,* (Letters to the Editor), 33, 1141–1142, 1961.

Raab, D. H., and Taub, H. B. Click-intensity discrimination with and without a background masking noise. *Journal of the Acoustical Society of America,* 46, 965–968, 1969.

Rochester, S. Detection and duration discrimination of noise increments. *Journal of the Acoustical Society of America,* 49, 1783–1789, 1971.

Ronken, D. A. Intensity discrimination of Rayleigh noise. *Journal of the Acoustical Society of America,* 45, 54–57, 1969.

Ronken, D. A. Monaural detection of a phase difference between clicks. *Journal of the Acoustical Society of America,* 47, 1091–1099, 1970.

Sandusky, A., and Ahumada, A. Contrast in detection with gated noise. *Journal of the Acoustical Society of America,* 49, 1790–1794, 1971.

Searle, C. L., Braida, L. D., Davis, M. F., and Colburn, H. S. Model for auditory localization. *Journal of the Acoustical Society of America,* 60, (5), 1164–1175, 1976.

Soderquist, D. R. Frequency analysis and the critical band. *Psychonomic Science,* 21, 117–119, 1970.

Srinivasan, R. Auditory critical bandwidth for short-duration signals. *Journal of the Acoustical Society of America,* 50, 616–622, 1971.

Taylor, M. M., and Clarke, D. P. J. Monaural detection with contra-lateral cue (MDCC). II. Interaural dela; of cue and signal. *Journal of the Acoustical Society of America,* 49, 1243–1253, 1971.

Taylor, M. M., Clarke, D. P. J., and Smith, S. M. Monaural detection with contralateral cue (MDCC). III. Sinusoidal signals at a constant performance level. *Journal of the Acoustical Society of America,* 49, 1795–1804, 1971.

Taylor, M. M., and Forbes, S. M. Monaural detection with contra-lateral cue (MDCC). I. Better than energy detector performance by human observers. *Journal of the Acoustical Society of America,* 46, 1519–1526, 1969.

Taylor, M. M., Smith, S. M., and Clarke, D. P. J. Monaural detection with contralateral cue (MDCC). IV. Psychometric functions with sinusoidal signals. *Journal of the Acoustical Society of America,* 50, 1151–1161, 1971.

Taylor, M. M., and Smith, S. M. Monaural detection with contralateral cue. V. Interstimulus interval in MDCC and amplitude discrimination. *Journal of the Acoustical Society of America,* 57, (6), 1500–1511, 1975.

Tucker, A., Williams, P. I., and Jeffress, L. A. Effect of signal duration on detection for gated and for continuous noise. *Journal of the Acoustical Society of America,* 44, 813–816, 1968.

Viemeister, N. F. Intensity discrimination of pulsed sinusoids: The effects of filtered noise. *Journal of the Acoustical Society of America,* 51, 1265–1269, 1972.

Watson, C. S., Franks, J. R., and Hood, D. C. Detection of tones in the absence of external masking noise. I. Effects of signal intensity and signal frequency. *Journal of the Acoustical Society of America,* 52, 633–643, 1972.

Wilbanks, W. A., and Whitmore, J. K. Detection of monaural signals as a function of interaural noise correlation and signal frequency. *Journal of the Acoustical Society of America,* 43, 785–797, 1968.

Woods, D. D., Sorkin, R. D., and Boggs, G. J. Stimulus context and duration discrimination. *Perception and Psychophysics,* 26, (2), 127–132, 1979.

CONCEPTUAL JUDGMENT

Hammerton, M. An investigation into changes in decision criteria and other details of a decision-making task. *Psychonomic Science,* 21, 203–204, 1970.

Hertzog, C. Applications of signal detection theory to the study of psychological aging: A theoretical review. Paper supported by a PHS Postdoctoral Fellowship from the National Institute on Aging. University of Washington, Seattle, Washington, 1–81.

Jagacinski, R. J., Isaac, P. D., and Burke, M. W. Application of signal detection theory to perceptual-motor skills: Decision processes in basketball shooting. *Journal of Motor Behavior,* 9, (3), 225–234, 1977.

Lieblich, A., and Lieblich, I. Arithmetical estimation under conditions of different payoff matrices. *Psychonomic Science,* 14, 87–88, 1969.

Martin, W. W., and Rovira, M. Signal detection theory: Its implications for social psychology. *Personality and Social Psychology Bulletin,* 7, (2), 232–239, 1981.

Miehle, W., and Siegel, A. I. Defect signal detection model based on variable confidence. *Human Factors,* 12, 409–420, 1970.

Pease, K., Tarling, R., and Meudell, P. Decision in the criminal justice process and signal detection theory: A note. *Quality and Quantity,* 11, 83–89, 1977.

Sattler, J. M., and Ryan, J. J. Scoring agreement on the Stanford-Binet. *Journal of Clinical Psychology, 29,* 35–39, 1973.

Schum, D. A., Goldstein, I. L., Howell, W. C., Southard, J. F. Subjective probability revisions under several cost-payoff arrangements. *Organizational Behavior and Human Performance,* 2, 84–104, 1967.

Segal, S. J., and Fusella, V. Effects of imaging on signal-to-noise ratio, with varying signal conditions. *British Journal of Psychology,* 60, 459–464, 1969.

Segal, S. J., and Fusella, V. Influence of imaged pictures and sounds on detection of visual and auditory signals. *Journal of Experimental Psychology,* 83, 458–464, 1970.

Segal, S. J., and Fusella, V. Effect of images in six sense modalities on detection of visual signal from noise. *Psychonomic Science,* 24, 55–56, 1971.

Segal, S. J., and Gordon, P. E. The Perky effect revisited: paradoxical threshold or signal detection error. *Perceptual and Motor Skills,* 28, 791–797, 1969.

Ulehla, Z. J., Canges, L., and Wackwitz, F. Signal detectability theory applied to conceptual discrimination. *Psychonomic Science,* 8, 221–222, 1967.

Ulehla, Z. J., Canges, L., and Wackwitz, F. Integration of conceptual information. *Psychonomic Science,* 8, 223–224, 1967.

Ulehla, Z. J., Little, K. B., and Weyl, T. C. Operating characteristics and realisms of certainty estimates. *Psychonomic Science,* 9, 77–78, 1967.

Williams, K. H., Williams, J. E., and Beck, R. C. Assessing children's racial attitudes via a signal detection model. *Perceptual and Motor Skills,* 36, 587–598, 1973.

EXTENDED THEORY

Allen, R. W., Schwartz, S. H., and Jex, H. R. Driver decision-making research in a laboratory simulation. Presented at NATO Conference on "Monitoring Behavior and Supervisory Control," Berchtesgaden (F.R.) Germany, March 8–12, Preprints pp. 49–59, 1976.

Ashby, F. G., and Townsend, J. T. Varieties of perceptual independence. *Psychological Review,* 93, (2), 154–179, 1986.

Baron, J. The threshold for successiveness. *Perception and Psychophysics,* 10, (4A), 201–207, 1971.

Berliner, J. E., and Durlach, N. I. Intensity perception. IV. Resolution in roving-level discrimination. *Journal of the Acoustical Society of America,* 53, 1270–1287, 1973.

Birdsall, T. G., and Gobien, J. O. Sufficient statistics and reproducing densities in simultaneous sequential detection and estimation. *IEEE Transactions on Information Theory,* IT-19, (6), 760–768, 1973.

Braida, L. D., and Durlach, N. I. Intensity perception. II. Resolution in one-interval paradigms. *Journal of the Acoustical Society of America,* 51, 1972.

Burkheimer, G. J., Stein, W. E., and Rapoport. A. A fixed observation boundary decision model for detection of change. Report No. 134, L. L. Thurstone Psychometric Laboratory, University of North Carolina, May, 1974.

Cohen, H. S., and Ferrell, W. R. Human operator decision-making in manual control. *IEEE Trans. on Man-Machine Systems,* 10, 41–47, 1969.

Divenyi, P. L., and Danner, W. F. Discrimination of time intervals marked by brief acoustic pulses of various intensities and spectra. *Perception and Psychophysics,* 21, (2), 125–152, 1977.

Durlach, N. I., and Braida, L. D. Intensity perception. I. Preliminary theory of intensity resolution. *Journal of the Acoustical Society of America,* 46, 372–383, 1969.

Frederiksen, J. R. Two models for psychophysical judgment: Scale invariance with changes in stimulus range. *Perception and Psychophysics,* 17, (2), 147–157, 1975.

Hodgkiss, W. S., and Nolte, L. W. Adaptive optimum array processing. *Journal of the Acoustical Society of America,* 61, (3), 763–775, 1977.

Jeffress, L. A. The logistic distribution as an approximation to the normal curve. *Journal of the Acoustical Society of America,* 53, 1296, 1973.

Kinchla, R. A., and Allan, L. G. A theory of visual movement perception. *Psychological Review,* 76, 537–558, 1969.

Kornbrot, D. E., Donnelly, M., and Galanter, E. Estimates of utility function parameters from signal detection experiments. Psychophysics Laboratory Report, Columbia University, New York.

Kristofferson, A. B. A real-time criterion theory of duration discrimination. *Perception and Psychophysics,* 21, (2), 105–117, 1977.

Kubovy, M., and Healy, A. F. Numerical decision and the ideal learner: A reply to Dorfman. *Journal of Experimental Psychology: General,* (in press).

Kubovy, M., and Healy, A. F. The decision rule in probabilistic categorization: What it is and how it is learned. *Journal of Experimental Psychology: General,* (in press).

Laming, D. Some principles of sensory analysis. *Psychological Review,* 92, (4), 462–485, 1985.

Laming, D. Analysis of variance of *d'*. To be submitted to the *Psychological Bulletin,* 1988.

Larkin, W. Response mechanisms in detection experiments. *Journal of Experimental Psychology,* 91, 140–153, 1971.

Nolte, L. W. Theory of signal detectability: Adaptive optimum receiver design. *Journal of the Acoustical Society of America,* 42, (4), 773–777, 1967.

Nolte, L. W., and Jaarsma, D. More on the detection of one of M orthogonal signals. *Journal of the Acoustical Society of America,* 41, (2), 497–505, 1967.

Nosofsky, R. M. Information integration and the identification of stimulus noise and criterial noise in absolute judgment. *Journal of Experimental Psychology: Human Perception and Performance,* 9, (2), 299–309, 1983.

Penner, M. J. The perception of offset: A problem of decision criteria. *Perception and Psychophysics,* 17, (6), 587–590, 1975.

Pynn, C. T., Braida, L. D., and Durlach, N. I. Intensity perception. III. Resolution in small-range identification. *Journal of the Acoustical Society of America,* 51, 559–566, 1972.

Rapoport, A., and Burkheimer, G. J. Models for deferred decision making. *Journal of Mathematical Psychology,* 8, 508–538, 1971.

Sorkin, R. D., and Robinson, D. E. Alerted monitors: Human operators aided by automated detectors. Final Report DOT/OST/P-34/85/021, W. Lafayette, IN: Purdue University, December 1984.

Sorkin, R. D. Sorkin, and Woods, D. D. Systems with human monitors: A signal detection analysis. In T. P. Moran (Ed.), *Human-Computer Interaction,* 1, (1), 49–75, 1985.

Spooner, R. L. Comparison of receiver performance: the ESP receiver. *Journal of the Acoustical Society of America,* 45, (1), 233–236, 1969.

Swensson, R. G., and Judy, P. F. Detection of noisy visual targets: Models for the effects of spatial uncertainty and signal-to-noise ratio. *Perception and Psychophysics,* 29, (6), 521–534, 1981.

Swets, J. A. Deferred decision in signal detection. In *Detection and Recognition of Signals,* B. F. Lomov (Ed.), Moscow University Press, Lenin Hills Moscow, 21–26, 1966.

Swets, J. A., and Birdsall, T. G. Deferred decision in human signal detection: A preliminary experiment. *Perception and Psychophysics,* 2, 15–28, 1967.

Tanner, W. P., Jr. Theory of recognition. *Journal of the Acoustical Society of America,* 28, (5), 882–888, 1956.

Thijssen, J. M., and Vendrik, A. J. H. Internal noise and transducer function in sensory detection experiments: Evaluation of psychometric curves and of ROC curves. *Perception and Psychophysics,* 3, 387–400, 1968.

Treisman, M. Relation between signal detectability theory and the traditional procedures for measuring thresholds: An addendum. *Psychological Bulletin,* 79, 45–47, 1973.

Treisman, M., and Leshowitz, B. The effects of duration, area, and background intensity on the visual intensity difference threshold given by the forced-choice procedure: Derivations from a statistical decision model for sensory discrimination. *Perception and Psychophysics,* 6, 281–296, 1969.

Treisman, M., and Watts, T. R. Relation between signal detectability theory and the traditional procedures for measuring sensory thresholds: Estimating d' from results given by the method of constant stimuli. *Psychological Bulletin,* 66, 438–454, 1966.

Treisman, M. On the use and misuse of psychophysical terms. *Psychological Review,* 83, (3), 246–256, 1976.

Treisman, M., and Faulkner, A. Can decision criteria interchange locations? Some positive evidence. *Journal of Experimental Psychology: Human Perception and Performance,* 11, (2), 187–208, 1985.

Treisman, M., and Williams, T. C. A theory of criterion setting with an application to sequential dependencies. *Psychological Review,* 91, 1, 68–111, 1984.

Wandell, B., and Luce, R. D. Pooling peripheral information: Averages versus extreme values. *Journal of Mathematical Psychology,* 17, (3), 220–235, 1978.

Wickelgren, W. A. Unidimensional strength theory and component analysis of noise in absolute and comparative judgments. *Journal of Mathematical Psychology,* 5, 102–122, 1968.

Wolfendale, G. L. An information-processing approach to human signal detection. *Perception and Psychophysics,* 45, 319–331, 1977.

Wolfendale, G. L. Decision times in signal detection. *Acta Psychologica*, 27, 154–159, 1967.

Zagorski, M. Perceptual independence of pitch and loudness in a signal detection experiment: A processing model for 2ATFC (2IFC) experiments. *Perception and Psychophysics*, 17, (6), 525–531, 1975.

GENERAL SURVEY

Beck, J. R., Pyle, K. I., Lusted, L. B. A citation analysis of the field of medical decision making, 1959–1982. *Medical Decision Making*, 4, (4), 449–468, 1984.

Beretta, A. *La Teoria della Detezione del Segnale*. University Degli Studi di Universita Milano, Instituto di psicologia Della Facolta Medica, 1968.

Brichacek, V. Matematicka psychologie 1972. *Activitas Nervosa Superior*, 15, (4), 278–286, 1973.

Green, D. M. Application of detection theory in psychophysics. *Proceedings of the IEEE*, 58, 713–723, 1970.

Greeno, J. G. An appraisal of mathematical psychology. MMPP 71–13, Michigan Mathematical Psychology Program, The University of Michigan, Department of Psychology, Ann Arbor, Michigan, 1971.

Hake, H. W., and Rodwan, A. S. Perception and recognition. In *Experimental Methods and Instrumentation in Psychology*, J. B. Sidowski (Ed.), McGraw-Hill Book Co., New York, 331–381, 1966.

Hutchinson, T. P. A review of some unusual applications of signal detection theory. *Quality and Quantity*, 15, 71–98, 1981.

Hutchinson, T. P. The usefulness of signal detection theory in the analysis of ordinal data from diverse fields. (Draft Report), Traffic Studies Group, University College, London. February, 1976.

Luce, R. D. What sort of measurement is psychophysical measurement? *American Psychologist*, 96–106, February 1972.

Swets, J. A. Theories of sensory thresholds. In *Sensory Evaluation of Food: Principles and Methods*, B. Drake (Ed.), A. Rydberg and Co., Gothenburg, Sweden, 17–18, 1969.

Swets, J. A. Theory of signal detection in psychology. In *Encyclopedia of Science and Technology*, McGraw-Hill, New York, 354–355, 1971.

Swets, J. A. The relative operating characteristic in psychology. *Science* (in press).

Tanner, W. P., Jr., and Sorkin, R. D. The theory of signal detectability. In *Foundations of Modern Auditory Theory*, J. V. Tobias (Ed.), Academic Press, Inc., New York, 63–98, 1972.

Watson, C. S. Psychophysics. In *Handbook of General Psychology*, B. B. Wolman (Ed.), Prentice-Hall, New York, 275–306, 1973.

IDEAL OBSERVER

Birdsall, T. G. The theory of signal detectability: ROC curves and their character. Ph.D. thesis, University of Michigan, Ann Arbor, Michigan, i–xxiii, 1–416, 1966.

Green, D. M., and McGill, W. J. On the equivalence of detection probabilities and well-known statistical quantities. *Psychological Review*, 41, 294–301, 1970.

Henning, G. B. A model for auditory discrimination and detection. *Journal of the Acoustical Society of America*, 42, 1325–1334, 1967.

Jeffress, L. A. Stimulus-oriented approach to detection re-examined. *Journal of the Acoustical Society of America,* 41, 480–488, 1967.

Jeffress, L. A. Mathematical and electrical models of auditory detection. *Journal of the Acoustical Society of America,* 44, 187–203, 1968.

Levison, W. H., and Tanner, R. B. A control-theory model for human decision-making. Report No. 2119, Bolt Beranek and Newman Inc., Cambridge, Mass., 1971.

Luce, R. D., and Green, D. M. A neural timing theory for response times and the psychophysics of intensity. *Psychological Review,* 79, 14–57, 1972.

McGill, W. J. A neural counting model with familiar outcomes in auditory detection. *Journal of Mathematical Psychology,* 4, 351–376, 1967.

McGill, W. J. Neural counting mechanisms and energy detection. *Journal of Mathematical Psychology,* 4, 351–376, 1968.

McGill, W. J. Variations on Marill's detection formula. *Journal of the Acoustical Society of America,* 43, 70–73, 1968.

McGill, W. J., and Goldberg, J. P. A study of the near-miss involving Weber's law and pure-tone intensity discrimination. *Perception and Psychophysics,* 4, 105–109, 1968.

Nolte, L. W. Theory of signal detectability: Adaptive optimum receiver design. *Journal of the Acoustical Society of America,* 42, 773–777, 1967.

Nolte, L. W. Adaptive optimum detection: Synchronous-recurrent transients. *Journal of the Acoustical Society of America,* 44, 224–239, 1968.

Nolte, L. W., and Jaarsma, D. More on the detection of one of *M* orthogonal signals. *Journal of the Acoustical Society of America,* 41, 497–505, 1967.

Siebert, W. M. Stimulus transformation in the peripheral auditory system. In *Recognizing Patterns,* P. A. Kolers and M. Eden (Eds.), MIT Press, Cambridge, Mass., 104–133, 1968.

Siebert, W. M. Signals and noise in sensory systems. *Technology Review,* 23–29, May, 1973.

Ward, L. M. Use of Markov-encoded sequential information in numerical signal detection. *Perception and Psychophysics,* 14, (2), 337–342, 1973.

Wilcox, G. W. Inter-observer agreement and models of monaural auditory processing in detection tasks. Report No. MMPP 68–4, Department of Psychology, The University of Michigan, 1968.

LEARNING

Aiken, E. G. Auditory discrimination learning: Prototype storage and distinctive features detection mechanisms. *Perception and Psychophysics,* 6, 95–96, 1969.

Bernbach, H. A., and Bower, G. H. Confidence ratings in continuous paired-associate learning. *Psychonomic Science,* 21, 252–253, 1970.

Colliver, J. A. "Confidence-rating" analysis on response amplitude scores of classical discrimination conditioning data. *Psychological Review,* 32, 79–84, 1973.

Cumming, G. D. Theoretical distribution of second choice scores in a paired-associate task if learning is all-or-none. *Journal of Mathematical Psychology,* 5, 463–469, 1968.

Dorfman, D. D., and Biderman, M. A learning model for a continuum of sensory states. *Journal of Mathematical Psychology,* 8, 264–268, 1971.

Dorfman, D. D., Saslow, C. F., and Simpson, J. C. Learning models for a continuum of sensory states reexamined. *Journal of Mathematical Psychology,* 12, (2), 178–211, 1975.

Eijkman, E. G. The measurement of fluctuation in perceptual and learning tasks. *IEEE Transactions on Man-Machine Systems,* 1, 11–19, 1970.

Estes, W. K. Global and local control of choice behavior by cyclically varying outcome probabilities. *Journal of Experimental Psychology: Learning, Memory, and Cognition,* 10, (2), 258–270, 1984.

Estes, W. K. Memory storage and retrieval processes in category learning. *Journal of Experimental Psychology: General,* 115, (2), 155–174, 1986.

Fishbein, H. D., and Engel, S. Human eyelid conditioning at detection threshold. *Psychonomic Science,* 4, 291–292, 1966.

Fishbein, H. D., and Rees, J. F. The interaction effects of CS intensity and CS-UCS interval in human eyelid conditioning. *British Journal of Psychology,* 60, 357–361, 1969.

Fried, L. S., and Holyoak, K. J. Induction of category distributions: A framework for classification learning. *Journal of Experimental Psychology: Learning, Memory, and Cognition,* 10, (2), 234–257, 1984.

Friedman, M. P., Carterette, E. C., Nakatani, L., and Ahumada, A. Comparisons of some learning models for response bias in signal detection. *Perception and Psychophysics,* 3, 5–11, 1968.

Grice, G. R. Stimulus intensity and response evocation. *Psychological Review,* 75, 359–373, 1968.

Grice, G. R. A threshold model for drive. (To be published in Kendler, H. H., and Spence, J. T. (Eds.), *Essays in Neobehaviorism: A Memorial Volume to Kenneth W. Spence,* Appleton-Century-Crofts.).

Grice, G. R. Conditioning and a decision theory of response evocation. (To be published in *Psychology of Learning and Motivation; Advances in Research and Theory,* G. H. Bower (Ed.), Academic Press.).

Hickson, R. H. Signal detection in a paired-associate learning task. *Psychonomic Science,* 12, 253–254, 1968.

Huff, E. M., and Nagel, D. C. Psychological aspects of aeronautical flight simulation. *American Psychologist,* 30, (3), 426–439, 1975.

Rees, J. F., and Fishbein, H. D. Test of the TSD model in human eyelid conditioning: A priori probability and payoff manipulations. *Journal of Experimental Psychology,* 83, 291–298, 1970.

MEDICAL DIAGNOSIS

Abrams, H. L., Siegelman, S. S., Adams, D. F., Sanders, R., Finberg, H. J., Hessel, S. J., and McNeil, B. J. Computed tomography versus ultrasound of the adrenal gland: a prospective study. *Radiology,* 143, (1), 121–128, 1982.

Ackerman, L. V. Computer classification of radiographs and xerograms of the breast. Ph.D. Thesis, Ann Arbor, Michigan, 1971.

Ackerman, L. V., and Gose, E. E. Breast lesion classification by computer and Xeroradiograph. *Cancer,* 30, (4), 1025–1035, 1972.

Alcorn, F. S., O'Donnell, E. Mammogram screeners: Modified program learning for nonradiologic personnel. *Radiology,* 90, (2), 336–338, 1968.

Alcorn, F. S., O'Donnell, E. The training of nonphysician personnel for use in a mammography program. *Cancer,* 23, 879–884, 1969.

Alcorn, F. S., O'Donnell, E., and Ackerman, L. V. The protocol and results of training nonradiologists to scan mammograms. *Radiology,* 99, (2), 523–529, 1971.

Anderson, T. McD., Jr., Mintzer, R. A., Hoffer, P. B., Lusted, L. B., Smith, V. C., and Pokorny, J. Nuclear image transmission by Picturephone evaluation by ROC curve method. *Investigative Radiology*, 8, (4), 244–250, 1973.

Andrus, W. S., and Bird, K. T. Radiology and the receiver operating characteristic (ROC) curve. *Chest*, 67, (4), 378–379, 1975.

Andrus, W. S., Dreyfuss, J. R., Jaffer, F., and Bird, K. T. Interpretation of roentgenograms via interactive television. *Radiology*, 116, (1), 25–31, 1975.

Andrus, W. S., Hunter, C. H., and Bird, K. T. Remote interpretation of chest roentgenograms. *Chest*, 67, (4), 463–468, 1975.

Bacus, J. W. The observer error in peripheral blood cell classification. *American Journal of Clinical Practice*, 59, 223–230, 1973.

Bacus, J. W., Wiley, E. L., Galbraith, W., Marshall, P. N., Wilbanks, G. E., and Weinstein, R. S. Malignant cell detection and cervical cancer screening. *Analytical and Quantitative Cytology*, 6, (2), 121–130, 1984.

Barnes, R., and Drury, C. G. An application of signal detection theory to EMS decision making. *Ethics in Science & Medicine*, 3, 187–193, 1976.

Beck, R. N. Current status of diagnostic counting and imaging techniques used in nuclear medicine: A sketch. Center for Radiologic Image Research (USPHS Grant GM 18940). Department of Radiology, The University of Chicago, 15–32, 1973.

Berbaum, K. S., Franken, E. A., Jr., Dorfman, D. D., Barloon, T., Ell, S. R., Lu, C. H., Smith W., and Abu-Yousef, M. M. Tentative diagnoses facilitate the detection of diverse lesions in chest radiographs. *Investigative Radiology*, 21, (7), 532-539, 1986.

Berbaum, K. S., Franken, E. A., Jr., and Smith W. L. The effect of comparison films upon resident interpretation of pediatric chest radiographs. *Investigative Radiology*, 20, 124–128, 1985.

Berbaum, K. S., Franken, E. A., Dorfman, D. D., Barloon, T., Ell, S. R., Lu, C. H., Smith, W., and Abu-Yousef, M. M. Tentative diagnoses facilitate the detection of diverse lesions in chest radiographs. *Investigative Radiology*, 21, (7), 532–539, 1986.

Berwick, D. M., and Thibodeau, L. A. Receiver operating characteristic analysis of diagnostic skill. *Medical Care*, 21, (9), 876–885, 1983.

Blackwell, R. J., Shirley, I., Farman, D. J., Michael, C. A. Ultra-sonic "B" scanning as a pregnancy test after less than six weeks amenorrhea. *British Journal on Obstetrics and Gynecology*, 82, 108–114, 1975.

Boom, R. A., Gil, D., Maass, R., and Manrique, G. The differential diagnosis of obstructive jaundice. *Medical Decision Making*, 1, (3), 225–237, 1981.

Bunch, P. C., Hamilton, J. F., Sanderson, G. K., and Simmons, A. H. A free response approach to the measurement and characterization of radiographic observer performance. *Optical Instrumentation in Medicine, VI*, 127, (22), 124–135, 1977.

Centor, R. M., Yarbrough, B., and Wood, J. P. Inability to predict relapse in acute asthma. *The New England Journal of Medicine*, 310, (9), 577–580, 1984.

Chakraborty, D. P., Breatnach, E. S., Yester, M. V., Soto, B., Barnes, G. T., Fraser, R. G. Digital and conventional chest imaging: A modified ROC study of observer performance using simulated nodules. *Radiology*, 158, (1), 35–39, 1986.

Cogill, B. Ranking anthropometric indicators using mortality in rural Bangladeshi children. Master Thesis, Cornell University, Ithaca, New York, 1982.

Crassini, B., and Broerse, J. Auditory-visual integration in neonates: A signal detection analysis. *Journal of Experimental Child Psychology*, 29, 144–155, 1980.

deDombal, F. T., and Horrocks, J. C. Use of receiver operating characteristic (ROC) curves to evaluate computer confidence threshold and clinical performance in the diagnosis of appendicitis. *Meth. Inform. Med.*, 17, (3), 157–161, 1978.

deDombal, F. T., Staniland Chir, B., J. R., and Clamp, S. E. Geographical variation in disease presentation. *Medical Decision Making*, 1, (1), 59–69, 1981.

Dowdy, A. H., LaGasse, L. D., Roach, P., and Wilson. D. Lay screeners in mammographic survey programs. *Radiology*, 94, (3), 619–621, 1970.

Eisenberg, J. M., and Sussman, E. J. (Editorial) Harder data for the soft science of quality assurance. *Medical Decision Making*, 2, (1), 7–11, 1982.

Elstein, A. S., Dawson-Saunders, B., and Belzer, L. J. Instruction in medical decision making. *Medical Decision Making*, 5, (2), 229–233, 1985.

Erdreich, L. S., and Lee, E. T. Use of relative operating characteristic analysis in epidemiology. *American Journal of Epidemiology*, 114, (5), 649–662, 1981.

Gohagan, J. K., Spitznagel, E. L., McCrate, M., and Frank, T. B. ROC analysis of mammography and palpation for breast screening. *Investigative Radiology*, 19, (6), 587–592, 1984.

Goin, J. E., and DeSmet, A. A. Diagnostic imaging system evaluation. *Medical Decision Making*, 2, (3), 311–321, 1982.

Goin, J. E., DeSmet, A. A., and Rosenthal, S. J. An expanded ROC analysis detection model. Department of Diagnostic Radiology. The University of Kansas College of Health Sciences and Hospital, Kansas City, KS.

Goin, J. E., Haberman, J. D., Linder, M. K., and Lambird, P. A. Analysis of mammography: A blind interpretation of BCDDP radiographs. *Radiology*, 148, (2), 393–396, 1983.

Goodenough, D. J. ROC Theory: Limitations and applications. *IEEE Transactions on Nuclear Science*, NS-29, (4), 1359–1367, 1982.

Goodenough, D. J. The use of ROC curves in testing the proficiency of individuals in classifying pneumoconiosis. *Radiology*, 114, (3), 472–473, 1975.

Goodenough, D. J., and Metz, C. E. Effect of listening interval on auditory detection performance. *Journal of the Acoustical Society of America*, 55, (1), 11–116, 1974.

Goodenough, D. J., Metz, C. E., and Lusted, L. B. Caveat on use of the parameter d' for evaluation of observer performance. *Radiology*, 106, (3), 565–566, 1973.

Goodenough, D. J., Rossmann, K., and Lusted, L. B. Radiographic applications of signal detection theory. *Radiology*, 105, (1), 199–200, 1972.

Goodenough, D. J., Weaver, K. E., and Davis, D. O. Development of a phantom for evaluation and assurance of image quality in CT scanning. *Optical Engineering*, 16, (1), 52–65, 1977.

Goodman, L. R., Foley, W. D., Wilson, C. R., Rimm, A. A., Lawson, T. L. Digital and conventional chest images: Observer performance with film digital radiography system. *Radiology*, 158, (1), 27–33, 1986.

Gray, J. E., Hanson, D. P., Herman, G. T., Lewitt, R. M., Reynolds, R. A., Robb, R. A., Smith B., and Tuy, H. Reconstruction algorithms for dose reduction in X-ray computed tomography. Final report, Department of Radiology, University of Pennsylvania, February, 1982.

Gray, R., Begg, C. B., and Greenes, R. A. Construction of receiver operating characteristic curves when disease verification is subject to selection bias. *Medical Decision Making*, 4, (2), 151–164, 1984.

Greenfield, S., Cretin, S., Worthman, L. G., and Dorey, F. The use of an ROC curve to express quality of care results. *Medical Decision Making*, 2, (1), 24–31, 1982.

Guignard, P. A., and Salehi, N. Validity of the Gaussian assumption in the analysis of ROC data obtained from scintigraphic-like images. *Physiological Medical Biology,* 28, (12), 1409–1417, 1983.

Hessel, S. J., Siegelman, S. S., McNeil, B. J., Sanders, R., Adams, D. F., Alderson, P. O., Finberg, H. J., Abrams, H. L. A prospective evaluation of computed tomography and ultrasound of the pancreas. *Radiology,* 143, (1), 129–133, 1982.

Hessel, S. J., Herman, P. G., and Swensson, R. G. Improving performance by multiple interpretations of chest radiographs: Effectiveness and cost. *Radiology,* 127, (3), 589–594, 1978.

Hoop, B., and Brandstetter, R. D. Evaluating diagnostic strategies for pulmonary embolism. (Letter to the Editors). *Medical Decision Making,* 399–404, 1983.

Hoop, B., and Metz, C. E. Operability of nuclear instruments for medical use in developing countries. *Medical Decision Making,* 1, (3), 247–263, 1981.

IAEA (International Atomic Energy Agency) Co-ordinated research program on the intercomparison of computer-assisted scintigraphic techniques. *Medical Radionuclide Imaging,* 1, 585–615, 1977.

Iinuma, T., Endo, M., Umegaki, Y. Quantitative evaluation for correct diagnosis in X-ray image interpretation-application of receiver operating characteristics (ROC) curve and information capacity. *The National Institute of Radiological Sciences,* Chiba, 51, (6), 24–30, 1976.

Ishida, M., Doi, K., Loo, L., Metz, C. E., Lehr, J. L. Digital image processing: Effect on detectability of simulated low-contrast radiographic patterns. *Radiology,* 150, (2), 569–575, 1984.

Ishida, M., Frank, P. H., Doi, K., Lehr, J. L. High quality digital radiographic images: Improved detection of low-contrast objects and preliminary clinical studies. *RadioGraphics,* 3, (2), 325–338, 1983.

Keeler, E. B. The value of a diagnostic test. The Rand Paper Series, P-5603, 1–15, 1976.

Kelsey, C. A., Moseley, R. D., Jr., Garcia, J. F., Mettler, F. A., Jr., Parker, T. W., and Juhl, J. H. ROC and contrast detail image evaluation tests compared. *Radiology,* 154, 629–631, 1985.

Kelsey, C. A., Moseley, R. D., Jr., Mettler, F. A., Jr., and Briscoe, D. E. Cost-effectiveness of stereoscopic radiographs in detection of lung nodules. *Radiology,* 142, (3), 611–613, 1982.

Kundel, H. L. Factors limiting roentgen interpretation—physical and psychologic. *Current Concepts in Radiology,* E. James Potchen, M. D. (ed.) St. Louis: The C. V. Mosby Company, 1–29, 1972.

Kundel, H. L. Images, image quality and observer performance. *Radiology,* 132, (2), 265–271, 1979.

Kundel, H. L., Revesz, G., and Stauffer, H. M. The electro-optical processing of radiographic images. *Radiological Clinics of North America,* 3, 447–460, 1969.

Lams, P. M., and Cocklin, M. L. Spatial resolution requirements for digital chest radiographs: An ROC study of observer performance in selected cases. *Radiology,* 158, (1), 11–19, 1986.

Ling, D., Ling, A. H., and Doehring, D. G. Stimulus, response, and observer variables in the auditory screening of newborn infants. *Journal of Speech and Hearing Research,* 13, 9–18, 1970.

Lusted, L. B. Receiver operating characteristic analysis and its significance in interpretation of radiologic images. *Current Concepts in Radiology, 2.* E. J. Potchen (ed.), C. V. Mosby Company, St. Louis, Missouri, 117–230, 1975.

Lusted, L. B. ROC Recollected. (Editorial), *Medical Decision Making,* 4, (2), 131–135, 1984.

Lusted, L. B. Twenty years of medical decision making studies. Presented at the *Third Annual Symposium for Computer Applications in Medical Care*, Silver Spring, Maryland, October, 1979. (To be published in the Conference Proceedings.)

Lusted, L. B. *Introduction to Medical Decision Making*. Springfield, Illinois: Charles C. Thomas, 1968.

Lusted, L. B. Perception of the roentgen image: applications of signal detectability theory. *Radiological Clinics of North America*, 3, 435–445, 1969.

Lusted, L. B. Signal detectability and medical decision making. *Science*, 171, 1217–1219, 1971.

Lusted, L. B. Decision making studies in patient management. *The New England Journal of Medicine*, 284, 416–424, 1971.

Lusted, L. B. Observer error, signal detectability, and medical decision making. In *Computer Diagnosis and Diagnostic Methods*, J. A. Jacquez (Ed.), C. C. Thomas, Springfield, Ill., 29–44, 1972.

MacMahon, H., Vyborny, C. J., Metz, C. E., Doi, K., Sabeti, V., and Solomon, S. L. Digital radiography of subtle pulmonary abnormalities: An ROC study of the effect of pixel size on observer performance. *Radiology*, 158, (1), 21–26, 1986.

McNeil, B. J. Pitfalls in and requirements for evaluations of diagnostic technologies. National Center for Health Services Research, Research Proceedings Services, DHEW Pub. No. (PHS) 79-3254, 33–39, September, 1979.

McNeil, B. J., and Adelstein, S. J. Measures of clinical efficacy. The value of case finding in hypertensive renovascular disease. *The New England Journal of Medicine*, 293, (5), 221–226, 1975.

McNeil, B. J., Hanley, J. A. Statistical approaches to the analysis of receiver operating characteristic (ROC) curves. *Medical Decision Making*, 4, (2), 139–150, 1984.

McNeil, B. J., Hanley, J. A., Funkenstein, H. H., and Wallman, M. D. Paired receiver operating characteristic curves and the effect of history on radiographic interpretation. *Radiology*, 149, (1), 75–77, 1983.

McNeil, B. J., Weber, E., Harrison, D., and Hellman, S. Use of signal detection theory in examining the results of a contrast examination: A case study using the lymphongiogram. *Radiology*, 123, (3), 613–618, 1977.

Metz, C. E. Basic principles of ROC analysis. *Seminars in Nuclear Medicine*, VIII, (4), 283–298, 1978.

Metz, C. E. ROC methodology in radiologic imaging. *Investigative Radiology*, 21, 9, 720–733, 1986.

Metz, C. E., and Goodenough, D. J. Quantitative evaluation of human visual detection performance using empirical receiver operating characteristic curves. In *Information Processing in Scintigraphy*. C. E. Metz, S. M. Prizer, and G. L. Brownell (eds.). Oak Ridge, Tenn.: USERDA Technical Information Center, 140–145, 1975.

Metz, C. E., and Goodenough, D. J. On failure to improve observer performance with scan smoothing: A rebuttal. Letter to the Editor. *Journal of Nuclear Medicine*, 14, (11), 873–876, 1973.

Metz, C. E., Goodenough, D. J., and Rossman, K. Evaluation of receiver operating characteristic curve data in terms of information theory, with applications in radiography. *Radiology*, 109, (2), 297–303, 1973.

Metz, C. E., Hoffer, P. B., Lusted, L. B., and McCartney, W. H. Diagnosis of colon malignancy from measurement of serum carcinoembryonic antigen (CEA): Effects of threshold of abnormality and an alternative approach based upon likelihood ratio estimates. Center for Radiologic Image Research. Department of Radiology, The University of Chicago. (Submitted to *Cancer*, 1975.) (no publishing date)

Metz, C. E., Hoffer, P. B., McCartney, W. H., and Lusted, L. B. Likelihood ratios for diagnosis of colon malignancy from measurements of serum carcinoembryonic antigen. (Abstract) *Journal of Nuclear Medicine,* 16, 550, 1975.

Metz, C. E., Rossman, K., and Lusted, L. B. ROC analysis: A bridge between physical and diagnostic image quality? Presented at the Symposium of the Society of Photography Scientists and Engineers, Washington, D. C., October, 1974.

Metz, C. E., Starr, S. J., and Lusted, L. B. Observer performance in detecting multiple radiographic signals: Prediction and analysis using a generalized ROC approach. *Radiology,* 121, (2), 337–347, 1976.

Metz, C. E., Starr, S. J., and Lusted, L. B. Quantitative evaluation of medical imaging. In *Medical Radionuclide Imaging,* Vol. 1. Vienna, International Atomic Energy Agency, 491–504, 1977.

Metz, C. E., Starr, S. J., and Lusted, L. B. Quantitative evaluation of visual detection performance in medicine: ROC analysis and determination of diagnostic benefit. In *Medical Images,* G. A. Hayes (ed.). London: John Wiley and Sons, 220–241, 1977.

Metz, C. E., Starr, S. J., Lusted, L. B., and Rossman, K. Progress in evaluation of human observer visual detection performance using the ROC curve approach. In *Information Processing in Scintigraphy,* C. Raynaud and A. E. Todd-Pokropek, (eds.), Orsay, France: Commissariat a l'Energie Atomique, Departement de Biologie, Service Hospitalier Frederic Joliot, 420–439, 1975.

Metz, C. E., Tokars, R. P., Kronman, H. B., and Griem, M. L. Maximum likelihood estimation of dose-response parameters for therapeutic operating characteristic (TOC) analysis of carcinoma of the nasopharynx. *International Journal of Radiation Oncology, Biology, and Physics,* 8, (7), 1185–1192, 1982.

Mobley, W. H., Goldstein, I. L. The effects of payoff on the visual processing of dental radiographs. *Human Factors,* 20, (4), 385–390, 1978.

Morgan, R. H., Donner, M. W., Gayler, B. W., Margulies, S. I., Rao, P. S., and Wheeler, P. S. Decision processes and observer error in the diagnosis of pneumoconiosis by chest roentgenography. *American Journal Roentgenology, Radiology Therapy and Nuclear Medicine,* 117, 757–764, 1973.

Moskowitz, M., Milbrath, J., Gartside, P., Zermeno, A., and Mandel, D. Lack of efficacy of thermography as a screening tool for minimal and Stage I breast cancer. *The New England Journal of Medicine,* 295, 249–252, 1976.

Murakski, B. J. Psychological approaches to study the uremic state. Presented at The Conference on Adequacy of Dialysis, Monterey, California, March, 1974; sponsored by the Artificial Kidney-Chronic Uremia Program of the National Institute of Arthritis, Metabolism and Digestive Diseases, International Society of Nephrology, 1975.

Nishiyama, H., Lewis, J. T., Ashare, A. B., and Saenger, E. L. Interpretation of liver images: Do training and experience make a difference? *Journal of Nuclear Medicine,* 16, 11–16, 1975.

Oster, Z. H., Larson, S. M., Strauss, H. W., and Wagner, H. N., Jr. Analysis of liver scanning in a general hospital. *Journal of Nuclear Medicine,* 16, 450–453, 1975.

Panzer, R. J., Suchman, A. L., and Griner, P. F. Workup bias in prediction research. *Medical Decision Making,* 7, (2), 115–119, 1987.

Pozen, M. W., Lerner, D. J., D'Agostino, R. B., Belanger, A. J., and Buckley, S. A. differential effects of experience on house officers' admission diagnoses for patients with possible myocardial infarction. *Medical Decision Making,* 2, (1), 13–21, 1982.

Pullan, B. R., Ritchings, R. T., Isherwood, I., and Adams, J. E. Effect of smoothing brain scans: A study using receiver operating characteristic curves. *Journal of Computer Assisted Tomography*, 4, (1), 91–93, 1980.

Revesz, G., and Haas, C. Television display of radiographic images with superimposed simulated lesions. *Radiology*, 102, (1), 197–199, 1972.

Revesz, G., and Kundel, H. L. Effects of non-linearities on the television display of X-ray images. *Investigative Radiology*, 6, 315–320, 1971.

Revesz, G., and Kundel, H. L. Videodisc storage of radiographs. *Radiology*, 106, (1), 91–93, 1973.

Revesz, G., Kundel, H. L., and Graber, M. A. The influence of structured noise on the detection of radiologic abnormalities. Twenty-Second Annual Meeting of the Association of University Radiologists, New York, 479–486, May 1974.

Revesz, G., Shea, F. J., and Kundel, H. L. The effects of kilovoltage on diagnostic accuracy in chest radiography. *Radiology*, 142, (3), 615–618, 1982.

Ritchings, R. T., Isherwood, I., Pullan, B. R., and Kingsley, D. Receiver operating characteristic curves in the evaluation of hard copies of computed tomography scans. *Journal of Computer Assisted Tomography*, 3, (3), 423–425, 1979.

Swets, J. A. Signal detection in medical diagnosis. In *Computer Diagnosis and Diagnostic Methods*, J. A. Jacquez (Ed.), C. C. Thomas, Springfield, Ill., 8–28, 1972.

Rose, C. C., Murphy, J. G., and Schwartz, J. S. Performance of an index predicting the response of patients with acute bronchial asthma to intensive emergency department treatment. *The New England Journal of Medicine*, 310, (9), 573–577, 1984.

Sanderink, G. C. H. *Imaging characteristics in rotational panoramic radiography. Journal of the International Association of Dento-Maxillo-Facial Radiology*, Supplementum 9, ISSN 0349–490X, 1987.

Sheft, D. J., Jones, M. D., Brown, R. E., and Ross, S. E. Screening of chest roentgenograms by advanced roentgen technologists. *Radiology*, 94, (2), 427–429, 1970.

Simon, T. R., Neumann, R. L., Gorelick, F., Riley, C., Hoffer, P., and Gottschalk, A. Scintigraphic diagnosis of cirrhosis: A receiver operator characteristic analysis of the common interpretative criteria. *Radiology*, 138, (3), 723–726, 1981.

Starr, S. J., and Metz, C. E. ROC analysis of the efficacy of breast thermography when disease localization is required. Unpublished letter to the editor. *The New England Journal of Medicine*, 1976. (Moskowitz et al. July 1976 article.)

Starr, S. J., Metz, C. E., and Lusted, L. B. Comments on the generalization of receiver operating characteristic analysis to detection and localization tasks. *Physics in Medicine and Biology*, 22, 376–381, 1977.

Starr, S. J., Metz, C. E., Lusted, L. B., and Goodenough, D. J. Visual detection and localization of radiographic images. *Radiology*, 116, (3), 533–538, 1975.

Swensson, R. G. A two-stage detection model applied to skilled visual search by radiologists. *Perception and Psychophysics*, 27, (1), 11–16, 1980.

Swensson, R. G., Hessel, S. J., and Herman, P. G. Omissions in radiology: Faulty search or stringent reporting criteria? *Radiology*, 123, (3), 563–567, 1977.

Tierney, W. M., Fitzgerald, J., McHenry, R., Roth, B. J., Psaty, B., Stump, D. L., and Anderson, F. K. Physicians' estimates of the probability of myocardial infarction in emergency room patients with chest pain. *Medical Decision Making*, 6, (1), 12–17, 1986.

Tierney, W. M., McDonald, C. J., and McCabe, G. Serum potassium testing in diuretic-treated outpatients. A multivariate approach. *Medical Decision Making*, 5, 1, 89–104, 1985.

Tolles, W. E., Horvath, W. J., and Bostrom, R. C. A study of the quantitative characteristics of exfoliated cells from the female genital tract. I. Measurement methods and results. *Cancer*, 14, 437–454, 1961.

Tolles, W. E., Horvath, W. J., and Bostrom, R. C. A study of the quantitative characteristics of exfoliated cells from the female genital tract. II. Suitability of quantitative cytological measurements for automatic prescreening. *Cancer*, 14, 455–468, 1961.

Turner, D. A. An intuitive approach to receiver operating characteristic curve analysis. *Journal of Nuclear Medicine*, 19, (2), 213–220, 1978.

Turner, D. A. Scintillation camera versus rectilinear scanner for liver imaging. Letter to the Editor. *Journal of Nuclear Medicine*, 17, (5), 419–421, 1975.

Turner, D. A., Fordham, E. W., Pagano, J. V., Ali, A. A., Ramos, M. V., and Ramachandran, P. C. Brain scanning with the Anger multiplane tomographic scanner as a second examination. *Radiology*, 121, (1), 115–124, 1976.

Turner, D. A., Ramachandran, P. C., Ali, A. A., Fordham, E. W., and Ferry, T. A. Brain scanning with the Anger multiplane tomographic scanner as a primary examination. *Radiology*, 121, (1), 125–129, 1976.

Turner, R. G., Frazer, G. J., and Shepard, N. T. Formulating and evaluating audiological test protocols. *Ear and Hearing*, 5, 6, 321–330, 1984.

Turner, R. G., and Nielsen, D. W. Application of clinical decision analysis to audiological tests. *Ear and Hearing*, 5, 3, 125–133, 1984.

Turner, R. G., Shepard, N. T., and Frazer, G. J. Clinical performance of audiological and related diagnostic tests. *Ear and Hearing*, 5, 4, 187–194, 1984.

Uchida, I., Onai, Y., Ohashi, Y., Tomaru, T., and Irifune, T. Quantitative diagnosis of breast thermograms by a computer. *Nippon Acta Radiologica*, 30, 401–411, 1979.

Warren, R. C. Contrast and latitude of CT hard copy: An ROC study. *Radiology*, 141, (1), 139–145, 1981.

Winter, J. Computer assessment of observer performance by receiver operating characteristic curve and information theory. *Computers and Biomedical Research*, 15, 555–562, 1982.

MEMORY

Ackroff, J. M., and Rouse, R. O., Jr. TSD and coding in STM. *Psychonomic Science*, 21, 231–232, 1970.

Allen, L. R., and Garton, R. F. Detection and criterion change associated with different test contexts in recognition memory. *Perception and Psychophysics*, 6, 1–4, 1969.

Allen, L. R., and Garton, R. F. The influence of word-knowledge on the word-frequency effect in recognition memory. *Psychonomic Science*, 10, 401–402, 1968.

Allen, L. R., and Garton, R. F. Manipulation of study trials in recognition memory. *Perception and Psychophysics*, 7, 215–217, 1970.

Anderson, J. R., and Bower, G. H. Recognition and retrieval processes in free recall. *Psychological Review*, 79, 97–123, 1972.

Atkinson, R. C., and Wickens, T. D. Human memory and the concept of reinforcement. In *The Nature of Reinforcement*, Robert Glaser (Ed.), Academic Press, Inc., New York, 66–119, 1971.

Banks, W. P. Criterion change and response competition in unlearning. *Journal of Experimental Psychology*, 82, 216–223, 1969.

Banks, W. P. Signal detection theory and human memory. *Psychological Bulletin,* 74, 81–99, 1970.

Banks, W. P. Confidence-rated recall, d_r, and tests of Bernbach's finite-state theory in recall. *Psychological Bulletin,* 76, 151–152, 1971.

Barr-Brown, M., and White, M. J. Sex differences in recognition memory. *Psychonomic Science,* 25, 75–76, 1971.

Bartlett, J. C., Hurry, S., and Thorley, W. Typicality and familiarity of faces. *Memory and Cognition,* 12, (3), 210–228, 1984.

Berch, D. B. Effects of stimulus probability and information feedback on response biases in children's recognition memory. *Bulletin of the Psychonomic Society,* 10, (4), 328–330, 1977.

Bernbach, H. A. Processing strategies for recognition and recall. *Journal of Experimental Psychology,* 99, (3), 409–412, 1973.

Bernbach, H. A. Decision processes in memory. *Psychological Review,* 74, 462–480, 1967.

Bernbach, H. A. Invariance of d* in memory: response to Banks. *Psychological Bulletin,* 76, 149–150, 1971.

Blick, K. I. Decision and decay processes in the short-term memory for length. *Journal of Experimental Psychology,* 82, 224–230, 1969.

Chechile, R. A. Is d' a suitable measure of recognition memory "strength"? *Bulletin of the Psychonomic Society,* 12, (2), 152–154, 1978.

Clark, W. C., and Greenberg, D. B. Effect of stress, knowledge of results, and proactive inhibition on verbal recognition memory (d') and response criterion (L_X). *Journal of Personality & Social Psychology,* 17, 42–47, 1971.

Crowder, R. G. A common basis for auditory sensory storage in perception and immediate memory. *Perception and Psychophysics,* 31, (5) 477–483, 1982.

DaPolito, F., Barker, D., and Wiant, J. Context in semantic information retrieval. *Psychonomic Science,* 24, 180–182, 1971.

Divenyi, P. L., and Hirsh, I. J. The effect of blanking on the identification of temporal order in three-tone sequences. *Perception and Psychophysics,* 17, (3), 246–252, 1975.

Donaldson, W., and Glathe, H. Signal-detection analysis of recall and recognition memory. *Canadian Journal of Psychology/Review of Canadian Psychology,* 24, (1), 42–56, 1970.

Donaldson, W., and Murdock, B. B. Jr. Criterion change in continuous recognition memory. *Journal of Experimental Psychology,* 76, 325–330, 1968.

Dosher, B. A. The retrieval of sentences from memory: A speed-accuracy study. *Cognitive Psychology,* 8, 291–310, 1976.

Dusoir, T. Isobias curves in some detection tasks. *Perception and Psychophysics,* 33, (5) 403–412, 1983.

Elias, C. S., and Perfetti, C. A. Encoding task and recognition memory: The importance of semantic encoding. *Journal of Experimental Psychology,* 99, (2), 151–156, 1973.

Fischler, I., and Juola, J. F. Effects of repeated tests on recognition time for information in long-term memory. *Journal of Experimental Psychology,* 91, 54–58, 1971.

Fisk, A. D., and Schneider, W. Memory as a function of attention, level of processing, and automatization. *Journal of Experimental Psychology: Learning, Memory, and Cognition,* 10, (2), 181–197, 1984.

Freund, R. D., Brelsford, J. W., Jr., and Atkinson, R. C. Recognition vs. recall: storage or retrieval differences? *Quarterly Journal of Experimental Psychology,* 21, 214–224, 1969.

Freund, R. D. Loftus, G. R., and Atkinson, R. C. Applications of multiprocess models for memory to continuous recognition tasks. *Journal of Mathematical Psychology,* 6, 576–594, 1969.

Friedman, M. P., Reed, S. K., and Carterette, E. C. Feature saliency and recognition memory for schematic faces. *Perception and Psychophysics,* 10, 47–50, 1971.

Gibson, K. L. Criterion shifts and the determination of the memory operating characteristic. *Psychonomic Science,* 9, 207–208, 1967.

Gillund, G., and Shiffrin, R. M. A retrieval model for both recognition and recall. *Psychological Review,* 91, (1), 1–67, 1984.

Grasha, A. F. Detection theory and memory processes: Are they compatible? *Perceptual and Motor Skills,* 30, 123–135, 1970.

Healy, A. F., and Kubovy, M. A comparison of recognition memory to numerical decision: How prior probabilities affect cutoff location. *Memory and Cognition,* 5, (1), 3–9, 1977.

Healy, A. F., and Kubovy, M. The effects of payoffs and prior probabilities on indices of performance and cutoff location in recognition memory. *Memory and Cognition,* 6, (5), 544–553, 1978.

Hockley, W. E., and Murdock, B. B., Jr. A decision model for accuracy and response latency in recognition memory. *Psychological Review,* 94, (3), 341–358, 1987.

Hopkins, R. H., and Schulz, R. W. Meaningfulness in paired-associate recognition learning. *Journal of Experimental Psychology,* 79, 533–539, 1969.

Kausler, D. H., Pavur, E. J., Jr., and Yadrick, R. M. Single-item recognition following a verbal discrimination study trial. *Memory and Cognition,* 3, (2), 135–139, 1975.

Kinchla, R. A., and Smyzer, F. A diffusion model of perceptual memory. *Perception and Psychophysics,* 2, (6), 219–229, 1967.

Kinchla, R. A. Selective processes in sensory memory: A probe-comparison procedure. In *Attention and Performance IV,* S. Kornblum (Ed.), Academic Press, New York, 87–99, 1973.

Kintsch, W. Memory and decision aspects of recognition learning. *Psychological Review,* 74, 496–504, 1967.

Kintsch, W. An experimental analysis of single stimulus tests and multiple-choice tests of recognition memory. *Journal of Experimental Psychology,* 76, 1–6, 1968.

Klatzky, R. L., and Loftus, G. R. Recognition memory as influenced by number of reinforcements and type of test. *Psychonomic Science,* 16, 302–303, 1969.

Kolers, P. A. Addendum to "Remembering operations." *Memory and Cognition,* 3, (1), 29–30, 1975.

Kolers, P. A. Remembering operations. *Memory and Cognition, 1,* 347–355, 1973.

Kounios, J., Osman, A. M., and Meyer, D. E. Structure and process in semantic memory: New evidence based on speed-accuracy decomposition. *Journal of Experimental Psychology: General,* 116, (1), 3–25, 1987.

Loftus, G. R. Comparison of recognition and recall in a continuous memory task. *Journal of Experimental Psychology,* 91, 220–226, 1971.

Lockhart, R. S., and Murdock, B. B., Jr. Memory and the theory of signal detection. *Psychological Bulletin,* 74, 100–109, 1970.

Marley, A. A. J. An observable property of a generalization of Kinchla's diffusion model of perceptual memory. *Journal of Mathematical Psychology,* 8, 481–488, 1971.

Massaro, D. W. The role of the decision system in sensory and memory judgments. *Perception and Psychophysics,* 5, 270–272, 1969.

McCormack, P. D., and Swenson, A. L. Recognition memory for common and rare words. *Journal of Experimental Psychology*, 95, (1), 72–77, 1972.

McNicol, D., and Ryder, L. A. Sensitivity and response bias effects in the learning of familiar and unfamiliar associations by rote or with mnemonic. *Journal of Experimental Psychology*, 90, 81–89, 1971.

Miller, J. D., and Tanis, D. C. Recognition memory for common sounds. *Psychonomic Science*, 23, 307–308, 1971.

Murdock, B. B., Jr. Serial order effects in short-term memory, *Journal of Experimental Psychology*, Monograph supplement, 76, 1–15, 1968.

Murdock, B. B., Jr. A theory for the storage and retrieval of item and associative information. *Psychological Review*, 89, 6, 609–626, 1982.

Murdock, B. B., Jr., and Duffy, P. O. Strength theory and recognition memory. *Journal of Experimental Psychology*, 94, (3), 284–290, 1972.

Nicol, E. H., Roby, T. B., Farrell, F. M. Confidence in recall in paired-associate learning experiments. Technical Report No. ESD-TR-67-457, Decision Sciences Lab., Electronic Systems Div., U.S. Air Force, Hanscom Field, Bedford, Mass., 1967.

Norman, D. A. Acquisition and retention in short-term memory. *Journal of Experimental Psychology*, 72, 369–381, 1966.

Norman, D. A., and Wickelgren, W. A. Strength theory of decision rules and latency in retrieval from short-term memory. *Journal of Mathematical Psychology*, 6, 192–208, 1969.

Pappas, B. A., Hepburn, L. K., and Suboski, M. D. A comparison of recall and binary recognition. *American Journal of Psychology*, 80, 398–404, 1967.

Pike, R., Dalgleish, L., and Wright, J. A multiple-operations model for response latency and the latencies of correct and incorrect responses in recognition memory. *Memory and Cognition*, 5, (5), 580–589, 1977.

Raser, G. A. Meaningfulness and signal-detection theory in immediate paired-associate recognition. *Journal of Experimental Psychology*, 84, 173–175, 1970.

Ratcliff, R., and Murdock, B. B., Jr. Retrieval processes in recognition memory. *Psychological Review*, 83, (3), 190–214, 1976.

Rundle, S. A. An experimental and theoretical study of recognition memory. Tech. Report No. 33, Department of Psychology, University of California, Los Angeles, July, 1970.

Schulman, A. I. Word length and rarity in recognition memory. *Psychonomic Science*, 9, 211–212, 1967.

Schulman, A. I. Recognition memory for targets from a scanned word list. *British Journal of Psychology*, 62, 335–346, 1971.

Schulman, A. I., and Lovelace, E. A. Recognition memory for words presented at a slow or rapid rate. *Psychonomic Science*, 21, 99–100, 1970.

Smith, P. T. The non-monotonicity of the psychometric function in recognition memory. *Perception and Psychophysics*, 5, 329–337, 1969.

Snodgrass, J. G., and Burns, P. M. The effect of repeated tests on recognition memory for pictures and words. *Bulletin of the Psychonomic Society*, 11, (4), 263–266, 1978.

Soli, S. D., and Balch, W. R. Performance biases and recognition memory for semantic and formal changes in connected discourse. *Memory and Cognition*, 4, (6), 673–676, 1976.

Sperling, G. A signal-to-noise theory of the effects of luminance on picture memory: Comment on Loftus. *Journal of Experimental Psychology: General*, 115, (2), 189–192, 1986.

Suboski, M. D. Signal detection analysis of recall paired-associates learning. *Psychonomic Science,* 7, 357–358, 1967.

Swets, J. A. Signal detection as a model of information retrieval. In *The Simulation of Human Behavior,* F. Bresson and M. deMontmollin, (Eds.), Dunod, Paris, 253–264, 1969.

Treisman, M., and Rostron, A. B. Brief auditory storage: A modification of Sperling's paradigm applied to audition. *Acta Psychologica,* 36, 161–170, 1972.

Tulving, E., and Madigan, S. A. Memory and verbal learning. *Annual Review of Psychology,* 21, 437–484, 1970.

Vorberg, D., and Schmidt, R. Theoretical Note: A testable property of some discrete-state models for recognition memory. *Psychological Review,* 82, (4), 316–342, 1975.

Welford, A. T. Signal, noise, performance, and age. *Human Factors,* 23, (1), 97–109, 1981.

Wickelgren, W. A. Consolidation and retroactive interference in short-term recognition memory for pitch. *Journal of Experimental Psychology,* 72, 250–259, 1966.

Wickelgren, W. A. Numerical relations, similarity, and short-term recognition memory for pairs of digits. *British Journal of Psychology,* 57, 263–274, 1966.

Wickelgren, W. A. Exponential decay and independence from irrelevant associations in short-term recognition memory for serial order. *Journal of Experimental Psychology,* 73, 165–171, 1967.

Wickelgren, W. A. Sparing of short-term memory in an amnexic patient: implications for strength theory of memory. *Neuropsychologica,* 6, 235–244, 1968.

Wickelgren, W. A. Associative strength theory of recognition memory for pitch. *Journal of Mathematical Psychology,* 6, 13–61, 1969.

Wickelgren, W. A. Time, interference, and rate of presentation in short-term recognition memory for items. *Journal of Mathematical Psychology,* 7, 219–235, 1970.

Wickelgren, W. A. Trace resistance and the decay of long-term memory. *Journal of Mathematical Psychology,* 9, 418–455, 1972.

Wickelgren, W. A., and Berian, K. M. Dual trace theory and the consolidation of long-term memory. *Journal of Mathematical Psychology,* 8, 404–417, 1971.

Wickelgren, W. A., and Norman, D. A. Invariance of forgetting rate with number of repetitions in verbal short-term recognition memory. *Psychonomic Science,* 22, 363–364, 1971.

Wickelgren, W. A., and Whitman, P. T. Visual very-short-term memory is non-associative. *Journal of Experimental Psychology,* 84, 277–281, 1970.

Wood, L. E. An objective test of goodness of fit of the continuous strength model in STM. *Perception and Psychophysics,* 9, 424–426, 1971.

Young, R. K., Saegert, J., and Linsley, D. Retention as a function of meaningfulness. *Journal of Experimental Psychology,* 78, 89–94, 1968.

METHODS AND MEASURES

Abramson, I. G., and Levitt, H. Statistical analysis of data from experiments in human signal detection. *Journal of Mathematical Psychology,* 6, 391–417, 1969.

Altham, P. M. A non-parametric measure of signal discriminability. *British Journal of Mathematical and Statistical Psychology,* 26, (1), 1–12, 1973.

Anderson, C. M. B., and Stephens, S. D. G. Automated psychophysical signal detection equipment. Report No. Ac36, National Physical Laboratory, Teddington, Middlesex, U. K., March, 1969.

Baker, E. M., and Schuck, J. R. Theoretical Note: Use of signal detection theory to clarify problems of evaluating performance in industry. *Organizational Behavior and Human Performance,* 13, 307–317, 1975.

Bamber, D. The area of the ordinal dominance graph and the area below the receiver operating characteristic graph. *Journal of Mathematical Psychology,* 12, (4), 387–415, 1975.

Bell, D. W., and Nixon, J. C. Reliability of ratings in an auditory signal-detection experiment. *Journal of the Acoustical Society of America,* 49, 435–439, 1971.

Bookstein, A. The anomalous behavior of precision in the Swets' model, and its resolution. *Recall and Precision,* 30, (4), 374–380, 1974.

Brookes, B. C. The measures of information retrieval effectiveness proposed by Swets. *Journal of Documentation,* 24, 41–54, 1968.

Brown, J., and Routh, D. A. Recognition assessed by d' and by a nonparametric alternative (the A-index) as a function of the number of choices. *Quarterly Journal of Experimental Psychology,* 22, 707–719, 1970.

Bunch, P. C., Hamilton, J. F., Sanderson, G. K., and Simmons, A. H. A free-response approach to the measurement and characterization of radiographic-observer performance. *Journal of Applied Photographic Engineering,* 4, (4), 166–171, 1978.

Caldeira, J. D. Parametric assumptions of some "nonparametric" measures of sensory efficiency. *Human Factors,* 22, (1), 119–120, 1980.

Calfee, R. C. Effects of payoff on detection in a symmetric auditory detection task. *Perceptual and Motor Skills,* 31, 895–901, 1970.

Carmon, J. L. A discriminant function index for information system evaluation. *Journal of the American Society for Information Sciences,* 118–122, 1974.

Centor, R. M. A visicalc program for estimating the area under a receiver operating characteristic (ROC) curve. *Medical Decision Making,* 5, (2), 139–148, 1985.

Centor, R. M., and Schwartz, J. S. An evaluation of methods for estimating the area under the receiver operating characteristic (ROC) curve. *Medical Decision Making,* 5, (2), 149–156, 1985.

Clark, W. C. The effect of information feedback and reference tones on d' and L_X: A further analysis of Nash and Adamson's data. *Psychonomic Science,* 16, 93–94, 1969.

Clark, W. C., and Mehl, L. Signal detection theory procedures are not equivalent when thermal stimuli are judged. *Journal of Experimental Psychology,* 97, 148–153, 1973.

Cooper, W. S. On selecting a measure of retrieval effectiveness. *Journal of the American Society for Information Sciences,* 87–100, 1974.

Cooper, W. S. On selecting a measure of retrieval effectiveness. Part II. Implementation of the philosophy. *Journal of the American Society for Information Sciences,* 413–424, 1974.

Dorfman, D. D., Beavers, L. L., and Saslow, C. Estimation of signal detection theory parameters from rating-method data: A comparison of the method of scoring and direct search. *Bulletin of the Psychonomic Society, 1,* 207–208, 1973.

Dorfman, D. D., and Berbaum, K. S. Computer technology: RSCORE-J: Pooled rating-method data: A computer program for analyzing pooled ROC curves. *Behavior Research Methods, Instruments, & Computers,* 18, (5), 452–462, 1986.

Dorfman, D. D., and Alf, E., Jr. Maximum likelihood estimation of parameters of signal detection theory—a direct solution. *Psychometrika,* 33, 117–124, 1968.

Dorfman, D. D., and Alf, E., Jr. Maximum likelihood estimation of parameters of signal-detection theory and determination of confidence intervals—rating method data. *Journal of Mathematical Psychology*, 6, 487–496, 1969.

Dorosh, M. E., Tong, J. E., and Boissonneault, D. R. White noise, instructions, and two-flash fusion with two signal-detection procedures. *Psychonomic Science*, 20, 98–99, 1970.

Dusoir, A. E. Treatments of bias in detection and recognition models: A review. *Perception and Psychophysics*, *17*, (2), 167–178, 1975.

Dusoir, T. Isobias curves in some detection tasks. *Perception and Psychophysics*, 33, (5), 403–412, 1983.

Egan, J. P. Two types of ROC curves. (Paper), Hearing and Communication Laboratory, Indiana University, Bloomington, Indiana, 1–17, 1960.

Emmerich, D. S. Receiver-operating characteristics determined under several interaural conditions of listening. *Journal of the Acoustical Society of America*, 43, 298–307, 1968.

Emmerich, D. S. ROCs obtained with two signal intensities presented in random order, and a comparison between yes-no and rating ROCs. *Perception and Psychophysics*, 3, 35–40, 1968.

Farradane, J. The evaluation of information retrieval systems. *Journal of Documentation*, 30, (2), 195–209, 1974.

Friedman, M. P., Carterette, E. C., Nakatani, L., and Ahumada, A., Jr. Feedback and frequency variables in signal detection. Technical Report No. 30, Department of Psychology, Human Communication Laboratory, University of California, Los Angeles, 1968.

Frijters, J. E. R. Three-stimulus procedures in olfactory psychophysics: An experimental comparison of Thurstone-Ura and three-alternative forced-choice models of signal detection theory. *Perception and Psychophysics*, 28, (5), 390–397, 1980.

Galanter, E., and Holman, G. L. Some invariances of the isosensitivity function and their implications for the utility function of money. *Journal of Experimental Psychology*, 73, 333–339, 1967.

Gardner, R. M., MacFee, M., and Krinsky, R. A comparison of binary and rating techniques in the signal detection analysis of recognition memory. *Acta Psychologica*, *39*, 13–19, 1975.

Gescheider, G. A., Herman, D. D., and Phillips, J. N. Criterion shifts in the measurement of tactile masking. *Perception and Psychophysics*, 8, 433–436, 1970.

Goodenough, D. J., and Metz, C. E. Effect of listening interval on auditory detection performance. *Journal of the Acoustical Society of America*, 55, (1), 111–116, 1974.

Goolkasian, P., and Dorfman, D. Discrimination measures in an ROC analysis of pain reactions. *Perception and Psychophysics*, 35, (3), 291–292, 1984.

Goranson, R. E., and Theodor, L. H. Optimal percent correct measures in recognition memory. *Perceptual and Motor Skills*, 31, 848, 1970.

Gourevitch, V., and Galanter, E. A significance test for one-parameter isosensitivity functions. *Psychometrika*, 32, 25–34, 1967.

Green, D. M., and Luce, R. D. Detection of auditory signals presented at random times. *Perception and Psychophysics*, 2, (19), 441–450, 1967.

Green, D. M., and Luce, R. D. Detection of auditory signals presented at random times: III. *Perception and Psychophysics*, 9, (3a), 257–268, 1971.

Green, D. M., and Weber, D. L. Detection of temporally uncertain signals. *Journal of the Acoustical Society of America*, 67, (4), 1304–1311, 1980.

Greenes, R. A., Begg, C. B., Cain, K. C., Swets, J. A., Feehrer, C. E., and McNeil, B. J. Patient-oriented performance measures of diagnostic tests. *Medical Decision Making*, 4, (1), 17–31, 1984.

Grey, D. R., and Morgan, B. J. T. Some aspects of ROC curve-fitting: Normal and logistic models. *Journal of Mathematical Psychology*, 9, 128–139, 1972.

Grier, J. B. Nonparametric indexes for sensitivity and bias: Computing formulas. *Psychological Bulletin*, 75, 424–429, 1971.

Gummerman, K. A response-contingent measure of proportion correct. *Journal of the Acoustical Society of America*, 52, 1645–1647, 1972.

Hacker, M. J., and Ratcliff, R. A revised table of d' for M-alternative forced choice. *Perception and Psychophysics*, 26, (2), 168–170, 1979.

Hammerton, M., and Altham, P. M. E. A non-parametric alternative to d'. *Nature*, 234, 487–488, 1971.

Hanley, J. A., and McNeil, B. J. The meaning and use of the area under a receiver operating characteristic (ROC) curve. *Radiology*, 143, (1), 29–36, 1982.

Healy, A. F. Can subjects maintain a constant criterion in a memory task? *Memory and Cognition*, 3, (3), 233–238, 1975.

Healy, A. F., and Jones, C. Criterion shifts in recall. *Psychological Bulletin*, 79, 335-340, 1973.

Heine, M. H. The inverse relationship of precision and recall in terms of the Swets model. *Journal of Documentation*, 29, 81–84, 1973.

Heine, M. H. distance between sets as an objective measure of retrieval effectiveness. *Information Storage and Retrieval*, 9, 181–198, 1973.

Heine, M. H. Design equations for retrieval systems based on Swets model. *Journal of the American Society for Information Sciences*, 183–198, 1974.

Heine, M. H. Measures of language effectiveness and Swetsian hypotheses. *Journal of Documentation*, 31, (4), 283–287, 1975.

Hershman, R. L., and Small, D. Tables of d' for detection and localization. *Perception and Psychophysics*, 3, 321–323, 1968.

Herzog, T. R. Effects of amount and kind of prior target-uncertainty reduction in the repeated presentations paradigm. *Perception and Psychophysics*, 10, 273–277, 1971.

Hochhaus, L. Correct response discrimination as a function of multiple recognition choices: effect of correct guessing on type II d'. *Journal of Experimental Psychology*, 84, 458–461, 1970.

Hochhaus, L. A table for the calculation of d' and β. *Psychological Bulletin*, 77, 375–376, 1973.

Hochhaus, L. A table for the calculation of d' and beta'. *Psychological Bulletin*, 77, (5), 375–376, 1972.

Hodos, W. Nonparametric index of response bias for use in detection and recognition experiments. *Psychological Bulletin*, 74, 351–354, 1970.

Holloway, C. M. The effects of response bias in two-alternative-forced-choice discrimination matrices. *Behavioral Research Methods and Instrumentation*, 1, 175–178, 1969.

Hutchinson, T. P. An extension of the signal detection model of information retrieval. *Journal of Documentation*, 34, (1), 51–54, 1978.

Hutchinson, T. P. On the relevance of signal detection theory to the correction for guessing. *Contemporary Educational Psychology*, 2, 50–54, 1977.

Ingham, J. G. Individual differences in signal detection. *Acta Psychologica*, 34, 39–51, 1970.

Ingleby, J. D. Further studies of the human observer as statistical decision maker. *Organizational Behavior and Human Performance,* 12, 299–314, 1974.

Johnson, D. M., Watson, C. S., and Kelly, W. J. Performance differences among the intervals in forced-choice tasks. *Perception and Psychophysics,* 35, (6), 553–557, 1984.

Kaplan, H. L., Macmillan, N. A., and Creelman, C. D. Tables of d' for variable-standard discrimination paradigms. *Behavioral Research Methods and Instrumentation,* 10, (6), 796–813, 1978.

Katz, L. A. A comparison of type II operating characteristics derived from confidence ratings and from latencies. *Perception and Psychophysics,* 8, 65–68, 1970.

Kay, E., and Weber, J. Detection in a four-observation two-channel task. *Perception and Psychophysics,* 17, (4), 425–428, 1975.

Keen, E. M. Evaluation parameters. *The Smart Retrieval System: Experiments in Automatic Document Processing.* Salton, G., (Ed.). New Jersey, Englewood: Prentice Hall, 74–111, 1971.

King, D. W., and Bryant, E. C. (eds.). The evaluation of information services and products. In *Measures for Evaluating Identification Systems.* Washington, D. C.: Information Resources Press, 20–35, 1971.

Kraft, D. H. A decision theory view of the information retrieval situation: An operations research approach. *Journal of the American Society for Information Science,* 368–376, 1973.

Kraft, D. H., and Bookstein, A. Evaluation of information retrieval systems: A decision theory approach. *Journal of the American Society for Information Science,* 31–40, 1978.

Kraft, D. H., and Hill, T. W., Jr. A journal selection model and its implications for a library system. *Information Storage and Retrieval,* 9, 1–11, 1973.

LaBerge, D. Effect of type of catch trial upon generalization gradients of reaction time. *Journal of Experimental Psychology,* 87, 225–228, 1971.

Leshowitz, B. Receiver operating characteristics and psychometric functions determined under simple- and pedestal-detection conditions. *Journal of the Acoustical Society of America,* 45, 1474–1484, 1969.

Leshowtiz, B. Comparison of ROC curves from one- and two-interval rating-scale procedures. *Journal of the Acoustical Society of America,* 46, 399–402, 1969.

Lippmann, R. P., Braida, L. D., and Durlach, N. I. Intensity perception versus effect of payoff matrix on absolute identification. *Journal of the Acoustical Society of America,* 59, (1), 129–134, 1976.

Long, G. M. Limitations on the practical applicability of d' and beta measures. *Human Factors,* 23, (3), 285–290, 1981.

Luce, R. D. A model for detection in temporally unstructured experiments with a poisson distribution of signal presentation. *Journal of Mathematical Psychology,* 3, 48–64, 1966.

Luce, R. D., and Green, D. M. Detection of auditory signals presented at random times, II. *Perception and Psychophysics,* 7, (1), 1–14, 1970.

Macmillan, N. A., and Kaplan, H. L. Detection theory analysis of group data: Estimating sensitivity from average hit and false alarm rates. *Psychological Bulletin,* 98, (1), 185–199, 1985.

Marascuilo, L. A. Extensions of the significance test for one-parameter signal detection hypotheses. *Psychometrika,* 35, 237–243, 1970.

McCarthy, D., and Davison, M. Towards a behavioral theory of bias in signal detection. *Perception and Psychophysics,* 29, (4), 371–382, 1981.

McFadden, D. Three computational versions of proportion correct for use in forced-choice experiments. *Perception and Psychophysics*, 8, 336–342, 1970.

Metz, C. E., and Kronman, H. B. Statistical significance tests for binormal ROC curves. *Journal of Mathematical Psychology*, 22, (3), 218–243, 1980.

Miles, J. Eliminating the guessing factor in the multiple choice test. *Educational and Psychological Measurement*, 33, 637–651, 1973.

Miller, H. The FROC curve: A representation of the observer's performance for the method of free response. *Journal of the Acoustical Society of America*, 46, 1473–1476, 1969.

Morgan, B. J. T. Measurement of signal detectability. *Nature*, 239, 174, 1973.

Morgan, B. J. T., Woodhead, M. M., and Webster, J. C. On the recovery of physical dimensions of stimuli, using multidimensional scaling. *Journal of the Acoustical Society of America*, 60, (1), 186–189, 1976.

Nachmias, J. Effects of presentation probability and number of response alternatives on simple visual detection. *Perception and Psychophysics*, 3, 151–155, 1968.

Nash, A., and Adamson, R. Effects of information feedback and reference tones on signal detection. *Psychonomic Science*, 13, 301–302, 1968.

Ogilvie, J. C., and Creelman, C. D. Maximum likelihood estimation of receiver operating characteristic curve parameters. *Journal of Mathematical Psychology*, 5, 377–391, 1968.

Pastore, R. E., and Sorkin, R. D. Adaptive auditory signal processing. *Psychonomic Science*, 23, 259–260, 1971.

Penner, M. J. The effect of payoffs and cue tones on detection of sinusoids of uncertain frequency. *Perception and Psychophysics*, 11, 198–202, 1972.

Pollack, I., and Hsieh, R. Sampling variability of the area under the ROC-curve and of d'_e. *Psychological Bulletin*, 71, 161–173, 1969.

Polzella, D. J., and Gouse, A. S. Psychic: A BASIC game to test ESP as d'. *Behavioral Research Methods and Instrumentation*, 10, (3), 426–428, 1978.

Reed, C. M., and Bilger, R. C. A comparative study of S/N_0 and E/N_0. *Journal of the Acoustical Society of America*, 53, 1039–1044, 1973.

Richardson, J. T. E. Nonparametric indexes of sensitivity and response bias. *Psychological Bulletin*, 78, (6), 429–432, 1972.

Robertson, S. E. A statistical analysis of retrieval tests: A Bayesian approach. *Journal of Documentation*, 30, (3), 273–282, 1974.

Robertson, S. E. the parametric description of retrieval tests. I. The basic parameters. *Journal of Documentation*, 25, 1–27, 1969.

Robertson, S. E. The parametric description of retrieval tests. II. Overall measures. *Journal of Documentation*, 25, 93–107, 1969.

Robinson, D. E., and Watson, C. S. Psychophysical methods in modern psychoacoustics. In *Foundations of Modern Auditory Theory*, J. V. Tobias (Ed.), Academic Press, New York, 101–131, 1972.

Rose, R. M., Teller, D. Y., and Rendleman, P. Statistical properties of staircase estimates. *Perception and Psychophysics*, 8, 199–204, 1970.

Sakitt, B. Canonical ratings. *Perception and Psychophysics*, 16, (3), 478–488, 1974.

Sakitt, B. Indices of discriminability. *Nature*, 241, 133, 1973.

Schulman, A. I., and Greenberg, G. Z. Operating characteristics and a priori probability of the signal. *Perception and Psychophysics*, 8, 317–320, 1970.

Schulman, A. I., and Mitchell, R. R. Operating characteristics from yes-no and forced-choice procedures. *Journal of the Acoustical Society of America*, 40, 473–477, 1966.

Semb, G., and Saslow, M. G. Conformity to experimenter-determined payoff-enforced criterion levels in the method of random staircases. *Perception and Psychophysics*, 2, 396–398, 1967.

Shipley, E. F. A signal detection theory analysis of a category judgment experiment. *Perception and Psychophysics*, 7, 38–42, 1970.

Simpson, A. J., and Fitter, M. J. What is the best index of detectability? *Psychological Bulletin*, 80, (6), 481–488, 1973.

Smith, J. E. K. Simple algorithms for M-alternative forced-choice calculations. *Perception and Psychophysics*, 31, (1), 95–96, 1982.

Smith, J. E. K. Some simplified indices of sensitivity and bias. Michigan Mathematical Psychology Program: MMPP 74-5, University of Michigan, Ann Arbor, Michigan, 1974.

Smith, K. A note on the standard error of the estimates of TSD parameters from "Yes-No" experiments. Michigan Mathematical Psychology Program: MMPP 69-8, University of Michigan, Ann Arbor, Michigan, 1969.

Swanson, D. R. On indexing depth and retrieval effectiveness. Proceedings of the 2nd Congress on Information Systems Sciences, Washington, D. C.: Spartan, 311–319, 1965.

Swets, J. A., and Markowitz, J. Factors affecting the slope of empirical ROC curves: Comparison of binary and rating response. *Perception and Psychophysics*, 2, 15–28, 1967.

Thomas, E. A. C. Sufficient conditions for monotone hazard rate: An application to latency-probability curves. *Journal of Mathematical Psychology*, 8, 303–332, 1971.

Tostesan, A. N. A., and Begg, C. B. A general regression methodology for ROC curve estimation. Technical Report 525z. Department of Biostatistics, Dana-Farber Cancer Institute, Boston, MA, February 1987.

Treisman, M. On the use and misuse of psychophysical terms. *Psychological Review*, 83, (3), 246–256, 1976.

Uebersax, J. S. Diversity of decision making models and the measurement of interrater agreement. *Psychological Bulletin*, 101, (1), 140–146, 1987.

Veldon, M., and Clark, W. C. Reduction of rating scale data by means of signal detection theory. *Perception and Psychophysics*, 25, (6), 517–518, 1979.

Viemeister, N. F. Intensity discrimination: Performance in three paradigms. *Perception and Psychophysics*, 8, 417–419, 1970.

von Winterfeldt, D., and Edwards, W. Costs and payoffs in perceptual research. *Psychological Bulletin*, 91, (3), 609–622, 1982.

Watson, C. S., Kellogg, S. C., Kawanishi, D. T., and Lucas, P. A. The uncertain response in detection-oriented psychophysics. *Journal of Experimental Psychology*, 99, (2), 180–185, 1973.

Watson, C. S., and Clopton, B. M. Motivated changes of auditory sensitivity in a simple detection task. *Perception and Psychophysics*, 5, 281–287, 1969.

Weir, C. C., Jesteadt, W., and Green, D. M. A comparison of method-of-adjustment and forced-choice procedures in frequency discrimination. *Perception and Psychophysics*, 19, (1), 75–79, 1976.

Winter, J. Computer assessment of observer performance by receiver operating characteristic curve and information theory. *Computers and Biomedical Research*, 15, 555–562, 1982.

Zimmerman, J., and Kimble, G. A. Effects of incentive on false recognition. *Journal of Experimental Psychology*, 97, (2), 264–266, 1973.

MINOR SENSES

Angus, R. C., and Daniel, T. C. Applying theory of signal detection in marketing: Product development and evaluation. *American Journal of Agricultural Economics*, 56, 573–577, 1974.

Berglund, B., Berglund, U., and Lindvall, T. A psychological detection method in environmental research. *Environmental Research*, 7, 342–352, 1974.

Berglund, B., Berglund, U., Engen, T., and Lindvall, T. The effect of adaption on odor detection. *Perception and Psychophysics*, 9, 435–438, 1971.

Boyer, W. N., Cross, H. A., Guyot, G. W., and Washington, D. M. A TSD determination of a DL using two-point tactual stimuli applied to the back. *Psychonomic Science*, 21, 195–196, 1970.

Berlin, F. S., Bartlett, R. L., and Black, J. D. Acupuncture and placebo: Effects on delaying the terminating response to a painful stimulus. *Anesthesiology*, 42, (5), 527–531, 1975.

Cain, W. S. Differential sensitivity for smell: "Noise" at the nose. *Science*, 195, 796–798, 1977.

Chapman, C. R. An alternative to threshold assessment in the study of human pain. In *Advances in Neurology*. New York: Raven Press, 115–126, 1974.

Chapman, C. R. Sensory decision theory methods in pain research: A reply to Rollman. *Pain*, 3, 295–305, 1977.

Chapman, C. R., Chen, A. C., and Bonica, J. J. Effects of intrasegmental electrical acupuncture on dental pain: Evaluation by threshold estimation and sensory decision theory. *Pain*, 3, 213–227, 1977.

Chapman, C. R., and Feather, B. W. Effects of diazepam on human pain tolerance and pain sensitivity. *Psychological Medicine*, 35, (4), 330–340, 1973.

Chapman, C. R., Murphy, T. M., and Butler, S. H. Analgesic strength of 33 percent nitrous oxide: A signal detection theory evaluation. *Science*, 179, 1246–1248, 1973.

Clark, W. C. Pain sensitivity and the report of pain: An introduction to sensory decision theory. *Anesthesiology*, 40, (3), 272–286, 1974.

Clark, W. C., and Goodman, J. S. Effects of suggestion on d' and Cx for pain detection and pain tolerance. *Journal of Abnormal Psychology*, 83, (4), 364–372, 1974.

Clark, W. C., and Yang, J. C. Acupunctural analgesia? Evaluation by signal detection theory. *Science*, 184, 1096–1098, 1974.

Clark, W. C. Sensory-decision theory analysis of the placebo effect on the criterion for pain and thermal sensitivity (d'). *Journal of Abnormal Psychology*, 74, 363–371, 1969.

Clark, W. C., and Dillon, D. J. SDT analysis of binary decisions and sensory intensity ratings to noxious thermal stimuli. *Perception and Psychophysics*, 13, 491–493, 1973.

Clark, W. C., and Mehl, L. A sensory decision theory analysis of the effect of age and sex on d', various response criteria, and 50% pain threshold, *Journal of Abnormal Psychology*, 78, 202–212, 1971.

Corbit, T. E., and Engen, T. Facilitation of olfactory detection. *Perception and Psychophysics*, 10, 433–436, 1971.

Cox, R. H., and Hawkins, H. L. Application of the theory of signal detectability to kinesthetic discrimination tasks. *Journal of Motor Behavior*, 8, (3), 225–232, 1976.

Craig, J. C. Vibratory temporal integration as a function of pattern discriminability. *Perception and Psychophysics*, 35, (6), 579–582, 1984.

Cross, H. A., Boyer, W. N., and Guyot, G. W. Determination of a DL using two-point tactual stimuli: A signal-detection approach. *Psychonomic Science*, 21, 198–199, 1970.

Dyhre-Poulsen, P. Increased vibration threshold before movements in human subjects. *Experimental Neurology*, 47, 516–522, 1975.

Engen, T., Kuisma, J. E., and Eismas, P. D. Short-term memory of odors. *Journal of Experimental Psychology*, 99, (2), 222–225, 1973.

Feather, B. W., Chapman, C. R., and Fisher, S. B. The effect of a placebo on the perception of painful radiant heat stimuli. *Psychological Medicine*, 34, (4), 290–303, 1972.

Fergenson, P. E., Moss, S., Dzendolet, E., Sawyer, F. M., and Moore, J. W. The effect of signal probability, food intake, sex, and smoking on gustation, as measured by the theory of signal detection. *Journal of General Psychology*, 92, 109–127, 1975.

Gescheider, G. A., Sager, L. C., and Ruffolo, L. J. Simultaneous auditory and tactile information processing. *Perception and Psychophysics*, 18, (3), 209–216, 1975.

Gescheider, G. A., Barton, G., Bruce, M. R., Goldberg, J. H., and Greenspan, M. J. Effects of simultaneous auditory stimulation on the detection of tactile stimuli. *Journal of Experimental Psychology*, 81, 120–125, 1969.

Gescheider, G. A., Wright, J. H., Weber, B. J., and Barton, W. G. Absolute thresholds in vibrotactile signal detection. *Perception and Psychophysics*, 10, 413–417, 1971.

Goolkasian, P. An ROC analysis of pain reactions in dysmenorrheic and non-dysmenorrheic women. *Perception and Psychophysics*, 34, (4), 381–386, 1983.

Goolkasian, P. Cyclic changes in pain perception: An ROC analysis. *Perception and Psychophysics*, 27, (6), 499–504, 1980.

Grossberg, J. M., and Grant, B. F. Clinical psychophysics: Applications of ratio scaling and signal detection methods to research on pain, fear, drugs, and medical decision making. *Psychological Bulletin*, 84, (5), 1154–1176, 1978.

Harkins, S. W., and Chapman, C. R. The perception of induced dental pain in young and elderly women. *Journal of Gerentology*, 32, (4), 428–435, 1977.

Hayes, R. L., Bennett, G. J., and Mayer, D. J. Acupuncture, pain, and signal detection theory. *Science*, 189, 65–66, 1975.

Liebeskind, J. C., and Paul, L. A. Psychological and physiological mechanisms of pain. *Annual Review of Psychology*, 28, 41–60, 1977.

McBurney, D. H. Acupuncture, pain, and signal detection theory. *Science*, 189, 66, 1975.

McFadden, D., Barr, E. A., and Young, R. E. Audio analgesia: Lack of a cross-masking effect on taste. *Perception and Psychophysics*, 10, 175–179, 1971.

Narbed, P. G., Marcer, D., and Howell, J. B. L. The contribution of the accelerating phase of inspiratory flow to resistive load detection in man. *Clinical Science*, 62, 367–372, 1982.

Narbed, P. G., Marcer, D., Howell, J. B. L., and Spencer, E. A signal detection theory analysis of the effect of chest cage restriction upon the detection of inspiratory resistive loads. *Clinical Science*, 64, 417–421, 1983.

Pursell, E. D., Sanders, R. E., and Haude, R. H. Sensitivity to sucrose in smokers and nonsmokers: A comparison of TSD and percent correct measures. *Perception and Psychophysics*, 14, 34–36, 1973.

Rabin, M. D., and Cain, W. S. Odor recognition: Familiarity, identifiability, and encoding consistency. *Journal of Experimental Psychology: Learning, Memory, and Cognition*, 10, (2), 316–325, 1984.

Rollman, G. B. Signal detection theory assessment of pain modulation: A critique. In *Advances in Pain Research and Therapy, Vol. I.* J. J. Bionica, and D. Albe-Fessard (eds.). New York: Raven Press, 355–362, 1976.
Rollman, G. B. Signal detection theory measurement of pain: A review and critique. *Pain,* 3, 187–211, 1977.
Rollman, G. B. Signal detection theory pain measures: Empirical validation studies and adaptation-level effects. *Pain,* 6, 9–21, 1979.
Rollman, G. B. Detection models: Experimental tests with electrocutaneous stimuli. *Perception and Psychophysics,* 5, 377–380, 1969.
Sekuler, R., Nash, D., and Armstrong, R. Sensitive objective procedure for evaluating response to light touch. *Neurology,* 23, 1282–1291, 1973.
Semb, G. The detectability of the odor of butanol. *Perception and Psychophysics,* 4, 335–340, 1969.
Steinmetz, G., Pryor, G. T., and Stone, H. Effect of blank samples on absolute odor threshold determinations. *Perception and Psychophysics,* 6, 142–144, 1969.
Swets, J. A., Markowitz, J., and Franzen, O. Vibrotactile signal detection. *Perception and Psychophysics,* 6, 83–88, 1969.
Stevens, J. C., Okulicz, W. C., and Marks, L. E. Temporal summation at the warmth threshold. *Perception and Psychophysics,* 14, (2), 307–312, 1973.
Stone, H., Sidel, J., Oliver, S., Woolsey, A., and Singleton, R. C. Sensory evaluation by quantitative descriptive analysis. *Food Technology,* 24–34, 1974.
Yang, J. C., Clark, W. C., Ngai, S. H., Berkowitz, B. A., and Spector, S. Analgesic action and pharmacokinetics of morphine and diazepam in man. *Anesthesiology,* 51, (6), 495–502, 1979.

NONDESTRUCTIVE EVALUATION

Feagin, F. J. Seismic data display and reflection perceptibility. *Geophysics,* 46, (2), 106–120, 1981.

PERSONALITY

Bernstein, I. H., and Eriksen, C. W. Effects of "subliminal" prompting on paired-associate learning. *Journal of Experimental Research In Personality,* 1, 33–38, 1965.
Clark, W. C. The psyche in psychophysics: A sensory-decision theory analysis of the effect of instructions on flicker sensitivity and response bias. *Psychological Bulletin,* 65, 358–366, 1966.
Clark, W. C., Brown, J. C., and Rutschmann, J. Flicker sensitivity and response bias in psychiatric patients and normal subjects. *Journal of Abnormal Psychology,* 72, 35–42, 1967.
Dandeliker, J., and Dorfman, D. D. Receiver-operating characteristics curves for taboo and neutral words. *Psychonomic Science,* 17, 201–202, 1969.
DiVesta, F. J., and Bartoli, A. The relation of field dependence to signal detection while imaging. *Perception and Psychophysics,* 31, (3), 219–226, 1982.
Dorfman, D. D. Recognition of taboo words as a function of a priori probability. *Journal of Personality of Social Psychology,* 7, 1–10, 1967.
Dorfman, D. D., Grossberg, J. M., and Kroeker, L. Recognition of taboo stimuli as a function of exposure time. *Journal of Personality of Social Psychology,* 2, 552–562, 1965.

Dorfman, D. D., Keeve, S., and Salow, C. Ethnic identification: A signal detection analysis. *Journal of Personality of Social Psychology,* 18, (3), 373–379, 1971.

Goldner, J., Reuder, M. E., Riba, B., and Jarmon, D. Neutral vs. ego-orientating instructions: Effects on judgments of magnitude estimation. *Perception and Psychophysics,* 9, 84–88, 1971.

Johnson, F. N. Depression: Some proposals for future research. *Diseases of the Nervous System,* 38, (5), 228–232, 1975.

Jones, B., and Alexander, R. Cross-modal matching by spastic children. *Developmental Medicine and Child Neurology,* 16, 40–46, 1974.

Koh, S. D., Kayton, L., and Berry, R. Mnemonic organization in young nonpsychotic schizophrenics. *Journal of Abnormal Psychology,* 81, (3), 299–310, 1973.

Koh, S. D., and Peterson, R. A. Perceptual memory for numerousness in "nonpsychotic schizophrenics." *Journal of Abnormal Psychology,* 83, (3), 215–226, 1974.

Poortinga, Y. H. Signal-detection experiments as tests for risk-taking: A pilot study. *Psychonomic Science,* 14, 185–188, 1969.

Price, R. H. Signal-detection methods in personality and perception. *Psychological Bulletin,* 66, 55–62, 1966.

Price, R. H., and Eriksen, C. W. Size constancy in schizophrenia: A reanalysis. *Journal of Abnormal Psychology,* 71, 155–160, 1966.

Rappaport, M., and Hopkins, H. K. Signal detection and chlorpromazine. *Human Factors,* 13, 387–390, 1971.

Rappaport, M., Silverman, J., Hopkins, H. K., Hall, K. Penothiazine effects on auditory signal detection in paranoid and nonparanoid schizophrenics. *Science,* 174, 723–725, 1971.

Schuck, J. R., Cross, H. A., and Mills, D. H. A signal detection analysis of the rod and frame test. *Perception and Psychophysics,* 7, (5), 276–280, 1970.

Silverman, W. P. High-speed scanning of nonalphanumeric symbols in cultural-familiarly retarded and nonretarded children. *American Journal of Mental Deficiency,* 79, (1), 44–51, 1974.

Stenson, H., Kleinmuntz, B., and Scott, B. Personality assessment as a signal detection task. *Journal of Consulting and Clinical Psychology,* 43, (6), 794–799, 1975.

Stephens, S. D. G. Auditory threshold variance, signal detection theory and personality, *International Audiology,* VII, 131–137, 1969.

Strickland, B. R., and Rodwan, A. S. Relation of certain personality variables to decision-making in perception. *Perceptual and Motor Skills,* 18, 353–359, 1964.

Ulehla, Z. J., and Adams, D. K. Detection theory and expectations for social reinforcers: An application to aggression. *Psychological Review,* 80, (6), 439–445, 1973.

Zubin, J., Salzinger, K., Fleiss, J. L., Gurland, B., Spitzer, R. L., Endicott, J., and Sutton, S. Biometric approach to psychopathology: Abnormal and clinical psychology—statistical, epidemiological, and diagnostic approaches. *Annual Review of Psychology,* 26, 621–671, 1975.

PHYSIOLOGY

Brown, J. L. Drug effects on vision: Strategies for study and selected results. *Human Factors,* 16, (4), 354–367, 1974.

Cohn, T. E., Green, D. G., and Tanner, W. P., Jr. Receiver Operating Characteristic Analysis: Application to the study of quantum fluctuation effects in optic nerve of Rana pipiens. *The Journal of General Physiology,* 66, 583–616, 1975.

Donchin, E., and Sutton, S. The "psychological significance" of evoked responses: A comment on Clark, Butler, and Rosner. *Communications in Behavoral Biology*, 5, 111–114, 1970.

Dore, D., and Sutton, S. Evoked potential correlates of response criterion in auditory signal detection. *Science*, 177, 362–364, 1972.

Harcum, E. R., and Monti, P. M. Cognitions and "placebos" in behavioral research on ambient noise. *Perceptual and Motor Skills*, 37, 75–99, 1973.

Hillyard, S. A., Hink, R. F., Schwent, V. L., and Picton, T. W. Electrical signs of selective attention in the human brain. *Science*, 182, 177–180, 1973.

Loveless, N. E. The effect of warning interval of signal detection and event-related slow potentials of the brain. *Perception and Psychophysics*, 17, (6), 565–570, 1975.

Moulin, L. K. The effects of physiological noise on the auditory threshold. *Journal of Speech and Hearing Research*, 15, 837–844, 1972.

Parasuraman, R. Response bias and physiological reactivity. *Journal of Psychology*, 91, 309–313, 1974.

Parasuraman, R., and Beatty, J. Brian events underlying detection and recognition of weak sensory signals. *Science*, 210, (3), 80–83, 1980.

Shakhar, G. B., Lieblich, I., and Kugelmass, S. Detection of information and GSR habituation: An attempt to derive detection efficiency from two habituation curves. *Psychophysiology*, 12, (3), 283–288, 1975.

Shakhar, G. B., Lieblich, I., and Kugelmass, S. Guilty-knowledge technique: Application of signal detection measures. *Journal of Applied Psychology*, 54, (5), 409–413, 1970.

Squires, K. C., Hillyard, S. A., and Lindsay, P. H. Vertex potentials evoked during auditory signal detection: Relation to decision criteria. *Perception and Psychophysics*, 14, (2), 265–272, 1973.

Squires, K. C., Squires, N. K., and Hillyard, S. A. Decision-related cortical potentials during an auditory signal detection task with cued observation intervals. *Journal of Experimental Psychology: Human Perception and Performance*, 1, (3), 268–279, 1975.

Squires, K. C., Squires, N. K., and Hillyard, S. A. Vertex evoked potentials in a rating-scale detection task: Relation to signal probability. *Behavioral Biology*, 13, (Abstract 4209), 21–34, 1975.

Squires, K. C., Hillyard, S. A., and Lindsay, P. H. Cortical potentials evoked by confirming and disconfirming feedback following an auditory discrimination. *Perception and Psychophysics*, 13, 25–31, 1973.

Szucko, J. J., and Kleinmuntz, B. Statistical versus clinical lie detection. *American Psychologist*, 36, (5), 488–496, 1981.

Van Voorhis, S., and Hillyard, S. A. Visual evoked potentials and selective attention to points in space. *Perception and Psychophysics*, 22, (1), 54–62, 1977.

REACTION TIME

Audley, R. J. Some observations on theories of choice reaction time: Tutorial review. In *Attention and Performance IV*, S. Kornblum (Ed.), Academic Press, New York, 509–545, 1973.

Audley, R. J. Tutorial review: Some observations on theories of choice reaction time. Conference on *Attention and Performance IV*, Boulder, Colorado, 1–47, 1971.

Bindra, D., Williams, J. A., and Wise, J. S. Judgments of sameness and difference: Experiments on decision time. *Science*, 150, 1625–1627, 1965.

Carterette, E. D., Friedman, M. P., and Cosmides, R. Reaction-time distributions in the detection of weak signals in noise. *Journal of the Acoustical Society of America,* 38, 531–542, 1965.

Debecker, J., and Desmedt, J. E. Maximum capacity for sequential one-bit auditory decisions. *Journal of Experimental Psychology,* 83, 366–372, 1970.

Emmerich, D. S., Gray, J. L., Watson, C. S., and Tanis, D. C. Response latency, confidence, and ROCs in auditory signal detection. *Perception and Psychophysics,* 11, 65–72, 1972.

Gescheider, G. A., Wright, J. H., and Evans, M. B. Reaction time in the detection of vibrotactile signals. *Journal of Experimental Psychology,* 77, 501–504, 1968.

Gescheider, G. A., Wright, J. H., Weber, B. J., Kirchner, B. M., and Milligan, E. A. Reaction time as a function of the intensity and probability of occurrence of vibrotactile signals. *Perception and Psychophysics,* 5, 18–20, 1969.

Green, D. M., and Luce, R. D. Speed-accuracy trade off in auditory detection. In *Attention and Performance IV,* S. Kornblum (Ed.), Academic Press, New York, 547–569, 1973.

Koppell, S. The latency function hypothesis and Pike's multiple-observations model for latencies in signal detection. *Psychological Review,* 83, (4), 308–309, 1976.

Lappin, J. S., and Disch, K. The latency operating characteristic: I. Effects of stimulus probability on choice reaction time. *Journal of Experimental Psychology,* 92, (3), 419–427, 1972.

Lappin, J. S., and Disch, K. The latency operating characteristic: II. Effects of visual stimulus intensity on choice reaction time. *Journal of Experimental Psychology,* 93, (2), 367–372, 1972.

Lappin, J. S., and Disch, K. Latency operating characteristic: III. Temporal uncertainty effects. *Journal of Experimental Psychology,* 98, (2), 279–285, 1973.

Link, S. W. Applying RT deadlines to discrimination reaction time. *Psychonomic Science,* 25, (6), 355–358, 1971.

Navon, D. A simple method for latency analysis in signal detection tasks. *Perception and Psychophysics,* 18, (1), 61–64, 1975.

Navon, D., and Gopher, D. On the economy of the human-processing system. *Psychological Review,* 86, (3), 214–255, 1979.

Navon, D., and Gopher, D. Task difficulty, resources, and dual-task performance. In R. S. Nickerson (ed.), *Attention and Performance VIII.* Hillsdale, New Jersey: Lawrence Erlbaum Associates, 297–315, 1980.

Proctor, R. W. A unified theory for matching task phenomena. *Psychological Review,* 88, (4), 291–326, 1981.

Proctor, R. W. Response bias, criteria settings, and the fast-*same* phenomenon: A reply to Ratcliff. (Theoretical Note) *Psychological Review,* 93, (4), 473–477, 1986.

Proctor, R. W., and Rao, K. V. Evidence that the *same-different* disparity is not attributable to response bias. *Perception and Psychophysics,* 34, (1), 72–76, 1983.

Proctor, R. W., Rao, K. V., and Hurst, P. W. An examination of response bias in multiletter matching. *Perception and Psychophysics,* 35, (5), 464–476, 1984.

Ratcliff, R. More on the speed and accuracy of positive and negative responses. (Theoretical Note) *Psychological Review,* 94, (2), 277–280, 1987.

Ratcliff, R. Theoretical interpretations of the speed and accuracy of positive and negative responses. *Psychological Review,* 92, (2), 212–225, 1985.

Reed, C. Reaction times for a same-different discrimination of vowel-consonant syllables. *Perception and Psychophysics,* 18, (2), 65–70, 1975.

Zinnes, J. L., and Kurtz, R. Matching, discrimination, and payoffs. *Journal of Mathematical Psychology,* 5, 392–421, 1968.

RECOGNITION

Auerbach, C., and Leventhal, G. Evidence for all-or-none preperceptual processing in perceptual set. *Perception and Psychophysics,* 14, (1), 24–30, 1973.

Broadbent, D. E., and Broadbent, M. H. P. Some further data concerning the word frequency effect. *Journal of Experimental Psychology: General,* 104, (4), 297–308, 1975.

Buckhout, R. Eyewitness testimony. *Scientific American,* 231, (6), 23–31, 1974.

Cutting, J. E. Plucks and bows are categorically perceived, sometimes. *Perception and Psychophysics,* 31, (5), 462–476, 1982.

Egan, J. P. Monitoring task in speech communication. *Journal of the Acoustical Society of America,* 29, (4), 482–489, 1957.

Erdelyi, M. H. A new look at the new look: Perceptual defense and vigilance. *Psychological Review,* 81, 1–25, 1974.

Green, D. M., and Birdsall, T. G. Detection and recognition. *Psychological Review,* 85, (3), 192–206, 1978.

Green, D. M., Weber, D. L., and Duncan, J. E. Detection and recognition of pure tones in noise. *Journal of the Acoustical Society of America,* 62, (4), 948–954, 1977.

Guth, S. L. A new color model. Paper presented at the A.I.C. Helmholtz Memorial Symposium on Color-Metrics, Driebergen, Holland, 1–20, September 1, 1971.

Guth, S. L., and Lodge, H. R. Heterochromatic additivity, foveal spectral sensitivity, and a new color model. *Journal of the Optical Society of America,* 63, (4), 450–462, 1973.

Haggard, M. Selectivity for distortions and words in speech perception. *British Journal of Psychology,* 65, (1), 69–83, 1974.

Ingleby, J. D. The separation of bias and sensitivity in multiple-choice tasks. *Perception,* 2, 295–305, 1973.

Johnston, J. C., and Halle, B. L. The influence of prior context on word identification: Bias and sensitivity effects. In R. S. Nickerson (ed.), *Attention and Performance VIII.* New Jersey: Lawrence Erlbaum Associates, 243–255, 1980.

Kopp, J., and Livermore, J. Differential discriminability or response bias? A signal detection analysis of categorical perception. *Journal of Experimental Psychology,* 101, (1), 179–182, 1973.

Ladan, C. J., Heron, R. M., and Nelson, T. M. A signal-detection evaluation of flat vs. curved marker performance. *Perceptual and Motor Skills,* 39, 355–358, 1974.

Lindner, W. A. Recognition performance as a function of detection criterion in a simultaneous detection-recognition task. *Journal of the Acoustical Society of America,* 44, (1), 204–211, 1968.

Malpass, R. S., Lavigueur, H., and Weldon, D. E. Verbal and visual training in face recognition. *Perception and Psychophysics,* 14, (2), 285–292, 1973.

Morgan, B. J. T. On Luce's choice axiom. *Journal of Mathematical Psychology,* 11, (2), 107–123, 1974.

Newell, K. M. Decision processes of baseball batters. *Human Factors,* 16, (5), 520–527, 1974.

Parasuraman, R., Richer, F., and Beatty, J. Detection and recognition: Concurrent processes in perception. *Perception and Psychophysics,* 31, (1), 1–12, 1982.

Swets, J. A., Green, D. M., Getty, D. J., and Sets, J. B. Signal detection and identification at successive stages of observation *Perception and Psychophysics,* 23, (4), 275–289, 1978.

Townsend, J. T., Hu, G. G., and Ashby, F. G. Perceptual sampling of orthogonal straight line features. *Psychological Review,* 43, 259–275, 1981.

Treisman, M. A theory of the identification of complex stimuli with an application to word recognition. *Psychological Review*, 85, (6), 525–570, 1978.

Walker, J. H. Pronounceability effects on word-nonword encoding in categorization and recognition tasks. *Journal of Experimental Psychology*, 99, (3), 318–322, 1973.

Weintraub, D. J., and Fidell, L. S. A signal-detection approach to subception: Concomitant verbal and finger-latency responses in metacontrast. *Perception and Psychophysics*, 26, (2), 143–152, 1979.

SPEECH

Corcoran, D. W. J., Dorfman, D. D., and Weening, D. L. Perceptual independence in the perception of speech. *Quarterly Journal of Experimental Psychology*, XX, (4), 336–350, 1968.

Wood, C. C. Discriminability, response bias, and phoneme categories in discrimination of voice onset time. *Journal of the Acoustical Society of America*, 60, (6), 1381–1389, 1976.

VIGILANCE

Adams, S. K. Decision making in quality control: Some perceptual and behavioral considerations. In *Human Reliability in Quality Control*, C. G. Drury and J. G. Fox (eds.). New York: Halsted Press, 55–69, 1975.

Baddeley, A. D., and Colquhoun, W. P. Signal probability and vigilance: A reappraisal of the 'signal-rate' effect. *British Journal of Psychology*, 60, 169–178, 1969.

Baker, E. M. Signal detection theory analysis of quality control inspector performance. *Journal of Quality Technology*, 7, (2), 62–71, 1975.

Benedetti, L. H., and Loeb, M. A comparison of auditory monitoring performance in blind subjects with that of sighted subjects in light and dark. *Perception and Psychophysics*, 11, (1A), 10–16, 1972.

Blignaut, C. J. H. The perception of hazard II. The contribution of signal detection to hazard perception. *Ergonomics*, 22, (11), 1177–1183, 1979.

Bloomfield, J. R. Theoretical approaches to visual search. In *Human Reliability in Quality Control*, C. G. Drury and J. G. Fox (eds.). New York: Halsted Press, 19–29, 1975.

Buck, J. R. Dynamic visual inspection: Task factors, theory and economics. In *Human Reliability in Quality Control*, C. G. Drury and J. G. Fox (eds.). New York: Halsted Press, 165–187, 1975.

Chapman, D. E., and Sinclair, M. A. Ergonomics in inspection tasks in the food industry. In *Human Reliability in Quality Control*, C. G. Drury and J. G. Fox (eds.). New York: Halsted Press, 231–251, 1975.

Coates, G. D., Loeb, M., and Alluisi, E. A. Influence of observing strategies and stimulus variables on watchkeeping performances. *Ergonomics*, 15, (4), 379–386, 1972.

Colquhoun, W. P. Training for vigilance: A comparison of different techniques. *Human Factors*, 8, 7–12, 1966.

Colquhoun, W. P. Sonar target detection as a decision process. *Journal of Applied Psychology*, 51, 187–190, 1967.

Colquhoun, W. P. Effects of raised ambient temperature and event rate on vigilance performance. *Aerospace Medicine*, 40, 413–417, 1969.

Colquhoun, W. P., and Edwards, R. S. Practice effects on a visual vigilance task with and without search. *Human Factors,* 12, 537–545, 1970.

Craig, A. Broadbent and Gregory revisited: Vigilance and statistical decision. *Human Factors,* 19, (1), 25–36, 1977.

Craig, A. Is the vigilance decrement simply a response adjustment towards probability matching? *Human Factors,* 20, (4), 441–446, 1978.

Craig, A. Discrimination, temperature, and time of day. *Human Factors,* 21, (1), 61–68, 1979.

Craig, A. Monitoring for one kind of signal in the presence of another: The effects of signal mix on detectability. *Human Factors,* 23, (2), 191–197, 1981.

Craig, A. Nonparametric measures of sensory efficiency for sustained monitoring tasks. *Human Factors,* 21, (1), 69–78, 1979.

Craig, A. Vigilance for two kinds of signal with unequal probabilities of occurrence. *Human Factors,* 21, (6), 647–653, 1979.

Craig, A., and Colquhoun, W. P. Vigilance: A review. In *Human Reliability in Quality Control,* C. G. Drury and J. G. Fox (eds.). New York: Halsted Press, 71–87, 1975.

Crider, A., and Augenbraun, C. B. Auditory vigilance correlates of electrodermal response habituation speed. *Psychophysiology,* 12, (1), 36–40, 1975.

Davenport, W. G. Auditory vigilance: The effects of costs and values on signals. *Australian Journal of Psychology,* 20, 213–218, 1968.

Davenport, W. G. Vibrotactile vigilance: The effects of costs and values on signals. *Perception and Psychophysics,* 5, 25–28, 1969.

Davies, D. R., Hockey, G. R. J., and Taylor, A. Varied auditory stimulation, temperament differences and vigilance performance. *British Journal of Psychology,* 60, (4), 453–457, 1969.

Davies, D. R., Lang, L., and Shackleton, V. J. The effects of music and task difficulty on performance at a visual vigilance task. *British Journal of Psychology,* 64, (3), 383–389, 1973.

Davies, D. R., and Parasuraman, R. Cortical evoked potentials and vigilance: A decision theory analysis. In R. R. Mackie (ed.), *Vigilance II: Relationships among Theory, Physiological Correlates and Operational Performance.* New York: Plenum, 285–306, 1977.

Deaton, M., Tobias, J. S., and Wilkinson, R. T. The effect of sleep deprivation on signal detection parameters. *Quarterly Journal of Experimental Psychology,* 23, 449–452, 1971.

DeMaio, J., Parkinson, S. R., and Crosby, J. V. A reaction time analysis of instrument scanning. *Human Factors,* 20, (4), 467–471, 1978.

Drury, C. G. The effect of speed working on industrial inspection accuracy. *Applied Ergonomics,* 4, (1), 2–7, 1973.

Drury, C. G. Human decision making in quality control. In *Human Reliability in Quality Control,* C. G. Drury and J. G. Fox (eds.). New York: Halsted Press, 45–53, 1975.

Drury, C. G., and Addison, J. L. An industrial study of the effects of feedback and fault density on inspection performance. *Ergonomics,* 16, (2), 159–169, 1973.

Drury, C. G., and Fox, J. G. The imperfect inspector. In *Human Reliability in Quality Control,* C. G. Drury and J. G. Fox (eds.). New York: Halsted Press, 11–16, 1975.

Embrey, D. E. Training the inspector's sensitivity and response strategy. In *Human Reliability in Quality Control,* C. G. Drury and J. G. Fox (eds.). New York: Halsted Press, 189–195, 1975.

Fox, J. G., and Haslegrave, C. M. Industrial inspection efficiency and the probability of a defect occurring. *Ergonomics,* 12, (5), 713–721, 1969.

Geyer, L. H., Patel, S., and Perry, R. F. Detectability of multiple flaws. *Human Factors,* 21, (1), 7–12, 1979.

Geyer, L. H., and Perry, R. F. Variation in detectability of multiple flaws with allowed inspection time. *Human Factors,* 23, (3), 361–365, 1982.

Guralnick, M. J. Effects of event rate and signal difficulty on observing responses and detection measures in vigilance. *Journal of Experimental Psychology,* 99, (2), 261–265, 1973.

Guralnick, M. J., and Harvey, K. C. Response requirements and performance in a visual vigilance task. *Psychonomic Science,* 20, (4), 215–217, 1970.

Guralnick, M. J. Observing responses and decision processes in vigilance. *Journal of Experimental Psychology,* 93, 239–244, 1972.

Hatfield, J. L., and Loeb, M. Sense mode and coupling in a vigilance task. *Perception and Psychophysics,* 4, 29–36, 1968.

Hatfield, J., and Soderquist, D. R. Practice effects and signal detection indices in an auditory vigilance task. *Journal of the Acoustical Society of America,* 46, 1458–1463, 1969.

Hatfield, J. L., and Soderquist, D. R. Coupling effects and performance in vigilance tasks. *Human Factors,* 12, 351–359, 1970.

Jerison, H. J. Signal detection theory in the analysis of human vigilance. *Human Factors,* 9, 285–288, 1967.

Johnston, W. A., Howell, W. C., and Williges, R. C. The components of complex monitoring. *Organizational Behavior and Human Performance,* 4, 112–124, 1969.

Levine, J. M. The effects of values and costs on the detection and identification of signals in auditory vigilance. *Human Factors,* 8, 525–537, 1966.

Loeb, M., and Alluisi, E. A. Influence of display task, and organismic variables on indices of monitoring behavior. *Acta Psychologica,* 33, 343–366, 1970.

Loeb, M., and Binford, J. R. Variation in performance on auditory and visual monitoring tasks as a function of signal and stimulus frequencies. *Perception and Psychophysics,* 4, 361–367, 1968.

Loeb, M., and Binford, J. R. Examination of some factors influencing performance on an auditory monitoring task with one signal per session. *Journal of Experimental Psychology,* 83, 40–44, 1970.

Loeb, M., Hawkes, G. R., Evans, W. O., and Alluisi, E. A. The influence of d-amphetamine, benactyzene, and chlorapromazine on performance in an auditory vigilance task. *Psychonomic Science,* 3, 29–30, 1965.

Loeb, M. On the analysis and interpretation of vigilance: Some remarks on two recent articles by Craig. *Human Factors,* 20, (4), 447–451, 1978.

Loeb, M., and Binford, J. R. Modality, difficulty, and 'coupling' in vigilance behavior. *American Journal of Psychology,* 84, (4), 529–541, 1971.

Lucas, P. Human performance in low-signal-probability tasks. *Journal of the Acoustical Society of America,* 42, 158–178, 1967.

Mackworth, J. F. Performance decrement in vigilance, threshold, and high-speed perceptual motor tasks. *Canadian Journal of Psychology,* 18, 209–223, 1964.

Mackworth, J. F. The effect of true and false knowledge of results on the detectability of signals in a vigilance task. *Canadian Journal of Psychology,* 18, 106–117, 1964.

Mackworth, J. F. Deterioration of signal detectability during a vigilance task as a function of background event rate. *Psychonomic Science,* 3, 421–422, 1965.

Mackworth, J. F. Effect of amphetamine on the detectability of signals in a vigilance task. *Canadian Journal of Psychology,* 19, 104–110, 1965.

Mackworth, J. F. Decision interval and signal detectability in a vigilance task. *Canadian Journal of Psychology,* 19, 111–117, 1965.

Mackworth, J. F. The effect of signal rate on performance in two kinds of vigilance task. *Human Factors*, 10, 11–18, 1968.

McCann, P. H. Variability of signal detection measures with noise type. *Psychonomic Science*, 15, 310–311, 1969.

Milosevic, S. Detection du signal en fonction due critere de response. *Le Travail Humain*, 32, 81–86, 1969.

Milosevic, S. Changes in detection measures and skin resistance during an auditory vigilance task. *Ergonomics*, 18, (1), 1–8, 1975.

Milosevic, S. Effect of time and space uncertainty on a vigilance task. *Perception and Psychophysics*, 15, (2), 331–334, 1974.

Moraal, J. The analysis of an inspection task in the steel industry. In *Human Reliability in Quality Control*. C. G. Drury and J. G. Fox (eds.). New York: Halsted Press, 217–230, 1975.

Murrell, G. A. A reappraisal of artificial signals as an aid to a visual monitoring task. *Ergonomics*, 18, (6), 693–700, 1975.

Nuechterlein, K. H., Parasuraman, R., and Jiang, Q. Visual sustained attention: Image degradation produces rapid sensitivity decrement over time. *Science*, 220, 327–329, 1983.

Parasuraman, R. Memory load and event rate control sensitivity decrements in sustained attention. *Science*, 205, 924–927, 1979.

Parasuraman, R., and Davies, D. R. A taxonomic analysis of vigilance performance. In R. R. Mackie (ed.), *Vigilance II: Relationships among Theory, Physiological Correlates and Operational Performance*, New York: Plenum, 559–574, 1977.

Parasuraman, R., and Mouloua, M. Interaction of signal discriminability and task type in vigilance decrement. *Perception and Psychophysics*, 41, (1), 17–22, 1987.

Poulton, E. C., and Edwards, R. S. Interactions and range effects in experiments on pairs of stresses. *Journal of Experimental Psychology*, 102, (4), 621–628, 1974.

Sheehan, J. J., and Drury, C. G. The analysis of industrial inspection. *Applied Ergonomics*, 2, (2), 74–78, 1971.

Smith, G. L., Jr. Inspector performance on microminiature tasks. In *Human Reliability in Quality Control*. C. G. Drury and J. G. Fox, (eds.). New York: Halsted Press, 149–163, 1975.

Smith, L., and Barany, J. W. An elementary model of human performance on paced visual inspection tasks. *Association of International Industrial Engineers*, 2, (4), 298–308, 1970.

Swets, J. A. Comment: Adaptation-level theory and signal-detection theory and their relation to vigilance experiments. In *Adaptation-Level Theory*, M. H. Appley (Ed.), Academic Press, Inc., New York, 49–53, 1971.

Swets, J. A. Signal detection theory applied to vigilance. In *Vigilance: Theory, Operational Performance and Physiological Correlates*, R. R. Mackie, (ed.). New York: Plenum Press, 705–718, 1977.

Taub, J. M., and Berger, R. J. Performance and mood following variations in the length and timing of sleep. *Psychophysiology*, 10, (6), 559–570, 1973.

Taub, J. M., and Berger, R. J. Acute shifts in the sleep-wakefulness cycle: Effects on performance and mood. *Psychosomatic Medicine*, 36, (2), 164–173, 1974.

Taylor, M. M. The effect of the square root of time in continuing perceptual tasks. *Perception and Psychophysics*, 1, 113–119, 1966.

Taylor, M. M. Detectability theory and the interpretation of vigilance data. *Acta Psychologica*, 27, 390–399, 1967.

Teichner, W. H. The detection of a simple visual signal as a function of time of watch. *Human Factors*, 16, (4), 339–353, 1974.

Thurmond, J. B., Binford, J. R., and Loeb, M. Effects of signal to noise variability over repeated sessions in an auditory vigilance task. *Perception and Psychophysics,* 7, 100–102, 1970.

Tickner, A. H., and Poulton, E. C. Monitoring up to 16 synthetic television pictures showing a great deal of movement. *Ergonomics,* 16, (4), 381–401, 1973.

Tsao, Y-C, Drury, C. G., and Morawski, T. B. Human performance in sampling inspection. *Human Factors,* 21, (1), 99–105, 1979.

Tyler, D. M., Waag, W. L., and Halcomb, C. G. Monitoring performance across sense modes: An individual differences approach. *Human Factors,* 14, (6), 539–547, 1972.

Vickers, D., and Leary, J. N. Criterion control in signal detection. *Human Factors,* 25, (3), 283–296, 1983.

Wallack, P. M., and Adams, S. K. A comparison of inspector performance measures. *Association of International Industrial Engineers Transactions,* 2, (2), 97–105, 1970.

Wallack, P. M., and Adams, S. K. The utility of signal-detection theory in the analysis of industrial inspector accuracy. *Association of Industrial Engineers Transactions,* 1, (1), 33–44, 1969.

Watson, C. S., and Nichols, T. L. Detectability of auditory signals presented without defined observation intervals. *Journal of the Acoustical Society of America,* 59, (3), 655–668, 1976.

Weiner, E. L. Individual and group differences in inspection. In *Human Reliability in Quality Control.* C. G. Drury and J. G. Fox (eds.). New York: Halsted Press, 101–122, 1975.

Williams, P. S. Processing demands, training and the vigilance decrement. *Human Factors,* 28, (5), 567–579, 1986.

Williges, R. C. Manipulating the response criterion in visual monitoring. *Human Factors,* 15, (2), 179–185, 1973.

Williges, R. C., and North, R. A. Knowledge of results and decision making performance in visual monitoring. *Organizational Behavior and Human Performance,* 8, 44–57, 1972.

Williges, R. C. Within-session criterion changes compared to an ideal observer criterion in a visual monitoring task. *Journal of Experimental Psychology,* 81, 61–66, 1969.

Williges, R. C. The role of payoffs and signal ratios in criterion changes during a monitoring task. *Human Factors,* 13, 261–267, 1971.

Zunzanyika, X. K., and Drury, C. G. Effects of information on industrial inspection performance. In *Human Reliability in Quality Control.* C. G. Drury and J. G. Fox (eds.). New York: Halsted Press, 189–195, 1975.

VISION

Allan, L. G. Visual position discrimination: A model relating temporal and spatial factors. *Perception and Psychophysics,* 4, 267–278, 1968.

Allan, L. G., Kristofferson, A. B., and Wiens, E. W. Duration discrimination of brief light flashes. *Perception and Psychophysics,* 9, 327–334, 1971.

Banks, M. S. The effect of head tilt on meridional differences in acuity: Implications for orientation constancy. *Perception and Psychophysics,* 17, (1), 17–22, 1975.

Baron, J. Temporal ROC curves and the psychological moment. *Psychonomic Science,* 15, 299–300, 1969.

Blake, R., and Fox, R. The psychophysical inquiry into binocular summation. *Perception and Psychophysics,* 14, 161–185, 1973.

Bruder, G. E., and Kietzman, M. L. Visual temporal integration for threshold, signal detectability, and reaction time measures. *Perception and Psychophysics,* 13, 293–300, 1973.

Caelli, T. M., and Finlay, D. C. Pattern discrimination of Gaussian distributions of orientation and line length parameters. *Perception and Psychophysics,* 16, (3), 489–493, 1975.

Campbell, F. W., Nachmias, J., and Jukes, J. Spatial-frequency discrimination in human vision. *Journal of the Optical Society of America,* 60, 555–559, 1970.

Clement, D. E., and Hosking, K. E. Scanning strategies and differential sensitivity in a visual signal detection task: Intrasubject reliability. *Psychonomic Science,* 22, 323–324, 1971.

Cogan, A. I., Silverman, G., and Sekuler, R. Binocular summation in detection of contrast flashes. *Perception and Psychophysics,* 31, (4), 330–338, 1982.

Cohn, T. E. A new hypothesis to explain why the increment threshold exceeds the decrement threshold. *Vision Research,* Letter to the Editor, 14, 1277–1279, 1974.

Cohn, T. E. Detection of 1-of-M orthogonal signals: Asymptotic equivalence of likelihood ratio and "multiband" models. Submitted to *Optics Letters,* 1982.

Cohn, T. E. Detectability of a luminance increment: Effect of superimposed random luminance fluctuation. *Journal of the Optical Society of America,* Pu[66], 12, 1426–1428, 1976.

Cohn, T. E. Quantum fluctuation limit in foveal vision. *Vision Research,* 16, 573–579, 1976.

Cohn, T. E. Receiver operating characteristic analysis of sensitivity in neural systems. *Proceedings of the IEEE,* 65, (5), 781–786, 1977.

Cohn, T. E., and Lasley, D. J. Binocular Vision: Two possible central interactions between signals from two eyes. *Science,* 192, 561–563, 1976.

Cohn, T. E., and Lasley, D. J. Detectability of a luminance increment: Effect of spatial uncertainty. *Journal of the Optical Society of America,* 64, 12, 1715–1719, 1974.

Cohn, T. E., and Lasley, D. J. Spatial summation of foveal increments and decrements. *Vision Research,* 15, 389–399, 1975.

Cohn, T. E., Thibos, L. N., and Kleinstein, R. N. Detectability of a luminance increment. *Journal of the Optical Society of America,* 64, (10), 1321–1327, 1974.

Cormack, R. H., and Blake, R. Do the two eyes constitute separate visual channels? *Science,* 207, 1100–1102, 1980.

Cox, S. T., and Dember, W. N. Effects of target-field luminance, interstimulus interval and target-mask separation on extent of visual backward masking. *Psychonomic Science,* 22, 79–80, 1971.

Creelman, C. D., and Donaldson, W. ROC curves for discrimination of linear extent. *Journal of Experimental Psychology,* 77, 514–516, 1968.

Glorioso, R. M., ánd Levy, R. M. Operator behavior in a dynamic visual signal detection task. *Perception and Psychophysics,* 4, 5–9, 1968.

Green, M. Masking by light and the sustained-transient dichotomy. *Perception and Psychophysics,* 35, (6), 519–535, 1984.

Guth, S. L. Nonadditivity and inhibition among chromatic luminances at threshold. *Vision Research,* 7, 319–328, 1967.

Guth, S. L., Donley, N. J., and Marrocco, R. T. On luminance additivity and related topics. *Vision Research,* 9, 537–575, 1969.

Halpern, J., and Ulehla, J. Z. The effect of multiple responses and certainty estimates on the integration of visual information. *Perception and Psychophysics,* 7, 129–132, 1970

Handel, S., and Christ, R. E. Detection and identification of geometric forms using peripheral and central viewing. *Perception and Psychophysics,* 6, 47–49, 1969.

Harvey, L. O., and Michon, J. A. Detectability of relative motion as a function of exposure duration, angular separation, and background. *Journal of Experimental Psychology,* 103, (2), 317–325, 1974.

Keller, W., and Kinchla, R. A. Visual movements discrimination. *Perception and Psychophysics,* 3, 233–236, 1968.

Kinchla, R. A. Visual movement perception: A comparison of absolute and relative movement discrimination. *Perception and Psychophysics,* 9, 165–171, 1971.

Kinchla, R. A., and Allan, L. G. Visual movement perception: A comparison of sensitivity to vertical and horizontal movement. *Perception and Psychophysics,* 8, 399–405, 1970.

Klein, S., and Stromeyer, C. F., III., and Ganz, L. The simultaneous spatial frequency shift: A dissociation between the detection and perception of gratings. *Vision Research,* 14, 1421–1432, 1974.

Kosnik, W., Fikre, J., and Sekuler, R. Improvement in direction discrimination: No role for eye movements. *Perception and Psychophysics, 38,* (6), 554–558, 1985.

Leshowitz, B., Taub, H. B., and Raab, D. H. Visual detection of signals in the presence of continuous and pulsed backgrounds. *Perception and Psychophysics,* 4, 207–213, 1968.

Lowe, G. Interval of time uncertainty in visual detection. *Perception and Psychophysics,* 2, 278–280, 1967.

Mansfield, R. J. W. Visual adaptation: Retinal transduction, brightness and sensitivity. *Vision Research,* 16, 679–690, 1976.

Massof, R. W., and Starr, S. J. Vector magnitude operation in color vision models: Derivation from signal detection theory. *Journal of the Optical Society of America,* 70, (7), 870–872, 1980.

Matin, E., and Drivas, A. Acuity for orientation measured with a sequential recognition task and signal detection methods. *Perception and Psychophysics,* 25, (3), 161–168, 1979.

Nachmias, J. On the psychometric function for contrast detection. *Vision Research,* 21, 215–223, 1981.

Nachmias, J., and Kocher, E. G. Visual detection and discrimination of luminance increments. *Journal of the Optical Society of America,* 60, 382–389, 1970.

Poulton, E. C., and Edwards, R. S. Percpetual load in searching for sloping colored lines camouflaged by colored backgrounds: A separate-groups investigation. *Journal of Experimental Psychology: Human Perception and Performance,* 3, (1), 136–150, 1977.

Schneider, B., Trehub, S. E., and Bull, D. High-frequency sensitivity in infants. *Science,* 207, 1003–1004, 1980.

Stromeyer, C. F., III, and Klein, S. Evidence against narrow-band spatial frequency channels in human vision: The detectability of frequency modulated gratings. *Vision Research,* 15, 899–910, 1975.

Stromeyer, C. F., III, and Klein, S. Spatial frequency channels in human vision as asymmetric (EDGE) mechanisms. *Vision Research,* 14, 1409–1420, 1974.

Theodor, L. H. The detectability of a brief gap in a pulse of light as a function of its temporal location within the pulse. *Perception and Psychophysics,* 12, 168–170, 1972.

Thijssen, J. M., and Vendrik, J. H. Differential luminance sensitivity of the human visual system. *Perception and Psychophysics,* 10, 58–63, 1971.

Tieger, T., and Ganz, L. Recognition of faces in the presence of two-dimensional sinusoidal masks. *Perception and Psychophysics,* 26, (2), 163–167, 1979.

Tyson, P. D. Perceptual modification of sensitivity (d'): Modifying temporal resolution by the consistency of the spatial configuration. *Perception and Psychophysics,* 12, 45–49, 1972.

Vogels, R., and Orban, G. A. Decision factors affecting line orientation judgments in the method of single stimuli. *Perception and Psychophysics,* 40, (2), 74–84, 1986.

Vogels, R., and Orban, G. A. Decision processes in visual discrimination of line orientation. *Journal of Experimental Psychology: Human Perception and Performance,* 12, (2), 115–132, 1986.

Womersley, M. A contextual effect in feature detection with application of signal detection methodology. *Perception and Psychophysics,* 21, (1), 88–92, 1977.

Westendorf, D. H., Blake, R. R., and Fox, R. Binocular summation of equal-energy flashes of unequal duration. *Perception and Psychophysics,* 12, 445–448, 1972.

White, M. J. Signal-detection analysis of laterality differences: Some preliminary data, free of recall and report-sequence characteristics. *Journal of Experimental Psychology,* 83, 174–176, 1970.

Wickelgren, W. A. Strength theories of disjunctive visual detection. *Perception and Psychophysics,* 2, 331–337, 1967.

Winnick, W. A., and Bruder, G. E. Signal detection approach to the study of retinal locus in tachistoscopic recognition. *Journal of Experimental Psychology,* 78, 528–531, 1968.

Wong, E., and Weisstein, N. Sharp targets are detected better against a figure, and blurred targets are detected better against a background. *Journal of Experimental Psychology: Human Perception and Performance,* 9, (2), 194–202, 1983.

Yellott, J. I., Jr., and Curnow, P. F. Second choices in a visual span of apprehension task. *Perception and Psychophysics,* 2, 307–311, 1967.

VISION AND AUDITION

Baker, E. M., and Schuck, J. R. A signal detection analysis of the effects of hearing on the visual recognition of two-digit numbers. *Perception and Psychophysics,* 12, (2B), 239–240, 1972.

Bothe, G. G., and Marks, L. E. Absolute sensitivity to white noise under auxiliary visual stimulation. *Perception and Psychophysics,* 8, (3), 176–178, 1970.

Brown, A. E., and Hopkins, H. K. Interaction of the auditory and visual sensory modalities. *Journal of the Acoustical Society of America,* 41, 1–6, 1967.

Carterette, E. C., and Jones, M. H. Visual and auditory information processing in children and adults. *Science,* 156, 986–988, 1967.

Choe, C. S., Welch, R. B., Gilford, R. M., and Juola, J. F. The "ventriloquist effect": Visual dominance or response bias? *Perception and Psychophysics,* 18, (1), 55–60, 1975.

Craig, A., Colquhoun, W. P., and Corcoran, D. W. J. Combining evidence presented simultaneously to the eye and the ear: A comparison of some predictive models. *Perception and Psychophysics,* 19, (6), 473–484, 1976.

Dougherty, W. G., Jones, G. B., and Engel, G. R. Sensory integration of auditory and visual information. *Canadian Journal of Psychology,* 25, 476–485, 1971.

Earle, D. C., and Lowe, G. Channel, temporal, and composite uncertainty in the detection and recognition of auditory and visual signals. *Perception and Psychophysics,* 9, 177–181, 1971.

Fidell, S. Sensory function in multimodal signal detection. *Journal of the Acoustical Society of America,* 47, 1009–1015, 1970.

Fidell, S. Comments on Mulligan and Shaw's "Multimodal signal detection: Independent decisions vs. integration." *Perception and Psychophysics,* 31, (1), 90, 1982.

Forbes, S. M., Taylor, M. M., and Lindsay, P. H. cue timing in a multi-dimensional detection task. *Perceptual and Motor Skills,* 25, 113–120, 1967.

Gunn, W. J., and Loeb, M. Correlation of performance in detecting visual signals. *American Journal of Psychology,* 80, 236–242, 1966.

Jones, B. Visual facilitation of auditory localization in schoolchildren: A signal detection analysis. *Perception and Psychophysics,* 17, (3), 217–220, 1975.

Jones, B., and Kabanoff, B. Eye movements in auditory space perception. *Perception and Psychophysics,* 17, (3), 241–245, 1975.

Kinchla, R. A., Townsend, J., Yellott, J. I., Jr., and Atkinson, R. C. Influence of correlated visual cues on auditory signal detection. *Perception and Psychophysics,* 1, 67–73, 1966.

Loveless, N. E., Brebner, J., and Hamilton, P. Bisensory presentation of information. *Psychological Bulletin,* 73, 161–199, 1970.

Morton, J. Comments on "Interaction of the auditory and visual sensory modalities" (*Journal of the Acoustical Society of America,* 41, 1–6, 1967). *Journal of the Acoustical Society of America,* 42, 1342–1343, 1967.

Mulligan, R. M., and Shaw, M. L. Multimodal signal detection: Independent decisions vs. integration. *Perception and Psychophysics,* 28, (5), 471–478, 1980.

Seif, T. F., and Howard, J. H., Jr. Stimulus compatibility effects of an accessory visual stimulus on auditory sensitivity. *Perception and Psychophysics,* 17, (5), 504–510, 1975.

Shaw, M. L., and Mulligan, R. M. Models for bimodal signal detection: A reply to Fidell. *Perception and Psychophysics,* 31, (1), 91–92, 1982.

Watkins, W. H., and Feehrer, C. E. Acoustic facilitation of visual detection. *Journal of Experimental Psychology,* 70, 332–333, 1965.

Welch, Gilford, and Juola. *Perception and Psychophysics,* 19, (6), 531–535, 1976.

WEATHER FORECASTING

Hess, G. D. Notes on the prediction of fog and low cloud. (Paper left with I. Mason and dated 13/11/87.)

Mason, I. A model for assessment of weather forecasts. *Australian Meteorological Magazine,* 30, 291–303, 1982.

Mason, I. On scores for yes/no forecasts. Preprints of papers delivered at the Ninth Conference on Weather Forecasting and Analysis, the American Meteorological Society, Seattle, Washington, 169–174, 1982.

McCoy, M. C. Severe-storm-forecast results from the PROFS 1983 forecast experiment. *Bulletin American Meteorological Society,* 67, (2), 155–164, 1986.

McCoy, M. C. An application of signal detection theory in scoring severe storm forecasts. Ninth Conference on Probability and Statistics in Atmospheric Sciences, Virginia Beach, VA. *American Meteorological Society,* 423–427, 1985.

Williams, G. M. An evaluation of precipitation probability forecasts using signal detection theory. Ninth Conference on Probability and Statistics in Atmospheric Services, Virginia Beach, VA. *American Meteorological Society,* 214–217, 1985.

index

Synopses of Reprint Classics by Peninsula Publishing

Books can be ordered by mail or telephone. See last page for instructions.

Ambient Noise in the Sea —Robert J. Urick. Ambient noise is the residual, unwanted noise after all other noise sources have been identified. This book encapsulates the body of knowledge on the subject. It discusses the sources of ambient noise, its variability and dependence on receiver depth, directionality and coherence. A ***must*** for engineers of dealing with active and passive sonars, underwater sensor and weapons systems and underwater signal processing.

Hardcover. 205 pages. Order Book No. P114. $27.95 USA, $29.95 Int'l.

An Introduction to Statistical Communication Theory — David Middleton. Written by the pioneer in statistical communication theory, this classic established a unified approach to the basic theory and applications of random signals in communication systems. The book provides a detailed account of systems and their elements as operations and changes on signal and noise ensembles; it addresses the adaptation of satatistical *decision theory* to communication problems. The book emphasizes system optimization and evaluation of threshold detection and extraction, system design, comparison between theoretical optimum and actual suboptimum systems, and structure of optimum systems in terms of existing elements.

Hardcover. 1100 pages. Order Book No. P107. $58.95 USA, $60.95 Int'l.

Applied Acoustics — G. Porges. This book develops the basic theory of sound from first principles and applies the theory to obtain practical formulae for the transmission and absorption of sound, sound levels in enclosures and the radiation of sound from common noise sources. The behavior of sound waves in enclosures is explained, leading to practical formulae for predicting sound levels in closed spaces. The transmission of waves through solids is discussed to show how real-life problems of noise and vibration isolation can be tackled. The final chapters introduce the radiation of sound from solids into fluids and describe the major sources of unwanted noise experienced today. The mathematics used is relatively elementary in keeping with the practical orientation of the book.

Hardcover. 190 pages. Order Book No. P115. $22.95 USA, $24.95 Int'l.

Digital Communications with Space Applications — This classic defined an entire new technology for space communications. Subjects addressed include: C^3, data telemetry, tracking and ranging, coding, sequences and synchronization techniques. The authors, Solomon W. Golomb, Andrew J. Viterbi, Leonard Baumert, Mahlon Easterling and Jack Stiffer are among the foremost experts in the communications field.

Hardcover. 210 pages. Order Book No. P109. $18.95 USA, $19.95 Int'l.

ECM and ECCM Techniques for Digital Communication Systems — Ray H. Pettit. This re-release presents an overview of contemporary concepts and techniques in the area of ECM and ECCM for digital communications. Focuses on applicable models and procedures, and gains and losses in systems performance, graphic illustrations and practical examples. Written in concise survey style for engineering and management professionals.

Hardcover. 178 pages. Order Book No. P105 $20,00 USA, $22.00 Int'l.

Electronic Countermeasures — Originally published as a secret reference in the 1960s by the U.S. Army Signal Corps, the book is now declassified. It covers signal intercept, jamming and deception fundamentals that are as valid today as when first written. Other subjects include intercept probabilities, receiver parameters, detection and analysis, direction finding, jamming techniques, IR and acoustic countermeasures. More than 600 references and a list of authors that reads like Who's Who in Electronic Warfare.

Hardcover. 1100 pages. Order Book No. P103. $37.50 USA, $40.00 Int'l.

Instruments of Darkness —The History of Electronic Warfare — Alfred Price. Previous accounts of electronic warfare may have left the impression that the subject is shrouded in secrecy and too complex to be understood by the layman. This impression is misleading. *Instruments of Darkness* provides an excellent guide to electronic warfare from its beginnings and makes fascinating reading. First published in 1967, this book is regarded as the standard reference work on World War II radar battle. It was Alfred Price's first book and the one on which his reputation as a historian was founded. In 1977 the book was enlarged and updated to include air actions over North Vietnam and the Middle East.

Hardcover. 284 pages. Order Book No. P101. $18.95 USA, $20.95 Int'l.

Introduction to the Theory and Design of Sonar Transducers — Oscar Bryan Wilson. Written in 1985 as a text at the Naval Postgraduate School, this book provides a complete treatment of the fundamentals of transducer theory and design using equivalent circuit techniques. The book contains ten chapters, each with a list of literature references and a set of problems for the student. Subjects addressed include: introductory baseline and definitions, equivalent circuits, properties of piezoelectric and magnetorestrictive materials, design of hydrophones and transducer arrays. *Introduction to the Theory and Design of Sonar Transducers* will be useful not only to the sonar transducer designer but also to underwater acousticians and sonar system engineers who need an appreciation of the problems of transducer design.

Hardcover. 202 pages. Order Book No. P122. $27.95 USA, $29.95 Int'l.

Mechanics of Underwater Noise — Donald Ross. Originally published in 1976, this book continues to be the most authoritative work on the fundamentals of underwater noise radiated by ships, submarines and torpedoes. It features physical explanations of the basic mechanisms by which noise is generated, transmitted by structures and radiated into the sea. These complex phenomena are explained in a straightforward manner that stresses the dominant mechanisms.

Hardcover. 375 pages. Order Book No. P112. $44.95 USA, $46.95 Int'l.

Methods of Operation Research — Kimball and Morse. One of the first books exclusively devoted to Operations Research (OR). It examines the application of OR to decision-making problems in military operations. Topics include: probability; measures of effectiveness; tactical analyses; Lanchester equations; evaluation of equipment performance; mini-max; exchange rate; sweep rates; operations involving men and equipment; and search theory. A highly articulate work that has special value to Systems Engineers and Operations Researchers.

Hardcover. 158 pages. Order Book No. P118. $21.95 USA, $23.95 Int'l.

Microwave Receivers and Related Components — James Tsui. Seven chapters devoted to receiver technology: crystal video and superheterodyne receivers, IFM, channelized, compressive and Bragg cell receivers. Discusses characteristics, receiver capabilities and limitations, basic design and principles of operation, mathematical analysis, probability of intercept, applications, and receiver evaluation. Another eight chapters provide an overview of the fundamental components of microwave receivers: transmission lines; delay lines; directional couplers; hybrid couplers and power dividers; attenuators, circulators and phase shifters; filters; linear and logarithmic amplifiers and limiters; mixers and detectors; oscillators and frequency synthesizers.

Hardcover. 530 pages. Order Book No. P106. $33.95 USA, $35.95 Int'l.

Microwave Scanning Antennas — R. C. Hansen. Three-volumes bound into a single hardcover book. This classic reference covers all types of narrow beam antennas with emphasis on those that scan the beam. Comprehensively treats phased arrays and quasi-optical antennas. Includes multiple-beam arrays, time domain and synthetic apertures and adaptive antennas. Concentrates on narrow beam antennas, both mechanically steered and electronically scanned. Constraining equations and design tradeoffs along with practical examples.

Hardcover. 1200 pages. Order Book No. P110. $49.95 USA, $51.95 Int'l.

Physics of Sound in the Sea — Classic work on underwater sound propagation resulting from the World War II program of studies organized by the National Defense Research Committee. Parts I and II deal with propagation of sound in the absence of a target. Part I discusses the transmission loss of sound sent out from a projector while Part II deals with sound which has been scattered back. Part III deals with target strengths and echoes returned from submarines and surface ships. Part IV discusses the transmission of sound through wakes and the echoes received.

Hardcover. 577 pages. Order Book No. P126. $44.95 USA, $46.95 Int'l.

Principles of Electronic Warfare — Robert J. Schlesinger. Provides an overview of EW technology and tactics in the space age. Written from an overall systems viewpoint, the book focuses on EW's contribution in the accomplishment of a military aircraft mission. Highlights are: radar countermeasure techniques; electronic intelligence (ELINT); elements of space environment; payload optimization between weapons and ECM; and air combat analysis.

Softcover. 213 pages. Order Book No. P104. $14.95 USA, $15.95 Int'l.

Principles of High-Resolution Radar — August Rihaczek. Presents a step-by-step development of the theory of radar resolution. Begins with basic measurements on single targets and proceeds through an analysis of the nature of the resolution problem. Capabilities and limits of radar and details of waveform design are discussed. Synthetic aperture radar is used to illustrate the practical application of principles and derivations are carefully supported by extensive reasoning. Principles are stressed without resorting to advanced mathematics. Topics include: measurements; ambiguities; target resolution and the limits on resolution performance; target detection in various forms of clutter and the relation to resolution; waveform design; Doppler distortions; wideband signals; and general types of target motion.

Hardcover. 500 pages. Order Book No. P111. $38.95 USA, $40.95 Int'l.

Propagation of Short Radio Waves — Donald E. Kerr. The best known classic of the prestigious MIT Radiation Laboratory Series. Still today's most authoritative reference despite being written more than forty years ago. The book characterizes the phenomena of radio propagation of radar, communication and navigation systems from 100 MHz to 300 GHz. The first chapter introduces the reader to basic definitions and concepts. Ensuing chapters address: Theory of Propagation in a Horizontally Stratified Atmosphere; Refraction and Its Meteorological Characterization; Reflections from the Earth's Surface; Diffraction; Scattering; Atmospheric Attenuation; Radar Cross Section Theory and Measurements; Radar Targets and Meteorological Echoes; and Clutter. The text in

Propagation is logical and easy to understand. Its techical information, data and formulas constitute a bedrock of theory and measurements.

Hardcover. 756 pages. Order Book No. P120. $42.95 USA, $44.95 Int'l.

Proposal Management Using the Modular Technique — Manning and Rugh. The *Modular Technique* can help you achieve effective proposal results. It establishes a vehicle for the communication of complex ideas between manager and authors. It facilitates a large group of authors documenting ideas in a cohesive, easily-read proposal. The *Modular Technique*, based on storyboarding procedures as outlined in this book, provides the manager with the methodology for planning the work, assigning design and writing tasks, implementing author-to-manager feedback and effecting document review in a timely manner.

Hardcover. 111 pages. Order Book No. P119. $23.95 USA, $25.95 Int'l.

Radar Signal Simulation — Richard L. Mitchell. Addresses modeling of radar signals including waveform modulation function, interaction of the scattering environment with the waveform and receiver processing. Presents radar environment model structures for simulation, mapping procedures, transformation, sampled signals and generation techniques.

Hardcover. 200 pages. Order Book No. P116. $36.95 USA, $38.95 Int'l.

Signal Detection and Recognition by Human Observers — John A. Swets. This book, written in 1964, was the first to bring together into one volume a broad discussion of modern signal detection theory applications to human performance, specifically in auditory and visual sensory tasks. Applications in the book address several substantive problems in psychology including the integration of sensory information, signal uncertainty, auditory frequency analysis, speech communication, vigilance and recognition memory. *Signal Detection and Recognition* outlines how decision factors are centrally involved in even the simplest detection task and how sensory capacity can by assessed. The bibliography in this reprint edition has been updated to 1988.

Hardcover. 734 pages. Order Book No. P124. $44.95 USA, $46.95 Int'l.

Signal Detection Theory and Psychophysics — David M. Green and John A. Swets. This classic, written in 1966, summarizes the application of signal detection theory to the analysis and measurement of the human observer's sensory system. The theory provides a way to analyze the threshold or sensory limen, the basic unit of all discrimination studies, whether human or animal. The book outlines the theory of statistical decision making and its application to a variety of common psychophysical activities. It shows how signal detection theory can be used to separate sensory and decision aspects of discrimination responses. The concepts of the ideal observer and energy detector are presented and compared with human auditory detection data. Signal detection theory is applied to a variety of other substantive problems in a sensory psychology. *Signal Detection Theory and Psychophysics* is an invaluable book for psychologists dealing with sensory perception, especially auditory, and for human factors engineers dealing with man/machine interfaces.

Hardcover. 521 pages. Order Book No. P125. $41.95 USA, $46.95 Int'l.

Sound Propagation in the Sea — Robert J. Urick. Subjects addressed: basic theory; speed of sound in the ocean; attentuation and absorption; surface duct; the deep sound channel; caustics and convergence zones; computer models of sound propagation; shallow-water ducts; reflections and scattering by the sea surface; reflections and scattering by the sea bottom; temporal coherence; spatial coherence; and multipath in the sea.

Hardcover. 225 pages. Order Book No. P113. $28.95 USA, $30.95 Int'l.

Space-Time Information Processing — Loda and Winder. Indispensable reference tool for audio signal processing and data analysis. Oriented to acoustics and sonar engineering. Features Fourier transforms, statistical analyses, correlation and spectra. Especially valuable chapters address measurement of spatially and temporally-limited functions, optimal filtering procedures and interpretation of results.

Hardcover. 192 pages. Order Book No. P117. $19.95 USA, $21.95 Int'l.

The Strategy of Electromagnetic Conflict — Written by the Air Force Academy faculty. Contents include: electronic countermeasures and counter-countermeasures; electronic reconnaissance; tradeoffs in air defense; use of chaff for aircraft self-protection; communications intelligence, security and cryptoloty; vulnerability of space stations; countermeasures in the millimeter, IR, optical, laser and UV regions. Required reading for engineering and analysis dealing with design and development of military electronic systems and the planning of air operations.

300 pages. Order Book No. P102. $21.95 USA, $23.95 Int'l

Topics in Communication Theory —David Middleton. Provides a concise treatment of basic problems in statistical communication theory. Concepts are discussed and illustrated with simple but important examples. Chapter headings are: Communication from the Viewpoint of Decision Theory; Detection of Signals in Noise; Extraction of Signals from Noise; Structure of Optimum Systems; and Critique, Extensions and Future Problems.

Hardcover. 125 pages. Order Book No. P108. $13.95 USA, $14.95 Int'l.

Understanding Chaff — Wilfred N. Carson. This preliminary edition covers chaff history, antenna fundamentals applicable to chaff, chaff's physical and electrical characteristics, and packaging, loading and dispensers. This typewritten book is the first part of a text which, when completed, will also address chaff manufacture, testing and tactics for the protection of aircraft, ships and land vehicles. This book concentrates on the basic theory of chaff design. Explanations are aided by more than 40 pages of step-by-step mathematical exercises for designing chaff. These exercises provide a clear basis of understanding for the systems planner who must address the specifications for chaff against future threats.

Softcover. 217 pages. Order Book No. P121. $22.95 USA, $24.95 Int'l.

Underwater Electroacoustic Measurements — Robert J. Bobber. Addresses the theory and practice of measuring electroacoustic parameters in sonars such as response, sensitivity, directivity, impedance, efficiency, linearity and noise limits of transducers. Discussed in detail are wide band transducers used as measurement instruments, near field and far field measurement methods, and measurements on acoustic windows, reflectors, baffles and absorbers.

Hardcover. 341 pages. Order Book No. P123. $31.95 USA, $33.95 Int'l.

ORDERING INFORMATION

You can order by postcard, personal letter or telephone, (415)948-2511. For orders by letter, pay by check or money order. Book order numbers and prices for each book are listed in the synopses. Add $1.50 per copy for postage and handling. California residents add 6 1/2% sales tax. Make remittance payable to: **Peninsula Publishing, P.O. Box 867, Los Altos, CA 94023 USA.**

Enter my order as follows:

Book No.	Quantity	Unit Price	Total Cost

Total of Book Purchases ________

Calif. Residents add 7% sales tax ________

Postage & handling @ $1.50 per book ________

GRAND TOTAL OF ORDER US$ ________

Peninsula Publishing
PO Box 867
Los Altos, CA 94022 USA

Charge to: ☐ Mastercard ☐ Visa

Account Number: ________

Expiration Date: ________

____
signature as it appears on charge card

____
name (please print)

____
organization (if required for shipment)

____
address

____
city state zip

____

Air Mail Service (surcharges per copy):
US priority mail, $3.00
Canada, $5.00
Europe, $12.50
Asia/Africa/Oceana, $15.00
South & Central America, $6.00

Enter my order as follows:

Book No.	Quantity	Unit Price	Total Cost

Total of Book Purchases ________

Calif. Residents add 7% sales tax ________

Postage & handling @ $1.50 per book ________

GRAND TOTAL OF ORDER US$ ________

Peninsula Publishing
PO Box 867
Los Altos, CA 94022 USA

Charge to: ☐ Mastercard ☐ Visa

Account Number: ________

Expiration Date: ________

____
signature as it appears on charge card

____
name (please print)

____
organization (if required for shipment)

____
address

____
city state zip

____

Air Mail Service (surcharges per copy):
US priority mail, $3.00
Canada, $5.00
Europe, $12.50
Asia/Africa/Oceana, $15.00
South & Central America, $6.00

NO POSTAGE
NECESSARY
IF MAILED
IN THE
UNITED STATES

BUSINESS REPLY MAIL

First Class PERMIT No. 722 Los Altos, CA 94022

POSTAGE WILL BE PAID BY ADDRESSEE

PENINSULA PUBLISHING
P.O. Box 867
Los Altos, California 94022

NO POSTAGE
NECESSARY
IF MAILED
IN THE
UNITED STATES

BUSINESS REPLY MAIL

First Class PERMIT No. 722 Los Altos, CA 94022

POSTAGE WILL BE PAID BY ADDRESSEE

PENINSULA PUBLISHING
P.O. Box 867
Los Altos, California 94022